THE SEPSIS TEXT

THE SEPSIS TEXT

edited by

Jean-Louis Vincent, M.D.
Department of Intensive Care
Erasme University Hospital
Brussels ,Belgium

Jean Carlet, M.D.
Service de Réanimation Polyvalente
Hôpital Saint-Joseph
Paris, France

Steven M. Opal, M.D.
Division of Infectious Diseases
The Memorial Hospital of Rhode Island
Pawtucket, RI

KLUWER ACADEMIC PUBLISHERS
Boston / Dordrecht / London

Distributors for North, Central and South America:
Kluwer Academic Publishers
101 Philip Drive
Assinippi Park
Norwell, Massachusetts 02061 USA
Telephone (781) 871-6600
Fax (781) 681-9045
E-Mail <kluwer@wkap.com>

Distributors for all other countries:
Kluwer Academic Publishers Group
Distribution Centre
Post Office Box 322
3300 AH Dordrecht, THE NETHERLANDS
Telephone 31 78 6392 392
Fax 31 78 6392 254
E-Mail <services@wkap.nl>

 Electronic Services <http://www.wkap.nl>

Library of Congress Cataloging-in-Publication Data

The sepsis text / edited by Jean-Louis Vincent, Jean Carlet, Steven M. Opal.
    p. cm.
    Includes bibliographical references and index.
    ISBN 0-7923-7620-X (alk. paper)
    1. Septicemia. I. Vincent, J. L. II. Carlet, Jean. III. Opal, Steven M.

RC182.S4 S457 2002
616.9'44--dc21

    2001050762

Printed on acid-free paper.

Printed in the United States of America

*The Publisher offers discounts on this book for course use and bulk purchases.
For further information, send email to melissa.ramondetta@wkap.com.*

CONTENTS

PATHOPHYSIOLOGY

MONITORING SYSTEMS

COMPLICATIONS

ANTI-SEPSIS THERAPIES

CONTRIBUTORS

Abraham E
Division of Pulmonary and Critical
Care Medicine
Health Science Center
Denver, CO
USA

Adib-Conquy M
Dept of Physiopathology
Institut Pasteur
Paris
France

Albair BB
Dept of Medicine
University of Arkansas Medical
School
Little Rock, AR
USA

Alberti C
Dept of Biostatistics
Hôpital Saint-Louis
Université de Paris VII
Paris
France

Anaissie EJ
Dept of Medicine
University of Arkansas Medical
School
Little Rock, AR
USA

Angele MK
Dept of Surgery
Ludwig Maximilians University
Grosshadern Hosp
Munich
Germany

Angus DC
Dept of Anesthesiology and
Critical Care Medicine
University of Pittsburgh School of
Medicine
Pittsburgh, PA
USA

Annane D
Service de Réanimation Médicale
Hôpital Raymond Poincarré
Faculté de Médecine Paris-Ouest
Université Paris V
Garches
France

Astiz M
Dept of Medicine
St Vincent's Hospital
New York, NY
USA

Beaton RK
Dept of Infectious Diseases and
Microbiology
Imperial College School of
Medicine
Hammersmith Hospital
London
United Kingdom

Bellingan GJ
Centre for Respiratory Research
Rayne Institute
University College London
Hospitals
London
United Kingdom

Bellissant E
Labo of Clinical and Experimental
Pharmacology
Faculté de Médecine
Université de Rennes
Rennes
France

Bennett D
Dept of Intensive Care
St George's Hospital
London
United Kingdom

Bernard GR
Division of Allergy, Pulmonary
and Critical Care Medicine
Vanderbilt University Medical
Center
Nashville, TN
USA

Bhattacharjee AK
Dept of Bacterial Diseases
Walter Reed Army Institute
Silver Spring, MA
USA

Bochud P Y
Division of Infectious Diseases
CHU Vaudois
Lausanne
Switzerland

Boulain T
Medical Intensive Care Unit
CHU Bicêtre
Université Paris XI
Le Kremlin-Bicêtre
France

Brun-Buisson C
Medical Intensive Care Unit
Hôpital Henri Mondor
Créteil
France

Calandra T
Division of Infectious Diseases
Centre Hospitalier Universitaire
Vaudois
Lausanne
Switzerland

Carlet J
Service de Réanimation
Polyvalente
Hôpital Saint Joseph
Paris
France

Castelain V
Medical Intensive Care Unit
CHU Bicêtre
Université Paris XI
Le Kremlin-Bicêtre
France

Cavaillon JM
Dept of Physiopathology
Institut Pasteur
Paris
France

Cohen J
Dept of Infectious Diseases and
Microbiology
Imperial College Medical School
Hammersmith Hospital
London
United Kingdom

Cross AS
Division of Infectious Diseases
Greenbaum Cancer Center
University of Maryland School of
Medicine
Baltimore, MA
USA

Cruz K
Dept of Critical Care Medicine
St Luke's Medical Center
Chicago, IL
USA

Cunha BA
Infectious Disease Division
Winthrop-University Hospital
Mineola, NY
USA

Dasta JF
College of Pharmacy
Ohio State University
Colombus, OH
USA

Dellinger P
Dept of Critical Care Medicine
St Luke's Medical Center
Chicago
USA

Döcke WD
Institute of Medical Immunology
Charité Humboldt-University
Berlin
Germany

Eggimann P
Dept of Internal Medicine
Medical Intensive Care Unit
University of Geneva Hospitals
Geneva
Switzerland

Evans TW
Unit of Critical Care
Imperial College School of
Medicine
Royal Brompton Hospital
London
United Kingdom

Faist E
Dept of Surgery
Ludwig Maximilians University
Grosshadern Hospital
Munich
Germany

Fevereiro T
Unidade de Cuidados Intensivos
Polivalente
Hospital de Santo Antònio dos
Capuchos
Lisboa
Portugal

Fink MP
Dept of Critical Care
University of Pittsburgh Medical
School
Pittsburgh, PA
USA

Finney SJ
Unit of Critical Care
Imperial College School of
Medicine
Royal Brompton Hospital
London
United Kingdom

Glauser MP
Division of Infectious Diseases
CHU Vaudois
Lausanne
Switzerland

Groeneveld ABJ
Medical Intensive Care Unit
Free University Hospital
Amsterdam
The Netherlands

Grütz G
Institute of Medical Immunology
Charité Humboldt-University
Berlin
Germany

Hack E
Central Laboratory of the
Netherlands Red Cross Blood
Transfusion Service
Amsterdam
The Netherlands

Hebert PC
Dept of Medicine
Ottawa General Hospital
Ottawa, Ontario
Canada

Heyland DK
Dept of Medicine and Surgery
Kingston General Hospital
Kingston, Ontario
Canada

Höflich C
Institute of Medical Immunology
Charité Humboldt-University
Berlin
Germany

Hollenberg SM
Dept of Cardiology and Critical
Care
Rush Medical College
Chicago, IL
USA

Hubert CE
Infectious Disease Division
Brown University School of
Medicine
Providence, RI
USA

Huettemann E
Klinik für Anästhesiologie und
Intensivtherapie
Klinikum der Friedrich-Schiller-
Universität Jena
Jena
Germany

Knaus W
Health Evaluation Sciences
University of Virginia Health
System
Charlottesville, VA
USA

Kruse JA.
Dept of Medicine
Detroit Receiving Hospital
Detroit
USA

Kudsk K
Dept of Surgery
University of Tennessee
Health Science Center
Memphis, TN
USA

Kvietys P
A.C Burton Vascular Biology
Laboratory
University of Western Ontario
London, Ontario
Canada

Lukan JK.
Dept of Medicine and Surgery
University of Louisville School of
Medicine
Louisville, KY
USA

Marshall JC
Dept of Surgical Intensive Care
Toronto General Hospital
University Health Network
Toronto, Ontario
Canada

Martin C
Réanimation Médicale
Hôpital Nord
Marseille
France

Martin GS
Division of Pulmonary and Critical
Care Medicine
Emory University
Atlanta, GA
USA

Matos R
Unidade de Cuidados Intensivos
Polivalente
Hospital de Santo Antònio dos
Capuchos
Lisboa
Portugal

McClave SA
University of Louisville School of
Medicine
Dept of Medicine and Surgery
Louisville, KY
USA

Mebazaa A
Département d'Anesthésie-
Réanimation
Hôpital Lariboisière
Paris
France

Meier-Hellmann A.
Klinik für Anästhesiologie und
Intensivtherapie
Klinikum der Friedrich-Schiller-
Universität Jena
Jena
Germany

Moreno R
Unidade de Cuidados Intensivos
Polivalente
Hospital de Santo Antònio dos
Capuchos
Lisboa
Portugal

Morrison DC
Office of Research Administration
Saint-Lukes Hospital
Kansas City, MI
USA

Neilipovitz D
Dept of Medicine
Ottawa General Hospital
Ottawa, Ontario
Canada

Opal SM
Infectious Disease Division
Memorial Hospital of Rhode Island
Pawtucket, RI
USA

Papasian C
Dept of Basic Medical Science
School of Medicine
University of Missouri
Kansas City, MI
USA

Philips B
Dept of Anaesthesia and Intensive
Care
St George's Hospital
London
United Kingdom

Piepot HA
Medical Intensive Care Unit
Free University Hospital
Amsterdam
The Netherlands

Pittet D
Dept of Internal Medicine
Infection Control Program
University of Geneva Hospitals
Geneva
Switzerland

Poli de Figueiredo LF
Intensive Care Unit
Hospital Israelita Albert Einstein
São Paulo
Brazil

Redl H
Ludwig Boltzmann Institute for
Experimental and Clinical
Traumatology
Vienna
Austria

Reinhart K.
Klinik für Anästhesiologie und
Intensivtherapie
Klinikum der Friedrich-Schiller-
Universität
Jena
Germany

Reinke P
Dept of Nephrology and Internal
Intensive Medicine
Charité Humboldt-University
Berlin
Germany

Rogiers P
Dept of Intensive Care
Middleheim General Hospital
Antwerp
Belgium

Rubinovitch B
Dept of Internal Medicine
Infection Control Program
University of Geneva Hospitals
Geneva
Switzerland

Sakka SG
Klinik für Anästhesiologie und
Intensivtherapie
Klinikum der Friedrich-Schiller-
Universität Jena
Jena
Germany

Sibbald WJ
Dept of Medicine
Sunnybrook & Women's College
Health Sciences Centre
Toronto, Ontario
Canada

Sielenkämper W
Dept of Anesthesiology and
Intensive Care Medicine
Westfälische Wilhelms-Universität
Münster
Germany

Silva E
Intensive Care Unit
Hospital Israelita Albert Einstein
São Paulo
Brazil

Slutsky AS
Critical Care Division
St Michael Hospital
Toronto, Ontario
Canada

Solomkin JS
Dept of Surgery
University of Cincinnati
College of Medicine
Cincinnati, OH
USA

Spittler A
Surgical Research Laboratory
University Clinic of Vienna
Vienna
Austria

Strohmaier W
Ludwig Boltzmann Institute for
Experimental and Clinical
Traumatology
Vienna
Austria

Stüber F
Klinik und Poliklinic für
Anästhesiologie
Friedrich-Wilhems-Universität
Bonn
Germany

Susla GM
Pharmacy Dept
National Institutes of Health
Bethesda, MA
USA

Suter PM
Dept of Surgical Intensive Care
Hôpital Cantonal Universitaire
Geneva
Switzerland

Tavernier B
Département d'Anesthésie-
Réanimation
Hôpital Huriez
CHU Lille
Lille
France

Teboul JL
Medical Intensive Care Unit
CHU Bicêtre
Université Paris XI
Le Kremlin-Bicêtre
France

Thijs LG
Dept of Intensive Care
University Hospital
Amsterdam
The Netherlands

Timsit JF
Service de Réanimation
Hôpital Saint Joseph
Paris
France

Vallet B
Dépt d'Anesthésie-Réanimation
CHU Lille
Lille
France

Vervloet MG
Medical Intensive Care Unit
Free University Hospital
Amsterdam
The Netherlands

Villar J
Critical Care Division
Mount Sinai Hospital
Toronto
Canada

Vincent JL
Dept of Intensive Care
Erasme University Hospital
Brussels
Belgium

Volk HD
Institute of Medical Immunology
Charité Humboldt-University
Berlin
Germany

Wax RS
Critical Care Unit
Mt. Sinai Hospital
Toronto, Ontario
Canada

Webb A.
Dept of Intensive Care
The Middlesex Hospital
London
United Kingdom

Zarzaur BL
Dept of Nutrition Research
University of Tennessee
Memphis, TN
USA

INTRODUCTORY COMMENTS

Jean-Louis Vincent   *Jean Carlet*   *Steven M. Opal*

This book is written at the dawn of a new era in the management of sepsis. Recent achievements in the clinical management of septic shock are the culmination of decades of basic and applied research by innovative researchers and clinical investigators worldwide. The contributing authors to this book have spearheaded much of this research, and, as editors, we have endeavored to create a textbook that is comprehensive in nature while maintaining a specific focus upon the multitude of work that constitutes the spectrum of sepsis research.

It has been over a century since Pfeiffer and Koch first isolated the most important microbial mediator of sepsis, endotoxin. Since that time, experimental and clinical research has revealed the complex nature of the sepsis response, which, although an essential and necessary part of innate defense, can become deleterious, leading to organ failure and death. It has become abundantly clear that the intricacies of the molecular pathogenesis of sepsis, and the multitude of immunologic and physiologic processes that interact into the final expression of clinically evident severe sepsis will not yield to simple solutions. Indeed, sepsis may be considered as a syndrome, rather than a disease per se; the term 'sepsis' is associated with many different disease processes, as, for example, the term 'cancer' can include leukemia, malignant melanoma, or brain tumor, all very different diseases requiring different treatment regimes. Techniques that will enable the physician to characterize the immune response in individual septic patients are being developed and will allow therapies to be directed more appropriately.

The management of sepsis can be considered in three parts, each important to patient outcome, and no one being sufficient alone:

1. Anti-infection – sepsis is, after all, a battle against an invading microorganism, and appropriate antimicrobial therapy is essential. Removal of the source of infection, by surgical drainage, if necessary is also a vital aspect of management.

2. Hemodynamic stabilization – septic shock is associated with an imbalance in the oxygen supply/demand ratio, and the restoration of blood flow, cardiac function, and adequate oxygenation are key factors in the treatment of sepsis and in the prevention of further organ dysfunction.

Administration of oxygen and of fluids, with vasoactive agents as needed, remain essential first line strategies in the septic patient.

3.   Anti-sepsis therapies – since the earliest discoveries of the pathways and mediators involved in sepsis, researchers have struggled, for many years seemingly in vain, to develop an effective anti-sepsis therapy. As we enter the 21st century, however, there is a great sense of excitement and anticipation as recent clinical trials with innovative therapies for sepsis, including activated protein C, have proven to be remarkably successful.

With the recent positive results from clinical trials and innovative anti-sepsis therapies, our basic understanding of the molecular pathogenesis of sepsis has moved forward at an accelerated pace. The precise molecular definition of the signaling mechanisms involved in lipopolysaccharide interactions is now increasingly understood with the discovery of the Toll-like receptors. The similarity between the Toll-like receptors and interleukin-1 is one of the most remarkable recent discoveries in the evolution of the host innate immune response to microbial pathogens.

The delicate and dynamic interactions between pro-inflammatory cytokines, anti-inflammatory cytokines, procoagulants, natural anticoagulants, the complement system, lipid mediators, the neuro-endocrine system, the innate and acquired immune response, is now appreciated in considerable detail. The basic elements of microvascular physiology, and the metabolic processes essential for survival and repair of damaged tissue in sepsis are increasingly understood at the molecular level. Similarly, advances in the understanding of mechanisms by which microbial pathogens evade host responses and cause disease, and the integration of humoral and cellular immune antimicrobial defenses has been clarified over the last two decades. Advances in respiratory care and ventilator equipment, diagnostic and interventional radiology, refinements in the use of blood products, vasopressors, fluid management, immunonutrition, oxygen delivery, and renal replacement therapy, have contributed greatly to the improved survival in patients with sepsis in modern intensive care units. Many of these topics are explored in great detail within the contents of this book.

We feel privileged to be working as intensivists in such exciting times. After so many years of seemingly endless frustration and disappointment, there is light at the end of the tunnel, and we believe that we will soon be able to offer our patients effective anti-sepsis therapies. We hope this book will convey some of our enthusiasm and provide encouragement to all working in the field of sepsis.

1

SEPSIS: THE MAGNITUDE OF THE PROBLEM

Jean-Louis Vincent

Sepsis is 'simply' defined as the host response to an infection. However, medicine is rarely simple, and sepsis is no exception. The various definitions which exist to describe sepsis demonstrate the complexities of the septic process, and lead to problems in assessing accurately the incidence of, and mortality from, sepsis. However, regardless of the definitions used, there is no doubt of the magnitude of the problem, with sepsis affecting some 3-5% of intensive care unit (ICU) admissions, with mortality rates of 35-50%. In this chapter we will discuss some of the general problems with definitions, before elaborating further on some of the larger studies focusing on the incidence of, and mortality from, sepsis.

DEFINITIONS

Despite vast improvements in our understanding of the mechanisms underlying the sepsis process, we have made little progress in establishing universal agreements on the terminology and definition of sepsis. Indeed, even the key issue, that sepsis is the response to an infection, has become clouded, and various, often confusing, definitions have been developed and employed to categorize patients.

One of the reasons for problems in definition is that sepsis is such a complex process; although typical signs and symptoms exist, these may not occur in all patients, or indeed in the same patient at all times during the sepsis response. For example, although fever is a typical sign of sepsis, not all patients will be febrile and some may be hypothermic, which is, in fact, associated with a worse prognosis. There are many so-called signs of sepsis which could be used in developing a 'sepsis' definition or to aid diagnosis (Table 1), but none on their own are specific for sepsis.

Fever (sometimes hypothermia)
Increased C-reactive protein (CRP)
Increased heart rate
Increased cardiac output, low systemic vascular resistance
Increased oxygen consumption
Tachypnea (with respiratory alkalosis)
Increased procalcitonin concentration
Increased interleukin 6 (Il-6), Il-8, …
Otherwise unexplained alterations in coagulation parameters
Otherwise unexplained alterations in mental status
Otherwise unexplained hyperbilirubinemia
Increased insulin requirements

Table 1. Most common signs of sepsis

Roger Bone and colleagues [1] developed the term the sepsis syndrome in the late 1980s to describe patients with severe sepsis. The sepsis syndrome is defined as:
- hypothermia (temperature less than 96°F [35.6°C]) or hyperthermia (greater than 101° F [38.3°C]),
- tachycardia (heart rate greater than 90 beats/min)
- tachypnea (respiratory rate greater than 20 breath/min)

with clinical evidence of an infection site, and at least one end-organ demonstrating inadequate perfusion or dysfunction expressed as poor or altered cerebral function, hypoxemia (PaO_2 less than 75 torr), elevated plasma lactate, or oliguria (urine output less than 30 ml/h or 0.5 ml/kg body weight/h without corrective therapy).

The main problem with this definition was that the criteria are fairly easily met by a large number of ICU patients. In addition, some found the criteria frustratingly limiting; for example, a patient who is clearly septic and fulfils all the criteria but has a temperature of just 38.2°C would not fit the definition. The sepsis syndrome is now rarely used.

A North American consensus conference [2] attempted to create a simple definition, but the criteria adopted were too sensitive, and the resultant systemic inflammatory response syndrome (SIRS) approach was not very helpful [3]. Indeed, to meet the SIRS criteria, one needs to have alterations in just two of four simple variables:
- body temperature

- heart rate
- respiratory rate
- white blood cell count.

By their definition, sepsis is the association of the SIRS criteria with an infection. Unfortunately, since virtually every ICU patient meets the SIRS criteria [4-6], such an approach minimizes the difference between infection and sepsis.

Infection is an essential pre-requisite for a diagnosis of sepsis; it is important to remember that even simple 'flu is typically associated with a septic response. However, it may not always be possible to document the infection, particularly in ICU patients who are frequently already on antibiotic therapy that interferes with microbiological culture results. This does not mean that such patients do not have sepsis, and indeed this group of patients have a higher mortality than patients in whom infection is clearly identified [7], presumably because a diagnosis of sepsis may be delayed if no obvious source of infection presents itself, and without microbiological data, it is not possible to target antibiotic therapy.

Infection	Microbial phenomenon characterized by the invasion of tissues by organisms inducing an inflammatory response (or the invasion of normally sterile host tissue with or without inflammatory response).
Bacteremia	Presence of viable bacteria in the blood
Sepsis	The systemic response to infection (see Table 1)
Septicemia	Association of bacteremia with sepsis
Severe sepsis	Sepsis associated with organ dysfunction such as oliguria, alterations in mental status, coagulation abnormality, hypoxemia or renal dysfunction.
Septic shock	Sepsis with hypotension along with the presence of perfusion abnormality and lactic acidosis. Arterial hypotension persists despite adequate fluid resuscitation so that vasopressor therapy is required.

Table 2. Commonly used terminology in sepsis

Although definitions of sepsis are varied and little universal agreement exists, there is a greater consensus regarding the definition of septic shock (Table 2). For severe sepsis, the associated organ dysfunction can be quantified using an organ dysfunction score such as the sequential organ failure assessment (SOFA) score [8] (Table 3). This enables more homogeneous groups of patients to be identified for epidemiological and clinical trial purposes.

SOFA score	0	1	2	3	4
Respiratory PaO$_2$/FiO$_2$, mm Hg	> 400	≤ 400	≤ 300	≤ 200	≤ 100
				--with respiratory support---	
Coagulation Platelets x10^3/mm^3	> 150	≤ 150	≤ 100	≤ 50	≤ 20
Liver Bilirubin, mg/dl (μmol/l)	< 1.2 (< 20)	1.2-1.9 (20-32)	2.0-5.9 (33-101)	6.0-11.9 (102-204)	> 12.0 (> 204)
CVS Hypotension	No hypo-tension	MAP < 70 mm Hg	dop ≤ 5, or dob (any dose)*	dop > 5, epi ≤ 0.1, or norepi ≤ 0.1*	dop > 15, epi > 0.1, or norepi > 0.1*
CNS Glasgow coma score	15	13-14	10-12	6-9	< 6
Renal Creatinine, mg/dl (μmol/l)	< 1.2 (< 110)	1.2-1.9 (110-170)	2.0-3.4 (171-299)	3.5-4.9 (300-440)	> 5.0 (> 440)
or urine output				or < 500 ml/d	or < 200 ml/d

adrenergic agents administered for at least one hour (doses given are in μg/kg/min). Norepi: norepinephrine; Dob: dobutamine; Dop: dopamine; Epi: epinephrine. CNS: central nervous system; CVS: cardiovascular

***Table 3**. The SOFA score [8]*

SOURCE OF SEPSIS AND CAUSATIVE ORGANISM

The source of infection is important for clinical purposes, as it can aid in the selection of appropriate antibiotic therapy, and certain sources, for example, the urinary tract are associated with a lower mortality. Over recent years, there has been a change in the etiology of septic shock with chest-related infections becoming more important than abdominal infections, possibly related to increased, and often prolonged use of mechanical ventilation [9]. The lungs are now the most common source of infection [10-12]. The most commonly isolated organisms in nosocomial infections, an important cause of sepsis in ICU patients, are listed in Table 4. In many cases, the infection will be polymicrobial [10, 12]. Gram-positive organisms are playing an increasingly important role in the etiology of septic shock [9].

Staphylococcus aureus
Coagulase negative Staphylococcus
Pseudomonas aeruginosa
Escherichia coli
Enterobacter
Klebsiella
Acinetocbacter
Serratia
Candida

Table 4. Most common microbial isolates in nosocomial infections

IMPACT OF SEPSIS

Allowing for the above problems in definition, there are about 500,000 cases of sepsis each year in the United States based on soft data from the Center for Disease Control (CDC) [13]. The incidence of sepsis has increased over time, with CDC statistics reporting a 139% increase over a ten year period. While many risk factors for sepsis have remained stable over time, for example presence of diabetes mellitus, malignancy, alcoholism, malnutrition, etc.) some have increased and it is this that likely accounts for the increase in incidence (Table 5).

Progress of medicine
Increased proportion of patients at both extreme of age
Increased used of invasive devices and procedures
Increased use of immunosuppression (therapy of cancer, auto-immune disease, organ transplant)
Immunosuppression in chronically ill and debilitated patients

Table 5. Some factors that may explain the increase in the incidence of sepsis overtime

Sepsis is associated with increased hospital and ICU stays, expensive antimicrobial therapies, and prolonged duration of mechanical ventilation. As such, the economic impact of sepsis is considerable, accounting for some $5-

10 billion of health care expenditure in the US each year [13]. In the UK, the average daily costs of treating a patient with sepsis on admission to the ICU were recently assessed at $930, compared to $750 for a patient without sepsis [14]. Given the longer ICU stay for a septic patient, the total ICU costs for a patient with sepsis on admission were two times greater than those for a patient without sepsis. For a patient who developed sepsis while on the ICU these costs were considerably greater, some ten times the costs of a non-septic patient.

PREVALENCE OF SEPSIS IN THE ICU

Sands et al. [11] prospectively evaluated the incidence of sepsis, using a modified version of the sepsis syndrome as their definition, in eight academic hospitals in the US over a four month period. A total of 12,759 patients were included in the study, and 1342 septic episodes were documented in 1166 patients. Overall the authors calculated that there were two episodes of sepsis per hundred hospital admissions, 2.8 episodes of sepsis per 1000 patient days. Fifty-five percent of these episodes originated in an ICU. From a larger patient population of 192,980 patients, Angus et al. (unpublished data) found slightly higher estimates of 2.26 episodes of sepsis/100 admissions, and estimated that 750,000 cases of sepsis occur per year in the US. Again, about half of the septic episodes occurred in the ICU.

In Europe, Brun-Buisson et al. [12], in a study involving 11,828 patients from 170 ICUs in France, reported an incidence for sepsis, using sepsis syndrome definitions, of 6.3% of ICU admissions. In Italy, Salvo and colleagues [5] used the ACCP/SCCM SIRS definitions [2] and noted, in a population of 1101 critically ill patients from 96 ICUs, an incidence of sepsis of 4.5%, of severe sepsis 2.1%, and of septic shock 3%. Other studies have reported similar rates [15]. The European Prevalence of Infection in Intensive Care study [10], involved more than 10,000 patients, and focused on infection rather than specifically on sepsis. The EPIC study was a prevalence study investigating the number of infected patients on one given day in 1417 European ICUs. The data showed that 45% of the patients were infected, 24% being infected on admission (14% community acquired, 10% hospital acquired) and another 21% had developed an infection during their ICU stay. Similar data were obtained in the SOFA study [8] that involved 14,049 patients followed throughout their ICU stay: this study revealed that 44% of ICU patients were infected. For those patients who stayed on the ICU for more than 7 days, 75% were infected.

The EPIC study also revealed some interesting international differences. The proportion of patients with ICU acquired infections was greatest in

Greece, Italy, Portugal and Spain, where the mortality rate was also the highest (22.3%). It is known that southern European countries usually have smaller ICUs where very severely ill patients are admitted. There is a clear parallel between the severity of disease and the incidence of sepsis. This is not really surprising when one considers the bilateral relation between sepsis and organ failure. On the one hand, patients with severe sepsis (e.g., severe pneumonia, peritonitis) are at high risk of developing organ failure, particularly when the sepsis is severe enough to lead to septic shock. On the other hand, risk factors for infection include chronic morbidity, high severity scores, high degree of invasiveness, use of mechanical ventilation, administration of immunosuppressive drugs.

PROGNOSIS

While definitions of sepsis vary between studies, mortality rates are also difficult to compare, as some studies use ICU mortality, others choose hospital mortality, some choose a 28-day rate and others select different time spans. However, regardless of the definition of sepsis or mortality used, sepsis is clearly associated with high morbidity and mortality. Importantly, the prognosis of septic patients is influenced not only by the severity of infection, but also by the previous health status and the host response (degree of immunocompetence). Sands et al. [11] reported a 34% 28-day mortality rate in their study of 12,759 patients. The Italian study [5] noted ICU mortality rates of 36, 52, and 82% for patients with sepsis, severe sepsis, and septic shock, respectively. In France, Brun-Buisson and co-workers [12] found 28-day mortality rates of 56% for their patients with severe sepsis. Interestingly, a diagnosis of sepsis affects not only immediate mortality, but has an effect on longer-term death rates as well. Quartin et al. [16] reported that sepsis increased the risk of death for up to five years after the septic episode.

A recent review of the literature [9] indicates that the mortality from septic shock varies widely between studies, no doubt related to differences in definition, with figures ranging from 18 to 91%. Interestingly, this study also revealed that the mortality rates may have somewhat decreased overtime despite a probable increase in the severity of illness of the patients treated. Armstrong et al. [17] have also reported a fall in mortality rates from infectious disease; from 797 deaths per 100,000 in 1900 to 59 deaths per 100,000 in 1996, although these authors note considerable year-to-year variations.

CONCLUSION

The magnitude of sepsis is considerable, affecting some 2-14% of ICU patients depending on the definition used. The impact of this disease process is considerable with mortality rates of around 50% depending on the definition used, and increasing with the degree of sepsis, from sepsis through sever sepsis to septic shock. With the associated morbidity, the economic costs of sepsis are also large. As the numbers of older, more debilitated patients being treated in our ICUs continues to increase, so the incidence of sepsis is increasing. While recent studies have shown some possible reductions in the mortality from sepsis, we cannot afford to be complacent. Definitions based on syndromes need to be replaced by more specific, mechanism-based entities reflecting the immunologic or biochemical changes seen in sepsis [18]; using such definitions to select more homogeneous patient populations for clinical trials, in combination with organ dysfunction scores to assess outcome, will lead to the development of effective new therapies, and the high costs of sepsis, in terms of mortality and finance, will be reduced.

REFERENCES

1. Bone RC, Fisher CJ, Clemmer TP, Slotman GJ, Metz CA, Balk RA. Sepsis syndrome: A valid clinical entity. Crit Care Med 1989; 17:389-393
2. ACCP-SCCM Consensus Conference. Definitions of sepsis and multiple organ failure and guidelines for the use of innovative therapies in sepsis. Crit Care Med 1992; 20:864-874
3. Vincent JL. Dear SIRS, I'm sorry to say that I don't like you... Crit Care Med 1997; 25:372-374
4. Rangel-Frausto MS, Pittet D, Costigan M, Hwang T, Davis CS, Wenzel RP. The natural history of the systemic inflammatory response syndrome (SIRS). A prospective study. JAMA 1995; 273:117-123
5. Salvo I, de cian W, Musicco M, et al. The Italian sepsis Study: preliminary results on incidence and evolution of SIRS, sepsis, severe sepsis and septic shock. Intensive Care Med 1995; 21 (suppl 2):S244-S249
6. Bossink AW, Groeneveld J, Hack CE, Thijs LG. Prediction of mortality in febrile medical patients: How useful are systemic inflammatory response syndrome and sepsis criteria? Chest 1998; 113:1533-1541
7. Reyes WJ, Brimioulle S, Vincent JL. Septic shock without documented infection: an uncommon entity with a high mortality. Intensive Care Med 1999; 25:1267-1270
8. Vincent JL, de Mendonça A, Cantraine F, et al. Use of the SOFA score to assess the incidence of organ dysfunction/failure in intensive care units: Results of a multicenter, prospective study. Crit Care Med 1998; 26:1793-1800
9. Friedman G, Silva E, Vincent JL. Has the mortality of septic shock changed with time? Crit Care Med 1998; 26:2078-2086

10. Vincent JL, Bihari D, Suter PM, et al. The prevalence of nosocmial infection in intensive care units in Europe. JAMA 1995; 274:639-644

11. Sands KE, Bates DW, Lanken PN, et al. Epidemiology of sepsis syndrome in 8 academic medical centers. JAMA 1997; 278:234-240

12. Brun-Buisson C, Doyon F, Carlet J, et al. Incidence, risk factors, and outcome of severe sepsis and septic shock in adults. JAMA 1995; 247:968-974

13. Anonymous. Increase in National Hospital Discharge Survey rates for septicemia--United States, 1979-1987. MMWR Morb Mortal Wkly Rep 1990; 39:31-34

14. Edbrooke DL, Hibbert CL, Kingsley JM, Smith S, Bright NM, Quinn JM. The patient-related costs of care for sepsis patients in a United Kingdom adult general intensive care unit. Crit Care Med 1999; 27:1760-1767

15. Pittet D, Thiévent B, Wenzel RP, Li N, Auckenthaler R, Suter PM. Bedside prediction of mortality from bacteremic sepsis: A dynamic analysis of ICU patients. Am J Respir Crit Care Med 1996; 153:684-693

16. Quartin AA, Schein RMH, Kett DH, Peduzzi PN. Magnitude and duration of the effect of sepsis on survival. JAMA 1997; 277:1058-1063

17. Armstrong GL, Conn LA, Pinner RW. Trends in infectious disease mortality in the united States during the 20th century. JAMA 1999; 281:61-66

18. Abraham E, Matthay MA, Dinarello CA, et al. Consensus conference definitions for sepsis, septic shock, acute lung injury, and acute respiratory distress syndrome: time for a reevaluation. Crit Care Med 2000; 28:232-235

2

DIAGNOSIS AND SOURCE OF SEPSIS: THE UTILITY OF CLINICAL FINDINGS

Kenneth Cruz
R. Phillip Dellinger

Sepsis continues to be one of the leading causes of mortality in hospitals today [1,2]. While the advent of intensive care units (ICUs) equipped with sophisticated monitoring systems and specially trained critical care physicians has likely reduced the mortality associated with this crippling syndrome, sepsis still remains an impressive medical foe. Therefore, early recognition of this clinical syndrome prompting empiric medical therapy likely improves patient outcome. Many signs, symptoms, and laboratory abnormalities may suggest the presence of sepsis, although their sensitivity and specificity vary considerably.

History, first and foremost, may suggest a source of infection as well as pre-existing breaches in the immune system that put the patient at risk. Identifying the immunocompromised state intensifies the search for subtle signs of sepsis. Patients with compromised immune systems include individuals at the extremes of age, the neonatal, and the geriatric populations. Other common immunocompromised states including the human immunodeficiency virus (HIV), chemotherapy for cancer, post-transplant; chronic renal and liver failure patients also have suboptimal immune systems. There are also a number of uncommon congenital immunodeficiency syndromes that predispose individuals to infection. Our integumentary system maintains a vital barrier to infection, but, when compromised, either through severe, widespread burns, or by iatrogenic interventions such as central venous catheters, may hide subtle sources of infection.

The history can also provide clues to the type of causative organism allowing empiric antibiotic therapy that targets likely organisms, potentially improving outcomes. Recent hospitalization or long-term care suggests the possibility of virulent Gram-negative organisms. Gram-positive organisms should be entertained by the presence of recently implanted prosthetic devices such as heart valves, joints, pacemakers/defibrillators, and indwelling catheters (urinary or vascular). Fungal infection is more likely in patients with T-cell dysfunction, long term steroid use, and broad-spectrum antibiotic use.

Organ	Clinical Findings	Organ	Clinical Findings
Central nervous system	Altered mental status Seizure Nuchal rigidity Brudzinski's sign Kernig's sign CSF pleocytosis	Gastrointestinal	Hematochezia Grey-Turner's/Cullen's signs Jaundice Abdominal tenderness Rebound/guarding Murphy's sign Elevated liver enzymes
Ears, nose, throat	Discharge Pain Photophobia Erythema Conjunctivitis Endophthalmitis Thrush	Genitourinary	CVA tenderness Hematuria/pyuria Elevated BUN/creatinine Cervical motion/adnexal tenderness
Cardiovascular	Murmur Rub Osler nodes Janeway lesions Splinter hemorrhages	Skin	Papules/macules Vesicles Abscesses Purpura/ecchymoses Erythema Furuncles/carbuncles
Pulmonary	Crackles/wheeze Egophany Bronchophony Rub Percussion, dullness Chest radiographic infiltrates		

Table 1. Organ-specific clinical findings suggesting the source of sepsis

A complete review of system symptomology can procure diagnostic clues to the source of infection (Table 1). These include, of course, general clues such as fever and chills, which suggest bacteremia or endotoxemia. Central nervous system (CNS) symptoms include headache, dizziness, and visual changes. Eye pain and discharge, ear pain and discharge, nasal discharge that is either purulent or bloody implies possible upper respiratory tract infection. Cough, especially with thickened or colored sputum, sore throat, dyspnea, chest pain/pleurisy, hemoptysis can suggest a cardiorespiratory infection. Nausea/vomiting, diarrhea, jaundice, abdominal pain or distention, may suggest an abdominal source. Dysuria or hematuria indicates possible urinary tract infection. Also, dermatologic clues such as rashes, bullae, vesicles, and their distribution is important. Patient symptoms allow a more directed physical examination.

History and review of systems when combined with physical examination and laboratory findings may point the way to the radiographic identification of niduses of infection that require source control (Figures 1 and 2).

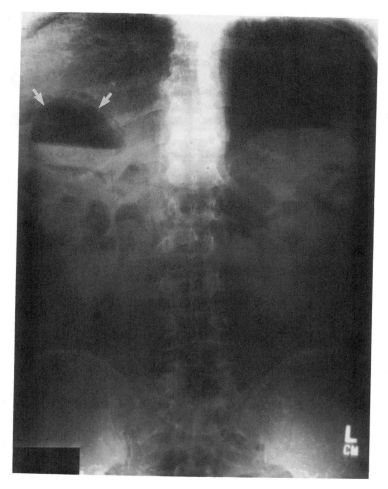

Figure 1. Plain film demonstration of emphysematous cholecystitis. Note the enlarged gallbladder with air demonstrated diffusely throughout the gallbladder wall (arrows).

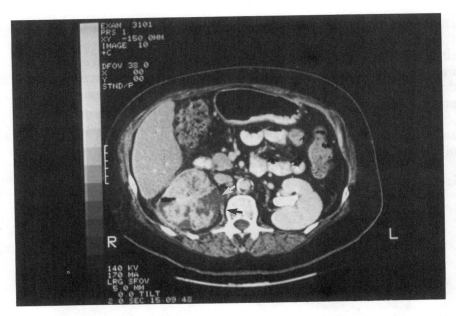

Figure 2. *Computed tomographic demonstration of emphysematous pyelonephritis. Note the air throughout the infected kidney (arrow).*

VITAL SIGNS

In all patients, vital signs are the initial focus of the evaluation.

Fever

One of the cardinal signs associated with sepsis is fever. Fever is defined as a temperature greater then 38 °C. Hypothermia may also suggest sepsis. Temperature is usually obtained with an oral thermometer. However, in the hyperventilating patient, this method may be misleading and underestimate the actual core temperature [3]. When infection is suspected, a core temperature, such as rectal, should be obtained to more accurately assess the presence of hyper- or hypothermia.

Bacterial products trigger the production of endogenous cytokines [1]. Tumor necrosis factor (TNF) and interleukin (IL)-1 are pyrogens known to be released by macrophages during sepsis [4], which, through the production of prostaglandin E_2 and cyclic AMP, increase the baseline temperature by interacting with the thermoregulatory center of the hypothalamus [5]. Animal models suggest that fever protects the host species in sepsis. Classic studies with poikilotherms in the past have suggested the benefits of hyperthermia during sepsis. In these experiments, cold-blooded animals were placed in separate environments during infection – with a heat source or without. Animals that moved closer to the heat source had reduced mortality most likely because they were able to elevate their body temperature [6]. In addition, salicylate-induced antipyresis has been linked to increased mortality in animal models. These studies, while simple, suggest the benefits of fever, or hyperthermia, during sepsis and how elevated temperatures may serve as a physiologic defense mechanism.

The reported incidence of hypothermia in sepsis varies. In a study by LeGall and colleagues, hypothermia, defined as a temperature less than 36 °C, was found in 15% of intensive care unit patients [8]. However, in another multi-institutional study by Clemmer et al, hypothermia, defined in their study as a temperature <35.5 °C, occurred in only 9% of cases of sepsis. Summarizing the literature as it relates to hypothermia is difficult due to a lack of a standard definition. Prior studies have linked hypothermia to poor prognosis in Gram-negative septicemia [9]. Detrimental physiologic effects of hypothermia include decreased immune function. At the onset of sepsis, hypothermic patients have greater physiologic derangements when compared with febrile patients, including central nervous dysfunction and circulatory shock. Renal function and need for mechanical ventilation were reported to be similar in both groups [10]. Hypothermia, therefore, identifies a group of septic patients with more severe physiologic abnormalities and increased mortality.

Respiratory Rate

While fever remains the most frequent diagnostic clue for sepsis, tachypnea is commonly exhibited in the early stages of sepsis [11]. Hyperventilation has multiple possible explanations. Sepsis may directly induce central hyperventilation and respiratory alkalemia by a mechanism that is not clearly defined. Another mechanism for tachypnea is as compensation for metabolic (lactic) acidosis. Lactate production may be related to oxygen debt, or other metabolic abnormalities such as abnormal glycolysis related to liver dysfunction in sepsis [12].

Hypotension associated with sepsis has also been postulated as an explanation for tachypnea. Sepsis-induced hypotension can potentially produce acute respiratory alkalosis through decreased blood flow to aortic and carotid baroreceptors. Decreased pressure at these sites triggers the body to increase its respiratory rate in order to compensate. This has also been hypothesized to account for the similar responses seen in cardiogenic and hypovolemic shock [13].

As the mechanistic theory of sepsis has evolved, the elucidation of cytokine-mediated damage has become clearer. Cytokines, such as TNF and IL-1, may be responsible for the tachypnea observed during sepsis through direct stimulation of the brainstem. There is, however, a lack of literature support for this theory.

Hypoxemia-induced tachypnea provides another possible physiologic explanation for the respiratory alkalosis observed in sepsis. Early in sepsis, ventilation/perfusion mismatching in the absence of any evidence of acute lung injury (ALI) might induce hypoxemia and associated tachypnea. ALI could also be associated with tachypnea, both as a response to hypoxemia and due to increased interstitial water stimulation of J-receptors.

Tachycardia and Hypotension

Hemodynamic derangements are commonly associated with sepsis. Tachycardia is an early clue to the diagnosis of sepsis and, as in exercise, is triggered to increase cardiac output. The average initial heart rate in septic individuals was approximately 120 beats per minute (bpm) in one study. In septic patients with tachycardia, a reduction below 106 bpm within the first twenty-four hours predicted improved survival [14]. Tachycardia is also observed despite the absence of hypotension.

Numerous mediators have been implicated in the pathogenesis of hypotension during sepsis. Throughout the years, a significant amount of research has been dedicated to finding one single culprit. However, as more mediators are identified, the presumption that one single endogenous mediator is primarily responsible for the pathogenesis of shock becomes less likely. Endogenous substances implicated in the endothelial dysfunction associated with sepsis include predominantly cytokines, nitric oxide (NO, previously referred to as endothelial derived relaxation factor [EDRF]), arachidonic acid metabolites, neutrophils and their interactions with endothelial cells, opioids, complement, and bradykinins [15]. The physiologic actions of these substances will be explained in more detail later in this text.

Septic hemodynamic parameters are described as 'hyperdynamic', alluding to the increased cardiac index (CI) and reduced systemic vascular resistance (SVR) [16]. Severe sepsis may be associated with a reduction in systemic vascular resistance (SVR) through the induction of NO synthase (NOS). This reduction in SVR initiates compensatory increases in heart rate to maintain adequate blood pressure. The following equations demonstrate the mechanisms involved:

$$SVR \times cardiac\ output = mean\ arterial\ pressure\ (MAP)$$
$$cardiac\ output = stroke\ volume\ (SV) \times heart\ rate\ (HR)$$

Therefore, the body attempts to compensate for the reduction in SVR by increasing cardiac output. Compensatory mechanisms available in the septic patient to maintain adequate cardiac output include: 1) increasing heart rates; and 2) in the presence of decreased ejection fraction, increasing left end diastolic volumes. In severe sepsis, myocardial function is depressed and left ventricular preload is compromised secondary to capillary leak and venodilation. Therefore, increasing left ventricular end diastolic volumes and increasing heart rate is necessary to maintain adequate blood pressure [17]. However, in time, as the mediators of sepsis and inflammation progress, the reduction in SVR may outpace the ability of the body to compensate. Therefore hypotension, and eventually shock, ensue. Shock is defined as vasopressor requirements to maintain blood pressure and compromised tissue perfusion leading to cellular dysfunction.

SYSTEMIC MANIFESTATIONS OF SEPSIS (TABLE 2)

Central Nervous System Findings

Encephalopathy, a common sepsis-induced CNS presentation, is defined as any mental dysfunction due to the systemic manifestations of sepsis. Manifestations of this disorder include lethargy, somnolence, agitation, disorientation, confusion, and at the extreme, obtundation. Sepsis has been demonstrated to produce brain dysfunction [18]. Patients with acute, sepsis-induced altered mental status have increased mortality when compared to those with normal mental capabilities or prior mental status changes [19]. Although altered mental status has been used as a criterion for enrolment in sepsis clinical trials, it is often difficult to define a constant threshold as well as to separate out altered mental status due to other causes.

Several theories have been proposed to explain the CNS abnormalities of sepsis. Causes may be direct (circulating toxins and inflammatory mediators) and indirect (hypotension and hypoglycemia). Abnormal amino acid metabolism is known to be a cause of encephalopathy as well as abnormal amino acid transport across the blood-brain barrier [20]. This cause of altered mental status is more related to hepatic dysfunction than to CNS dysfunction. Altered cerebral perfusion has also been implicated in the pathophysiology of

CNS dysfunction in sepsis. Other theories implicate a breakdown of the blood-brain barrier, which allows the crossing of inflammatory cytokines as well as other humoral mediators into the CNS. The migration into the CNS of these inflammatory mediators, which affect astrocytes and neurons, causes encephalopathy irrespective of other confounding factors [21]. It remains unclear whether encephalopathy associated with sepsis contributes to the mortality or does the encephalopathy merely indicate the presence of severe global organ dysfunction?

Vital signs
        Fever, chills/rigors, hypothermia
        Tachypnea
        Tachycardia
Central nervous system
        Encephalopathy
Cardiopulmonary
        Increased cardiac output
        Decreased systemic vascular resistance
        Hypotension
        Metabolic acidosis hyperlactatemia
        Acute lung injury (ALI), hypoxemia
Renal
        Decreased urinary output (oliguria, anuria)
        Elevated BUN and creatinine
Gastrointestinal
        Ileus
        Elevated bilirubin, predominantly direct fraction
Dermatology
        Ecthyma gangrenosum
        Symmetrical peripheral gangrene
        Acrocyanosis
        Purpura fulminans
        Toxic erythema
        Rash-maculopapular, vesicular, bullous
Other
      Metabolic
        Hyperglycemia, hypoglycemia
      Hematologic
        Leukocytosis, leukopenia
        Thrombocytopenia
        Disseminated intravascular coagulation

Table 2. *Systemic manifestations of sepsis*

Cardiopulmonary Findings

As previously mentioned, the hemodynamic findings during sepsis include a reduced SVR and an elevated CI. The compensatory increase in cardiac output functions to maintain an adequate blood pressure despite increased oxygen extraction. However, should the physiologic abnormalities associated with sepsis continue, overwhelming the cardiovascular compensatory mechanisms initiated, then hypotension and shock ensue.

Metabolic acidosis due to increased lactate production and decreased clearance is one of the hallmark manifestations of severe sepsis and septic shock. The overproduction of lactate created by global organ hypoperfusion (distributive shock) was initially thought to be the primary cause for acidosis with ensuing anaerobic glycolysis, producing energy in the absence of oxygen with the by-product being lactate [22]. Several additional theories regarding the level of cellular dysfunction have arisen to explain the metabolic abnormalities of sepsis. Hypotheses regarding dysfunction at the regional level, microcirculatory level, cellular metabolic level, and the level of liver metabolism have arisen. The NADH/NAD$^+$ ratio, which can be measured indirectly using the lactate/pyruvate ratio, is a marker of global hypoperfusion. The lactate/pyruvate (L/P=) ratio increases (>10) during cellular hypoxia and coincides with a poor prognosis [23]. The presence of circulatory dysfunction, demonstrated at the gastrointestinal level with tonometry, has been used to indicate regional hypoperfusion, allowing the translocation of endotoxin and bacteria that fuel sepsis. Low intramucosal pH has been shown to correlate with systemic hypoperfusion and with increased morbidity and mortality [24]. Alternatively, microcirculatory changes leading to cellular dysoxia may underlie the hemodynamic and metabolic changes seen during hypoperfusion in sepsis [25]. However, there has been some question raised as to whether elevated lactate levels correlate with oxygen debt, or rather suggest a metabolic abnormality. Recently, there has been some interest in the hypothesis that hyperlactatemia may not symbolize global organ hypoperfusion during sepsis. Instead, metabolic abnormalities may produce such levels. There has been some suggestion in the past that pyruvate dehydrogenase dysfunction in sepsis may lead to hyperlactatemia [26]. Another hypothesis argues that lactate production by an adrenergically stimulated Na$^+$, K$^+$ATPase increases despite evidence of normal oxygen delivery and consumption by skeletal muscles [27]. Other studies have shown that despite increased oxygen consumption, pyruvate oxidation, and lactate production during sepsis, the production of excess pyruvate accounts for the hyperlactatemia seen [28].

Findings of parenchymal lung diseases include adventitious breath sounds such as crackles. The chest X-ray may provide radiographic evidence of ALI.

In early literature, sepsis-induced lung disease was seen pathologically with increased interstitial edema and bronchopneumonia/lung inflammation. Physiologically, an increased shunt fraction likely related to increased parenchymal atelectasis, and decreased compliance primarily related to non-cardiogenic lung edema was observed. This lung disease initially was termed "shock lung" [29]. This was later termed acute respiratory distress syndrome (ARDS), or ALI, produced by lung inflammation related to the inflammatory-mediated injury as a result of a septic insult. This entity is defined by the presence of new bilateral infiltrates on the chest radiograph, PaO_2/FiO_2 ratio less than or equal to 300 in ALI or a PaO_2/FiO_2 ratio less than equal to 200 in ARDS, and no evidence of left atrial hypertension.

Renal Findings

Sepsis-induced renal dysfunction is evidenced by decreased urine output, elevated blood urea nitrogen (BUN) and creatinine, and uremia. In previous studies of bacteremic patients, approximately 24% developed acute renal failure, defined as a doubling of their creatinine. The mortality for bacteremic patients who developed acute renal failure was 50% [30]. Causes of sepsis-induced renal dysfunction include decreased glomerular filtration. Systemic hypotension and vasodilatation may contribute to some of this dysfunction by decreasing renal perfusion. However, afferent and efferent vasoconstriction also occurs as the renin-angiotensin system upregulates during sepsis-induced hypovolemia. Cortical ischemia (anuria suggests bilateral kidney involvement) secondary to sepsis-induced disseminated intravascular coagulation (DIC) thrombosis may also play a role [31]. A direct mediator effect on kidney function is also possible. Documentation of acute tubular necrosis as a cause of renal dysfunction is not supported by the literature.

Some causes of sepsis such as endocarditis can produce independent renal injury. Other pyogenic foci have been shown less frequently to produce glomerular disease. However, this glomerulopathy does not correlate with the immune complex disease that has been demonstrated in endocarditis [32].

Gastrointestinal Findings

Ileus (intestinal obstruction secondary to neuromuscular bowel dysfunction) may be adynamic and occur in the critically ill, including sepsis. Although usually benign, this obstruction may delay feeding, decrease medication absorption or cause aspiration or perforation [33]. The causes are usually multifactorial, but medications and electrolyte abnormalities (e.g., hypokalemia) must be considered.

Liver dysfunction during sepsis is, in some reports, as low as 0.6%, or as high as 50-60% [34]. Higher percentages of liver dysfunction are seen in post-surgical patients with peritonitis. Commonly, a cholestatic picture emerges with hyperbilirubinemia. While Gram-negative sepsis is frequently the cause, hyperbilirubinemia was initially described in patients with *Streptoccocus pneumoniae* infection [35]. The pediatric population is more prone to develop liver dysfunction with sepsis. Neonates are believed to have decreased rates of bile salt formation and a smaller pool of biliary salts. Speculation exists that Gram-negative sepsis may also cause decreased biliary flow through its interaction with membrane bound Na^+-K^+ ATPase [36]. Pathologically, there appears to be no evidence of macroscopic parenchymal necrosis. However, microscopically, intrahepatic cholestasis, Kupffer cell hyperplasia, focal liver cell necrosis, portal tract inflammation, and venous congestion are found in many cases [37].

The laboratory abnormalities reflect the intrahepatic cholestasis observed under the microscope and are manifested primarily by rises in direct bilirubin. Commonly, there may be a minor increase in transaminases, but usually no more than two to three times normal, not approaching the rise seen in hepatitis or ischemic liver disease. Alkaline phosphatase typically rises, again not more than three times that of normal values. These altered values will return to normal, usually within two to six weeks with the resolution of sepsis [34]. Hyperbilirubinemia, predominantly direct in nature, is found on laboratory evaluation. The indirect fraction is usually low implying liver dysfunction as the cause of hyperbilirubinemia. Hemolysis however may occur with sepsis, as evidenced by an elevated indirect bilirubin. *Clostridium perfringens* infection for example has been linked to severe intravascular hemolysis [38].

Dermatologic Findings

Dermatologic manifestations of infection are plentiful. The causes of dermatologic manifestations include: 1) DIC and associated coagulopathy; 2) direct invasion of blood vessels by circulating bacteria; 3) immune complex formation and vasculitis; and 4) emboli from endocarditis [39]. Toxic shock syndrome also produces a characteristic blanching diffuse malar rash (Figure 3).

The skin changes associated with DIC include acrocyanosis, defined as peripherally located grayish cyanosis of the extremities, symmetrical peripheral gangrene (SPG), and purpura fulminans [39]. Commonly caused by Gram-negative bacteria, especially *Neisseria meningitidis*, these skin changes include purpura, ecchymoses, or acrocyanosis (Figure 4). Progression to SPG may occur with ischemic necrosis of the peripheral extremities. Purpura fulminans is characterized by coagulopathic hemorrhage into necrotic skin lesions. All these changes are related to DIC with no histologic evidence of bacterial invasion.

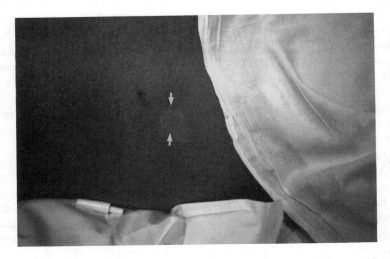

Figure 3. 25-year-old female with toxic shock syndrome due to a staphylococcal buttock abscess. Note blanching produced on lateral abdomen by thumb impression (arrow).

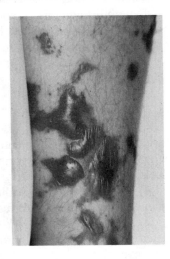

Figure 4. Demonstration of classic skin findings of purpura fulminans in a patient with meningococcemia.

Direct vascular infiltration by circulating bacteria can also occur. This can result in similarly purpuric lesions that were initially macular. These purpuric lesions can be seen in meningococcemia as well as in overwhelming *Pseudomonas* bacteremia with invasion of the medial and adventitious walls of veins resulting in hemorrhage into the dermis. These hemorrhagic vesicular lesions soon rupture, leaving an ulcer with a necrotic base. Ecthyma gangrenosum, as these lesions are known, typically develop with bacterial invasion of the endothelium and minimal presence of inflammatory cells. The lack of inflammatory reaction can be explained by the fact that most of the victims are neutropenic. Gram-negative bacteria may be isolated from these lesions on biopsy. Candida infections can produce lesions similar to ecthyma gangrenosum [40].

There are also vasculitic skin lesions that develop from immune complex formation. These lesions are seen in more chronic forms of *N. meningitidis* as well as *N. gonorrhea*. Arthritis, nephritis, and myocarditis may be associated with these skin lesions. Lesions usually form seven days or more after infection, with antibiotic therapy already instituted. In disseminated gonococcemia, lesions develop in association with polyarthritis. Routinely, these lesions are maculopapular in nature, but can also be purpuric, pustular or ulcerated. On biopsy, microorganisms are rarely found in these lesions. Instead, antigens and antibodies can be isolated in the vessel walls. Immune complex formation may be found with endocarditis, manifesting with Osler nodes, Janeway lesions, purpura, and erythematous lesions.

Finally, toxins such as those found with *Staphylococcus* and *Streptococcus* can generate well-characterized dermatologic lesions. Toxic shock syndrome exhibits a diffuse, macular erythroderma that blanches with pressure, subsequently fading, and desquamating in three to four days [41]. Histologically, these lesions reveal perivascular edema and lymphatic perivascular cuffing. Immune complex deposition is rarely present.

Metabolic Findings

Both hypoglycemia and hyperglycemia may be seen in sepsis. Low blood sugar occurs early and, as previously mentioned, may be a cause of mental status changes such as confusion, obtundation and seizures. While the possible mechanisms of this abnormality are diverse, a common theme in the literature involves both impaired production by the liver and increased uptake at the tissue level. Carbohydrate metabolism as influenced by counterregulatory hormones may also play a role. Recent studies in septic rats have shown increased uptake of glucose at several sites (liver, spleen, lung and ileum) in both euglycemic and hypoglycemic rats as well as insulopenic rats, the latter suggesting that factors other than insulin affect glucose uptake [42]. In other studies, the suggestion has been made that impaired gluconeogenesis in the liver coupled with increased peripheral uptake accounts for the hypoglycemia observed in sepsis [43].

Hyperglycemia is seen commonly during sepsis. Because of the stress state associated with infection, increased epinephrine, corticosteroids, and glucagon drive the production of glucose, overwhelming the counterregulatory hormone insulin. Specifically, the elevated glucagon/insulin ratio drives hepatic gluconeogenesis and insulin resistance peripherally, leading to an overall overproduction of glucose. This excess glucose production counteracted by decreased peripheral utilization leads to hyperglycemia. Epinephrine both inhibits insulin release through the interruption of insulin exocytosis, an α-adrenergic mediated action, while also increasing hepatic production through β-adrenergic stimulation [44]. In addition, the peripheral lactate production funnels into the liver, producing glucose through the Cori cycle further contributing to the hyperglycemia observed. In addition, increased protein catabolism leads to the production of amino acids, which provide substrate in the liver for gluconeogenesis as well [45].

Hematologic Findings

The most common hematologic manifestation of sepsis is leukocytosis. However, the absence of abnormalities in white blood cell (WBC) count cannot be used to reliably exclude sepsis. The rise in WBC count is commonly over 10,000 cells/mm^3. Infection by bacterial source may further be identified by a left shift in the WBC count. Left shift refers to neutrophil predominance in the WBC count, or a rise in the immature form of neutrophils, called 'bands'. Bandemia indicates a shift in marrow production towards neutrophil formation to combat infection. With the stress of infection, some of the WBCs may transit into the intravascular compartment before full maturation, thus increasing the number of bands in the peripheral circulation. On the other end of the spectrum, one can also see leukopenia as a presenting sign of sepsis. Leukopenia represents sepsis-mediated marrow suppression, leading to a paradoxical decrease in WBC count. An ominous sign, leukopenia is also associated with increased mortality during sepsis.

Thrombocytopenia is another hematologic manifestation of sepsis. Thrombocytopenia occurs in 18%-50% of septic patients [46,47]. There are two possible causes for this manifestation: the evolution of platelet-associated immunoglobulins, or the development of DIC. Immune-mediated thrombocytopenia is associated with higher levels of platelets (> 50,000/ml) than are found in DIC (< 50,000/ml) [48]. DIC, on the other hand, indicates severe disease. Other laboratory signs of DIC include an elevated prothrombin time, an elevated D-dimer (indicating clot formation with increased fibrin split products), and a decreased fibrinogen (signaling consumption of clotting factors). Small quantities of thrombin production may be triggered by sepsis and produce thrombocytopenia without other manifestations of DIC.

SPECIAL CONSIDERATIONS IN THE GERIATRIC POPULATION

The geriatric population represents the most rapidly growing segment in the medical community. Of greater concern, sepsis has become the third leading cause of death in the elderly [49]. The elderly are at great infection risk due to immune system compromise, increased number of comorbid illnesses, and residence in chronic care facilities. Commonly, the geriatric population lacks the appropriate increase in WBC count making the diagnosis of sepsis in this population very difficult. Atypical presentation of infection is often observed.

Fever may be absent or blunted in the elderly, and may infer poor prognosis. The inability of the elderly to mount a febrile response may be related to: 1) the presence of older macrophages unable to release endogenous pyrogens; 2) an anterior hypothalamus that cannot respond appropriately to pyrogens; or 3) an individual who cannot mount the proper physiologic response to endogenous pyrogens such as cytokines [50]. Therefore, the presence or absence of fever is unreliable in ruling in or out the diagnosis of sepsis in the elderly.

SPECIAL CONSIDERATIONS IN THE PEDIATRIC POPULATION

As with the elderly, identification of sepsis in the neonatal and pediatric populations can perplex the best of physicians. In this instance, relying on parental observation becomes critical in the history. Once again, vital signs play a critical role in diagnosing sepsis in the infant. From studies done in neonatal meningitis, the most important clinical signs coinciding with severe infection included respiratory status, mental affect, and decreased peripheral perfusion [51]. Good quantitation of urine output, and judicious use of arterial blood gases assist the clinician in assessing perfusion status. Decreased urine output, metabolic acidosis or respiratory alkalosis are all signs of hypoperfusion and may occur despite maintenance of normal blood pressure. This is more likely to occur in the pediatric population than in adults.

DIFFERENTIAL DIAGNOSIS OF SEPSIS AND SEPTIC SHOCK

In treating the patient with sepsis, the physician must generate a differential diagnosis to include clinical entities that present similarly to sepsis [52]. This differential diagnosis includes illnesses that may also manifest some combination of tachypnea, tachycardia, hyperthermia, hypothermia, and leukocytosis. Non-infectious causes of fever include toxins such as cocaine or salicylates, thyroid storm, adrenal insufficiency, neuroleptic malignant syndrome, environmental heat injury, and hypothalamic injury. Systemic illnesses that can present similarly to sepsis include collagen vascular disease or vasculitic syndromes, solid and blood borne neoplasms, and drug overdose and toxins. Those disease syndromes associated with shock and acidosis include acute myocardial infarction, pulmonary embolism, acute hemorrhage, adrenal insufficiency, and anaphylaxis or drug reaction.

CONCLUSION

In conclusion, the best diagnostic tool for sepsis remains suspicion. Other than fever, many of the other commonplace signs of sepsis have a broad differential; therefore, the clinician's intuition, history, and physical examination provide important clues to the diagnosis of sepsis. In addition, laboratory evaluation provides clues that may be hidden from the physical examination. Accurate early diagnosis and institution of empiric medical therapy is critical. Vital signs are important clues and must be combined with history, physical examination, and laboratory values to guide the clinician in the diagnosis and early treatment of sepsis.

REFERENCES

1. Harris RL, Musher DM, Bloom K, et al. Manifestations of sepsis. Arch Intern Med 1987; 147:1895-1906
2. Parker MM, Parillo JE. Septic shock: hemodynamics and pathogenesis. Arch Intern Med 1987; 147:1895-1906
3. Tandberg D, Sklar D. Effect of tachypnea on the estimation of body temperature by an oral thermometer. N Engl J Med 1983; 308:945-6

4. Dinarello CA, Cannon JG, Wolff SM, et al. Tumor necrosis factor is an endogenous pyrogen and induces the production of interleukin-1. J Exp Med 1986; 163:1433-1446
5. Dinarello CA, Wolff SM. Pathogenesis of fever in man. N Engl J Med 1978; 298:607-612
6. Kluger MJ, Ringler DH, Anuer MR. Fever and survival. Science 1975; 188:166-168
7. Vaughn LK, Veale WL, Cooper KE. Antipyresis: Its effect on mortality rate of bacterially infected rabbits (abstract). Fed Proc 1980; 39:1077
8. LeGall J, Lemeshow S,Leleu G, et al. Customized probability models for early severe sepsis in adult intensive care patients. JAMA 1995; 273:644-650
9. Bryant RE, Hood AF, et al. Factors affecting mortality of gram negative rod bacteremia. Arch Intern Med 1971; 127:120-128
10. Clemmer TP, Fisher CJ, Bone RC, et al. Hypothermia in the sepsis syndrome and clinical outcome. Crit Care Med 1992; 20:1395-1401
11. Simmons DH, et al. Hyperventilation and respiratory alkalosis as signs of gram negative bacteremia. JAMA 1960; 174:2196-2199
12. Astiz, ME, Rackow EC. Septic Shock. Lancet 1998;351:1501-5
13. Kaehny WD. Respiratory acid-base disorders. Med Clin North Am 1983; 67:915-928
14. Parker MM, et al. Serial cardiovascular variables in survivors and nonsurvivors of human septic shock: heartrate as an early predictor of prognosis. Crit Care Med 1987; 15:923-9
15. Parrillo JE. Shock syndromes related to sepsis. In: RL Cecil, L. Goldman, JC Bennett (eds) Cecil Textbook of Medicine. WB Saunders, Philadelphia, 1970, pp. 496-501
16. Parrillo JE. Pathogenetic mechanisms of septic shock. N Engl J Med 1993; 328:1471-77
17. Abraham E, Shoemaker WC, Bland RD, et al. Sequential cardiorespiratory patterns in septic shock. Crit Care Med 1983; 11:799-803
18. Eidelman LE, Putterman D, Putterman C, et al. The spectrum of septic encephalopathy: definitions, etiologies, and mortalities. JAMA 1996; 275:470-473
19. Sprung CL, Peduzzi PN, Shatney CH, et al. Impact of encephalopathy on mortality in sepsis syndrome. Crit Care Med 1990; 18: 801-806
20. Freund HR, et al. Amino acid derangements in patients with sepsis: Treatment with branched chain amino acid rich infusions. Ann Surg 1978; 188:423
21. Papadopoulos MC, Davies DC, Moss RF. Pathophysiology of septic encephalopathy: a review. Crit Care Med 2000; 28:3019-3024
22. Vincent JL, Dufaye P, Barre J, et al. Serial lactate determinations during circulatory shock. Crit Care Med 1983; 11:449-451
23. Levy B, Sadoune LO, Gelot AM, et al. Evolution of lactate/pyruvate and arterial ketone body ratios in the early course of catecholamine-treated septic shock. Crit Care Med 2000; 28 114-119
24. Essen F, Lutfi T, Cakar N, et al. Comparison of gastric intramucosal pH measurements with oxygen supply, oxygen consumption, and arterial lactate in patients with severe sepsis. Adv Exp Med & Biology 1996; 388:521-531
25. Ince C, Sinaasappel M. Microcirculatory oxygenation and shunting in sepsis and shock. Crit Care Med 1999; 27:1369-1377
26. Vary TC, Siegel JH, et al. Effect of sepsis on activity of pyruvate dehydrogenase complex in skeletal muscle and liver. Am J Physiol 1986; 250:E634-640
27. James HJ, Luchette FA, McCarter FD, et al. Lactate is an unreliable indicator of tissue hypoxia in injury or sepsis. Lancet 1999; 354:505-508
28. Gore DC, Jahoor F, Hibbert JM, et al. Lactic acidosis during sepsis is related to increased pyruvate production, not deficits in tissue oxygen availability. Ann Surg 1996; 224:97-102
29. Clowes GH. Pulmonary abnormalities in sepsis. Surg Clin North Am 1974; 54:993-1011
30. Rayner BL, Willcox PA, Pascoe MD. Acute renal failure in community-acquired bacteraemia. Nephron 1990; 54:32-35

31. Coratelli P, Passavanti G, Giannattasio M, et al. Acute renal failure after septic shock. Adv Exp Med Bio 1987; 212:233-243
32. Beaufils M, Morel-Maroger L, Sraer JD, et al. Acute renal failure of glomerular origin during visceral abscesses. N Engl J Med 1976; 295:185-9
33. Liolios A, Oropello JM, Benjamin E. Gastrointestinal complications in the intensive care unit. Clin Chest Med 1999; 20:329-345
34. Ledgerwood A. Hepatobiliary complications of sepsis. Heart Lung 1976; 5:621-623
35. Zimmerman HJ, Thomas LD. The liver in pneumococcal pneumonia: Observations in 94 cases of liver function and jaundice in pneumonia. J Lab Clin Med 1950; 35:556-567
36. Zimmerman HJ, Fang M, et al. Jaundice due to bacterial infection. Gastroenterology 1979; 77:362-374
37. Banks JG, Foulis AK, Ledingham IM, et al. Liver function in septic shock. J Clin Pathol 1982; 35:1249-52
38. Batge B, Filejski W, Kurowski V. Clostridial sepsis with massive intravascular hemolysis: rapid diagnosis and successful treatment. Intensive Care Med 1992; 18:488-490
39. Kingston ME, Mackey D. Skin clues in the diagnosis of life-threatening infections. Rev Infect Dis 1986; 8:1-11
40. Bodey GP, Luna M. Skin lesions associated with disseminated candidiasis. JAMA 1997; 229: 1466-1468
41. Tofte RW, Williams DN. Clinical and Laboratory manifestations of toxic shock syndrome. Ann Intern Med 1982; 96:843-7
42. Lang CH, Dobrescu C. Sepsis-induced increases in glucose uptake by macrophage-rich tissues persist during hypoglycemia. Metabolism 1991; 40:585-593
43. Fikins JP, Figlewicz DP. Increased insulin responsiveness in endotoxicosis. Circ Shock 1979; 6:1-6
44. Weissman C. The metabolic response to stress: an overview and update. Anesthesiology 1990; 73:308-327
45. Barton R, Cerra FB. The hypermetabolism multiple organ failure syndrome. Chest 1989; 96:1153-1160
46. Poskitt TR, Poskitt PK. Thrombocytopenia of sepsis: the role of circulating IgG-containing immune complexes. Arch Intern Med 1985; 145:891-894
47. Kelton JG, Neame PB, Gauldie J, et al. Elevated platelet-associated IgG in the thrombocytopenia of septicemia. N Engl J Med 1979; 300:760-764
48. Neane PB, Kelton JG, Walker IR, et al. Thrombocytopenia in septicemia: the role of disseminated intravascular coagulation. Blood 1980; 56:88-92
49. Krieger BP. Sepsis and Multiorgan Failure: Sepsis in the Geriatric Age Group. Williams and Wilkins, Baltimore 1997
50. Cunha B. Infectious Diseases in the Elderly. PSG Publishing Company, Littleton, 1988
51. Bonadio WA, Hennes H, Smith D, et al. Reliability of observation variable in distinguishing infectious outcome of febrile young infants. Pediatr Infect Dis J 1993; 12:111-14
52. Dellinger RP. Current therapies for sepsis. Infect Dis Clin North Am 1999; 13:495-509

3

ORGAN FAILURE

Rui Moreno
Ricardo Matos
Teresa Fevereiro

> *The organism possesses certain contrivances*
> *by means of which the immune reaction, so*
> *easily produced by all kinds of cells, is*
> *prevented from acting against the organism's*
> *own elements and so giving raise to*
> *autotoxins. Further investigations made by*
> *us have confirmed this view so that one*
> *might be justified in speaking of a "horror*
> *autotoxicus" of the organism. The formation*
> *of tissue autotoxins would, therefore,*
> *constitute a danger threatening the*
> *organism.*
>
> Ehrlich and Morgenroth (1901)

When challenged by an invading microorganism, such as a bacteria, a fungus or a virus, the human body starts a series of defense mechanisms, aimed at confining the invaders, controlling the damage and repairing the injured organs and tissues. Such a reaction, that involves a series of cells of the immune system and the liberation of pro and anti-inflammatory cytokines, is in most cases beneficial, allowing the survival of the patient with a minimum of residual injuries.

In some cases, due to poorly understood mechanisms, probably influenced by the type of microorganism involved [1], an imbalance occurs between the degree of injury and the host reaction, resulting in a process of generalized autodestructive inflammation with widespread tissue injury [2]. The clinical manifestation of this process is the multiple organ dysfunction syndrome (MODS), also termed multiple organ failure (MOF) syndrome, the sequential and progressive dysfunction/failure of diverse organs and systems in an acutely ill patient such that homeostasis cannot be maintained without intervention [3].

The pathogenesis of this syndrome, that is responsible for a large number of deaths in critically ill patients, is still poorly understood. There are no doubts, however, that its incidence is increasing. An older population, at least in the western world, an increasing prevalence of chronic diseases, and a greater use of aggressive therapies all contribute to an increasing severity of illness in the patients admitted to general intensive care units (ICUs). The advances in our knowledge of the etiological and physiopathological mechanisms of severe diseases, and in the technologic possibilities for organ support also result in the initial survival of patients who, until a few years ago, would have died before reaching the hospital or within the first hours of hospital stay. MODS/MOF has emerged as one of the consequences of these advances. The initial survival of those patients, after severe insults, usually with very long stays in the ICU, results in an increasing number of complications during the ICU stay. At the same time, we still do not have any therapeutic approach to the status of immunological imbalance that is responsible, or at least occurs, in this syndrome. Consequently, our interventions are mainly preventive, trying to avoid the development of MODS/MOF and supporting homeostasis during the course of the disease. These factors result in considerable morbidity, mortality and resource consumption.

The objective of this chapter is to review the definition, epidemiology, and prognosis of MODS/MOF, with particular attention to sepsis and septic shock.

DEFINITION

Most of the patients with sepsis die in the ICU as a consequence of the sequential and progressive dysfunction/failure of several organs and systems, MODS [4-8]. Described initially by Tilney e al. after severe hemorrhage and shock in major aortic surgery [9], MODS/MOF was subsequently described in association with infection [10,11], acute pancreatitis [12], burns [13], shock [14] and trauma [15].

Over recent years, several definitions of MODS/MOF have been used. A consensus conference organized by the American College of Chest Physicians/Society of Critical Care Medicine Consensus Conference in 1992, defined MODS as the presence of altered organ function in an acutely ill patient such that homeostasis cannot be maintained without intervention [3]. The MODS was also divided into primary or secondary. In primary MODS, organ dysfunction occurs as the result of a well-defined direct insult in which organ dysfunction occurs early and can be directly attributable to the insult itself, such as acute renal failure due to rhabdomyolisis in trauma. In secondary MODS, the organ dysfunction/failure is not a direct consequence of the initial insult, but secondary to the host response to a primary insult such as infection. In this case, the generalized activation of the inflammatory cascade leads to the injury of normal tissues, remote from the initial site of injury.

In both cases, it should be noted that MODS/MOF represents a continuum of organ dysfunction, modulated by numerous factors at different time periods, both process and host related and in which changes in organ function over time are an important element in prognosticating the outcome of the syndrome.

EPIDEMIOLOGY

Sepsis and MOF represents the largest cause of mortality in the ICU [16-18]. Its increasing prevalence and the emergence of new pathogens has been related to changes in the characteristics of the populations and in the use of immunosuppressive therapies and invasive procedures [3]. We are currently treating older patients, with more severe underlying pathology and subjected to more aggressive therapy.

The relationship between the development of MODS/MOF and infection was postulated several years ago [10,11], although, only recently, has accurate data become available on the relationship between these two processes and on the magnitude of the phenomenon.

Bacteremic sepsis was, in 1997, the 12th cause of death in the general population of the United States (US) [19], with an age-adjusted death rate of 4.2 cases per 100,000 standard population. This number is increasing, with a 2.4% increase from 1996 to 1997 and an 82.6% increase from 1979 to 1997. Sands et al. estimated that in large academic centers in the US, the incidence of sepsis was two cases per hundred hospital admissions, with more than 50% of all cases being admitted to the ICU [20].

In France, Brun-Buisson et al. [21], analyzing a large number of patients with the systemic inflammatory response syndrome (SIRS) admitted to 24 French hospitals, found incidence rates of bacteremia and of bacteremic severe sepsis of 9.8 and 2.6 per 1,000 adult admissions, respectively with rates 8 and 32 times higher in ICUs than in the wards. The probability of developing severe sepsis during bacteremia was higher in older patients, and in those with infections of intraabdominal, pulmonary, neuromeningeal, and multiple sources. The development of severe sepsis presented a large impact on mortality, with mortality ranging from 29% in bacteremic patients to 54% in those with bacteremic severe sepsis.

Rangel-Frausto et al. [22], analyzing data from patients admitted to three ICUs in a University Hospital, found in 2527 patients with SIRS, that 48% of them developed the sepsis continuum (sepsis 26%, severe sepsis 18%, and septic shock 4%), with a very important mortality (sepsis 16%, severe sepsis 20% and septic shock 46%) [22]. The number of bacteremic patients increased when patients progressed from SIRS to sepsis, severe sepsis and septic shock (sepsis 17%, severe sepsis 25%, septic shock 69%). No differences in prognosis were evident between patients with bacteremic and non-bacteremic sepsis and septic shock. The number of failing organ/systems, defined as the occurrence of the adult respiratory distress syndrome (ARDS), disseminated intravascular coagulation (DIC), acute renal failure and shock increased when patients progressed from SIRS to sepsis, severe sepsis and septic shock. The same finding was demonstrated by Pittet et al. who found that, in ICU patients with sepsis and positive blood cultures, outcome is mainly determined by the severity of illness at ICU admission and preexisting comorbidities, the need for mechanical ventilation, hypothermia and previous antibiotic therapy at onset of sepsis and the number of vital organ dysfunctions developing subsequently [23].

In the EPIC study, published in 1995, based on data from 1417 ICUs in 17 Western European countries, Vincent et al. estimated that 44.8% of the patients were infected (20.6% with ICU acquired infection) [24]. Clinical sepsis was associated with a 3.5 odds-ratio for mortality. These results are similar to those described before by Parrillo et al. in 1990, who found that when sepsis develops, mortality is close to 30%, reaching 50% in septic shock and up to 80% in the MODS/MOF syndrome [25].

This issue was studied also by the Outcome and Prognosis Working Groups of the Portuguese Society of Intensive Care and the Portuguese Society of Internal Medicine [26]. In this study, in 15 Portuguese ICUs, infection was present on admission in 33.6% of the patients, and significantly associated with a higher age, greater severity of disease, a longer ICU stay and a greater ICU and hospital mortality. The amount of organ dysfunction/failure present at admission, as evaluated by the SOFA score, was significantly related to the presence of infection (Figure 1) and with the presence of criteria for sepsis and septic shock [3], both on admission and during the ICU stay. Mortality in the ICU and in the hospital was significantly related to the development of sepsis and septic shock (patients without criteria 12.3% and 14.3%; SIRS 18.6% and 26.8%; sepsis 27.3% and 39.8%; septic shock 41.7% and 58.0%, respectively).

A similar impact on mortality was demonstrated in a multicenter study promoted in 40 ICUs by Vincent et al., with ICU mortality ranging from 3.2% in patients that never developed an organ failure during ICU stay to 91.3% in patients that presented failure of the 6 analyzed organ/systems at any time during the ICU stay (Figure 2). An impact on ICU mortality was demonstrated also for minor degrees of organ dysfunction (Figure 3), and for the degree of organ dysfunction/failure appearing during the ICU stay (Figure 4) [27].

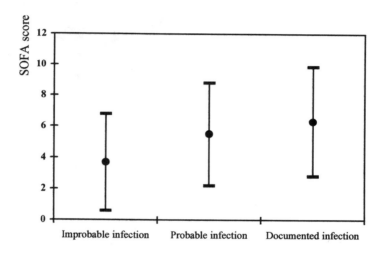

Figure 1. *Admission sequential organ failure assessment (SOFA) score on admission to the ICU and presence of infection in 15 Portuguese ICUs. Results are presented as mean ± standard deviation. Adapted from [26].*

These increases in the frequency and gravity were not accompanied by the emergence of new diagnostic or therapeutic approaches. After a decade of clinical trials with marginal or null results [28,29], mortality remains high, although some authors suggest a recent reduction [30]. It should be noted, however, that the absence of standard definitions for the definition of individual organ dysfunction/failure makes it almost impossible to compare different series. Also, most reports do not describe the presence and impact of other events in the evolution of the disease that influence the prognosis such as inadequate etiological treatment, late or inadequate surgery, and the appropriateness of concomitant therapeutics [31].

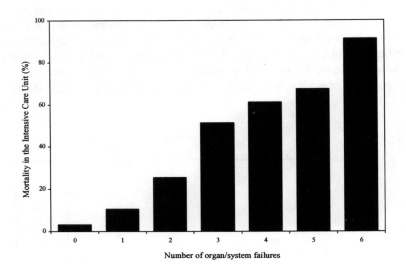

Figure 2. *Maximum number of organ failures during the stay in the ICU and mortality. Organ failure was defined as the occurrence of a SOFA score ≥ 3. Adapted from [27].*

THE QUANTIFICATION OF MODS/MOF

Since the publication by Knaus et al. of an objective scale for the quantification of MOF [4], several such systems have appeared in the literature. The last published systems are the Multiple Organ Dysfunction score (MODS), by Marshall et al. [32], the Logistic Organ Dysfunction (LOD) score by Le Gall et al. [33] and the Sequential Organ Failure Assessment (SOFA) score, developed by a panel of experts of the European Society of Intensive Care Medicine [34].

All these systems have been developed in order to be:
- able to quantify the increasing dysfunction of individual organs, evaluating MODS/MOF as a continuum of dysfunction/failure instead of an on/off phenomena;
- applied sequentially, since MODS/MOF is a dynamic process and the degree of dysfunction varies with time;
- using objective variables, easy to collect and register, available in all ICUs, for the evaluation of each organ. They should be specific for the

analyzed organ and independent from baseline characteristics of the patients;
- independent from local variations in therapeutic approaches;
- designed to describe morbidity and not to predict mortality;
- allowing the individualization of individual organ function instead of aggregated physiological status.

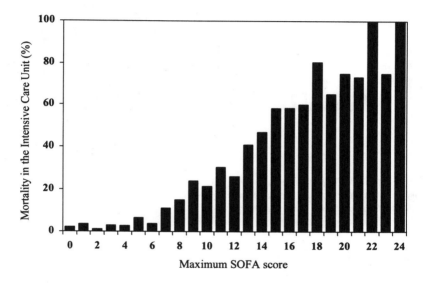

Figure 3. *Maximum SOFA score during the ICU stay, and mortality. Adapted from [27]*

This process of sequential, repeated evaluation of the MODS/MOF is quite new in intensive care medicine, and there is no consensus about which organ/systems should be monitored and quantified, or which is the best system to use. Several such systems have been proposed in the past [2,4,10,32-41], differing among them in the type of variables used: physiologic and/or therapeutic (Table 1) [42,43]. Most of the scores analyze six organ/systems: respiratory, cardiovascular, renal, hematological, neurological and hepatic.

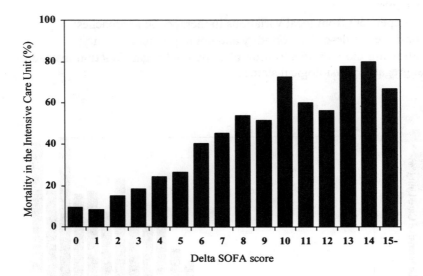

Figure 4*. Delta SOFA score during the ICU stay, and mortality. Delta SOFA, the degree of organ dysfunction/failure appearing during the ICU stay, was computed as maximum SOFA minus admission SOFA score. Adapted from [27]*

Organ System Failure (OSF) Score [4]

Published by Knaus et al. [4], the OSF score is the oldest of these systems in use. Describing MODS/MOF as a binary phenomenon (absent/present), it does not allow the quantification of smaller degrees of organ dysfunction. It should be applied daily, in consecutive periods of 24 hours, during the whole ICU stay. An extensive revision of the OSF was published recently by Zimmerman et al. [44], suggesting that mortality from MOF has decreased in recent years [45].

The OSF originally evaluated five organs/systems: respiratory, cardiovascular, renal, hematological, and neurological. Some modifications have been published, such as that by Garden et al., which added hepatic failure [46].

Organ/system	Physiologic variables	Therapeutic variables
Respiratory	PaO$_2$/FiO$_2$	Mechanical ventilation Level of PEEP
Cardiovascular	Blood pressure	Use of vasoactive drugs
Renal	Urinary output Blood urea Blood creatinine	Dialysis
Hematological	Platelets Leucocytes Hematocrit	Use of blood
Neurological	Glasgow coma score	Use of sedative drugs

PEEP: Positive pressure at end-expiration

Table 1. Types of variables used in multiple organ dysfunction/failure systems. Adapted from [71].

Multiple Organ Dysfunction Score (MODS) [32]

The MODS score was described in 1995 by Marshall et al [32]. Developed after an extensive critical review of the literature, it was later tested and validated in a sample of surgical critically ill patients. This system was subject recently to an external validation in patients with septic shock, revealing a good behavior in medical and surgical patients [47].

The MODS analyzes six organ/systems, assigning from 0 (normality) to 4 (failure) points to each of them: respiratory, renal, hepatic, cardiovascular, hematological and neurological, for a maximum of 24 points. The worst values for each organ or system in a certain period of 24 hours are added later for the calculation of total MODS score in a certain day.

This system differs significantly from the other modern systems in the method chosen for assessing the cardiovascular system. While in the other systems a group of physiologic and/or therapeutic parameters is evaluated, in MODS the evaluation of the cardiovascular dysfunction/failure is given by a composed variable, the pressure-adjusted heart rate (PAR). This fact leads to a more complex calculation, although it presents an excellent discriminative capability when compared with the other systems [48].

It was demonstrated that this system presents a better discriminative capacity than APACHE II or daily OSF [47] and it has been used in several studies [49-52].

Logistic Organ Dysfunction (LOD) System [53]

Proposed by Le Gall et al. [53], this system was developed with the use of complex statistical techniques to choose and weight the variables in a large sample of critical ill patients. The database used (the same as that used for the development of the SAPS II and MPM II) only had data collected during the first 24 hours of ICU stay, and no information exists about its performance later during the ICU stay.

The LODS comprises six organ/systems: neurological, cardiovascular, renal, respiratory, hematological and hepatic and it is the only one of the systems published to allow the calculation of the probability of hospital mortality, based on the amount of dysfunction/failure present at 24 hours on the ICU.

For the computation of the score, each organ or system receives a growing value between 0 and 5 points, this last possible of being just reached for the cardiovascular, neurological and renal systems (for the respiratory and hematological systems the maximum is 3 and for the hepatic system the maximum is 1). Maximum score is 22 points. All the variables should be measured at least once. The chosen value is the most abnormal in the period of 24 hours, missing values being considered normal for the calculation of the score.

In preliminary analyzes the LODS seems to present a deficient calibration and a lower discriminative capability than the other systems [48]. It has been used to date in just one published study [54], although it was the chosen system for European Sepsis Project, recently ended.

Sequential Organ Failure Assessment (SOFA) Score [34]

Developed in 1994 by a panel of experts of the European Society of Intensive Care (ESICM), based on a revision of the literature, the SOFA score was originally denominated sepsis-related organ failure assessment score.

The SOFA quantifies the dysfunction/failure of six organ/systems: respiratory, hematological, hepatic, cardiovascular, neurological and renal, punctuated from 0 (normal function) up to 4 points (severe failure). It presents therefore a maximum score of 24 points.

The SOFA has been validated in several contexts, presenting a good behavior in unselected critically ill patients [55], and in patients with trauma [56], renal failure [57], and cardiovascular disorders [58]. Recently we published derived measures based on this system, destined to a more detailed evolutionary patterns of the critically ill patient [27]. The used in several clinical studies [58-62].

ıns are Created Equal

gan dysfunction/failure is usually reached soon after ICU though some differences exist among the different organ and e ESICM study [27], the mean time to reach maximum failure th organ failure (SOFA score ≥ 3 points) was 2.9 ± 1.1 days, 1.6 days for the neurological score to 4.9 for liver failure (Table

Organ/System	Days in the ICU
	2.33 (2.03 – 2.63)
	2.54 (2.09 – 2.98)
	2.75 (2.10 – 3.41)
	3.09 (2.38 – 3.80)
	4.90 (3.91 – 5.89)
	1.57 (1.23 – 1.91)

each maximum organ failure in patients with organ failure (SOFA score ≥ ented as mean (95% confidence interval for the mean). Adapted from [27].

ıscular score was associated with the highest relative o outcome (odds-ratio for a one point change in the score 1.68, ence interval 1.49 to 1.91), followed by the renal (odds-ratio confidence interval 1.29 to 1.64), the neurological (odds-ratio ınfidence interval 1.28 to 1.55), the coagulation (odds-ratio 1.22, nce interval 1.06 to 1.40) and the respiratory (odds-ratio 1.18, ce interval 1.01 to 1.38) scores. No such contribution could be demonstrated for the hepatic score (odds-ratio 0.82, 95 % confidence interval 0.60 to 1.11). These findings corroborate what is known about the importance of hemodynamic derangements in sepsis [63]. This differential contribution to outcome of the several organ/systems is taken into account only by the LOD score.

The best discriminative power was shown for the cardiovascular score (are under ROC curve 0.802, standard error (SE) 0.015), the renal score (0.739, SE 0.016) and the respiratory score (0.736, SE 0.016). For the neurological score the value was intermediate (0.727, SE 0.016). Coagulation (0.684, SE 0.018) and hepatic scores (0.655, SE 0.019) had a lower discriminative power. The aggregated score (total maximum SOFA score) presented an area under ROC curve of 0.847 (SE 0.012) which was significantly higher (cardiovascular score p = 0.005, all others p < 0.001) than any of its individual components.

Which System to Use?

The systems for the quantification of MODS/MOF differ mainly in the way they evaluate the cardiovascular system: the SOFA score uses the mean blood pressure and the level of vasoactive support, the LOD score the systolic blood pressure and the heart rate and the MODS a composed variable, the pressure-adjusted heart rate(PAR). The only formal comparison among them, published as abstract, seems to indicate a better discriminative capability for MODS and of the SOFA systems than for LOD [48]. However, the low number of analyzed patients requires additional confirmation of these findings from other studies. From a theoretical point of view, the LOD score presents the advantage to assigning different points to different organ/systems based on empirical data, with ranges defined by multiple logistic regression.

The main similarities and differences among these methods are described in Table 3.

Currently, and in the absence of better recommendations, each ICU should use the system that:
-    is tested and validated in their population;
-    results in the smallest percentage of missing values;
-    is least time-consuming to register and compute.

Comparative to the general outcome prediction models, these systems are an important part in our evaluation of the critically ill patient, since they describe better the evolution of the individual patient and are more sensitive to changes due to the evolution of the disease, to the response to therapy or to the emergence of complications.

It should be noted that, independent of the system used, several doubts remain about their sensitivity, the best endpoint to be used in their evaluation (ICU versus hospital mortality), the best time to start evaluation (ICU admission versus start of the septic process) or their incorporation in more general systems (such as the daily APACHE II adjusted for organ-failure [37]).

Organ/system	SOFA [34]	MODS [32]	LOD [33]	OSF [4]
Respiratory	PaO_2/FiO_2 ratio Mechanical ventilation	PaO_2/FiO_2 ratio	PaO_2/FiO_2 ratio Mechanical ventilation	Respiratory rate $PaCO_2$ $AaDO_2$ Mechanical ventilation > 72 hours
Cardiovascular	Mean blood pressure Use of vasoactive agents	PAR	Systolic blood pressure Heart rate	Heart rate Mean arterial pressure Ventricular tachicardia Ventricular fibrillation pH
Renal	Creatinine Urinary output	Creatinine	Creatinine Urea Urinary output	Urinary output Urea Creatinine
Hematological	Platelets	Platelets	Leucocytes Platelets	Leucocytes Platelets Hematocrit
Neurological	Glasgow coma score	Glasgow coma score	Glasgow coma score	Glasgow coma score
Hepatic	Bilirubin	Bilirubin	Bilirubin Protgrombin time	---

$AaDO_2$: alveolo-arterial diference in oxigen; PAR: pressure-adjusted heart rate

Table 3. Comparison of the variables used in the systems for the quantification of MODS/MOF

The Application of MODS/MOF systems

The systems for the quantification of MODS/MOF are destined to the description of the critically ill patient. Several aggregated measures have been proposed for this effect [27,64,65]. The most important are:
-   Admission score: reflects the condition of the patient at ICU admission. Depends basically on the pre-ICU care and admission policies of each ICU, allowing the quantification of the severity at

admission. It can be used for instance as an entry criterion in clinical studies or to evaluate the baseline comparability of groups in clinical trials;

- Daily score: sum of the individual scores for the several organ/systems in a certain day. Evaluates therefore the degree of dysfunction/failure on a certain day. It is especially useful when analyzed in a serial way to monitor the evolution of a certain patient;
- Delta score: the difference between the maximum score and the admission score. Reflects the degree of dysfunction/failure that appears after admission in the ICU, being especially useful to monitor the impact of events occurring after ICU admission, such as the development of nosocomial infection;
- Total maximum scores: is the sum of the scores for each organ or appraised system during the whole ICU stay. Reflects the cumulative insult suffered by the patient, taking into consideration that the dysfunctions/failures of the organ systems appear in different periods of time;
- Organ failure free days: computed for a certain organ, counting, in a certain period of time (usually 28 days), the number of days in which that the patient was alive and without failure of the respective organ. It is especially useful for combining a measure of the morbidity of the surviving patients and of the mortality in the patients who died.

CONCLUSION

MODS/MOF continues to be associated with a poor survival rate. We are still unable to treat etiologically MODS/MOF or, at least, to modulate the immunological mechanisms underlying its installation and progression. Consequently, our best weapon to fight this disease is prevention. Unfortunately, this is not possible in many cases.

While we wait for the physiologists, immunologists, and geneticists to return from the drawing board, as Chernow once said [66], our clinical efforts should be directed especially at the early detection and treatment of sepsis and infection. Early diagnosis and the start of effective antimicrobial therapy have been proven to be associated with a better outcome [67-69]. Krager et al. demonstrated more than 20 years ago that appropriate antibiotic treatment reduced the fatality rate in patients with bacteremia by approximately 50% [67]. Additionally, they shown that early appropriate antibiotic therapy also reduced the frequency with which shock developed by 50%. Even after the development of shock, appropriate antibiotic therapy significantly reduced fatality rates. These are clinical lessons so often forgotten by those more concerned with microbial ecology and cost-saving at any price than with the lives of the human beings, critically ill, that are in our ICUs. Special attention should also be given to early surgery, aimed at the drainage of septic focus. As someone once said "there is no good medicine for bad surgery". Other factors are also probably important, such as the way we feed our patients [70].

All these factors should be taken into account and incorporated in future systems for risk stratification and description of septic patients. We need to learn better how to monitor our patients, how to decide in whom, and when, we must start anti-inflammatory therapy and in whom, and when, we must start immunostimulating therapy. In this complex decision-making process, instruments such as the organ dysfunction/failure scores will be certainly helpful.

Finally, it is very important to use standardized language, following the advice of Lewis Carroll "When I use a word, it means just what I choose it to mean – neither more or less" (Lewis Carroll, Alice's Adventures in Wonderland & Through the Looking Glass, 1965). If we look at the plethora of names we have been using in the past 30 years to describe this syndrome (sequential system failure; multiple, progressive, or sequential systems failure; multiple organ failure; multiple-systems organ failure; post-traumatic syndrome; hypermetabolism organ failure complex; gut origin septic state; multiple organ system failure; syndrome de insuficiencia multiple de organos y sistemas; multiple organ injury syndrome; post-traumatic organ system infection syndrome; multiple organ dysfunction syndrome), this is not what we have been doing.

REFERENCES

1. Opal SM, Cohen J. Clinical Gram-positive sepsis: does it fundamentally differ from Gram-negative bacterial sepsis? Crit Care Med 1999; 27:1608-1616
2. Goris RJA, te Boekhorst TP, Nuytinck JKS, Gimbrère JSF. Multiple-Organ Failure. Generalized autodestructive inflammation? Arch Surg 1985; 120:1109-1115
3. Members of the American College of Chest Physicians and the Society of Critical Care Medicine Consensus Conference Committee. American College of Chest Physicians/Society of Critical Care Medicine Consensus Conference: definitions of sepsis and multiple organ failure and guidelines for the use of innovative therapies in sepsis. Crit Care Med 1992; 20:864-874
4. Knaus WA, Draper EA, Wagner DP, Zimmerman JE. Prognosis in acute organ-system failure. Ann Surg 1985;202:685-693
5. Deitch EA. Multiple organ failure: pathophysiology and potential future therapy. Ann Surg 1992; 216:117-14
6. Tran DD. Age, chronic disease, sepsis, organ system failure and mortality in the elderly admitted to the intensive care medicine. Intensive Care Med 1994; 20:S110 (Abst)

7.   Beal AL, Cerra FB. Multiple organ failure syndrome in the 1990s. Systemic inflammatory response and organ dysfunction. JAMA 1994; 271:226-233
8.   Bone RC, Grodzin CJ, Balk RA. Sepsis: a new hypothesis for pathofenesis of the disease process. Chest 1997; 112:235-243
9.   Tilney NL, Baily GL, Morgan AP. Sequential system failure after rupture of abdominal aortic aneurisms: an unsolved problem in postoperative care. Ann Surg 1973; 178:117-122
10. Fry DE, Pearlstein L, Fulton RL, Polk HC. Multiple system organ failure. The role of uncontrolled infection. Arch Surg 1980;115:136-140
11. Bell RC, Coalson JJ, Smith JD, Johanson WG. Multiple organ failure and infection in adult respiratory distress syndrome. Ann Intern Med 1983; 99:293-298
12. Tran DD, Cuesta MA. Evaluation of severity in patients with acute pancreatitis. Am J Gastroenterol 1992; 87:604-608
13. Marshall WG, Dimick AR. Natural history of major burns with multiple subsystem failure. J Trauma 1983; 23:102-105
14. Henao FJ, Daes JE, Dennis RJ. Risk factors for multiorgan failure: a case-control study. J Trauma 1991; 31:74-80
15. Faist E, Baue AE, Dittmer H, Heberer G. Multiple organ failure in polytrauma patients. J Trauma 1983; 23:775-787
16. Manship L, McMillin RD, Brown JJ. The influence of sepsis and multisystemic organ failure on mortality in the surgical intensive care. Ann Surg 1984; 50:94-101
17. Niederman MS, Fein AM. Sepsis syndrome, the adult respiratory distress syndrome, and nosocomial pneumonia: a common clinical sequence. Clin Chest Med 1990; 11:633-650
18. Bernard G. Sepsis trials. Intersection of investigation, regulation, funding, and practice. Am J Respir Crit Care Med 1995; 152:4-10
19. Centers for Disease Control. Mortality patterns - United States 1997. Morb Mortal Wkly Rep 1999; 48:664-668
20. Sands KE, Bates DW, Lanken PN, et al. Epidemiology of sepsis syndrome in 8 academic medical centers. Academic Medical Center Consortium Sepsis Project Working Group. JAMA 1997;278:234-40.
21. Brun-Buisson C, Doyon F, Carlet J. Bacteremia and severe sepsis in adults: a multicenter prospective survey in ICUs and wards of 24 hospitals. French Bacteremia-Sepsis Study Group. Am J Respir Crit Care Med 1996; 154:617-624
22. Rangel-Frausto MS, Pittet D, Costigan M, Hwang T, Davis CS, Wenzel RP. The natural history of the systemic inflammatory response syndrome (SIRS). A prospective study. JAMA 1995; 273:117-23
23. Pittet D, Thiévent B, Wenzel RP, Li N, Auckenthaler R, Suter PM. Bedside prediction of mortality from bacteriemic sepsis. A dynamic analysis of ICU patients. Am J Respir Crit Care Med 1996; 153:684-693
24. Vincent J-L, Bihari DJ, Suter PM, et al. The prevalence of nosocomial infection in intensive care units in Europe. Results of the European Prevalence of Infection in Intensive Care (EPIC) Study. JAMA 1995; 1:639-644
25. Parrillo JE, Parker MM, Natanson C, et al. Septic shock in humans. Advances in the understanding of pathogenesis, cardiovascular dysfunction, and therapy. Ann Intern Med 1990; 113:227-242
26. Moreno R, Matos R, Fevereiro T, Pereira ME. À procura de um índice de gravidade na sépsis. Rev Port Med Intensiva 1999; 8:43-52
27. Moreno R, Vincent J-L, Matos R, et al. The use of maximum SOFA score to quantify organ dysfunction/failure in intensive care. Results of a prospective, multicentre study. Intensive Care Med 1999; 25:686-696
28. Eidelman LA, Sprung CL. Why have new therapies for sepsis not been developed? Crit Care Med 1994; 22:1330-1334

29. Bone RC. Why sepsis trials fail. JAMA 1996; 276:565-566
30. Friedman G, Silva E, Vincent J-L. Has the mortality of septic shock changed with time? Crit Care Med 1998; 26:2078-2086
31. Sprung CL, Finch RG, Thijs LG, Glauser MP. International sepsis trial (INTERSEPT): role and impact of a clinical evaluation committee. Crit Care Med 1996; 24:1441-1447
32. Marshall JC, Cook DA, Christou NV, Bernard GR, Sprung CL, Sibbald WJ. Multiple organ dysfunction score: a reliable descriptor of a complex clinical outcome. Crit Care Med 1995; 23:1638-1652
33. Le Gall JR, Klar J, Lemeshow S, et al. The logistic organ dysfunction system. A new way to assess organ dysfunction in the intensive care unit. JAMA 1996; 276:802-810
34. Vincent J-L, Moreno R, Takala J, et al. The SOFA (Sepsis-related organ failure assessment) score to describe organ dysfunction/failure. Intensive Care Med 1996; 22:707-710
35. Elebute EA, Stoner HB. The grading of sepsis. Br J Surg 1983;70:29-31.
36. Stevens LE. Gauging the severity of surgical sepsis. Arch Surg 1983; 118:1190-1192
37. Chang RW, Jacobs S, Lee B. Predicting outcome among intensive care unit patients using computerised trend analysis of daily Apache II scores corrected for organ system failure. Intensive Care Med 1988; 14:558-566
38. Meek M, Munster AM, Winchurch RA, et al. The Baltimore Sepsis Scale: measurement of sepsis in patients with burns using a new scoring system. J Burn Care Rehabil 1991;12:564-568
39. Baumgartner JD, Bula C, Vaney C, et al. A novel score for predicting the mortality of septic shock patients. Crit Care Med 1992; 20:953-960
40. Fagon J-Y, Chastre J, Novara A, Medioni P, Gilbert C. Characterization of intensive care unit patients using a model based on the presence or absence of organ dysfunctions and/or infection: the ODIN model. Intensive Care Med 1993; 19:137-144
41. Bernard GR, Doig BG, Hudson G, et al. Quantification of organ failure for clinical trials and clinical practice. Am J Respir Crit Care Med 1995; 151:A323 (Abst)
42. Bertleff MJ, Bruining HA. How should multiple organ dysfunction syndrome be assessed? A review of the variations in current scoring systems. Eur J Surg 1997; 163:405-409
43. Marshall JD, Bernard G, Le Gall J-R, Vincent J-L. The measurement of organ dysfunction/failure as an ICU outcome. Sepsis 1997; 1:41
44. Zimmerman JE, Knaus WA, Sun X, Wagner DP. Severity stratification and outcome prediction for multisystem organ failure and dysfunction. World J Surg 1996; 20:401-405
45. Zimmerman JE, Knaus WA, Wagner DP, Sun X, Hakim RB, Nystrom P-O. A comparison of risks and outcomes for patients with organ failure: 1982-1990. Crit Care Med 1996; 24:1633-1641
46. Garden OJ, Motyl H, Gilmour WH, Utley RJ, Carter DC. Prediction of outcome following acute variceal haemorrhage. Br J Surg 1985; 72:91-95
47. Jacobs S, Zuleika M, Mphansa T. The multiple organ dysfunction score as a descriptor of patient outcome in septic shock compared with two other scoring systems. Crit Care Med 1999; 27:741-744
48. Moreno R, Pereira E, Matos R, Fevereiro T. The evaluation of cardiovascular dysfunction/failure in multiple organ failure. Intensive Care Med 1997; 23:S153 (Abst)
49. Gonçalves JA, Hydo LJ, Barie PS. Factors influencing outcome of prolonged norepinephrine therapy for shock in critical surgical illness. Shock 1998; 10:231-236
50. Maziak DE, Lindsay TF, Marshall JC, et al. The impact of multiple organ dysfunction on mortality following ruptured abdominal aortic aneurysm repair. Ann Vasc Surg 1998; 12:93-100
51. Pinilla JC, Hayes P, Laverty W, et al. The C-reactive protein to prealbumin ratio correlates with the severity of multiple organ dysfunction. Surgery 1998; 124:799-805

52. Staubach KH, Schroder J, Stuber F, et al. Effect of pentoxifylline in severe sepsis: Results of a randomized, double-blind, placebo-controlled study. Arch Surg 1998; 133:94-100
53. Le Gall J-R, Klar J, Lemeshow S. How to assess organ dysfunction in the intensive care unit? The logistic organ dysfunction (LOD) system. Sepsis 1997; 1:45-47
54. Soufir L, Timsits JF, Mahe C, et al. Attributable morbidity and mortality of catheter-related septicemia in critically ill patients: a matched, risk-adjusted, cohort study. Infect Control Hosp Epidemiol 1999; 20:396-401
55. Vincent J-L, de Mendonça A, Cantraine F, et al. Use of the SOFA score to assess the incidence of organ dysfunction/failure in intensive care units: results of a multicentric, prospective study. Crit Care Med 1998; 26:1793-800
56. Antonelli M, Moreno M, Vincent J-L, et al. Application of SOFA score to trauma patients. Intensive Care Med 1999; 25:389-394
57. Mendonça A, Vincent J-L, Suter PM, et al. Acute renal failure in the ICU: risk factors and outcome evaluated by the SOFA score. Intensive Care Med 2000; 26:915-921
58. Janssens U, Graf C, GGraf J, et al. Evaluation of the SOFA score: a single center experience of a medical intensive care unit in 303 consecutive patients with predominantly cardiovascular disorders. Intensive Care Med 2000; 26:1037-1045
59. Di Filippo A, De Gaudio AR, Novelli A, et al. Continuous infusion of vancomycin in methicillin-resistant staphylococcus infection. Chemotherapy 1998; 44:63-68
60. Fiore G, Donadio PP, Gianferrari P, et al. CVVH in postoperative care of liver transplantation. Minerva Anestesiol 1998; 64:83-87
61. Briegel J, Forst H, Haller M, et al. Stress doses of hydrocortisone reverse hyperdynamic septic shock: a prospective, randomized, double-blind, single-center study. Crit Care Med 1999; 27:723-732
62. Hynninen M, Valtonen M, Markkanen H, et al. Interleukin 1 receptor antagonist and E-selectin concentrations: a comparison in patients with severe acute pancreatitis and severe sepsis. J Crit Care 1999; 14:63-68
63. Marik PE, Varon J. The hemodynamic derangements in sepsis. Implications for treatment strategies. Chest 1998; 113:854-860
64. Bernard GR. Quantification of organ dysfunction: seeking standardization. Crit Care Med 1998; 26:1767-1768
65. Marshall J. Charting the course of critical illness: prognostication and outcome description in the intensive care unit. Crit Care Med 1999; 27:676-678
66. Chernow B. Back to the drawing board. Crit Care Med 1996; 24:1097-1098
67. Kreger BE, Craven DE, McCabe WR. Gram-negative bacteremia. IV. Re-evaluation of clinical features and treatment in 612 patients. Am J Med 1980; 68:344-355
68. Bryan CS, Reynolds KL, Brenner ER. Analysis of 1186 episodes of gram-negative bacteremia in non-university hospitals: the effects of antimicrobial therapy. Rev Infect Dis 1983; 5:629-638
69. Weinstein MP, Murphy JR, Reller LB, Lichtenstein KA. The clinical significance of positive blood cultures: a comprehensive analysis of 500 episodes of bacteremia and fungemia in adults. II. Clinical observations, with special reference bto factors influencing prognosis. Rev Infect Dis 1983; 5:54-70
70. Beale RJ, Bryg DJ, Bihari DJ. Immunonutrition in the critically ill: a systematic review of clinical outcome. Crit Care Med 1999; 27:2799-2805
71. Marshall JD, Bernard G, Le Gall J-R, Vincent J-L. Conclusions. Sepsis 1997; 1:55-57

4

MARKERS OF SEPSIS

Heinz Redl
Andreas Spittler
Wolfgang Strohmaier

Sepsis related organ failures are among the major causes of prolonged intensive care, placing a heavy burden upon health care. It is, therefore, imperative to monitor biochemical/immunological markers and to identify those predicting isolated or multiple organ failure. Traditionally the term 'sepsis' has been used to describe the process of infection accompanied by the host's systemic inflammatory response. Based upon that understanding, previous clinical studies have been designed to include only patients with positive blood cultures [1]. However, the frequent occurrence of an inflammatory response without detection of microorganisms in the circulation has led to a new understanding and definition of sepsis, mainly as the systemic host response to a microbiological, event which is often undetectable as such, or non-microbiological, process, with detectable levels of cytokines independent of the presence of documented infection [2]. Initially, a hyperinflammatory stage is present, which can be rapidly replaced by a hypoinflammatory phase with considerable overlap and then may lead to immunoparalysis if no recovery has taken place. In fact pro- and anti-inflammatory stimuli exist simultaneously in every patient [3]. Therefore, it is often difficult to identify the status of a patient. Despite this lack of knowledge and the limited monitoring possibilities, enormous resources have been invested into therapeutic studies.

Basically, there are two approaches for biochemical/immunological monitoring (Figure 1):

1) to study *body fluids*, mainly plasma, since the sepsis response can be highly compartmentalized, e.g., broncho-alveolar lavage (BAL) fluid may be more relevant [4] in certain situations;

2) to study *cells*, usually blood derived peripheral cells, but local cells, e.g., pulmonary macrophages could be more relevant on some occasions.

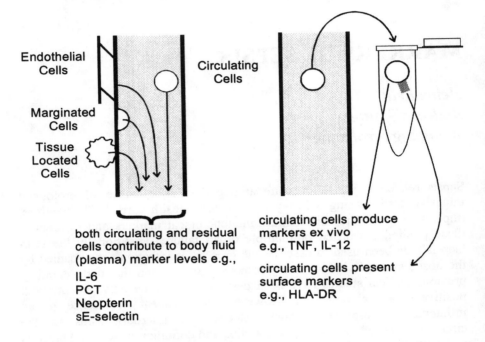

Figure 1: Possible approaches in sepsis monitoring

Body fluids are usually easier to obtain. The measured markers are products of both circulating and resident cells (e.g., polymorphonuclear leukocytes [PMN], Kupffer, or endothelial cells). Apart from the rates of product synthesis and release or shedding of surface molecules, clearance and iatrogenic dilution are factors affecting concentrations. On the other hand *ex vivo* measurements of cells are dependent on the mode of collection (separation) and represent the non-resident fraction of cells only. However, such measurements probably reflect the activation potential and the receptor status of the peripheral immune system. For each of the two approaches some examples will be discussed below.

BODY FLUID (PLASMA) MARKERS

The spectrum of markers to be measured in plasma comprises: a) sepsis inducers such as lipopolysaccharide (LPS) and related molecules; b) products of responding cells; and c) products of humoral activation cascades.

Inducers

Endotoxin (and associated LPS binding protein [LBP], LPS-Ab)

Bacterial endotoxin (LPS) is a primary inducer in the pathophysiology of gram-negative bacterial sepsis. Therefore, LPS is considered an important monitoring parameter. However, there are several obstacles to LPS measurements. A single measurement of endotoxin may be misleading. The often transient appearance of bacteria/LPS in the circulation makes it difficult to document the occurrence in patients and this might be one possible explanation for conflicting clinical results [5], although in a recent study Opal et al. [6] were able to demonstrate in > 250 sepsis patients that median LPS levels at study entry were more highly elevated in non-survivors. A Kaplan-Meier survival plot revealed a 28 day mortality of 35 % in LPS positive, and 22 % in LPS negative, patients. From a practical point of view LPS assays using current techniques cannot be recommended for routine use.

In the same study LBP, the principle protein responsible for transporting endotoxin to effector cells, was measured. While there was no correlation between LPS and LBP, LBP levels were less highly elevated in non-survivors [6]. Plasma levels of LBP correlate with outcome in sepsis and other patients [7].

Beside LPS and LBP, the levels of anti-LPS core antibodies in plasma have been considered for monitoring with the rationale of identifying those sepsis patients who might benefit from endotoxin-neutralizing therapy. Decreased levels of anti-LPS core antibodies were associated with increased mortality [8, 9].

No routinely applicable analytical tools are available for Gram-positive cell components.

Products of Responding Cells

One important aspect in the understanding of the pathophysiological network in sepsis is the ability to detect and measure cytokines. This is a difficult task due to local production and action, low levels and short half-lives [4]. The short half-life in plasma results partly from binding to receptors, including circulating soluble cytokine receptors. Not only can these soluble receptors neutralize cytokines, they are diagnostic tools in themselves [9].

An approach to avoiding difficulties associated with cytokine monitoring is the use of so-called surrogate markers for sepsis monitoring, of which the macrophage activation marker neopterin [10] and procalcitonin [11] are the most well-known.

Plasma Cytokines

From the large pool of cytokines, IL-6 has been most widely used, due to favorable characteristics such as fast kinetic response, independence of soluble receptor-binding in most assays, and relative independence of kidney function. Relevant concentrations in the low nanogram range are suitable for reliable commercial immunoassays. Elevated levels of interleukin (IL-)-6 were found to be associated with fatal outcome, while tumor necrosis factor (TNF) levels did not prove to be a prognostic indicator [12], thus indicating that IL-6 is a reliable marker of sepsis [12-14]. Furthermore, plasma IL-8 [15], IL-10 [16], IL-18 [17], and natural antagonists such as IL-1 receptor antagonist (IL-1ra) and soluble TNF receptors [9] have been repeatedly used for monitoring purposes in sepsis patients.

Plasma IL-6 levels have also given useful information regarding therapy. In some anti-TNF trials, the overall study population showed no increase in survival after sepsis upon treatment. Retrospective stratification of patients by IL-6 concentrations suggested beneficial effects of the drug for patients with baseline circulating IL-6 concentrations of > 1000 pg/ml [18]. Interestingly, the administration of an anti-TNF antibody resulted in a decrease in IL-6 and not in TNF-α [14]. As a result of these findings, two prospective studies (RAMSES in Europe, MONARCS in North America) were set up to evaluate the effect of anti-TNF antibody therapy in patients presenting with a hyperinflammatory state based on IL-6 plasma levels at the time of study entry. In the MONARCS study, of the 2,634 patients enrolled, 998 had IL-6 levels > 1000 pg/ml and 1,636 did not. Patients with IL-6 > 1000 pg/ml had a significantly higher mortality (47.7 vs. 28.6 %) (Panacek et al. unpublished data). In those with elevated IL-6 levels, TNF antibody reduced risk-adjusted 28-day mortality (6.9 %) compared to placebo (41.5 % vs. 48.4 %, p = 0.041). Mortality at 28-days was also reduced (3.6 %) in the overall population (32.3 % vs. 35.9 %, p = 0.049). In other words, anti-TNF therapy was twice as effective in patients with IL-6 > 1000 pg/ml indicating the potential of markers of sepsis. Anti-TNF therapy also significantly reduced serum IL-6 levels (p > 0.05).

One of the most recently identified substances acting as a cytokine is high mobility group 1 (HMG-1) [19], which does not appear in the plasma of endotoxic animals until 8 hours after endotoxin administration. However, even late therapeutic blockade is associated with improved survival. Although currently there are only limited data, HMG-1 could become a valuable marker in the future, since sepsis patients who succumb to infection have increased serum HMG-1 levels [19].

Neopterin

Neopterin (NEO), a member of the ubiquitous family of unconjugated pteridines, is derived from guanosine triphosphate (GTP) [20] and released from monocyte/macrophages upon stimulation with interferon (IFN)-γ and LPS [21]. Related molecules such as biopterins have gained widespread interest since tetrahydrobiopterin is the essential co-factor for aromatic amino acid monoxygenases and thus for neurotransmitter synthesis, as well as for nitric oxide synthases (NOS) [22].

After previous use in graft versus host disease, a strong correlation between NEO levels and the occurrence of septic events in intensive care patients was first described in 1987 [10] with discrimination between survivors and non-survivors among these 21 patients as early as day one. An investigation on 56 patients [23] was in agreement; in that study NEO testing (96% sensitivity and 73% specificity for NEO < 40 nmol/l) yielded an overall accuracy of 83%. NEO also predicted the Goris multiple organ failure (MOF) score (if > 5) when measured one day before the evaluation. In this study NEO always differentiated between septic and non-septic survivors and non-survivors as well. Increased NEO concentrations were also reported [24] in parallel with demonstrating that freshly isolated monocytes stimulated *ex vivo* with LPS are exhausted to produce NEO in surgical patients. The authors concluded that resident, tissue-bound macrophages are responsible for the high serum levels. In another study [25] a clear discrimination between survivors and non-survivors starting as early as day two post trauma in a 14 day observation period could be observed. One hundred patients with severe polytrauma (mean injury severity score [ISS] = 37) were studied. Both NEO and soluble IL-2 receptor were identified by Delogu et al. as significant predictors of shock states in Gram-negative sepsis [26]. Slightly divergent data were presented in a prospective study of 56 patients, evaluating various inflammatory mediators as predictors of MOF after blunt trauma (ISS > 33) with significant changes in the later course of sepsis [27]. The authors used the NEO/creatinine ratio in their calculations to compensate for kidney dysfunction, since NEO is cleared via the kidneys in a creatinine-like fashion [28].

For well over ten years now, NEO has been assessed routinely in the ICU at the Lorenz Böhler Trauma Hospital and has gained acceptance as part of monitoring. Moreover, it has turned out that NEO lends itself to a number of additional applications. First, selective puncture of corresponding veins and arteries allows a comparison of their respective NEO concentrations. The resulting arterio-venous difference may be an indication for the existence, or absence, of septic foci [29], the latter information often being of more importance. Second, in 1996, Strohmaier et al. [30] showed that NEO blood levels can provide a reliable basis for the decision on whether or not to use antibiotics in our ICU. After a two-year evaluation period with 536 patients enrolled and the definition of a few exceptions (e.g., open head fracture), we ultimately adopted the present procedure: In cases of suspected infection, antibiotics are given only if serum NEO levels exceed 40 nmol/l. This approach is supported by bedside infection screening using Gram-stained smears [31]. The cut-off value of 40 nmol/l serves as a discriminator between colonization, which remains untreated, and systemic infection. The main results of this strategy have been a marked reduction in infectious episodes and isolated microorganisms, particularly *Pseudomonas* spp. and staphylococci, as well as in the cost of therapy.

Procalcitonin

Procalcitonin (PCT) is a 116-amino acid propeptide, which undergoes proteolysis into the hormone calcitonin. PCT has been suggested as an excellent early and discriminating marker of bacteria-associated sepsis in patients (with low levels in virus-induced infection) [32]. An increasing number of clinical studies have been performed, since a commercial assay has become available (for review see Meisner [33]. Although the source of calcitonin has been generally considered to be the thyroid cell (and other neuroendocrine cells), this cell is probably not the source of PCT, as an infection-associated rise in PCT has also been shown in thyroidectomized sepsis patients [11]. The source of PCT in sepsis is currently unclear. Some of the inducers of PCT, such as endotoxin and *E. coli* are known. Given to chimpanzees and volunteers [34], and to baboons [35], these agents resulted in increased serum PCT concentrations.

Reith et al. [36] reported significant falls in plasma PCT concentrations in patients with peritonitis after successful focal ablation. When surgical removal of septic foci failed and patients died, mean PCT levels remained high. Brunkhorst et al. [37] clearly discriminated between an infectious and a non-infectious etiology of acute respiratory distress syndrome (ARDS) using PCT levels. In a series of 17 consecutive patients with very similar Murray scores, PCT distinguished between the septic and the non-septic origin of ARDS. TNF and NEO yielded equivalent results, while IL-6 and C-reactive protein (CRP) proved inadequate. Scoring the patients by means of the APACHE II also clearly discriminated septic from non-septic etiology. Another group highly vulnerable to infection are burns victims. Nylen et al. [38] investigated 41 patients and demonstrated a preferential release of PCT from the lung; these authors concluded that serum PCT levels might have prognostic power regarding the severity of inhalational injury. Circulating PCT was measured in 40 burns patients with total body surface area (TBSA) > 30% by Carsin et al. [39] up to one week after admission and compared to levels of IL-6, TNF-α and endotoxin. PCT levels proved to be of prognostic value for mortality and to correlate with IL-6 and the severity of skin burn injury, but were not associated with inhalation injury. The finding that mortality was decreased when septic animals were treated with an antiserum reactive to PCT, suggests that PCT is more than a marker of bacterial sepsis and can actually be regarded as an active player in inflammatory processes [40].

Endothelial Markers

Since it is difficult to obtain the few circulating endothelial cells [41], plasma measurement is the method of choice. Amongst many other events during sepsis is an activation of endothelial cells with an up-regulation of cell surface adhesion molecules such as P-selectin, E-selectin and intercellular adhesion molecule (ICAM)-1. This up-regulation increases leukocyte adherence. A small proportion of these adherence molecules is shed into plasma and thus is accessible for plasma analysis. In a polytrauma study, from the 4th day onwards sE-selectin and sICAM-1 were different in three outcome groups, namely lethal, reversible, and no organ failure (Jochum et al., unpublished data). Endothelial cells are also considered to be a possible source of increased IL-6 production observed in situations such as stress or septic shock, in which catecholamines are elevated due to endogenous production or exogenous application [42].

It is not only interesting to monitor endothelial activation but also endothelial damage. One factor is thrombomodulin. Besides being present on the endothelial surface, a soluble form of thrombomodulin (in reality, several fragments) has been found in plasma and urine of normal subjects. *In vitro* [43] and *in vivo* [44] experiments in rabbits suggest that soluble thrombomodulin is not shed from the endothelial surface but is the result of cellular damage. Several investigators have reported that plasma thrombomodulin levels are elevated in disease states commonly associated with perturbation of the vascular endothelium, such as ARDS [45] and sepsis [46]. Experimental results provide evidence for an *E. coli* dose-related and TNF-dependent thrombomodulin release into the plasma of septic baboons and suggest a possible role of anti-TNF for the protection of the endothelium [47].

Apart from thrombomodulin, plasma levels of soluble endothelial cell protein C receptor are elevated in patients with sepsis. However, there is lack of correlation with thrombomodulin, which suggests the involvement of different pathological processes [48].

Humoral Factors

Humoral cascades become activated in the plasma of sepsis patients partly as a direct reaction with sepsis inducers (e.g., during opsonization), but mainly upon reaction with activated cells (e.g., monocytes and tissue factor). These reactions lead to the induction of coagulation, fibrinolysis, and the complement cascade (for review see Hack [49]). Since clinical intervention trials are underway or completed (antithrombin [AT]III, tissue factor pathway inhibitor [TFPI], activated protein C [APC]), the obvious question is whether plasma levels of elements of the humoral cascades can be of use in monitoring sepsis. Two examples worth pointing out in this context are the good correlation of low ATIII [50] and low protein C [46, 51] with higher risk in sepsis patients. ATIII levels < 70 % at the onset of fever predicted a lethal outcome with 85 % sensitivity and 85 % specificity [50].

Kinetics of Plasma Markers

One must be aware that different plasma markers have different appearance kinetics. This is easily demonstrated in a non-human primate sepsis model (Figure 2). While TNF or IL-10 follow short time kinetics, NEO exhibits a slow but stable response. Other parameters such as IL-6 or PCT occur between these extremes. On the one hand, although a fast response is desirable for the early detection of sepsis complications, a fast response is usually associated with unstable plasma levels. Thus, the time of sampling is a possible source of inaccurate results. One of the slow reacting markers is CRP. Since CRP is elevated in all inflammatory conditions, however, its value as a sepsis marker is limited.

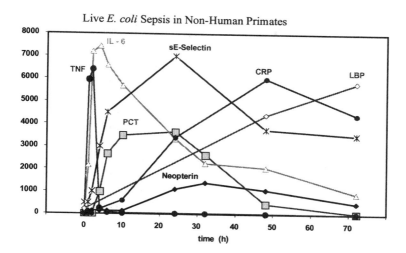

Figure 2: *Kinetics of plasma markers. Data are displayed with the following dimension and correction factors: TNF, IL-6, PCT (pg/ml); NEO x 10 (nmol/l); LBP, CRP x 20 (mg/l); sE-Selectin x 500 (pg/ml).*

CELL ASSOCIATED MARKERS

To define inflammatory stages, several cell surface molecules on various cell types have been investigated and functional assays performed to determine the *ex vivo* reactivity of immunocompetent cells after stimulation. Highly standardized methods (e.g., flow cytometry, ELISA), which are easily carried out, yield results in a short time. Immunological interventions and therapeutic strategies should now be applied depending on what immunological phase the patient exhibits.

HLA-DR expression as a prognostic and predictive parameter

The best characterized cell surface antigen in septic disease is the human leukocyte antigen (HLA) with its cluster DR. HLA-DR is part of the major histocompatibility class II antigen complex mainly expressed by antigen-presenting cells such as monocytes and macrophages but also by activated T and B cells. In this context, monocytes have been intensively studied since they play a central role in both specific and non-specific immunity against bacterial, viral, and fungal infection. As early as 1986, Polk and co-workers correlated the percentage of HLA-DR expressing monocytes with the appearance of infection [52]. The authors investigated patients who had sustained major trauma and showed a positive correlation between low monocyte HLA-DR expression and the development or presence of major infection at days 7-8 and days 10-12. Some years later, Hershman and co-workers investigated 60 trauma patients divided into three groups [53]. Monocyte HLA-DR expression in those patients with uneventful recovery returned to normal range after one week, whereas in patients with recovery from severe sepsis, normal levels were reached after 3 weeks. In those patients who died, HLA-DR expression never returned to normal levels. Similar results have been observed by other investigators. Döcke et al. demonstrated that a diminished MHC class II antigen expression (< 30 % HLA-DR+) on monocytes over a period of over 5 days strongly correlated with fatal outcome after septic disease [54]. Immune monitoring in cardiac transplant recipients performed by our group showed that patients with a reduced HLA-DR density on monocytes after 5-7 days following transplantation were at a high risk of developing infectious complications [55]. Those patients with an increased HLA-DR expression in comparison to their individual HLA-DR density preoperatively had a high rejection risk.

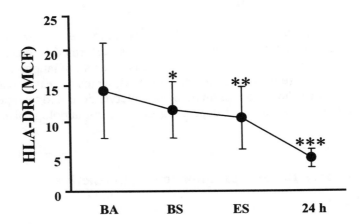

Figure 3. Expression of HLA-DR on CD14⁻ monocytes before anesthesia (BA), before surgery (BS), at the end of surgery (ES), and 1 day after surgery (24 h). *p<0.05, **p<0.01, ***p<0.001 vs baseline.

It must, however, also be pointed out that a decrease in density of HLA-DR on monocytes always occurs during surgery and that a significant decline takes place immediately after induction of anesthesia, even before surgical intervention [56]. In this study the density of HLA-DR at day 1 after thoracic surgery was reduced to 30% of baseline levels (Figure 3). Interestingly, all patients had an uncomplicated post-operative course despite such a large decrease in HLA-DR density. Patients with severe pancreatitis also showed a decrease in HLA-DR on monocytes after surgery. However, repeated surgical interventions did not further influence HLA-DR expression [57].

Various mediators have been shown to regulate the expression of HLA-DR. Among the main regulators are cytokines: e. g., IL-10 and transforming growth factor (TGF)-β are known to dramatically reduce HLA-DR expression on monocytes *in vitro,* whereas IFN-γ is a potent counter-regulator. The beneficial effect of IFN-γ was demonstrated in patients with severe sepsis [54]. Patients with a monocyte HLA-DR expression below 30% on two consecutive days were treated with IFN-γ until more than 50% of monocytes were HLA-DR$^+$ for three consecutive days. Recovery of monocyte HLA-DR expression led to clearance of sepsis in 8 out of 9 patients in this study.

An additional mediator which influences HLA-DR expression on human monocytes in cell culture experiments as well as *in vivo* is the amino acid glutamine (GLN). GLN is the most abundant amino acid in the blood and in the free amino acid pool of the body. During starvation and catabolic stress following trauma, surgical procedures or sepsis, GLN loss correlates with the severity of the disease and supplementation of GLN has beneficial effects in those patients. Low GLN concentrations have profound effects on cells of the immune system. These effects include the inhibition of mitogen-induced T-cell proliferation, a decrease in the capacity of macrophages to phagocytose opsonized particles, and the reduction of the differentiation of B-cells into plasma cells. Previously we have shown that GLN deprivation in the culture medium down-regulates HLA-DR antigen expression on monocytes and reduces their capacity to present tetanus-toxoid to CD4$^+$ T lymphocytes [58]. Recently we demonstrated that the treatment of patients with a GLN-containing solution in the postoperative phase reduced immunosuppression by partial prevention of the surgery induced decrease in HLA-DR expression on monocytes [59].

The regulatory capacities of mediators on the expression of HLA-DR on monocytes and macrophages raises the question whether the reduced number of MHC class II molecules determines the capacity to present antigen. In fact, in a previous study it was shown that occupancy of as few as 0.1% of all MHC class II molecules has been found to be sufficient for stimulation of quiescent T-cells [60]. Therefore, these data suggest that the capacity of circulating monocytes to present antigen and to stimulate proliferation of T-cells is not suppressed during uneventful recovery after major surgery, despite a significant loss of cell surface HLA-DR proteins. Thus, the correlation of HLA-DR reduction and clinical outcome are based on other mechanisms. However, since there is a well documented correlation between infectious complications, clinical outcome and the expression of HLA-DR on circulating monocytes, this antigen seems to be a reliable marker in the course of sepsis [52-54, 56, 57, 61].

Despite the well characterized expression of HLA-DR on monocytes, its expression on other cell types is only partly documented. Wakefield et al. described that in contrast to monocytes the level of T-cell HLA-DR expression rose significantly on the first day after surgery in non-septic patients to a level higher than in those who developed infection [62]. The investigators concluded that these findings have important implications for biological response modification in patients at risk of developing sepsis after surgery. However, in patients with septic shock Lin et al. observed no significant alterations in lymphocyte activation and they concluded that the study of lymphocyte cell surface marker expression during sepsis may be too insensitive to measure transient changes in lymphocyte activation [63]. Furthermore, HLA-DR expression on circulating B-cells from severely injured patients was investigated by Ditschkowski et al. [64]. In this study HLA-DR was significantly reduced from days 6-14 after admission in patients with subsequent severe sepsis compared to those who did not develop sepsis.

A recently published study by Ditschkowski et al. showed that the soluble form of HLA-DR in septic patients immediately after trauma was significantly lower then in non-septic patients. This was paralleled by a reduced expression of HLA-DR on circulating T-cells [65].

Additional Cell Associated Markers in Sepsis

Since monocytes play a decisive role in the development and course of sepsis and the expression of cell surface antigens is correlated with functional properties of these cells, numerous additional markers have been studied. One of these, the CD14 antigen, plays a central role in innate immune responses. CD14 is highly expressed on monocytes, binds bacterial LPS and LBP, and functions as an opsonin presenting LPS to CD14. Moreover, it is found as a soluble CD14 (sCD14) form in circulation, and the plasma level has been shown to be increased in some infectious diseases, including sepsis. The membrane-bound CD14 is down-regulated during sepsis and it has been suggested that decreased expression possibly indicates a poor prognosis [63, 66]. Recently, it has been shown that the signaling pathway of the complex LPS-LBP-CD14 is triggered by binding to Toll-like receptor (TLR) 4 and its co-factor MD2. So far, only limited data are available concerning the regulation of TLR4 on monocytes and further studies will clarify its role as a suitable sepsis marker in an immune monitoring system.

In addition, a subset of monocytes with weak expression of CD14 and increased CD16 expression has been described in healthy subjects. This subset is expanded up to 80 % in sepsis patients and is characterized with features of tissue macrophages [67]. Interestingly, the appearance of these cells was paralleled by a high concentration of IL-6 in those patients. As previously mentioned, IL-6 has a high predictive value in the course of sepsis. However, in contrast to recently published work which demonstrated a down-regulation of HLA-DR, these CD16 + monocytes express high levels of MHC class II products. These different findings may be explained by different time points of measurement. Patients with high levels of HLA-DR and IL-6 are possibly in a state of transition from the hyper-inflammatory phase to immunosuppression. Our own observations have confirmed these results, since we have demonstrated that patients in the very early phase of sepsis had high IL-6 levels and showed an increase in the expression of HLA-DR and the production of TNF-α as well as in their capacity to phagocytose [68]. Therefore, sepsis patients with low IL-6 and TNF-α plasma levels, in combination with a progressively reduced monocytic phagocytic capacity and HLA-DR expression are possibly in a later phase of septic disease eventually leading to immunoparalysis.

To characterize the systemic inflammatory status, additional markers on monocytes as well as on various other cells have been described. The CD11b/CD18 complex functions as an adhesive molecule in promoting cell interaction and mediates binding of iC3b-coated particles, leading to their ingestion and destruction. Takala et al. demonstrated that the expression of CD11b/CD18 increased with the severity of systemic inflammatory response syndrome (SIRS) and sepsis [69]. Since the increase in CD11b/CD18 expression does not require time-consuming *de novo* protein synthesis and occurs *in vivo* within minutes after stimulation, its expression may serve as an extremely early and sensitive cell-associated marker of phagocyte activation. On neutrophils the reduced expression of CD11b and CD16 after severe traumatic injury was correlated with the severity of injury and therefore possibly explains the increased incidence of septic complications seen in the more severely injured group after injury [70].

Ex vivo Inducible Sepsis Markers

Over the last few years techniques and measurements have been established to differentiate between the phases of the hyper-inflammatory phase of the sepsis disease and immunoparalysis. One of these techniques is the stimulation of peripheral blood with LPS to determine the ability of leukocytes to produce and release pro-inflammatory cytokines into the plasma. Ertel et al. demonstrated that the LPS induced release of TNF-α, IL-1β and IL-6 into whole blood from sepsis patients was significantly depressed when compared with a control group [71]. This depression persisted up to 10 days after study enrollment. Interestingly, the half-life and consequently the expression of TNF-α and IL-6 mRNA were strongly reduced in the septic group. Despite the well-documented fact that the excessive secretion of pro-inflammatory cytokines in the early phase of sepsis has detrimental effects upon the patient, the reduced capacity of peripheral blood mononuclear cells (PBMCs) to synthesize and secrete pro-inflammatory cytokines may result in immunodeficiency, since these cytokines are involved in the up-regulation of essential cellular and humoral immune functions. This hypothesis was confirmed by Döcke et al [54]. As previously described, the administration of IFN-γ to sepsis patients reconstituted the expression of HLA-DR on monocytes. Simultaneously, their capacity to produce TNF-α after LPS stimulation recovered to normal levels when patients were cured from sepsis [54]. Further results in the immunosuppressive perioperative phase were obtained by Weighardt et al. who demonstrated that sepsis after major visceral surgery is associated with sustained and IFN-γ-resistant defects of monocyte cytokine production [66]. In this study an immediate defect of endotoxin-stimulated monocyte production of IL-12, IL-1β, and IL-10 was detected in both surviving and non-surviving patients. However during the final phase of postoperative sepsis, a significant recovery of IL-12 and IL-1, though interestingly not of IL-10, production, correlated with survival. The authors concluded that because both the pro- and anti-inflammatory cytokine secretion was affected immediately, immunosuppression is a primary rather than a compensatory response to a septic challenge.

T lymphocytes play an important role in the septic disease since they are able to act as immunostimulators (Th1-cells) and as immunosuppressors (Th2-cells) as well. Both cell types are characterized by a specific cytokine pattern secreted under different immunological conditions. During the early postoperative course, reduced cytokine secretion is observed for IL-2, IFN-γ and TNF-α, which are associated with the Th1 phenotype of T helper lymphocytes [72].

IL-4 production indicating the Th2 phenotype is also suppressed after major surgery, which demonstrates that major surgery is associated with a severe but transient reduction of T-cells to secrete a large panel of cytokines. The persistence of a diminished ability of T-cell cytokine secretion possibly leads to susceptibility of infectious complications.

A further study from this group with purified and stimulated peripheral T-cells demonstrated that selective T-cell proliferation and production of IL-2 and TNF were severely suppressed in patients with lethal intra-abdominal infection as compared with survivors and healthy controls [73]. TNF suppression in survivors was less severe than in non-survivors. Defective T-cell functions were also observed at the onset of sepsis and persisted throughout the entire observation period. Interestingly, the production of IL-4 and IL-10 was not affected by post-operative intra-abdominal infection. Since the immune defects were evident at the onset of sepsis, the authors concluded that immunosuppression may develop as a primary response to sepsis without preceding immune hyperactivity.

The importance of the cytokine IL-12 as a predictive parameter has been investigated by several groups. IL-12, mainly produced from phagocytes, is required for the production of IFN-γ by natural killer (NK)-cells and T lymphocytes and strongly supports the development of the Th1 phenotype of CD4+ cells. Furthermore IL-12 is required for the immediate defense mechanisms of the innate immune system as well as for the induction of subsequent adaptive immune responses. Hensler et al. demonstrated that monocyte IL-12 secretion was significantly impaired before surgery in patients developing post-operative sepsis and indicated that IL-12 may be crucial for establishing a protective immune response against post-operative infection [74]. Additionally, Ertel et al. were able to show diminished secretion of both IL-12 and IFN-γ in trauma or sepsis patients [75]. Because IL-12 and IFN-γ up-regulate essential immune functions, the marked inhibition of IL-12 and IFN-γ release may be pivotal for high susceptibility of critically ill patients to infection. Supporting results for a protective role of IL-12 were reported by Haraguchi et al. [76]. In a case report the authors demonstrated that IL-12 deficiency is associated with recurrent infections and that IFN-γ production from isolated and stimulated PBMCs was reduced.

'THE FUTURE IS AT THE BEDSIDE'

Thanks to progress in technology, sepsis markers are becoming more readily available with the use of automatic machines equipped with luminometric technique (cytokine analysis $\approx$ 20 minutes, e.g., DPC Bierman, Germany) or rapid bedside methods - IL-6 strips (Knoll, Germany) $\pm$ decision only [68], PCT cassettes (Brahms, Germany) semiquantitative, neopterin semiquantitative [77].

CONCLUSION

Considering the range of options available, one must be aware of the fact that the increase in parameters and compartments included in diagnosis, is directly proportional to the uncertainties arising [78]. Therefore, on the one hand, more prospective studies on sepsis markers are required to identify the most relevant and predictive markers (not to mention the financial aspects of costly analysis). On the other, the use of new approaches of data mining to identify specific patterns in specific patient groups is warranted. These efforts need the support of extensive pathophysiological research, since more extensive knowledge regarding patients' underlying diseases may facilitate the finding and choice of an appropriate marker (or set of markers). In conclusion we suggest improved monitoring of sepsis patients to enable a better selection of the appropriate cases and more precise timing for therapeutic interventions; much as vasopressors are not administered without pressure monitoring. We recommend the measurement of IL-6, PCT, and neopterin in plasma, particularly to determine the hyper-inflammatory phase. The most suitable marker for the immunoparalytic phase seems to be a combination of HLA-DR measurement on peripheral blood monocytes and the determination of the capacity of whole blood to secrete pro-inflammatory cytokines after stimulation. The fact that the use of sepsis markers for monitoring – though the actual parameter may ultimately be different – can be beneficial for the therapeutic regimen has recently been nicely demonstrated within the MONARCS, IL-6 monitored anti-TNF study. Furthermore, the active approach using the ACTH response test with monitoring of cortisol in plasma to identify specific sepsis patients [79] is a promising step for the future of sepsis trials.

The most recent research results raise hopes that sepsis markers in combination with increasing knowledge on the influence of polymorphisms and gender may enable us to identify patients at high risk of infectious complications. These patients may be those who will profit most from immune/biochemical monitoring, since individualized therapeutic interventions supporting the immune and humoral systems are within reach.

REFERENCES

1. Bone RC, Fisher CJ, Jr., Clemmer TP, et al. A controlled clinical trial of high-dose methylprednisolone in the treatment of severe sepsis and septic shock. N Engl J Med 1987; 317:653-658
2. Casey LC, Balk RA, Bone RC. Plasma cytokine and endotoxin levels correlate with survival in patients with the sepsis syndrome. Ann Intern Med 1993; 119:771-778
3. Bone RC. Current topics in critical care medicine. Crit Care Int 1997; 7: 4

4. Cavaillon JM. Possibilities and problems of cytokine measurements. In: Redl H, Schlag G (eds) Cytokines in Severe Sepsis and Septic Shock. Birkhäuser, Basel, 1999, pp 95-119
5. Moore F, Poggetti R, McAnena O, et al. Gut bacterial translocation via the portal vein: a clinical perspective with major torso trauma. J Trauma 1991; 31:629-638
6. Opal SM, Scannon PJ, Withe M, et al. Relationship between plasma levels of lipopolysaccharide (LPS) and LPS-binding protein in patients with severe sepsis and septic shock. J Infect Dis 1999; 180:1584-1589
7. Carroll SF, Dedrick RL, White ML. Plasma levels of lipopolysaccharide binding protein (LBP) correlate with outcome in sepsis and other patients. Shock 1997; 8:35 (abstr)
8. Strutz F, Heller G, Krasemann K, et al. Relationship of antibodies to endotoxin core to mortality in medical patients with sepsis syndrome. Intensine Care Med 1999; 25:435-444
9. Goldie AS, Fearon KC, Ross JA, et al. Natural cytokine antagonists and endogenous antiendotoxin core antibodies in sepsis syndrome. The Sepsis Intervention Group. JAMA 1195; 274:172-177
10. Strohmaier W, Redl H, Schlag G, et al. D-erythro-neopterin plasma levels in intensive care patients with and without septic complications. Crit Care Med 1987; 15:757-760
11. Assicot M, Gendrel D, Carsin H, et al. High serum procalcitonin concentration in patients with sepsis and infection. Lancet 1993; 341:515-518
12. Patel RT, Deen KI, Youngs D, et al. Interleukin 6 is a prognostic indicator of outcome in severe intra-abdominal sepsis. Br J Surg 1994; 81:1306-1308
13. Moscovitz H, Shofer F, Mignott H, et al. Plasma cytokine determinations in emergency department patients as a predictor of bacteremia and infectious disease severity. Crit Care Med 1994; 22:1102-1107
14. Fisher CJ, Opal SM, Dhainaut JF, et al. Influence of an anti-tumor necrosis factor monoclonal antibody on cytokine levels in patients with sepsis. Crit Care Med 1993; 21:318-327
15. Marty C, Misset B, Tamion F, et al. Circulating interleukin-8 concentrations in patients with multiple organ failure of septic and nonseptic origin. Crit Care Med 1994; 22:673-679
16. Neidhardt R, Keel M, Steckholzer U, et al. Relationship of interleukin-10 plasma levels to severity of injury and clinical outcome in injured patients. J Trauma 1997; 42:863-870
17. Grobmyer SR, Lin E, Lowry SF, et al. Elevation of IL-18 in human sepsis. J Clin Immunol 2000; 20:212-215
18. Reinhart K, Wiegand-Lohnert C, Grimminger F, et al. Assessment of the safety and efficacy of the monoclonal anti-tumor necrosis factor antibody-fragment, MAK 195F, in patients with sepsis and septic shock: a multicenter, randomized, placebo-controlled, dose-ranging study. Crit Care Med 1996; 24:733-742
19. Wang H, Bloom O, Zhang M, et al. HMG-1 as a late mediator of endotoxin lethality in mice. Science 1999; 285:248-251
20. Brown GM. The biosynthesis of pteridines. Adv Enzymol 1971; 35:5-77
21. Fuchs D, Hausen A, Huber C, et al. Pteridinausscheidung als Marker für alloantigen-induzierte Lymphozytenproliferation. Hoppe Seyler's Z Physiol Chem 1982; 363:661-664
22. Kaufman S. The structure of phenylalanine hydroxylation cofactor. Proc Natl Acad Sci USA 1963; 50:1085-1093
23. Pacher R, Redl H, Frass M, et al. Relationship between neopterin and granulocyte elastase plasma levels and the severity of multiple organ failure. Crit Care Med 1989; 17:221-226
24. Faist E, Storck M, Hültner L, et al. Functional analysis of monocyte activity through synthesis patterns of proinflammatory cytokines and neopterin in patients in surgical intensive care. Surgery 1992; 112:562-572

25. Nast-Kolb D, Waydhas C, Jochum M, et al. Biochemical factors as objective parameters for assessing the prognosis in polytrauma. Unfallchirurg 1992; 95:59-66
26. Delogu G, Casula MA, Mancini P, et al. Serum neopterin and soluble interleukin-2 receptor for prediction of a shock state in gram-negative sepsis. J Crit Care 1995; 10:64-71
27. Roumen RMH, Redl H, Schlag G, et al. Scoring systems and blood lactate concentrations in relation to the development of adult respiratory distress syndrome and multiple organ failure in severely traumatized patients. J Trauma 1993; 35:349-355
28. Estelberger W, Weiss G, Petek W, et al. Determination of renal clearance of neopterin by a pharmacokinetic approach. FEBS Lett 1993; 329:13-16
29. Strohmaier W, Mauritz W, Gaudernak T, et al. Septic focus localized by determination of arterio-venous difference in neopterin blood levels. Circ Shock 1992; 38:219-221
30. Strohmaier W, Poigenfürst J, Mauritz W. Neopterin blood levels: a basis for deciding to use antibiotics in intensive care unit (ICU) patients. Pteridines 1996; 7:1-4
31. Huemer G, Graninger W, Mauritz W. Bed-side infection screening of ICU patients using Gram stained smears. Eur J Anaesthesiol 1992; 9:229-233
32. Gendrel D, Bohuon C. Procalcitonin, a marker of bacterial infection. Infection 1997; 25:133-134
33. Meisner M. Procalcitonin (PCT): Ein neuer, innovativer Infektionsparameter. Biochemische und klinische Aspekte. Thieme, Stuttgart, 2000
34. Dandona P, Nix D, Wilson MF, et al. Procalcitonin increase after endotoxin injection in normal subjects. J Clin Endocrinol Metab 1994; 79:1605-1608
35. Redl, H., Schlag, G., Paul, E., et al. Procalcitonin release patterns in baboon models of trauma and sepsis - relationship to cytokines and neopterin. Crit Care Med 2000; 28:3659-3663
36. Reith HB, Lehmkuhl R, Beier W, et al. Procalcitonin - ein prognostischer Infektionsparameter bei der Peritonitis. Chir Gastroenterol 1995; 11 (Suppl.2):47-50
37. Brunkhorst FM, Forycki ZF, Wagner J. Frühe Identifizierung der biliären akuten Pankreatitis durch Procalcitonin-Immunreaktivität - vorläufige Ergebnisse. Chir Gastroenterol 1995; 11 (Suppl. 2):42-46
38. Nylen ES, O'Nell WO, Jordan MH, et al. Serum procalcitonin as an index of inhalation injury in burns. Horm Metab Res 1992; 24:439-442
39. Carsin H, Assicot M, Feger F, et al. Evolution and significance of circulating procalcitonin levels compared with IL-6, TNF alpha and endotoxin levels early after thermal injury. Burns 1997; 23:218-224
40. Nylen ES, Whang KT, Snider RH, et al. Mortality is increased by procalcitonin and decreased by an antiserum reactive to procalcitonin in experimental sepsis. Crit Care Med 1998; 26:1001-1006
41. Lin Y, Weisdorf DJ, Solovey A, et al. Origins of circulating endothelial cells and endothelial outgrowth from blood. J Clin Invest 2000; 105:71-77
42. Gornikiewicz A, Sautner T, Brostjan C, et al. Catecholamines up-regulate lipopolysaccharide-induced IL-6 production in human microvascular endothelial cells. FASEB J 2000; 14:1093-1100
43. Ishii H, Uchiyama H, Kazama M. Soluble thrombomodulin antigen in conditioned medium is increased by damage of endothelial cells. Thromb Haemost 1991; 65:618-623
44. Sawada K, Yamamoto H, Matsumoto K, et al. Changes in thrombomodulin level in plasma of endotoxin-infused rabbits. Thromb Res 1992; 65:199-209
45. Takano S, Kimura S, Ohdama S, et al. Plasma thrombomodulin in health and diseases. Blood 1990; 10:2024-2029
46. Boldt J, Papsdorf M, Rothe A, et al. Changes of the hemostatic network in critically ill patients - is there a difference between sepsis, trauma, and neurosurgery patients? Crit Care Med 2000; 28:445-450

47. Redl H, Schlag G, Schiesser A, et al. Thrombomodulin release in baboon sepsis: its dependence on the dose of Escherichia coli and the presence of tumor necrosis factor. J Infect Dis 1995; 171:1522-1527

48. Kurosawa S, Stearns-Kurosawa DJ, Carson CW, et al. Plasma levels of endothelial cell protein C receptor are elevated in patients with sepsis and systemic lupus erythematosus: lack of correlation with thrombomodulin suggests involvement of different pathological processes. Blood 1998; 91:725-727

49. Hack CE. Cytokines, coagulation and fibrinolysis. In: Redl H, Schlag G (eds) Cytokines in Severe Sepsis and Septic Shock. Birkhäuser, Basel, 1999, pp 199-212

50. Mesters RM, Mannucci PM, Coppola R, et al. Factor VIIa and antithrombin III activity during severe sepsis and septic shock in neutropenic patients. Blood 1996; 88:881-886

51. Mesters RM, Helterbrand J, Utterback BG, et al. Prognostic value of protein C concentrations in neutropenic patients at high risk of severe septic complications. Crit Care Med 2000; 28:2209-2216

52. Polk HC, Jr., George CD, Wellhausen SR, et al. A systematic study of host defenses in badly injured patients. Ann Surg 1986; 204:282-299

53. Hershman MJ, Cheadle WG, Wellhausen SR, et al. Monocyte HLADR antigen expression characterizes clinical outcome in the trauma patient. Br J Surg 1990; 77:204-207

54. Döcke WD, Randow F, Syrbe U, et al. Monocyte deactivation in septic patients: restoration by IFN-gamma treatment. Nature Med 1997; 3:678-681

55. Kocher AA, Dockal M, Weigel G, et al. Immune monitoring in cardiac transplant recipients. Transplant Proc 1997; 29:2895-2898

56. Hiesmayr MJ, Spittler A, Lassnigg A, et al. Alterations in the number of circulating leukocytes, phenotype of monocyte and cytokine production in patients undergoing cardiothoracic surgery. Clin Exp Immunol 1999; 115:315-323

57. Götzinger, P., Sautner, T., Spittler, A., et al. Severe acute pancreatitis causes alterations in HLA-DR and CD14 expression on peripheral blood monocytes independently of surgical treatment. Eur J Surg 2000; 166:628-632

58. Spittler A, Winkler S, Götzinger P, et al. Influence of glutamine on the phenotype and function of human monocytes. Blood 1995; 86:1564-1569

59. Spittler, A., Sautner, T., Gornikiewicz, A., et al. Postoperative glycyl-glutamine infusion reduces immunosuppression: partial prevention of the surgery induced decrease in HLA-DR expression on monocytes. Clin Nutr 2001; 20:37-42

60. Demotz S, Grey HM, Sette A. The minimal number of class II MHC-antigen complexes needed for T cell activation. Science 2000; 249:1028-1030

61. Cheadle WG, Hershman MJ, Wellhausen SR, et al. HLA-DR antigen expression on peripheral blood monocytes correlates with surgical infection. Am J Surg 1991; 161:639-645

62. Wakefield CH, Carey PD, Foulds S, et al. Changes in major histocompatibility complex class II expression in monocytes and T cells of patients developing infection after surgery. Br J Surg 1993; 80:205-209

63. Lin RY, Astiz ME, Saxon JC, et al. Altered leukocyte immunophenotypes in septic shock. Chest 1993; 104:847-853

64. Ditschkowski M, Kreuzfelder E, Majerus PW, et al. Reduced B cell HLA-DR expression and natural killer cell counts in patients prone to sepsis after injury. Eur J Surg 1999; 165:1129-1133

65. Ditschkowski M, Kreuzfelder E, Rebmann V, et al. HLA-DR expression and soluble HLA-DR levels in septic patients after trauma. Ann Surg 1999; 229:246-254

66. Weighardt H, Heidecke CD, Emmanuilidis K, et al. Sepsis after major visceral surgery is associated with sustained and interferon gamma resistant defects of monocyte cytokine production. Surgery 2000; 127:309-315

67. Fingerle G, Pforte A, Passlick B, et al. The novel subset of CD14+/CD16+ blood monocytes is expanded in sepsis patients. Blood 1993; 82:3170-3176

68. Spittler, A., Razenberger, M., Kupper, H., et al. Relationship between IL-6 plasma concentration of septic patients, monocyte phenotype, their phagocytic properties, and cytokine production. Clin Infect Dis 2000; 31:1338-1342

69. Takala A, Jousela I, Olkkola KT, et al. Systemic inflammatory response syndrome without systemic inflammation in acutely ill patients admitted to hospital in a medical emergency. Clin Sci Colch 1999; 96:287-295

70. White-Owen C, Alexander JW, Babcock GF. Reduced expression of neutrophil CD11b and CD16 after severe traumatic injury. J Surg Res 1992; 52:22-26

71. Ertel W, Kremer JP, Kenney J, et al. Downregulation of proinflammatory cytokine release in whole blood from septic patients. Blood 1995; 85:1341-1347

72. Hensler T, Hecker H, Heeg K, et al. Distinct mechanisms of immunosuppression as a consequence of major surgery. Infect Immun 1997; 65:2283-2291

73. Heidecke CD, Hensler T, Weighardt H, et al. Selective defects of T lymphocyte function in patients with lethal intraabdominal infection. Am J Surg 1999; 178:288-292

74. Hensler T, Heidecke CD, Hecker H, et al. Increased susceptibility to postoperative sepsis in patients with impaired monocyte IL-12 production. J Immunol 1998; 161:3655-2659

75. Ertel W, Keel M, Neidhardt R, et al. Inhibition of the defense system stimulating interleukin-12 interferon gamma pathway during critical illness. Blood 1997; 89:1612-1620

76. Haraguchi S, Day NK, Nelson RPjr, et al. Interleukin-12 deficiency associated with recurrent infections. Proc Natl Acad Sci USA 1998; 95:13125-13129

77. Bührer-Sekula S, Hamerlinck FFV, Out TA, et al. Simple dipstick assay for semi quantitative detection of neopterin sera. J Immunol Method 2000; 238:55-58

78. Strohmaier W, Tatzber F. Relevance of surrogate tests in intensive care patients or "Heisenberg at the ICU". In: Redl H, Schlag G (eds) Cytokines in Severe Sepsis and Septic Shock. Birkhäuser, Basel, 1999, pp 133-147

79. Annane D, Sebille V, Troche G, et al. A 3-level prognostic classification in septic shock based on cortisol levels and cortisol response to corticotropin. JAMA 2000; 283:1038-1045

5

GENETIC PREDISPOSITION

Frank Stüber

The inflammatory response contributes as a major factor to morbidity and mortality on today's intensive care units (ICUs), and displays considerable interindividual variation [1]. Comparable amounts of infectious units of microbial organisms induce a wide range of severities of infectious diseases. The role of an individual's genetic background and predisposition for the extent of inflammatory responses is determined by genetic variabilities in endogenous mediators which constitute the pathways of endogenous mediators of inflammation.

Primary responses in inflammation are mediated by proinflammatory cytokines such as tumor necrosis factor (TNF) and interleukin 1 (IL-1) [2]. Recent evidence suggests that anti-inflammatory mediators have important effects on the host's immune system [3]. Anti-inflammatory mediators induce a state of immunosuppression in sepsis which has also been named immunoparalysis [4]. Pro- and anti-inflammatory responses contribute to the outcome of patients with systemic inflammation and sepsis. Therefore, all genes encoding proteins involved in the transduction of inflammatory processes are candidate genes to determine the human genetic background which is responsible for interindividual differences in systemic inflammatory responses to injury.

Genetically determined capacity for cytokine production and release, heat shock protein expression, nitric oxide synthase (NOS) activity, gene polymorphisms of coagulation factors and many other genes involved in inflammation, may contribute to a wide range of clinical manifestations of inflammatory disease: a patient with peritonitis, for example, may present without symptoms of sepsis and recover within days or may suffer from fulminant septic shock resulting in death within hours.

What is the benefit of having information on the genetic background of an individual's inflammatory response to infectious as well as non-infectious challenges? Besides the interest of basic science concerning role and interaction of mediators, there is a very practical and clinical purpose: Which groups of patients carry a high risk of developing severe sepsis and multiple organ dysfunction in the situation of a systemic inflammatory reaction? Is there a high risk group concerning non-survival? Will certain patients benefit more than others from anti-mediator strategies because of their genetic determination to high cytokine release in the inflammatory response?

CYTOKINES

Primary proinflammatory cytokines like TNF and IL-1 induce secondary pro- and anti-inflammatory mediators like IL-6 and IL-10. These have been shown to contribute substantially to the host's primary response to infection. Both TNF and IL-1 are capable of inducing the same symptoms and the same severity of septic shock and organ dysfunction as endotoxin in experimental settings as well as in humans [5]. Genetic variations in the TNF and IL-1 genes are of major interests concerning genetically determined differences in the response to infection.

Tumor Necrosis Factor (TNF)

TNF is considered as one of the most important mediators of endotoxin-induced effects. Interindividual differences in TNF release have been described [6,7]. The TNF locus consists of three functional genes. TNF is positioned between lymphotoxin-α (LT-α) in the upstream direction and lymphotoxin-β (LT-β) in the downstream direction. Genomic polymorphisms within the TNF locus have been under intense investigation. Genetic variation within the TNF locus is rare as the TNF gene is well conserved throughout evolution [8], particularly the coding region.

Most interest has been focused on the genomic variations of the TNF locus. Biallelic polymorphisms defined by restriction enzymes (NcoI, AspHI) or other single base changes (-308, -238) as well as multiallelic microsatellites (TNFa-e) have been investigated in experimental *in vitro* studies and also in various diseases in which TNF is considered as an important or possible pathogen. Functional importance for regulation of the TNF gene has been suggested for two polymorphisms within the TNF promoter region. Single base changes have been detected at position -850, -376, -308 and position -238 [9-12]. A G to A transition at position -308 has been associated with susceptibility to cerebral malaria [13]. These results could not be confirmed by another malaria study which showed fewer fever episodes in heterozygous carriers of the allele TNF2 [14].

The rare allele TNF2 (A at position -308) was suggested to be linked to high TNF promoter activity [13]. Autoimmune diseases like diabetes mellitus or lupus erythematosus did not show differences in allele frequencies or genotype distribution between patients and controls [15,16]. In addition, patients with severe sepsis and a high proportion of Gram-negative infections also did not display altered allele frequencies concerning both biallelic promoter polymorphisms (position -238 and -308) [17]. Analysis of the TNF promoter by means of reporter gene constructs revealed contradictory results: A first report supposed a functional importance of the -308 G to A transition [13]. Two papers could not confirm differences of TNF promoter activity in relation to the -308 polymorphism [17,18]. A recent paper reports on a possible influence on TNF promoter activity by the -308 G to A transition in a B cell line [19]. Data demonstrating an impact of this genomic polymorphism on transcription are rather weak as reports predominantly derive from one group [20], fndings seem to be restricted to few cell lines, and impaired or enhanced binding of transcription factors has not been shown. In addition, the difference in transcription rates in the responsive cell line seems to require a specific stimulus (PMA plus retinoic acid) [21]. Until September 2000 a total of 74 clinical studies had tried to associate the -308 TNF polymorphism with disease. Twenty-three (31%) studies showed positive results with regard to susceptibility or course of disease and detection of the rare allele TNF2 (Adenine at position -308). Studies comprised diverse entities ranging from acute to chronic inflammation as well as cancer or transplant rejection. The majority of studies did not find an association of this genetic variation with disease (n=51, 69%). Most of the negative studies (89%) contrast positive findings in the same disease entity. Association studies are questioned by concepts of genetic epidemiology because of their low statistical power. Study designs similar to the transmission disequilibrium test used in state of the art epidemiologic studies are needed.

Genotyping of this polymorphism in patients with severe sepsis does not contribute to risk assessment. The -308 polymorphism is neither a marker for susceptibility to, nor outcome from, severe sepsis caused by Gram-negative infection [17]. TNF plasma levels do not seem to be influenced by this polymorphism in patients with severe abdominal sepsis (Fig.1).

In contrast to these findings are the results of two recent studies which suggest an association of the rare allele TNF2 with non-survivors of septic shock [22,23]. These publications again open the discussion about functionality of the -308 TNF promoter polymorphism and its possible relevance for routine clinical use. In addition to the discussion about the relevance of association, formal standards of genotyping techniques have to be established. Are there typing techniques such as allele-specific amplification which imply over- or underestimation of certain alleles and genotypes?

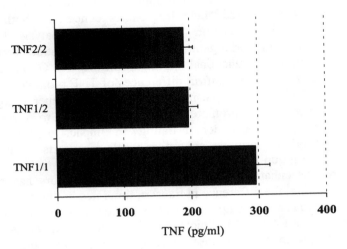

Figure 1. Median (median absolute deviation, MAD) of TNF plasma levels in 105 patients with severe sepsis (12 blood samples in each patient drawn in the first 96 hrs of severe sepsis) grouped according to their -308 TNF promoter genotype (TNF1: Guanine; TNF2: Adenine). (p<0.05, Kruskal Wallis Test)

In contrast to genomic variations located in the promoter region, intronic polymorphisms are more difficult to associate with a possible functional relevance. Two biallelic polymorphisms located within intron two of LT-α have been studied in autoimmune disease [24,25]. One polymorphism is characterized by absence or presence of a NcoI restriction site. First reports demonstrated genomic blots revealing characteristic 5.5 or 10.5 kb bands after genomic NcoI digest which hybridize to TNF specific probes [26]. These bands correspond to the presence and absence, respectively, of a NcoI restriction site within intron one of LT α.

The allele TNFB2 of this NcoI polymorphism (10.5 kb band) has been shown to be associated with high TNF-β release *ex vivo* [27]. Other studies showed no differences between genotypes in other models of *ex vivo* TNF induction, while another study suggests an increased LT-α response in TNFB2 homozygotes [7]. The question of which genotype is clearly associated with a high proinflammatory response in the clinical situation of severe Gram-negative infection and severe sepsis cannot yet be answered by *ex vivo* studies. Different conditions of cell culture and cytokine induction contribute to differing results. In addition, the genomic NcoI polymorphism within intron one of the LT-α gene may represent a genomic marker without evidence for own functional importance in gene regulation. This genomic marker may coincide with so far undetected genomic variations which are responsible for genetic determination of a high proinflammatory responses to infection. Results from studies in patients with severe intraabdominal sepsis suggest TNFB2 homozygotes are associated with a high TNF response (Fig. 2). In contrast, genotyping for another biallelic polymorphism within intron 1 of LT-α (AspHI) did not show significant association with TNF plasma levels (data not shown).

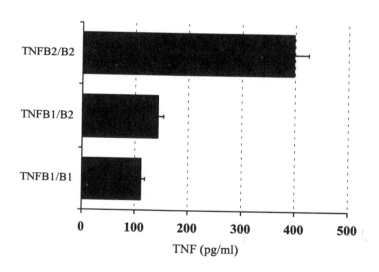

Figure 2. *Median (median absolute deviation, MAD) of TNF plasma levels in 105 patients with severe sepsis grouped according to their lymphotoxin-α (TNF-β) NcoI genotype (p<0.05, Kruskal-Wallis-Test).*

Several studies in chronic inflammatory autoimmune diseases suggest an association between TNFB2 and incidence or severity and outcome of the disease [24,25,28]. Studies in acute inflammatory diseases like severe sepsis in patients on surgical ICUs showed a correlation between TNFB2 homozygosity and mortality [17] or incidence of septic states in traumatized patients [29]. TNFB2 homozygotes displayed a relative risk of 2.9 of dying from severe sepsis when compared to corresponding genotypes.

Interleukin-1

Besides TNF, IL-1 is another potent proinflammatory cytokine released by macrophages in the systemic inflammatory response. IL-1 is capable of inducing the symptoms of septic shock and organ failure in animal models and is regarded as a primary mediator of the systemic inflammatory response. Antagonizing IL-1 in endotoxin-challenged animals including primates abrogates the lethal effects of endotoxin [30]. A biallelic TaqI polymorphism has been described within the coding region (exon 5) of IL-1β [31,32]. Despite the finding that a homozygous TaqI genotype correlates with high IL-1 β secretion [31], genotyping of patients with severe sepsis did not reveal any association with incidence or outcome of the disease.

Interleukin-1 Receptor Antagonist (IL-1ra)

Proinflammatory mediators comprise the hyperinflammatory side of the systemic inflammatory reaction. At the same time, anti-inflammatory mediators are induced by proinflammatory cytokines and try to counterbalance the overshoot of inflammatory activity. This physiologic process of limiting the extent of inflammation by release of anti-inflammatory proteins may escape the physiologic boundaries of local and systemic concentrations of these mediators. Proteins like IL-4, IL-10, IL-11 or IL-13 or IL-1ra contribute to a very powerful downregulation of cellular and humoral proinflammatory activities. This downregulation results in decreased expression of class II molecules in antigen presenting cells as well as in low *ex vivo* responses of immuncompetent cells to inflammatory stimuli. This state of imunosuppression has also been termed immunoparalysis [4], and it results in a situation of areactivity and diminished ability to fight infectious pathogens. A new term for this status, which is a consequence of the systemic inflammatory response, is the compensatory anti-inflammatory response syndrome (CARS) [33]. The outcome of patients with severe sepsis is not only influenced by hyperinflammation in fulminant situations of progressing organ dysfunction but may also be limited by immunosuppression and lack of restoration of immune function. In this view, an overwhelming anti-inflammatory response with a possible genetic background of interindividual differences in the release of anti-inflammatory mediators contributes to the human systemic inflammatory reaction to a similar extent as proinflammatory responses.

A genomic polymorphism of the anti-inflammatory cytokine IL-1ra is located within intron two and consists of variable numbers of a tandem repeat (VNTR) of a 86 bp motif. This 86 basepair motif contains at least three known binding sites for DNA binding proteins [34]. *Ex vivo* experiments suggest higher IL-1ra responses combined with alleles containing low numbers of the 86 bp repeat. *Ex vivo* studies also demonstrate a higher level of IL-1ra protein expression and protein release of A2 homozygous individuals compared to heterozygotes following stimulation with lipopolysaccharide (LPS) [35].

The allele A2 has been associated with increased incidence of autoimmune diseases like lupus erythematosus and insulin dependent diabetes mellitus [36,37]. In acute systemic inflammation, there is no difference between surviving or non-surviving patients with severe sepsis. This finding is in contrast to the results concerning the biallelic NcoI polymorphism within intron one of LTα: homozygotes for the TNFB2 genotype revealed a high mortality when compared to heterozygotes and TNFB1 homozygotes. The overall group of patients with severe sepsis did not show an increase in the TNFB2 allele frequency. For the IL-1ra polymorphism, however, an increase of the allele A2 was detected in the patients with severe sepsis. Patients carrying the haplotype TNFB2 homozygous and A2 homozygous did not survive in this study.

NON-CYTOKINE MEDIATORS

Major efforts have been made in cytokine research to disclose the mechanisms of endotoxin mediated effects. On the other hand, there are a number of non-cytokine mediators which contribute significantly to the toxicity of endotoxin. Interest has focussed on nitric oxide (NO) and the pathways controlling NO release [38]. Eicosanoids take part in the organism's inflammatory response as well as complex coagulation cascades that may lead to disseminated intravascular coagulation (DIC) followed by impaired organ perfusion and organ dysfunction. Platelet activating factor (PAF) is another mediator activating platelet aggregation and contributing to microvascular malperfusion [39].

Potential benefit and protection against cellular stress induced by endotoxin and its mediators is provided by intracellular heat shock proteins. These proteins are capable of playing a role as molecular chaperones facilitating protein synthesis and folding, as well as restructuring, partially denatured proteins [40].

Nitric Oxide and NO-Synthase

NO is suggested to contribute to the state of hypotension in severe sepsis and septic shock. Endotoxin and proinflammatory mediators like TNF and IL-1 induce an inducible form of NOS (iNOS2) in macrophages and the vasoendothelium [41]. In macrophages, NO is a potent radical and contributes to killing of invading pathogens. Excessive release of NO leads to severe hypotension in septic shock. Pharmacological antagonism of NO synthesis reverses hypotension in animal models of septic shock as well as in patients [42].

Constitutive and inducible isoforms of NOS exist which are regulated differently. Some constitutively expressed forms are tissue specific (brain, neuron, vessels), while inducible forms are expressed in endothelial cells and macrophages. A single base change has been discovered in the promoter region of the human endothelial NOS (NOS3). This polymorphism has been associated with the smoking-dependent risk of coronary artery disease [43]. Still, there is a lack of studies examining NOS3 promoter activities and NOS3 expression depending on allele and genoype. Associations of NOS polymorphisms and incidence of, or outcome from, septic shock have not been reported yet.

Heat Shock Protein Genes

Heat shock proteins (HSP) represent a physiologic response to cellular stress which is highly conserved in evolution. Expression of HSP as molecular chaperones facilitates intracellular folding of synthesized proteins [40]. Inhibition of the heat shock response worsens septic shock in animal models. On the other hand, induction of HSP prior to lethal endotoxin challenges reduces lethality of septic shock [40].

A well studied member of the HSP family is HSP 70. Two genomic polymorphisms have been described within the HSP 70-2 and the HSP 70 HOM gene. The first is an inducible form of HSP while the latter is expressed constitutively [44]. No study testing the relation between allele and HSP 70-HOM expression has been performed. The HSP 70-2 polymorphism has been related to variable expression of HSP 70-2 mRNA [45]. So, the functional relevance of these HSP polymorphisms still has to be elucidated.

Genotyping of patients with severe sepsis shows no significant differences in allele frequencies or genotype distribution compared to healthy controls. On the other hand, a significant linkage between HSP 70-2/2 homozygotes and TNFB2 homozygotes has been demonstrated (data not shown). In this view, the allele HSP 70-2/2 may be included in an extended haplotype comprising of alleles linked to each other and defining individuals at risk of developing or even dying from severe sepsis when challenged by Gram-negative infection and endotoxemia.

FROM FLIES TO MICE TO MAN

Transduction of the LPS signal into the cell has been an unknown mechanism until recently. An analogon of the so called Toll receptor in drosophila species which transduces signals for the elaboration of innate immune responses in flies directed against bacteria and fungi has been identified in mice and other species [46]. A single base pair change resulting in an amino acid change of the murine Toll-like receptor 4 (TLR4) renders the extensively studied mouse strain CH3/HeJ highly resistant to LPS challenge [47]. Nine TLR (1-9) [48] have been identified in mammals so far. TLR1, 3 and 5-9 have been found to be orphan receptors, whereas TLR2 has been identified to transduce peptidoglycan stimulation by Gram-positive organisms [49-51]. In contrast, TLR4 seems to play a key role in the LPS-induced signaling pathway [52-55].

Studies of sepsis have used animal models as surrogates for the septic human. These models are conveniently divided into toxic and microbial types. Each model type provides evidence of a genetic component. The canonical toxic (or 'endotoxic') model involves administration of bacterial LPS endotoxin to animals. The fidelity of the model with respect to authentic sepsis is disputed. The acute inflammatory response initiated by endotoxemia is one of several responses to clinical infection. From the historical perspective, the first evidence for genetic predisposition to sepsis emerged from an experiment of nature, the discovery of the endotoxin-resistant mouse. The genetic locus of this endotoxin resistance (denoted *lps*) has been mapped to mouse chromosome 4 (reference) and a functionally significant gene and product have been identified (TLR4).

Presence of a functional TLR4 gene and gene product appears to be one of several determinants of outcome in endotoxemia. Survey of inbred laboratory mice demonstrated a broad range of sensitivity to endotoxin, and genetic analysis of inbred recombinant mice (genetically defined crosses of the most and least sensitive of the laboratory strains) demonstrates five loci that appear to regulate endotoxin sensitivity. High resolution mapping is in progress. The data suggest that response to endotoxemia is a definable multigenic characteristic of laboratory mice. In humans, the work of Beutler and colleagues reveals several genomic variations within the coding region of human TLR4. It still remains to be evaluated, wether the function of the human TLR4 is affected by these polymorphisms. If this is the case, the gene for the human TLR4 is a most important candidate gene to determine the genomic contribution to variability of innate immunity.

CONCLUSION

Understanding the genetic determination of the inflammatory process includes the possibility of developing valuable diagnostic tools and new therapeutic approaches in severe sepsis. Evaluation of possible genomic markers for risk stratification of sepsis patients and individuals at high risk of developing organ failure, respectively, has just begun. Many candidate genes still have to be studied and the clinical significance of genomic markers will be tested. In addition, this new approach may provide valuable inclusion criteria for studies testing immunomodulatory agents in severe sepsis. Extension of single genomic markers to combined haplotypes including relevant alleles may reveal highest informativity and diagnostic relevance.

REFERENCES

1. Sasse KC, Nauenberg E, Long A, Anton B, Tucker HJ, Hu TW. Long-term survival after intensive care unit admission with sepsis. Crit Care Med 1995; 23:1040-1047
2. Blackwell TS, Christman JW. Sepsis and cytokines: current status. Br J Anaesth 1996; 77:110-117
3. van der Poll T, de Waal Malefyt R, Coyle SM, Lowry SF. Antiinflammatory cytokine responses during clinical sepsis and experimental endotoxemia: sequential measurements of plasma soluble interleukin (IL)-1 receptor type II, IL-10, and IL-13. J Infect Dis 1997; 175:118-122
4. Volk HD, Reinke P, Krausch D, et al. Monocyte deactivation--rationale for a new therapeutic strategy in sepsis. Intensive Care Med 1996; 22 (Suppl 4):S474-81:S474-S481
5. Weinberg JR, Boyle P, Meager A, Guz A. Lipopolysaccharide, tumor necrosis factor, and interleukin-1 interact to cause hypotension. J Lab Clin Med 1992; 120:205-211
6. Westendorp RG, Langermans JA, Huizinga TW, et al. Genetic influence on cytokine production and fatal meningococcal disease. Lancet 1997; 349:170-173
7. Whichelow CE, Hitman GA, Raafat I, Bottazzo GF, Sachs JA. The effect of TNF*B gene polymorphism on TNF-alpha and -beta secretion levels in patients with insulin-dependent diabetes mellitus and healthy controls. Eur J Immunogenet 1996; 23:425-435
8. Gray PW, Aggarwal BB, Benton CV, et al. Cloning and expression of cDNA for human lymphotoxin, a lymphokine with tumour necrosis activity. Nature 1984; 312:721-724

9. Kato T, Honda M, Kuwata S, et al. Novel polymorphism in the promoter region of the tumor necrosis factor alpha gene: No association with narcolepsy. Am J Med Genet 1999; 88:301-304

10. Knight JC, Udalova I, Hill AV, et al. A polymorphism that affects OCT-1 binding to the TNF promoter region is associated with severe malaria. Nat Genet 1999; 22:145-150

11. Wilson AG, di Giovine FS, Blakemore AI, Duff GW. Single base polymorphism in the human tumour necrosis factor alpha (TNF alpha) gene detectable by NcoI restriction of PCR product. Hum Mol Genet 1992; 1:353-353

12. Brinkman BM, Huizinga TW, Kurban SS, et al. Tumour necrosis factor alpha gene polymorphisms in rheumatoid arthritis: association with susceptibility to, or severity of, disease? Br J Rheumatol 1997; 36:516-521

13. McGuire W, Hill AV, Allsopp CE, Greenwood BM, Kwiatkowski D. Variation in the TNF-alpha promoter region associated with susceptibility to cerebral malaria. Nature 1994; 371:508-510

14. Stirnadel HA, Stockle M, Felger I, Smith T, Tanner M, Beck HP. Malaria infection and morbidity in infants in relation to genetic polymorphisms in Tanzania. Trop Med Int Health 1999; 4:187-193

15. Pociot F, Wilson AG, Nerup J, Duff GW. No independent association between a tumor necrosis factor-alpha promotor region polymorphism and insulin-dependent diabetes mellitus. Eur J Immunol 1993; 23:3050-3053

16. Wilson AG, Gordon C, di Giovine FS, et al. A genetic association between systemic lupus erythematosus and tumor necrosis factor alpha. Eur J Immunol 1994; 24:191-195

17. Stuber F, Udalova IA, Book M, et al. -308 tumor necrosis factor (TNF) polymorphism is not associated with survival in severe sepsis and is unrelated to lipopolysaccharide inducibility of the human TNF promoter. J Inflamm 1995; 46:42-50

18. Brinkman BM, Zuijdeest D, Kaijzel EL, Breedveld FC, Verweij CL. Relevance of the tumor necrosis factor alpha (TNF alpha) -308 promoter polymorphism in TNF alpha gene regulation. J Inflamm 1995; 46:32-41

19. Wilson AG, Symons JA, McDowell TL, McDevitt HO, Duff GW. Effects of a polymorphism in the human tumor necrosis factor alpha promoter on transcriptional activation. Proc Natl Acad Sci USA 1997; 94 :3195-3199

20. Abraham LJ, Kroeger KM. Impact of the -308 TNF promoter polymorphism on the transcriptional regulation of the TNF gene: relevance to disease. J Leukoc Biol 1999; 66:562-566

21. Kroeger KM, Steer JH, Joyce DA, Abraham LJ. Effects of stimulus and cell type on the expression of the -308 tumour necrosis factor promoter polymorphism. Cytokine 2000; 12:110 -119

22. Mira JP, Cariou A, Grall F, et al.Association of TNF2, a TNF-alpha promoter polymorphism, with septic shock susceptibility and mortality: a multicenter study. JAMA 1999; 282:561-568

23. Tang GJ, Huang SL, Yien HW, et al. Tumor necrosis factor gene polymorphism and septic shock in surgical infection. Crit Care Med 2000; 28:2733-2736

24. Pociot F, Molvig J, Wogensen L, et al. A tumour necrosis factor beta gene polymorphism in relation to monokine secretion and insulin-dependent diabetes mellitus. Scand J Immunol 1991; 33:37-49

25. Bettinotti MP, Hartung K, Deicher H, et al. Polymorphism of the tumor necrosis factor beta gene in systemic lupus erythematosus: TNFB-MHC haplotypes. Immunogenetics 1993; 37:449-454

26. Badenhoop K, Schwarz G, Trowsdale J, et al. TNF-alpha gene polymorphisms in type 1 (insulin-dependent) diabetes melltus. Diabetologia 1989; 32:445-448

27. Pociot F, Briant L, Jongeneel CV, et al. Association of tumor necrosis factor (TNF) and class II major histocompatibility complex alleles with the secretion of TNF- alpha and TNF-beta by human mononuclear cells: a possible link to insulin- dependent diabetes mellitus. Eur J Immunol 1993; 23:224-231

28. Vinasco J, Beraun Y, Nieto A, et al. Polymorphism at the TNF loci in rheumatoid arthritis. Tissue Antigens 1997; 49:74-78

29. Majetschak M, Flohe S, Obertacke U, et al. Relation of a TNF gene polymorphism to severe sepsis in trauma patients. Ann Surg 1999; 230:207-214

30. Boermeester MA, Van Leeuwen PA, Coyle SM, Wolbink GJ, Hack CE, Lowry SF. Interleukin-1 blockade attenuates mediator release and dysregulation of the hemostatic mechanism during human sepsis. Arch Surg 1995; 130:739-748

31. Pociot F, Molvig J, Wogensen L, Worsaae H, Nerup J. A TaqI polymorphism in the human interleukin-1 beta (IL-1 beta) gene correlates with IL-1 beta secretion in vitro. Eur J Clin Invest 1992; 22:396-402

32. Guasch JF, Bertina RM, Reitsma PH. Five novel intragenic dimorphisms in the human interleukin-1 genes combine to high informativity. Cytokine 1996; 8:598-602

33. Bone RC. Sir Isaac Newton, sepsis, SIRS, and CARS. Crit Care Med 1996; 24:1125-1128

34. Tarlow JK, Blakemore AI, Lennard A, et al. Polymorphism in human IL-1 receptor antagonist gene intron 2 is caused by variable numbers of an 86-bp tandem repeat. Hum Genet 1993; 91:403-404

35. Danis VA, Millington M, Hyland VJ, Grennan D. Cytokine production by normal human monocytes: inter-subject variation and relationship to an IL-1 receptor antagonist (IL-1Ra) gene polymorphism. Clin Exp Immunol 1995; 99:303-310

36. Blakemore AI, Tarlow JK, Cork MJ, Gordon C, Emery P, Duff GW. Interleukin-1 receptor antagonist gene polymorphism as a disease severity factor in systemic lupus erythematosus. Arthritis Rheum 1994; 37:1380-1385

37. Metcalfe KA, Hitman GA, Pociot F, et al. An association between type 1 diabetes and the interleukin-1 receptor type 1 gene. The DiMe Study Group. Childhood Diabetes in Finland. Hum Immunol 1996; 51:41-48

38. Fink MP, Payen D. The role of nitric oxide in sepsis and ARDS: synopsis of a roundtable conference held in Brussels on 18-20 March 1995. Intensive Care Med 1996; 22:158-165

39. Mathiak G, Szewczyk D, Abdullah F, Ovadia P, Rabinovici R. Platelet-activating factor (PAF) in experimental and clinical sepsis. Shock 1997; 7:391-404

40. Buchman TG. Manipulation of stress gene expression: a novel therapy for the treatment of sepsis? Crit Care Med 1994; 22:901-903

41. Spitzer JA. Cytokine stimulation of nitric oxide formation and differential regulation in hepatocytes and nonparenchymal cells of endotoxemic rats. Hepatology 1994; 19:217-228

42. Pfeilschifter J, Eberhardt W, Hummel R, et al. Therapeutic strategies for the inhibition of inducible nitric oxide synthase--potential for a novel class of anti-inflammatory agents. Cell Biol Int 1996; 20:51-58

43. Meier J, Affeldt M, Opitz C, Kleber FX, Speer A. A common base change in the promoter region of the human endothelial NO- synthase (NOS3) gene. Hum Mutat 1996; 8:394-394

44. Milner CM, Campbell RD. Polymorphic analysis of the three MHC-linked HSP70 genes. Immunogenetics 1992; 36:357-362

45. Pociot F, Ronningen KS, Nerup J. Polymorphic analysis of the human MHC-linked heat shock protein 70 (HSP70-2) and HSP70-Hom genes in insulin-dependent diabetes mellitus (IDDM). Scand J Immunol 1993; 38:491-495

46. Janeway-CA J, Medzhitov R. Lipoproteins take their toll on the host. Curr Biol 1999; 9:R879-R882

47. Poltorak A, He X, Smirnova I, et al. Defective LPS signaling in C3H/HeJ and C57BL/10ScCr mice: mutations in Tlr4 gene. Science 1998; 282:2085-2088

48. Takeuchi O, Kawai T, Sanjo H, et al. TLR6: A novel member of an expanding toll-like receptor family. Gene 1999; 231:59-65
49. Schwandner R, Dziarski R, Wesche H, Rothe M, Kirschning CJ. Peptidoglycan- and lipoteichoic acid-induced cell activation is mediated by toll-like receptor 2. J Biol Chem 1999; 274:17406-17409
50. Yoshimura A, Lien E, Ingalls RR, Tuomanen E, Dziarski R, Golenbock D. Cutting edge: recognition of Gram-positive bacterial cell wall components by the innate immune system occurs via Toll-like receptor 2. J Immunol 1999; 163:1-5
51. Takeuchi O, Kaufmann A, Grote K, et al. Cutting edge: preferentially the R-stereoisomer of the mycoplasmal lipopeptide macrophage-activating lipopeptide-2 activates immune cells through a toll-like receptor 2- and MyD88-dependent signaling pathway. J Immunol 2000; 164:554-557
52. Poltorak A, Smirnova I, He X, et al. Genetic and physical mapping of the Lps locus: identification of the toll-4 receptor as a candidate gene in the critical region. Blood Cells Mol Dis 1998; 24:340-355
53. Takeuchi O, Hoshino K, Kawai T, et al. Differential roles of TLR2 and TLR4 in recognition of gram-negative and gram-positive bacterial cell wall components. Immunity 1999; 11:443-451
54. Ohashi K, Burkart V, Flohe S, Kolb H. Cutting edge: heat shock protein 60 is a putative endogenous ligand of the toll-like receptor-4 complex. J Immunol 2000; 164:558-561
55. Cario E, Rosenberg IM, Brandwein SL, Beck PL, Reinecker HC, Podolsky DK. Lipopolysaccharide activates distinct signaling pathways in intestinal epithelial cell lines expressing Toll-like receptors. J Immunol 2000; 164:966-972

6

QUANTIFYING RISK IN SEPSIS: A REVIEW OF ILLNESS SEVERITY AND ORGAN DYSFUNCTION SCORING

Randy S. Wax
Derek C. Angus
William Knaus

Sepsis is a complicated entity composed of different etiologies, physiological abnormalities, and degrees of organ failure. Sepsis occurs in a wide variety of patients with broad differences in underlying diseases and demographic characteristics. Many of these demographic, clinical and pathophysiologic characteristics can strongly influence outcome. As such, accurate comparisons and prognosis of septic patients across and within therapeutic trials and observational cohorts requires assessment of the relative contribution of these risk factors. Fortunately, there are several sophisticated severity adjustment tools in the field of critical care that can be applied to sepsis. In this chapter we review some of these approaches to risk adjustment for sepsis, and discuss some concerns regarding the application of commonly used scoring systems.

THE NEED FOR GOOD PROGNOSTIC SYSTEMS FOR PATIENTS WITH SEPSIS

Patients, surrogate decision-makers, and clinicians are frequently faced with difficult decisions regarding the appropriateness of care in the intensive care unit (ICU). In theory, intensive care should prolong survival with reasonable quality of life. Prolongation of death, on the other hand, is not an acceptable goal for most. A prognostic system that could predict patients likely to benefit from intensive care would provide many advantages; in particular, this would enable patients and surrogate decision-makers to make more informed decisions regarding health care options.

Investigators, too, require scoring systems to aid measurement of severity of illness when comparing groups of patients within clinical studies. Ensuring that groups are similar prior to intervention is a key step in evaluating the effect of an intervention. A scoring system for prognosis can allow clinicians to compare their patient populations with those in studies to determine whether an intervention applies to their own group of patients. In addition, such systems could identify subgroups of patients more likely to benefit from an intervention (Panacek, unpublished data, [1]).

IDENTIFIED RISK FACTORS FOR MORTALITY IN SEPSIS

Many published studies have analyzed risk factors for mortality in cohorts of patients with sepsis. In general, logistic regression or Cox modeling techniques are used to identify those clinical factors that are independently associated with the probability of death. Clinical risk factors found recurrently in many studies include adequacy of antibiotics, presence of underlying disease, source and type of infection, presence of shock, need for vasopressors, multiple organ failure (MOF), and neutropenia [2].

A recent review of studies examining sepsis mortality differences due to microbiology has suggested that bacteremia due to *Candida* and *Enterococcus* species are associated with the highest attributable mortality (30-40%) and those due to coagulase-negative Staphylococcus are associated with the lowest attributable mortality (15-20%) [3]. The microbiologic etiology of sepsis may not only affect outcome from sepsis but also influence the response to intervention [4]. The site of infection leading to sepsis can also influence outcome, with increased mortality noted due to intra-abdominal or lower respiratory tract sources, or when no source of infection could be identified [5].

Recently, some authors have suggested that provocative tests of physiological reserve may also prove useful in identifying those patients at risk for death from sepsis. Rhodes et al demonstrated in patients with septic shock that a 15% increase in oxygen consumption (VO_2) after dobutamine challenge (10 µg/kg/min) was a strong predictor of survival [6]. Despite considerable controversy regarding the relationship between oxygen delivery (DO_2) and VO_2 in sepsis, further study of this approach to short-term risk prediction may be warranted [7].

DIFFERENCES BETWEEN EFFECTS ON SHORT- AND LONG-TERM RISK FOR MORTALITY AFTER SEPSIS

In a study of 1052 patients meeting criteria for severe sepsis, Brun-Buisson et al found that early mortality (<3 days after ICU admission) was associated with increasing number of failing organs, arterial blood pH < 7.33, presence of shock, multiple sources of sepsis, and higher SAPS II scores [8]. In contrast, mortality up to 28 days was additionally associated with severity of underlying disease and preexisting organ insufficiency. A study of long-term survival by Perl et al. found similar results in that severity of underlying illness and number of active comorbid illnesses were also found to be associated with death during periods of observation up to 6 months [9].

In another study of outcome up to one year after sepsis, Sasse et al noted that acute physiologic derangement, measured by the acute physiology score, remained strongly associated with mortality up to one month after hospital discharge [10]. However, at three months, acute physiology was no longer predictive, but rather the presence of human immunodeficiency virus (HIV) infection and malignancy were stronger predictors at later time-points. These data are not surprising – one would anticipate that the hazards associated with different risk factors would not be proportional over time. However, non-proportional hazard modeling is not trivial [1,8] and has received minimal attention in the sepsis literature to date.

INFLAMMATORY MOLECULES AS MARKERS OF ADVERSE OUTCOME

Attempts to understand the role of inflammation in sepsis have prompted studies of the impact of cytokines on outcome. Small studies have demonstrated associations between risk of death and cytokine levels, such as elevated measured interleukin (IL)-6 [11-13] or tumor necrosis factor (TNF) [13-15]. However, cytokine levels from survivors and non-survivors typically overlap, leading to poor discriminative value of such tests. Technical difficulties with cytokine assays have also contributed to the gap between measurement of cytokine levels and application to patient care. One should distinguish also between inflammatory markers that provide information about risk versus those that predict response to therapy. For example, recent data suggest that cytokine levels, such as IL-6, may help to identify patients who are likely to respond to specific anti-sepsis therapy (Panacek, unpublished data). It is possible that some cytokine levels may predict risk without enhancing decisions regarding therapy, and other inflammatory markers may identify subgroups of patients more likely to benefit from therapy but have no prognostic significance from an epidemiological perspective.

GENETIC PREDISPOSITION AS A RISK FACTOR FOR ADVERSE OUTCOME

A number of investigators have examined the contribution of genetic predisposition to the incidence and severity of sepsis. In particular, the presence of the TNF2 polymorphism in the promotor region of the gene for TNF has been associated with greater risk of death in septic populations [16]. A detailed discussion of the role of genetic risk in sepsis is presented elsewhere in this book. In the future, investigators may attempt to refine predictive models by adding genetic variables. However, if genetics influence physiological variables already accounted for by models, the addition of genotype to the system may not provide additional useful information.

The importance of gender in sepsis genetic predisposition has been emphasized recently. Experimentally, gender differences in the inflammatory response to hemorrhagic shock [17], including responses to immunomodulation therapy [18], have been noted. The incidence of sepsis requiring ICU admission and the development of septic shock appears to be lower in females [19]. Schroder et al demonstrated that mortality was higher in septic male patients homozygous for the TNFB2 single nucleotide polymorphism compared with male patients with TNFB1 [20]. However, female patients did not demonstrate any difference in mortality when considering TNFB2 status. This study demonstrates an interaction between factors that predispose for poor outcome and gender. Future research to determine the importance of gender as a risk factor in sepsis is required.

DETERMINING THE EXTENT TO WHICH RISK OF DEATH FROM SEPSIS CAN BE MODIFIED

One important aspect regarding risk factors is the extent to which they can be modified. For example, inappropriate initial antibiotics are associated with a worse outcome. Similarly, failure to provide appropriate surgical drainage increases mortality. Such risk factors obviously carry added clinical importance since efforts by the clinical team to address them can result in improved outcome. In contrast, there is nothing that can be done about a patient's age. With recent trials suggesting sepsis-specific therapies may also improve outcome (e.g., activated protein C [APC] replacement), it will be important to delineate those risk factors that reflect the septic process and are potentially modifiable, as distinct from factors that cannot be modified (Figure 1). Such delineation may improve patient selection both for clinical trials and in clinical practice.

THE ROLE OF SCORING SYSTEMS IN PREDICTING RISK OF DEATH FROM SEPSIS

A Brief Primer on Scoring Systems

Scoring systems are typically developed using multiple logistic regression models, which measure the association of independent patient characteristics with death prior to hospital discharge. Coefficients for each of the independent variables are generated using a model development set. Validation of generated models requires assessment of calibration and discrimination. Calibration measures the agreement between observed mortality and mortality expected from the model and is typically tested with the Hosmer-Lemeshow statistic. Discrimination represents the ability of a model to accurately identify patients who die and is measured with the c-index (calculated from the area under the receiver-operating characteristic curve [ROC]). Although calibration and discrimination are initially evaluated on the development dataset, model performance should also be tested on a validation dataset different from that used to generate the model (usually a portion of the initial dataset) as well as on an independent dataset. Mourouga et al. describe in further detail techniques for evaluating severity scoring models in ICU patients [21].

General Critical Care Scoring Systems used to Predict Risk for Mortality in Sepsis

In the early 1980s, the first general risk scoring systems for critically-ill patients were created, including the Acute Physiology and Chronic Health Evaluation (APACHE) [22], the Simplified Acute Physiologic Score (SAPS) [23], and the Mortality Probability Model (MPM) [24]. A number of methodologic concerns were addressed in the development of second and third generation versions of these commonly used systems. Calibration and discrimination of the newer systems have improved as compared to their predecessors, as demonstrated in an international general ICU database. Characteristics of the latest systems are summarized in Table 1.

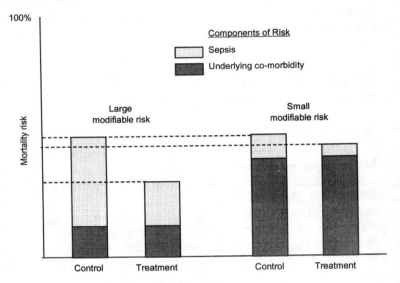

Alternative scenarios for sepsis study with
therapy that has strong effect on sepsis process.

Figure 1. *Hypothetical cohorts of patients with sepsis with different combination of risk factors. Although the mortality rate in both control arms is identical, the ability of a therapy to improve survival is considerably greater in the left treatment arm, where a large proportion of the risk of death is due to the septic process, and consequently modifiable by the therapy (modified from [65] with permission).*

APACHE II scores [25] have been applied for mortality prediction in multiple studies of patients with sepsis. Some studies found that APACHE II could predict mortality [26,27] while others eliminated the scoring system as an independent predictor [9,28]. SAPS II [29] was evaluated in the study by Brun-Buisson et al. and, although the model coefficient was statistically significant, the clinical significance of the effect was questionable (odds ratio 1.03) [8].

In a recent evaluation of APACHE III in a novel dataset, calibration of the scoring system for patients with urosepsis was suboptimal (p=0.006 for Hosmer-Lemeshow test, n=174 patients); in contrast, calibration for patients with non-urinary tract sepsis was better (p=0.330 for Hosmer-Lemeshow test, n=707 patients) [30].

Characteristics	APACHE III	SAPS II	MPM II
Year of publication	1991	1993	1993
Participating countries	1	12	12
Participating ICUs	40	137	140
Patients in development set (#)	17,440	12,997	19,124
Septic patients in development set (#)	519	unknown	unknown
Methodology	MLR	MLR	MLR
Variables			
Age	✓	✓	✓
Patient origin	✓		
Surgical status	✓	✓	✓
Chronic health status	✓	✓	✓
Physiology	✓	✓	✓
Acute diagnosis	✓		✓
Variables (#)	26	17	15
Score	✓	✓	
Equation to predict mortality	✓	✓	✓
Coefficients available in public domain		✓	✓

MLR - multiple logistic regression; # - number

Table 1. *Overview of most recent versions of severity scoring systems (Modified from [56] with permission)*

Modification of General ICU Scoring Systems for Sepsis

Some investigators have tried to refine the general scoring systems with modifications for septic patients. Combining APACHE II scores with results from delayed-type hypersensitivity skin-test responses in a cohort of patients with intra-abdominal sepsis resulted in improved calibration and discrimination when compared with APACHE II scores alone [31]. Presterl et al. reported that repeated APACHE III and MPM II sepsis scores correlated with various cytokine levels during different stages of illness, however the authors did not attempt to generate predictive mortality models by combining severity scoring with cytokine level data [32]. APACHE III scores (in addition to IL-6, IL-10 and phospholipase A levels) were not predictive of mortality in a small multivariate analysis of patients with sepsis, although multiple organ dysfunction scores and monocyte membrane TNF receptor levels were found to be independent predictors [33].

Le Gall et al. evaluated general SAPS II and MPM II$_{24}$ and found that both models had poor calibration within a cohort of patients with sepsis [34]. They then generated new sepsis-specific SAPS II and MPM II$_{24}$ models using a development sepsis dataset but the same variables as the original models and verified the models with a validation dataset. Calibration of the sepsis-specific models were improved, and discrimination as measured by area under the ROC curve ranged from 0.75 to 0.78 in all development and validation datasets.

Knaus et al. integrated aspects of the APACHE III scoring system (Acute Physiology Score [APS] variables) into a new survival model for patients with sepsis [1]. Additional variables included patient age, diagnostic category, number of days in hospital before scoring, and day of ICU care when the patient met criteria for entry into the study. The addition of other important variables to the usual APACHE III APS score improved discrimination (ROC curve area 0.71 increased to 0.76). This approach was tested by Fisher et al. in a sepsis therapy trial in which patients with predicted mortality 24% or greater could be shown to benefit from therapy, whereas those with predicted mortality less than 24% showed no benefit [35].

Modifying existing general ICU severity scoring systems for specific diseases may be a preferred approach to creating unique models with variables for each disease. In theory, using a constant data collection format may improve data gathering efficiency and accuracy for all patients in the ICU. Rather than generating new models for dozens of diseases in the ICU, new coefficients can be generated for patients or additional relevant variables can be explored, which can improve both calibration and discrimination.

Organ Failure Scoring Systems in Sepsis

An alternate approach to understanding risk of death in patients with sepsis focuses on quantification of organ failure. ICU mortality is correlated with increasing number of organs failing [36,37]. However, organ failure is not a discrete event. Most organ failure scores present failure as a spectrum. Compared to mortality prediction scores, organ failure scores tend to be simpler to calculate, provide information on individual organ function, and are designed for repeated measure to reflect fluctuations in organ function over time.

Historically, many authors developed measures of organ failure for both prognostication and measurement of outcome, many based on the number of organ systems failing [36,37]. In recent years, three scoring systems have been used predominantly: the Multiorgan Dysfunction Score (MODS) [38], the Logistic Organ Dysfunction System (LODS) [39], and the Sequential Organ Failure Assessment (SOFA) score [40]. Table 2 describes important features of these scoring systems. One important development in the new generation of organ dysfunction scoring systems is a measure of degree of organ failure rather than a simple 'yes/no' approach. In general, the worst value over a 24 hour period for a physiological parameter is used to calculate organ failure scores.

The MODS, created by Marshall et al., had excellent discrimination for ICU mortality in both development (ROC curve area = 0.936) and validation (ROC curve area = 0.928) datasets [38]. However, the datasets were derived from patients with mixed diagnoses. A recent paper by Jacobs et al. evaluated MODS in a cohort of patients with septic shock [41]. Maximum MOD scores and changes in MOD scores were different between survivors and non-survivors, although the scores could not be used to predict individual patient outcome. In contrast, maximum, and changes in, APACHE II scores were similar in survivors and non-survivors.

The LODS is more complicated than other organ failure scoring systems, and has been applied in a limited fashion for sepsis studies [42].

SOFA, although originally proposed as an organ failure scoring system for sepsis, was eventually recommended for expanded use with general ICU populations. High SOFA scores and increases in SOFA scores are associated with increases in mortality in mixed ICU populations [43,44]. The SOFA scoring system has been used to quantify organ dysfunction in infection and sepsis in a number of studies [45-47].

A consensus meeting organized by the European Society of Intensive Care Medicine (ESICM) [40] suggested that an ideal organ failure variable should have the following characteristics:
1) be objective
2) be simple, available and reliable,
3) be obtained routinely and regularly in every institution
4) be specific for the function of the organ considered
5) be continuous
6) be independent of the type of patients, and finally
7) be independent of the therapeutic interventions.

However, some concerns exist regarding all organ failure systems. Are we truly measuring organ dysfunction? For example, is serum creatinine a valid and sensitive marker of changes in renal function? Measures of organ dysfunction are not clearly independent of therapeutic intervention in many cases, such as the PaO_2/FiO_2 ratio reflecting changes in positive end-expiratory pressure (PEEP) [48]. Although organ failure is associated with mortality, should it serve as an intermediate end-point to mortality for efficacy in therapeutic trials? Mortality reduction is considered a gold-standard for effective therapy by many, however organ failure could theoretically impact on quality-of-life in survivors of ICU care, and therefore its importance may be underemphasized [49].

CONTROVERSIES IN SEPSIS RISK PREDICTION

Appropriate Validation

Despite methodologic improvements in scoring systems, there remain some challenges in better understanding the validity and appropriate application of these tools. To use these scoring systems in a particular population, their application should be validated in that population. A major effort has been underway to evaluate scoring systems in the international setting. Rowan et al. found that APACHE II was superior to MPM when applied to general intensive care patients (over 25% with suspected infection) in the United Kingdom [50]. APACHE II has demonstrated good discriminative ability in a Canadian mixed ICU population [51]. SAPS II and APACHE II were found to be poorly calibrated in mixed ICU patients in Portugal [52], and similarly multiple systems performed poorly in Tunisian ICUs [53]. Evaluation of APACHE III in Brazil demonstrated that calibration and discrimination were good in their overall sample of patients [54].

Calibration and discrimination may be improved by customizing general risk scoring systems to specific populations, with a customized APACHE III system successfully developed for ICUs in Spain as an example [55]. A number of explanations could explain performance differences between countries, including differences in health care systems, diagnostic case mix, underlying risk in patient populations (e.g., genetic factors), and in interpretation of definitions and procedures used for data collection [56].

Disease-specific vs. General Risk Prediction Models

Another area of debate regarding risk prediction relates to the use of disease-specific models instead of general models. Whether these combine disease-specific variables with general risk prediction systems (e.g., Ranson criteria plus APACHE III for pancreatitis [57]) or provide a unique set of variables for prediction (e.g., Pneumonia Severity Index by Fine et al. [58]), the potential for increased model performance must be balanced by increased complexity in data collection for multiple different systems in the ICU. A number of scoring systems specific for sepsis have been developed in the past but are not currently in common use [59-62]. Despite being disease specific, risk prediction scores developed using only patients with sepsis still face the challenge of adequate performance in different populations.

	MODS	LODS	SOFA
Organ failure measurements			
CNS	Glasgow Coma Scale	Glasgow Coma Scale	Glasgow Coma Scale
Respiratory	PaO_2/FiO_2 ratio	PaO_2/FiO_2 ratio on mechanical ventilation or CPAP	PaO_2/FiO_2 ratio
Cardiovascular	Pressure-adjusted heart rate (HR x RAP/MAP)	Heart rate, systolic blood pressure	MAP, need for inotrope/ vasopressor support
Renal	Serum creatinine	Serum urea, creatinine, urine output	Serum creatinine, urine output
Hepatic	Serum bilirubin	Serum bilirubin, prothrombin time	Serum bilirubin
Hematologic	Platelet count	White blood cell count, platelet count	Platelet count
Score per organ	0 to 4 points	Varies by organ system	1-4 points
Maximum score (most failure)	24	22	24
Pts in development dataset	Surgical ICU, pts admitted for >24 hours, 336 pts	Mixed ICUs, excluded pediatric/burn/ cardiac surgery, 10,547 pts	Developed at consensus meeting

Pts - Patients, MAP - mean arterial pressure, RAP - right atrial pressure, PaO2-Arterial partial pressure of oxygen, FiO2-Fraction of oxygen in inspired gas

Table 2. *Characteristics of organ failure scoring systems*

Timing

The timing of application of risk prediction systems has been studied. Given that sepsis is not a static process during an entire stay in the ICU, one might expect that taking multiple measures of illness severity or organ failure might increase the predictive value of models. Serial measurements of APACHE II scores in general ICU patients were superior to a single measure of APACHE II [63]. The role for repeated measures of organ failure or illness severity over time requires further study.

Individual Patient Predictions

Finally, a major issue that remains for scoring systems is their difficulty in making predictions about individual patients. Although accurate predictions of mortality at the bedside could be helpful for clinical care, some question remains as to whether it is appropriate to use scoring systems in this manner [64].

CONCLUSION

Well-established clinical risk factors in sepsis include adequacy of antibiotics, presence of underlying disease, source and type of infection, and the presence of shock with MOF. The heterogeneous nature of patients with sepsis and difficulty in reliably describing their disease burden has led to the development of illness severity scoring systems that can be a useful tool for clinicians and investigators.

Advances in illness severity and organ dysfunction scoring systems have allowed investigators and clinicians to use consistent measures of illness to allow comparison between patient populations. There remain a number of areas for potential refinement in this field. When using general risk prediction systems in a novel population of septic patients, one should verify that the models perform adequately for that specific population. Illness severity and organ dysfunction scores provide a useful tool for prognostication and comparison in septic patients, and have played an important role in the advancement of patient care and research in sepsis.

Continuing advances in our understanding of the inflammatory pathways of sepsis will hopefully lead to more effective use of biological markers in sepsis risk prediction. The integration of exciting research in genetic predisposition, coupled with advances in technology allowing more complex analyses (e.g., DNA microarray), will lead to better understanding of the importance of such factors as gender, ethnicity and race from a mechanistic rather than an epidemiological standpoint.

As with other areas of research in critical illness, prognostication in sepsis must take into account patient-centered outcome measures, such as long-term, quality-adjusted survival. Recent preliminary data suggesting that some anti-sepsis interventions may be effective in improving outcome will encourage the development of improved identification of patients likely to benefit from specific interventions. Thus, the near future will hopefully allow prediction of 'modifiable' risk, leading to a transition from fatalism in sepsis risk prediction to an environment wherein guided action leads to improved patient outcome.

REFERENCES

1. Knaus WA, Harrell FEJ, Fisher CJ, Jr., et al. The clinical evaluation of new drugs for sepsis. A prospective study design based on survival analysis. JAMA 1993; 270:1233-1241
2. Barriere SL, Lowry SF. An overview of mortality risk prediction in sepsis. Crit Care Med 1995; 23:376-393
3. Rangel-Frausto MS. The epidemiology of bacterial sepsis. Infect Dis Clin North Am 1999; 13:299-312
4. Opal SM, Cohen J. Clinical gram-positive sepsis: does it fundamentally differ from gram-negative bacterial sepsis? Crit Care Med 1999; 27:1608-1616
5. Rello J, Ricart M, Mirelis B, et al. Nosocomial bacteremia in a medical-surgical intensive care unit: epidemiologic characteristics and factors influencing mortality in 111 episodes. Intensive Care Medicine 1994; 20:94-98
6. Rhodes A, Lamb FJ, Malagon I, et al. A prospective study of the use of a dobutamine stress test to identify outcome in patients with sepsis, severe sepsis, or septic shock. Crit Care Med 1999; 27:2361-2366
7. Kumar A. The dobutamine oxygen flux test: a road map to outcome in sepsis? Crit Care Med 1999; 27:2571-2573
8. Brun-Buisson C, Doyon F, Carlet J, et al. Incidence, risk factors, and outcome of severe sepsis and septic shock in adults: a multicenter prospective study in intensive care units. JAMA 1995; 274:968-974
9. Perl TM, Dvorak L, Hwang T, et al. Long-term survival and function after suspected gram-negative sepsis. JAMA 1995; 274:338-345
10. Sasse KC, Nauenberg E, Long A, et al. Long-term survival after intensive care unit admission with sepsis. Crit Care Med 1995; 23:1040-1047
11. Casey LC, Balk RA, Bone RC. Plasma cytokine and endotoxin levels correlate with survival in patients with the sepsis syndrome. Ann Intern Med 1993; 119:771-778
12. Calandra T, Gerain J, Heumann D, et al. High circulating levels of interleukin-6 in patients with septic shock: evolution during sepsis, prognostic value, and interplay with other cytokines. The Swiss-Dutch J5 Immunoglobulin Study Group. Am J Med 1991; 91:23-29
13. Pinsky MR, Vincent JL, Deviere J, et al. Serum cytokine levels in human septic shock. Relation to multiple-system organ failure and mortality. Chest 1993; 103:565-575
14. Damas P, Reuter A, Gysen P, et al. Tumor necrosis factor and interleukin-1 serum levels during severe sepsis in humans. Crit Care Med 1989; 17:975-978
15. Marks JD, Marks CB, Luce JM, et al. Plasma tumor necrosis factor in patients with septic shock. Mortality rate, incidence of adult respiratory distress syndrome, and effects of methylprednisolone administration. Am Rev Respir Dis 1990; 141:94-97

94   *Quantifying risk in sepsis*

16. Mira JP, Cariou A, Grall F, et al. Association of TNF2, a TNF-a promoter polymorphism, with septic shock susceptibility and mortality. A multicenter study. JAMA 1999; 282:561-568
17. Angele MK, Schwacha MG, Ayala A, et al. Effect of gender and sex hormones on immune responses following shock. Shock 2000; 14:81-90
18. Kahlke V, Dohm C, Brotzmann K, et al. Gender-related therapy: early IL-10 administration after hemorrhage restores immune function in males but not in females. Shock 2000; 14:354-359
19. Wichmann MW, Inthorn D, Andress H-J, et al. Incidence and mortality of severe sepsis in surgical intensive care patients: the influence of patient gender on disease process and outcome. Intensive Care Med 2000; 26:167-172
20. Schroder J, Kahlke V, Book M, et al. Gender differences in sepsis: genetically determined? Shock 2000; 14:307-310
21. Mourouga P, Goldfrad C, Rowan KM. Does it fit? Is it good? Assessment of scoring systems. Curr Opin Crit Care 2000; 6:176-180
22. Knaus WA, Zimmerman JE, Wagner DP, et al. APACHE-acute physiology and chronic health evaluation: a physiologically based classification system. Crit Care Med 1981; 9:591-597
23. Le Gall JR, Loirat P, Alperovitch A, et al. A simplified acute physiology score for ICU patients. Crit Care Med 1984; 12:975-977
24. Lemeshow S, Teres D, Klar J, et al. Mortality probability models (MPM$_0$ and MPM$_{24}$) based on 19,124 patients. Crit Care Med 1993; 21:S175 (Abst)
25. Knaus WA, Draper EA, Wagner DP, et al. APACHE II: a severity of disease classification system. Crit Care Med 1985; 13:818-829
26. Bohnen JM, Mustard RA, Oxholm SE, et al. APACHE II score and abdominal sepsis. A prospective study. Arch Surg 1988; 123:225-229
27. Lundberg JS, Perl TM, Wiblin T, et al. Septic shock: an analysis of outcomes for patients with onset on hospital wards versus intensive care units. Crit Care Med 1998; 26:1020-1024
28. Cerra FB, Negro F, Abrams J. APACHE II score does not predict multiple organ failure or mortality in postoperative surgical patients. Arch Surg 1990; 125:519-522
29. Le Gall JR, Lemeshow S, Saulnier F. A new Simplified Acute Physiology Score (SAPS II) based on a European/North American multicenter study. JAMA 1993; 270:2957-2963
30. Zimmerman JE, Wagner DP, Draper EA, et al. Evaluation of acute physiology and chronic health evaluation III predictions of hospital mortality in an independent database. Crit Care Med 1998; 26:1317-1326
31. Poenaru D, Christou NV. Clinical outcome of seriously ill surgical patients with intra-abdominal infection depends on both physiologic (APACHE II score) and immunologic (DTH score) alterations. Ann Surg 1991; 213:130-136
32. Presterl E, Staudinger T, Pettermann M, et al. Cytokine profile and correlation to the APACHE III and MPM II scores in patients with sepsis. Am J Respir Crit Care Med 1997; 156:825-832
33. Calvano SE, Coyle SM, Barbosa KS, et al. Multivariate analysis of 9 disease-associated variables for outcome prediction in patients with sepsis. Arch Surg 1998; 133:1347-1350
34. Le Gall JR, Lemeshow S, Leleu G, et al. Customized probability models for early severe sepsis in adult intensive care patients. Intensive Care Unit Scoring Group. JAMA 1995; 273:644-650
35. Fisher CJ, Jr., Dhainaut JF, Opal SM, et al. Recombinant human interleukin 1 receptor antagonist in the treatment of patients with sepsis syndrome. Results from a randomized, double-blind, placebo-controlled trial. JAMA 1994; 271:1836-1843
36. Knaus WA, Draper EA, Wagner DP, et al. Prognosis in acute organ-system failure. Ann Surg 1985; 202:685-693

37. Hebert PC, Drummond AJ, Singer J, et al. A simple multiple system organ failure scoring system predicts mortality of patients who have sepsis syndrome. Chest 1993; 104:230-235

38. Marshall JC, Cook DJ, Christou NV, et al. Multiple organ dysfunction score: a reliable descriptor of a complex clinical outcome. Crit Care Med 1995; 23:1638-1652

39. Le Gall JR, Klar J, Lemeshow S, et al. The Logistic Organ Dysfunction system. A new way to assess organ dysfunction in the intensive care unit. JAMA 1996; 276:802-810

40. Vincent JL, Moreno R, Takala J, et al. The SOFA (Sepsis-related Organ Failure Assessment) score to describe organ dysfunction/failure. Intensive Care Med 1996; 22:707-710

41. Jacobs S, Zuleika M, Mphansa T. The Multiple Organ Dysfunction Score as a descriptor of patient outcome in septic shock compared with two other scoring systems. Crit Care Med 1999; 27:741-744

42. Soufir L, Timsit JF, Mahe C, et al. Attributable morbidity and mortality of catheter-related septicemia in critically ill patients: a matched, risk-adjusted, cohort study. Infect Control Hosp Epidemiol 1999; 20:396-401

43. Vincent JL, de Mendonca A, Cantraine F, et al. Use of the SOFA score to assess the incidence of organ dysfunction/failure in intensive care units: results of a multicenter, prospective study. Crit Care Med 1998; 26:1793-1800

44. Moreno R, Vincent JL, Matos R, et al. The use of maximum SOFA score to quantify organ dysfunction/failure in intensive care. Results of a prospective, multicentre study. Working Group on Sepsis related Problems of the ESICM. Intensive Care Med 1999; 25:686-696

45. Hynninen M, Valtonen M, Markkanen H, et al. Interleukin 1 receptor antagonist and E-selectin concentrations: a comparison in patients with severe acute pancreatitis and severe sepsis. J Crit Care 1999; 14:63-68

46. Alsous F, Khamiees M, DeGirolamo A, et al. Negative fluid balance predicts survival in patients with septic shock: a retrospective pilot study. Chest 2000; 117:1749-1754

47. Di Filippo A, De Gaudio AR, Novelli A, et al. Continuous infusion of vancomycin in methicillin-resistant staphylococcus infection. Chemotherapy 1998; 44:63-68

48. Vincent JL, Ferreira F, Moreno R. Scoring systems for assessing organ dysfunction and survival. Crit Care Clin 2000; 16:353-366

49. Petros AJ, Marshall JC, van Saene HK. Should morbidity replace mortality as an endpoint for clinical trials in intensive care? Lancet 1995; 345:369-371

50. Rowan KM, Kerr JH, Major E, et al. Intensive Care Society's Acute Physiology and Chronic Health Evaluation (APACHE II) study in Britain and Ireland: a prospective, multicenter, cohort study comparing two methods for predicting outcome for adult intensive care patients. Crit Care Med 1994; 22:1392-1401

51. Wong DT, Crofts SL, Gomez M, et al. Evaluation of predictive ability of APACHE II system and hospital outcome in Canadian intensive care unit patients. Crit Care Med 1995; 23:1177-1183

52. Moreno R, Morais P. Outcome prediction in intensive care: results of a prospective, multicentre, Portuguese study. Intensive Care Med 1997; 23:177-186

53. Nouira S, Belghith M, Elatrous S, et al. Predictive value of severity scoring systems: comparison of four models in Tunisian adult intensive care units. Crit Care Med 1998; 26:852-859

54. Bastos PG, Sun X, Wagner DP, et al. Application of the APACHE III prognostic system in Brazilian intensive care units: a prospective multicenter study. Intensive Care Med 1996; 22:564-570

55. Rivera-Fernandez R, Vazquez-Mata G, Bravo M, et al. The Apache III prognostic system: customized mortality predictions for Spanish ICU patients. Intensive Care Med 1998; 24:574-581

56. Moreno R. Outcome prediction in intensive care. In: Vincent JL (ed) Yearbook of Intensive Care and Emergency Medicine. Springer-Verlag, Berlin, Germany, 2000, pp 825-836
57. Williams M, Simms HH. Prognostic usefulness of scoring systems in critically ill patients with severe acute pancreatitis. Crit Care Med 1999; 27:901-907
58. Fine MJ, Auble TE, Yealy DM, et al. A prediction rule to identify low-risk patients with community-acquired pneumonia. N Engl J Med 1997; 336:243-250
59. Baumgartner JD, Bula C, Vaney C, et al. A novel score for predicting the mortality of septic shock patients. Crit Care Med 1992; 20:953-960
60. Meek M, Munster AM, Winchurch RA, et al. The Baltimore Sepsis Scale: measurement of sepsis in patients with burns using a new scoring system. J Burn Care Rehabil 1991; 12:564-568
61. Bosscha K, Reijnders K, Hulstaert PF, et al. Prognostic scoring systems to predict outcome in peritonitis and intra- abdominal sepsis. Br J Surg 1997; 84:1532-1534
62. Elebute EA, Stoner HB. The grading of sepsis. Br J Surg 1983; 70:29-31
63. Chang RW, Jacobs S, Lee B. Predicting outcome among intensive care unit patients using computerised trend analysis of daily Apache II scores corrected for organ system failure. Intensive Care Med 1988; 14:558-566
64. Lemeshow S, Klar J, Teres D. Outcome prediction for individual intensive care patients: useful, misused, or abused? Intensive Care Med 1995; 21:770-776
65. Angus DC. Discourse on method: Measuring the value of new therapies in intensive care. In: Vincent J-L (ed) Yearbook of Intensive Care and Emergency Medicine. Springer, Heidelberg, 1998, p: 265

7

THE PATHOGENESIS OF GRAM-NEGATIVE SEPSIS

Christopher Papasian
David C. Morrison

Microbial sepsis, and Gram-negative sepsis in particular, continues to serve as a major clinical problem throughout the world. While considerable advances have been realized not only in the treatment of this disease, but also in our understanding of the mechanisms involved in disease pathogenesis, Gram-negative sepsis continues to challenge both practicing physicians and basic scientists. A clear delineation of the events leading to Gram-negative sepsis, however, has been complicated by evolving definitions of the term 'sepsis', which have changed considerably over the past two decades [1,2]. The problem is further exacerbated by a failure of existing databases tracking nosocomial infections to include 'sepsis' as a trackable entity [3]. For example, statistics are maintained for the incidence and etiology of nosocomial bacteremia, but not for sepsis, and it has not been uncommon to utilize statistics on nosocomial bacteremia to draw conclusions about sepsis. In fact, much of the older literature utilized the terms 'bacteremia' and 'sepsis' interchangeably [4]. Yet, according to modern definitions of sepsis, approximately half of septic patients are not bacteremic, and a significant proportion of bacteremic patients are not septic [4]. Similarly, while Infection Control Practitioners track the incidence and etiology of pneumonia, urinary tract, surgical site, and other infections, the proportion of each of these that progress to sepsis is not monitored [3,5]. Even carefully conducted studies designed to determine the epidemiology of sepsis are consistently vague about the relative proportion of Gram-negative pneumonias, surgical site infections, urinary tract infections, etc. that progress to sepsis [4,6,7]. Often, such studies determine the overall proportion of infections in each category that ultimately progress to sepsis, and the relative proportion of each of these infection categories caused by specific etiologic agents. Unfortunately, the proportion of a given infection caused by a specific agent, or group of agents, that progress to sepsis is not easily discernible from the published literature (e.g., how often do patients with *Pseudomonas* pneumonia become septic, and what proportion of sepsis is attributable to *Pseudomonas* pneumonia?)

Allowing for the existing constraint on current data surrounding Gram-negative sepsis we shall, in the following paragraphs, attempt to review the key issues surrounding the pathogenesis of Gram-negative sepsis. It has been determined that approximately 40% of all septic patients are infected with Gram-negative bacilli, and about half of these patients are bacteremic [4]. Importantly, Gram-negative bacteremia is substantially more likely to result in septic shock (50-60 %) than is fungemia or Gram-positive bacteremia (5-10 %). Patients admitted to medical and surgical intensive care units (ICUs) are at substantially greater risk of developing sepsis than are patients on the general wards [2,4,6,7]. The increased risk of sepsis in ICU patients is likely to be explained, at least in part, by the finding that poor overall health as indicated by APACHE II or ASA scores is an independent risk factor for developing sepsis; ICU patients typically have the poorest overall health among hospitalized patients [4].

EPIDEMIOLOGY OF GRAM-NEGATIVE SEPSIS

A recent prospective study of sepsis syndrome at eight academic medical centers in the United States by Sands et al. has been particularly enlightening with respect to the incidence of sepsis [6]. Over a 15-month period, 1,342 episodes of sepsis syndrome were documented in a study of 12,759 patients. Approximately 55 % of those patients developing sepsis syndrome had been previously admitted to the ICU, 12 % were from Emergency Departments, and 33 % were from non-ICU patient care units. The most frequent sites of infection in patients with sepsis syndrome included the respiratory tract (42 %), primary bacteremia (12 %), genitourinary tract (11 %), and abdomen (10 %). In those patients where an etiologic agent was identified, Gram-negative bacteria accounted for approximately 40 % of the cases of sepsis syndrome. Of those 40%, approximately two thirds (67 %) were attributable to members of the family *Enterobacteriaceae* and 25 % to *Pseudomonas* spp. Bacteremia occurred in 45% of the patients with sepsis syndrome attributable to Gram-negative bacteria. Brun-Buisson's review of predominantly ICU patients yielded similar epidemiologic findings; in cases of microbiologically documented severe sepsis, the most common sites for infection were the lung (41 %), abdomen (32 %), bone and joints (13 %) and urinary tract (11 %) [2].

Of bacteremic patients with sepsis and severe sepsis, 44 % were infected with Gram-negative bacteria, and 85 % of these were *E. coli*. The extraordinarily high proportion of *E. coli* reported by Brun-Buisson probably reflects the restriction of his analysis to bacteremic patients as abdominal and urinary tract infections were the most common sources for bacteremia, and *E. coli* predominates in this setting.

ORIGIN OF INFECTION

Infections leading to sepsis may be either endogenous or exogenous in origin [8]. Exogenous infections usually are manifest shortly after microorganisms invade the patient from the immediate surrounding environment. While exogenous infections occasionally result in sepsis, they usually constitute only a small proportion of the overall contribution to this disease syndrome. Examples include meningococcal sepsis shortly after acquisition of the organism from another infected or colonized individual, and *Yersinia* sepsis following exposure to contaminated transfusion products. Endogenous infections may be divided into primary and secondary endogenous infections. Primary endogenous infections are those in which the infecting organism is part of the patient's normal colonizing flora, whereas secondary endogenous infections are those attributable to the patient's flora following modification, an event which, for a number of reasons, commonly occurs in hospitalized patients. Endogenous infections account for most cases of sepsis, and a significant proportion of these cases develop in hospitalized patients following modification of their normal flora.

The Gastrointestinal Tract

The major reservoir for Gram-negative bacterial colonization in the human host includes mucosal surfaces of the genitourinary tract of females, and the gastrointestinal and respiratory tracts of both sexes. It has been estimated that approximately 10^{14} bacterial organisms (about 100-200 g) representing more than 400 different species, many of which are Gram-negative, routinely inhabit the normal human gastrointestinal tract [9]. The stomach is normally sterile, and microbial colonization of the proximal small intestine is relatively sparse, but bacterial concentrations increase with increasing distance from the stomach. The colon is invariably the major site of endogenous bacterial colonization, with ubiquitous representation by members of the family *Enterobacteriaceae*, particularly *E. coli*, and substantially greater numbers of obligate anaerobes such as *Bacteroides* spp. Anaerobes generally are considered to be weak inducers of systemic inflammation, presumably due to a relatively low level of activity manifest by the endotoxin molecules expressed by these organisms [10]. In point of fact, these organisms actually appear to protect the host by preventing overgrowth with more virulent organisms, thereby decreasing the potential for subsequent translocation of these organisms or their components across the gut [11].

Unfortunately, one of the major consequences of antimicrobial therapy is that it rapidly alters the normal ecology of the gut. Anaerobic organisms are easily killed by antibiotics, and the ecological void established by their elimination is rapidly filled by increasing numbers of more virulent Gram-negative bacteria such as *E. coli*, *Klebsiella pneumoniae*, *Enterobacter* spp., and *Pseudomonas aeruginosa,* as well as by yeasts and Gram-positive bacteria such as staphylococci and *Enterococcus* spp. [8,11,12]. These new gut inhabitants frequently represent strains that are circulated from patient to patient primarily via the unwashed hands of hospital personnel. The end result is that hospitalized patients, particularly those inhabiting the ICU, manifest a markedly altered colonic flora which often includes increased numbers of Gram-negative aerobes. These latter organisms are often selected because of their resistance to antimicrobial agents that are commonly used within the hospital.

While a physiologically and anatomically intact intestinal mucosa usually provides a relatively effective barrier against bacterial translocation and invasion, the intestinal mucosa of many hospitalized patients has been compromised by factors related to their underlying illness, including alteration of gut flora due to prior antimicrobial therapy [13]. Colonization of the gastrointestinal tract is also often a precursor to genitourinary and probably less frequently, respiratory colonization [14-16]. Thus, enhanced colonization of the gastrointestinal tract by Gram-negative bacteria can lead to Gram-negative sepsis by direct invasion and/or translocation of bacteria or their constituents (e.g., endotoxin) across the gastrointestinal mucosa, and by serving as a source for colonization of the genitourinary and respiratory tracts with organisms that might subsequently produce genitourinary or respiratory infections.

The Respiratory Tract

The upper respiratory tract of healthy adults is heavily colonized by Gram-positive bacteria (e.g., *Streptococcus* and *Peptostreptococcus*), *Haemophilus* spp. (other than *H. influenzae*), *Neisseria* spp. (other than *N. meningitidis and N. gonorrhoeae)*, and obligately anaerobic Gram-negative bacteria such as

Bacteroides, *Porphyromonas*, *Fusobacterium*, and *Prevotella* spp. These microorganisms have little potential to produce serious infection. Other Gram-negative bacteria that sporadically colonize the upper respiratory tract include *Haemophilus influenzae*, *Neisseria meningitidis*, and *Moraxella catarrhalis*. These latter organisms are important human pathogens that can produce serious infection in the proper clinical setting.

As physical illness ensues, the normal flora of the upper respiratory tract is altered. Members of the family *Enterobacteriaceae*, which are not present in significant quantities in healthy individuals, begin to colonize the upper respiratory tract [8,11,17]. This transition in upper respiratory flora occurs in both hospitalized and non-hospitalized individuals, but the process is expedited in hospitalized patients by their frequent exposure to antimicrobial agents. The Gram-positive upper respiratory flora of healthy adults is extremely susceptible to most antimicrobial agents, and the void created by their elimination is filled rapidly by organisms such as *Enterobacter cloacae* and *Klebsiella pneumoniae*. As hospitalized patients are subjected to more aggressive antimicrobial therapy for putative infectious processes, this new selective pressure leads to colonization with progressively more resistant organisms such as *Pseudomonas aeruginosa* and *Acinetobacter lwoffi*. This transition in upper respiratory flora is a significant factor in the development of Gram-negative sepsis. Lower respiratory infections are among the most common infectious processes leading to sepsis, and a substantial proportion of these infections develop following microaspiration of respiratory secretions contaminated with Gram-negative bacteria from the upper respiratory tract of hospitalized patients [7,17].

ROLE OF ENDOTOXIN IN THE PATHOGENESIS OF GRAM-NEGATIVE SEPSIS

While, as will be clearly documented in other chapters in this volume, a very broad spectrum of microbes can contribute to the initiation of sepsis in human hosts, it is nevertheless generally recognized that Gram-negative bacteria occupy a unique and probably special position within the collection of sepsis-causing microorganisms. The primary reason for this is the fact that Gram-negative organisms possess a complex outer cell envelope that, in contrast to Gram-positive bacteria, contains a functionally important outer cell membrane that is exterior to the rigid peptidoglycan layer of the cell wall. This outer membrane contains a true lipid bilayer with the innermost lipid leaflet consisting of traditional phospholipids and the outer leaflet composed of lipopolysaccharide (LPS). The LPS molecules are structurally unique to the Gram-negative bacteria (with the possible exception of some blue green algae) and, as will be reviewed elsewhere in this volume, consist of covalent constructs of lipids and polysaccharide. It is the presence of these LPS structures and, in particular the very potent pluripotential ability of these macromolecules to interact with host innate and acquired immune cells and humoral mediators that imparts much of the clinical threat associated with Gram-negative infections [18]. It is important to point out that the presence of this LPS macromolecule is a general characteristic of virtually all Gram-negative microbes regardless of whether the organism is considered part of the host's normal flora or a newly acquired potential pathogen. Noteworthy in this respect is the fact that the biological activity of LPS derived from a variety of Gram-negative clinical isolates including *E. coli, Proteus, Klebsiella* and *Aeromonas* spp., all manifest roughly equivalent biological activity in terms of their proinflammatory potential [19]. In contrast, as pointed out earlier, LPS derived from certain obligate anaerobes (e.g., *Bacteroides* and *Porphyromonas* spp.) is remarkably less biologically active, and in some instances, such LPS has been shown to modulate the expression of activity of more potent LPS preparations

Based upon studies with temperature-conditional mutant strains of *E. coli* that fail to synthesize the minimal structural features of LPS at non-permissive temperatures, LPS was considered essential for viability of Gram-negative bacteria, but recently this view has been challenged by the isolation of a mutant *Neisseria meningitidis* strain which totally lacked LPS [20]. Although capable of replication, the LPS-deficient *N. meningitidis* mutant replicated more slowly and produced much smaller colonies on solid media than the wild type strain. Since it is established that LPS serves as a selective permeability barrier to potentially deleterious molecules in the external environment, it may be that this gatekeeper function contributes substantially to bacterial viability. Alternatively, the presence of LPS in the outer leaflet may serve to stabilize the lipid bilayer. In any case, it is clear that the presence of LPS on the outer proximal layer of the outer membrane places this microbial constituent in an optimal position to interface with the external environment. In the case of potentially pathogenic Gram-negative microbes, this external environment would include the repertoire of host defense systems, both innate and acquired, that the bacteria must confront in any effort to establish an infectious nidus within a host. In this respect, LPS is known to serve as a dominant immunogen for the generation of potentially protective antibody. This dominant microbial LPS antigen has been termed the O-antigen, in contrast to the less immunogenic lipid component of the LPS macromolecule, termed Lipid A. The latter is universally recognized as the 'toxic' component of this microbial constituent and is responsible for almost all of the biological activity of LPS.

Antibody to the O antigen is usually, although not always, found to convey antigen specific protection against infection with antigenically related Gram-negative microbes. The fact that the O-antigen structure of individual strains of Gram-negative bacteria are sufficiently diverse as to serve as unique identifying signatures, however, precludes their use as generalized vaccine candidates to provide prophylactic protection against infection with Gram-negatives. Nevertheless, LPS also contains highly conserved polysaccharide structural domains interior to the immunodominant O-antigen (termed core polysaccharide) as well as the highly conserved lipid A component. These conserved structural features of LPS have, during the past several decades, provided investigators with potential opportunities to develop protective immunotherapeutic strategies. The successes and failures of this particular approach is discussed in other chapters in this volume.

Perhaps equally as important to the concept of the interface between outer membrane LPS and the external environment is the almost ubiquitous ability of this bacterial constituent to be recognized as 'non-self' by the various constructs of the innate host defense system. In this respect, LPS is ubiquitous in its ability to interact effectively with essentially all of the host humoral and cellular pathways that trigger an inflammatory response. Indeed, this unique feature of LPS, which can be manifest *in vitro* at concentrations as low as 1-10 pg/ml, and *in vivo* at doses as low as 1-10 ng in a mouse, has allowed this molecule to be generally adopted as a prototype standard immunopathologic stimulus against which all other biologically active molecules can be compared. It is just such biological properties of LPS that prompted Ivan Bennett, almost fifty years ago, to comment "An investigator in almost any field who wishes to obtain a positive result should try endotoxin in his/her experimental system." [21]

It is precisely this plethora of biological activities of LPS *in vitro* and *in vivo* that prompted investigators early on to target this microbial constituent in the development of potentially novel therapeutic approaches for treatment of Gram-negative sepsis. Such studies were originally predicated upon early-published evidence suggesting that treatment of Gram-negative infections with antibiotics would in many patients lead to a temporary exacerbation of clinical symptoms [22,23]. This is, of course, the prototype response first observed more than a century ago by Jarisch who reported that treatment of syphilis patients with spirocheticidal drugs, such as arsenic, would lead to elevated temperatures [24]. These and other studies led to the formulation of the now well-documented Jarisch-Herxheimer reaction, the mechanism of which has been largely attributed to the release of microbial triggers of inflammation. Indeed, more recent evidence, that treatment of patients infected with *Borrelia recurrentis* with the antibiotic doxycycline manifest a number of consequent pathophysiological responses consistent with endotoxemia, would further support this concept [25]. It needs to be noted that there is no good evidence that spirochetes actually contain macromolecular structures identifiable as LPS. Nevertheless, the fact that treatment of microbes with agents that cause disruption or dissolution of bacterial structural integrity lends credence to the concept that release/exposure of microbial constituents to the external environment can potentiate inflammatory responses.

As a consequence, it has been an attractive hypothesis to consider endotoxic LPS synthesized by Gram-negative microbes, particularly when liberated from the microbial outer membrane structure, as a major contributing factor to the pathophysiology of sepsis caused by Gram-negative microbes. Consistent with this interpretation is the very impressive list of innate and acquired host defense and maintenance systems with which LPS has been documented to interact [26,27]. It would be far beyond the scope of this or any single chapter to delineate what is known about LPS-induced activation of host defense systems. Suffice it to say that it includes both the extrinsic and intrinsic pathways of the plasma coagulation system, the classical (antibody independent) and alternative pathways of serum complement, the activation of B-lymphocytes to both proliferate and differentiate, the activation of γ-δ T-cells, the activation of macrophages and monocytes for synthesis, secretion, and surface expression of an array of pro- and anti-inflammatory mediators, as well as activation of endothelial cells, epithelial cells, fibroblasts and hepatocytes. Collectively therefore, it is difficult to envision an infectious scenario with a Gram-negative microbe that would not involve endotoxin-induced production of host inflammatory mediators as contributors to the pathogenesis of disease.

As pointed out above, one of the more dominant themes surrounding the role of endotoxin in Gram-negative sepsis is the concept that it is the release of LPS from the microbial surface outer membrane that unleashes the full manifestation of endotoxin's inflammatory potential. From a structural perspective, this would appear to be a valid concept in that the biologically active component of LPS, lipid A, is precisely that part of the molecule that serves to anchor LPS within the lipid bilayer. Consequently, the majority of schematic renderings of the outer membrane of Gram-negative bacteria have not placed lipid A in a position where it could be easily envisioned to interact with host defense systems [28]. Further, the majority of the available data would suggest that LPS that has been liberated from the microbial envelope is at least twenty fold more active than an equivalent amount of microbe associated LPS, as assessed by induction of procoagulant activity or tumor necrosis factor (TNF)-α secretion in cultures of human monocytes [29]. This latter finding is consistent with the postulated relative inactivity of lipid A in the intact outer membrane.

In vitro data generated by a number of investigators, using a variety of microbial systems, collectively tend to confirm that antibiotic treatment of Gram-negative microorganisms promotes the release of LPS, resulting in enhanced production of proinflammatory cytokines [reviewed in 30, 31]. Importantly, antibiotics with different binding affinities for different penicillin binding proteins (PBPs) were found to differentially affect the resulting structural features of the organism (i.e., filaments vs spheroblasts vs lysis), which in turn affected both the quantity of LPS released into the external environment and the generation of proinflammatory cytokines. In parallel studies carried out in an experimental rodent model of sepsis, similar differential levels of protective efficacy were noted depending upon the type of antibiotic chosen (normalized to equivalent MIC). These experimental studies *in vitro, in vivo* and *ex vivo* would all support the hypothesis that antibiotics that manifest different modes of action/endotoxin release may differentially stimulate the pathophysiologic septic response to Gram-negative microbes.

The extrapolation of such hypotheses to antibiotic therapy in patients with Gram-negative sepsis, however, has unfortunately failed to yield findings that are fully in accord with these convincing experimental results. In this respect, an early study by Prins *et al* in patients with documented urosepsis strongly suggested that treatment with a PBP-3 binding third generation cepholosporin resulted in increased serum and urine concentrations of inflammatory cytokines compared to an equivalent population of patients treated with a PBP-2 binding carbapenem [32]. Unfortunately, a more comprehensive repeat of this earlier study did not confirm the initial findings. In the more recent study, virtually no detectable differences in endotoxin levels or inflammatory cytokines were noted over the first eight hours post antibiotic administration [33]. The conclusion reached in these later prospective studies were in accord with several earlier retrospective studies in which no correlations were observed between various antibiotic treatments and outcomes due to Gram-negative sepsis [34].

While noting these findings, it is important to remember that a number of additional factors, not considered in these analyses, could strongly influence the interpretation of the findings regarding the role of endotoxin and, perhaps more specifically, antibiotic released endotoxin, in the pathogenesis of Gram-negative sepsis. Among the most important of these are two factors that can profoundly influence the response of most inflammatory cells to endotoxin. Specifically, these two factors include: 1) the role of the specific genetic background of the host; and 2) the induction of endotoxin hyporesponsiveness/tolerance. An additional important factor that might be expected to be superimposed upon the endotoxin effect, is the potential contribution of additional microbial components that are either actively secreted by Gram-negative microbes or released from the microbe subsequent to exposure to bacteriolytic agents. There is, in this respect, considerable experimental evidence that each of these factors can significantly affect the pro-inflammatory potential of bacterial endotoxin in its interaction with host mediator systems. Since most analyses of patients with Gram-negative infections have not considered these potentially important variables, it would be reasonable to conclude that the establishment of precise correlations between endotoxin and disease outcome would be, in most instances, difficult if not impossible to establish.

Influence of Genetic Background

We will consider first the issue of differential responses of inflammatory cells to endotoxin stimulation as a function of genetic background. It has already been well established that most inflammatory cells from different inbred strains of mice manifest significantly different levels of responsiveness to stimulation *in vitro* with LPS, and that different doses of LPS are required *in vivo* to elicit 50% lethality. Indeed, studies comparing inbred and outbred mice for the ability of neutralizing anti-TNF-α antibody or soluble TNF-α receptor-Ig constructs to protect against a lethal dose of LPS would support these differences in endotoxin inflammatory potential [35]. In human peripheral blood monocytes, careful quantitative dose-response profiles have established differences in the relative ability of cells to respond to immunostimulation by LPS that are in the range of two orders of magnitude different among a population of healthy donors [30]. Careful genetic studies of relative LPS responsiveness in isolated peripheral blood monocytes of family members have provided convincing evidence for genetic inheritance of differential LPS responsiveness [36]. Therefore, it is difficult to conclude that it would be useful to seek correlation between endotoxin levels, inflammatory cytotine responses, and outcome, without knowledge of the genetically predetermined endotoxic potential of host inflammatory cells, if one were to accept the very reasonable concept that inflammatory mediator production is important in the pathogenesis of Gram-negative sepsis.

Induction of Endotoxin Hyporesponsiveness/Tolerance

Compounding the potential problems associated with genetic variability in responsiveness of host inflammatory mediator cells to the immunostimulatory actions of LPS is the fact that environmental factors, including LPS itself, can significantly influence the host response to LPS. This phenomenon of selective hyporesponsiveness to LPS was initially referred to as 'early endotoxin tolerance' and was first described in *in vivo* studies in experimental animals [37]. This feature was later shown to exist at the level of inflammatory cell responses themselves, and could be shown to involve a selective refractory state to subsequent exposure to LPS. Other studies have documented that this observed alteration in LPS responsiveness of macrophages can be induced *in vitro* using concentrations of LPS that are orders of magnitude lower (i.e., pg/ml of LPS) than those necessary to induce detectable macrophage cell activation [38]. Moreover, and perhaps more importantly, pretreatment of macrophages with these low substimulatory concentrations of LPS induces a biphasic differential profile of enhanced and suppressed responses to subsequent stimulation by LPS, depending upon which macrophage mediator is measured. For example, pretreatment of macrophages with LPS at 10-50 pg/ml profoundly upregulates the ability of these cells to synthesize and secrete TNF-α following subsequent exposure to higher stimulating concentrations of LPS (e.g., 100 ng/ml), while at the same time these cells are no longer able to synthesize inducible nitric oxide synthetase (iNOS) in response to LPS. Alternately, if macrophages are preexposed to higher substimulatory concentrations of LPS (0.5 – 1.0 ng/ml), TNF-α is not produced upon subsequent stimulation with 100 ng/ml, while levels of iNOS are markedly elevated. We have termed this plasticity in the differential responsiveness to LPS as 'reprogramming' and have postulated that reprogramming is a pivotal event in preparing the host to optimally respond to the presence of microbial antigens [39].

Studies designed to examine the molecular mechanisms involved in these reprogramming events have strongly suggested that autocrine/paracrine feedback mechanisms are most likely involved as key factors in regulating responses. In fact, the available evidence would indicate that differential regulation of IL-10 and IL-12 in response to substimulating concentrations of LPS is a key in directing outcome [39]. Of additional potential importance is very recent evidence demonstrating that the treatment of macrophages with pg/ml levels of LPS will upregulate the induction and synthesis of caveolin-1 in macrophages [40]. This cytoplasmic protein is well documented to regulate signal transduction by virtue of a conserved scaffolding domain that regulates binding of caveolin-1 to a variety of proteins involved in transmembrane signaling, including G proteins, kinases and the EGF-receptors. The fact that Toll-like receptor (TLR)-4, the membrane protein involved in LPS signaling, also expresses a caveolin-1 consensus scaffolding domain in its cytoplasmic tail would potentially implicate this regulatory mechanism as well.

Important to this concept is the finding that circulating leukocytes from either normal human volunteers previously administered endotoxin, or patients diagnosed with sepsis, also manifest reduced responsiveness to stimulation by LPS when examined *in vitro* [41]. With these two populations, there is considerable published evidence to support the conclusion that both monocytes and polymorphonuclear leukocytes synthesize less TNF-α, interleukin (IL)-1β, and other cytokines when stimulated with LPS, than comparable cells from normal individuals. In some instances this hyporesponsiveness appears to be stimulus (i.e., LPS) specific, whereas in other experimental protocols, the refractory state also extends to other microbial stimuli, such as staphylococcal enterotoxin B. Of potential importance is the finding that both LPS and IL-1β are able to induce a state of mutual cross-tolerance in which pretreatment with LPS reduced responsiveness to IL-1β and *vice versa*. These findings would strongly support the conclusion that both systems share a common pathway of signal transduction and a common factor involved in reprogramming. Pertinent to this finding are recent studies suggesting that the IL-1 receptor associated kinase (IRAK) may be a molecular candidate for the induction of the refractory state [42].

Collectively therefore, there is compelling evidence from *in vitro, in vivo* and clinical studies with peripheral blood cells from septic patients indicating that exposure to either endotoxin or other proinflammatory mediators can profoundly influence the phenotypic profile of inflammatory mediator production upon subsequent immunostimulation. It is reasonable to conclude that similar alterations in the potential responsiveness of other LPS-sensitive cell types (e.g., tissue macrophages, vascular endothelial cells, etc.) might also result from preexposure to their mediators. The subsequent pattern of responsiveness would then depend upon their prior history of exposure to immunostimulants, as well as the specific conditions of that exposure (concentration, time, genetics).

Involvement of other Proinflammatory Triggers

A third and undoubtedly important contributing factor to the overall host inflammatory response to infection with Gram-negative microbes is the potential collective contribution of all of the various proinflammatory triggers that would either be actively secreted from viable organisms, expressed and accessible on the microbial surface, or released from the microbe following bacteriolysis. Although, over the last several decades, much effort has justifiably focused on the role of endotoxin in the pathogenesis of Gram-negative sepsis, there has recently been considerable interest in the potential contributing role of other microbial constituents with known biological activity; in particular, those with documented proinflammatory activity. These constituents would include such diverse factors as peptidoglycan, lipoteichoic acid (LTA), lipoprotein, capsular polysaccharide and more recently, bacterial DNA. It is noteworthy that most of these microbial factors are either localized to the bacterial cell envelope or are readily released from the microbe following bacteriolysis.

Of potential importance to the consideration of these additional (non-LPS) microbial factors as important contributors to disease, is the recognition that the majority of surface membrane receptors implicated in inflammatory cell responses function through an initial association with the phosphatidyl inositol linked glycoprotein CD14 (discussed extensively in other chapters in this volume). This initial interaction is followed by signal transduction mediated through either TLR-2 (e.g., lipoprotein stimulation) or TLR-4 (e.g., LPS stimulation). Given this relatively high level of conservation in the molecular recognition and signal transduction pathways utilized by these various microbial constituents, it is likely that this would translate into a relatively similar panel of mediators secreted by inflammatory cells in response to these proinflammatory microbial stimuli.

Lipoprotein

Perhaps one of the more potent of these additional non-LPS microbial mediators is lipoprotein, which is either covalently bound to peptidoglycan or free in the outer membrane. Importantly, lipoprotein is generally recognized as the most abundant protein present in the outer membrane of Gram-negative bacteria and, in terms of percent by weight of the bacterium, is approximately equal to that of LPS [43]. Synthetic low molecular mass analogs of the lipoprotein, containing the active site in terms of immunostimulatory activity, have been synthesized and shown to possess almost all of the biological activities of the intact lipoprotein [44]. These include stimulation of B lymphocyte proliferation in *in vitro* culture and activation of macrophages to secrete inflammatory mediators such as TNF–α and IL-6. Given these properties of lipoprotein and its presence in high abundance in the bacterial cell, it is likely that this constituent is relevant in the pathogenesis of Gram-negative infections. It is noteworthy in this respect, that biologically active lipoprotein can readily be detected in the supernatants of actively growing *E. coli* with concentrations approximating those of soluble LPS ($\approx$1-10 ng/ml) [45]. This finding was not restricted to *E. coli* but was also observed with *Salmonella* and *Yersinia*. Of potential importance was the finding that treatment with the cell wall active antibiotic ceftazidime markedly increased the levels of lipoprotein found in culture supernatants, similar to that which have been described earlier for LPS.

Equally important, however, is the fact that lipoprotein also can manifest biological activity *in vitro* in the induction of proinflammatory cytokines, and *in vivo* in the induction of lethal shock in mice. Stimulation of macrophages to secrete TNF-α and IL-6 can be elicited at lipoprotein concentrations as low as 50 ng/ml and this has also been demonstrated in macrophages from the C3H/HeJ endotoxin-hyporesponsive mouse. This latter finding would strongly support the hypothesis that lipoprotein most likely signals through the TLR-2 membrane receptor, as C3H/HeJ mice appear to lack functional TLR-4 receptors. Further, purified lipoprotein induces lethality in *vivo* in D-galactosamine-treated mice at doses roughly equivalent to those used to induce lethality with LPS. Most interesting is the finding that lipoprotein and LPS appear to interact synergistically in the induction of lethality [46]. Somewhat unexpectedly, LPS will potentiate lipoprotein lethality in C3H/HeJ mice even though the LPS alone was completely nontoxic at the doses tested. Nevertheless, it is important that these two microbial factors, each proinflammatory in its own right, can function to potentiate the production of proinflammatory mediators leading to systemic inflammation and death. It appears likely that other microbial factors that function through TLR-2 will also synergize with LPS in the activation of inflammatory mediatory cells.

Bacterial DNA

Bacterial DNA has recently become the subject of considerable study because of its potent adjuvant and proinflammatory properties. This microbial constituent is distinguished from mammalian DNA by virtue of the fact that the latter is usually extensively methylated in the CpG residues, whereas bacterial DNA is not. Therefore, it is not surprising that the innate host immune system has developed mechanisms to differentiate between these two forms of nucleic acid. Importantly, DNA has been shown *in vitro* to also induce the production of inflammatory mediators, and like LPS and lipoprotein, to induce lethality in D-galactosamine-sensitized mice [47]. The observed activity of bacterial DNA is critically dependent upon the presence of CpG residues and can be reproduced by synthetic oligonucleotides containing CpG. *In vitro*, macrophages have been clearly demonstrated to be responsive to bacterial CpG-containing DNA as assessed by synthesis and secretion of inflammatory mediators, including TNF-α and NO. Perhaps most significant is the recently reported finding that CpG-DNA and LPS can interact synergistically in the induction of macrophage activity [48]. In this respect, substimulatory concentrations of either LPS or DNA can be potentiated in their ability to induce TNF-α and NO secretion *in vitro* by equally substimulatory concentrations of DNA or LPS, respectively. Since, in the absence of LPS, concentrations of DNA exceeding those required to effect macrophage activation directly would be unlikely to be present in an infectious locus, it can be anticipated that any significant contribution of CpG DNA to inflammation may well require some degree of synergy either with LPS or some other microbial constituent.

Lipoteichoic acid

It is actually not uncommon to find that microbial products will synergize with LPS in the induction of macrophage activation, given that this has been demonstrated with both CpG-DNA and liproprotein. Our own experiments have documented that LTA will also synergize with LPS, a finding that emerged from studies originally designed to assess the proinflammatory potential of LTA itself. In those studies, we found that much of the macrophage-inducing activity of commercial preparations of LTA was, in fact, the result of contamination with LPS [49]. Further, while LTA purified by affinity chromatography had markedly reduced activity relative to the unpurified preparation (with all of the direct biological activity on macrophages co-purifying with the LPS component) this purified LTA was, nevertheless, able to synergize with LPS in enhancing the induction of TNF-α and NO.

Collectively, therefore, these and other studies indicate that there are multiple microbial factors that can contribute both singularly and in concert to the induction of host inflammatory responses; endotoxin, though a well-recognized stimulus for Gram-negative sepsis, must be considered in concert with these additional microbe-derived mediators. This fact, in conjunction with other (e.g., host related) factors summarized above, may well explain, at least in part, the difficulty in correlating morbidity and/or mortality with circulating endotoxin levels *per se*. Given the undoubtedly important role of inflammatory mediators in the development of multiorgan dysfunction associated with Gram-negative sepsis, a more complete understanding and appreciation for the potential interplay of various microbe-derived factors in the induction of this inflammatory cascade will likely contribute to the development of additional novel therapeutic modalities.

CONCLUSION

In this chapter we have reviewed the various factors that contribute to the pathogenesis of Gram-negative sepsis. The major sources of Gram-negative bacteria inducing the septic response are most often patient flora that constitutively colonize the gastrointestinal, genitourinary, or respiratory mucosa. As a general rule, these organisms are likely to have existed as constituents of the patient's commensal microflora for prolonged periods of time preceding the septic episode. It is also possible, however, that the infection nidus might derive from a relatively recent microbial acquisition whose colonization is promoted by a disruption in normal mucosal ecology due to physiological alterations associated with illness, selective pressures of antimicrobial therapy, or both. Either way, these resident Gram-negative bacteria establish a mucosal presence which, under certain potentially adverse circumstances, predispose to deeper invasion and a more extensive interface with the host immune system. Infections in the lung, for example, induce the very rapid secretion of proinflammatory mediators such as TNF-α, IL-1, NO, and inteferon (IFN)-γ from alveolar macrophages, whereas invasion of the peritoneal cavity or blood induces similar responses from peritoneal macrophages and Kupffer cells, respectively. This early proinflammatory cascade can be, and often is, perpetuated and potentiated by many other cell types and proinflammatory mediators. The most potent proinflammatory stimulus derived from Gram-negative organisms appears to be LPS, but other microbial constituents (e.g., DNA, lipoprotein) are also proinflammatory, and may act synergistically with LPS. In the intact Gram-negative microbe, these constituents may not be ideally situated to provide an optimal inflammatory stimulus. Antimicrobial therapy, however, particularly with agents whose primary mode of action is dissolution of the cell wall, facilitates release of these constitutents, thereby enhancing the proinflammatory stimulus. In many situations, the host's inflammatory response has a substantially beneficial effect and the infectious process is contained, with or without antimicrobial therapy. Occasionally, however, the inflammatory response appears to far exceed that which would ordinarily be required to contain the infection. The resultant potentiated inflammatory response is designed to induce systemic vascular leakage, endothelial damage, and intravascular clotting which, in turn, produces the profound hemodynamic alterations that are the signature of severe septic shock and death. In this respect, the patients who would be at greatest risk for the sequence of events leading to sepsis are those with the poorest overall health, most notably those admitted to the various hospital ICUs. The reason for this, is that body defenses of such patients are either unable to contain localized infections before they induce systemic responses, or because the normal physiological processes which counter the detrimental effects of a proinflammatory stimulus are functionally impaired. In any event, the mortality rate associated with Gram-negative sepsis remains between 20 and 50%. Although our increased understanding of pathogenic mechanisms leading to Gram-negative sepsis remains to be fully translated into therapeutic strategies that would significantly impact this mortality, a number of important novel approaches are on the horizon. It is also inevitable that more such novel approaches will be discovered in the near future, all of which suggests that significant improvements in the management of Gram-negative sepsis will soon be forthcoming.

ACKNOWLEDGEMENT

Support from the National Institutes of Health through research grants R37 AI23447, R01 AI/HL 44936 (Morrison) and R15 AI46493 (Papasian), from the UMKC Sara Morrison Trust, the Saint Luke's Hospital Foundation, and from Merck and Co, Inc., Rahway, NJ is gratefully acknowledged.

REFERENCES

1. Bone RC, Grodzin CJ, Balk RA. Sepsis: a new hypothesis for pathogenesis of the disease process. Chest 1997; 112:235-243
2. Brun-Buisson C. The epidemiology of the systemic inflammatory response. Intensive Care Med 2000; 26: S64-S74
3. Anonymous. National Nosocomial Infections Surveillance (NNIS) System report, data summary from January 1990-May 1999, issued June 1999. Am J Infect Contr 1999; 27:520-532
4. Rangel-Frausto MS. The epidemiology of bacterial sepsis. Infect Dis Clin North Am 1999; 13:229-312
5. Fridkin SK, Welbel SF, Weinstein RA. Magnitude and prevention of nosocomial infections in the intensive care unit. Infect Dis Clin North Am 1997; 11:479-496
6. Sands KE, Bates DW, Lanken PN, et. al. Epidemiology of sepsis syndrome in eight academic medical centers. JAMA 1997; 278:234-240
7. Martin, MA. Epidemiology and clinical impact of Gram-negative sepsis. Infect Dis Clin North Am 1991; 5:739-754
8. Occhipinti DJ, Itokazu G, Danziger LH. Selective decontamination of the digestive tract as an infection-control measure in intensive care unit patients. Pharmacotherapy 1992; 12:50S-63S
9. Wells CL. Colonization and translocation of intestinal bacterial flora. Transplant Proc 1996; 28: 2653-2656
10. Poxton IR, Edmond DM. Biological activity of *Bacteroides* lipopolysaccharide—reappraisal. Clin Infect Dis 1995; 20 (Suppl. 2):S149-153
11. Jarvis WR. The epidemiology of colonization. Infection Control and Hospital Epidemiology 1996; 17:47-52
12. Norrby SR. Ecological consequences of broad spectrum versus narrow spectrum antimicrobial therapy. Scand J Infect Dis Suppl 1986; 49:189-195

13. Deitch EA. Bacterial translocation of the gut flora. J Trauma 1990; 30:S184-S189
14. Svanborg C, Godaly G. Bacterial virulence in urinary tract infection. Infect Dis Clin North Am 1997; 11:513-529
15. Bonten MJM, Gaillard CA, de Leeuw PW, Stobberingh EE. Role of colonization of the upper intestinal tract in the pathogenesis of ventilator-associated pneumonia. Clin Infect Dis 1997; 24:309-319
16. Niederman MS, Craven DE. Devising strategies for preventing nosocomial pneumonia – should we ignore the stomach? Clin Infect Dis 1997; 24:320-323
17. McEachern R, Campbell Jr GD. Hospital-acquired pneumonia: epidemiology, etiology, and treatment. Infect Dis Clin N Amer 1998; 12:761-779
18. Morrison DC, Ryan JL. Endotoxins and disease mechanisms. Annu Rev Med 1987; 38:417-32
19. Luchi M, Morrison DC. Comparable endotoxic properties of lipopolysaccharides are manifest in diverse clinical isolates of Gram-negative bacteria. Infect Immun 2000; 68:2301-2308
20. Steeghs L, den Hartog R, den Boer A, Zomer B, Roholl P, van der Ley P. Meningitis bacterium is viable without endotoxin. Nature 1998; 392:449-450
21. Bennett IL Jr. Approaches to the mechanism of endotoxin action. In: Landy M, Braun W (eds) Bacterial Endotoxins, Rutgers Univ Press, New Brunswick, NJ (xiii-xvi), 1964.
22. Patel JC, Banker DD, Modi JC. Chloramphenicol in typhoid fever: a preliminary report of clinical trial in six cases. Brit Med J 1949; 908-909
23. Spink WW, Hall WH, Shaffer JM, Braude AI. Human brucellosis: its specific treatment with a combination of streptomycin and sulfadizine. JAMA 1948;136:382-387
24. Jarisch A. Therapeutiche Veruche bei syphilis. Wien Med. Wochenschr 1895; 45:721-724
25. Galloway RE, Levin J, Butler T, Naff GB, Goldsmith GH, Saito H, Awoke S, Wallace CK. Activation of protein mediators of inflammation and evidence for endotoxemia in *Borrelia recurrentis* infection. Am J Med 1977; 63:933-938
26. Morrison DC, Ulevitch RJ. The effects of bacterial endotoxins on host mediation systems; A review. Am J Path 1978; 93:526-617
27. Morrison DC, Ryan JL. Bacterial endotoxins and host immune responses. Adv Immunol 1979; 28:293-450
28. Rietschel ET, Brade H. Bacterial endotoxins. Sci Am 1992; 267:54-61
29. Leeson MC, Morrison DC. Induction of proinflammatory responses in human monocytes by particulate and soluble forms of LPS. Shock 1994; 2:235-245
30. Morrison DC ed. Symposium on endotoxin/antibiotics and Gram-negative sepsis. J Endotoxin Res 1996; 3:171-279
31. Jackson JJ, Kropp H. Antibiotic-induced endotoxin release: important parameters dictating responses In: Brade H, Opal S, Vogel S, Morrison DC (eds) Endotoxin in Health and Disease. Marcel Dekker Pub, NY p 67-75, 1999
32. Prins JM, van Agtmael MA, Kujiper EJ, van Deventer SJH, Speelman P. Antibiotic-induced endotoxin release in patients with Gram-negative urosepsis: a double-blind study comparing imipenem and ceftazidime. J Infect Dis 1995; 172:886-891
33. Luchi M, Morrison DC, Opal S, et al. A comparative trial of imipenem vs. ceftazidime in the release of endotoxin and cytokine generation in patients with Gram-negative urosepsis. J Endotoxin Res 2000; 6:25-32.
34. Hurley JC. Bacteremia, endotoxemia, and mortality in Gram-negative sepsis. J Infect Dis 1993; 168:246-248.
35. Remick D, Manohar P, Bolgos G, Rodrigues J, Moldawer L, Wollenberg G. Blockage of tumor necrosis factor reduces lipopolysaccharide lethality, but not lethality of cecal ligation and puncture. Shock 1995; 4:89-95

36. Derks HHF, Bruin KF, Jongeneel CV,et al. Familial differences in endotoxin-induced TNF release in whole blood and peripheral blood mononuclear cells in vitro: relationship to TNF gene polymorphism. J Endotoxin Res 1995; 2:19-26

37. Greisman SE, Woodward WE. Mechanisms of endotoxin tolerance III. The refractory state during continuous intravenous infusions of endotoxin. J Exp Med 1965; 121:911-933

38. Zhang X, Morrison DC. Lipopolysaccharide-induced selective priming effects on tumor necrosis factor alpha and nitric oxide production in mouse peritoneal macrophages. J Exp Med 1993;177:511-516

39. Shnyra A, Brewington R, Alipio A, Amura CR, Morrison DC. Reprogramming of LPS-primed macrophages is controlled by a counterbalanced production of IL-10 and IL-12. J Immunol 1998; 160:3729-3736

40. Lei MG, Morrison DC. Differential expression of caveolin-1 in lipopolysaccharide-activated murine macrophages. Infect Immun 2000; 68:5084-5089

41. McCall EE, Grosso-Wilmoth LM, Larue KEA, Guzman R, Cousart SL. Dysregulation of in vitro cytokine production by monocytes during sepsis. J Clin Invest 1993; 88:1747-1757

42. Li L, Cousart S, Hu J, McCall CE. Characterization of interleukin-1 recepto-associated kinase in normal and endotoxin tolerant cells. J Biol Chem 2000; 275:23340-23345

43. Braun V, Hanktke K. Biochemistry of bacterial cell envelopes. Annu Rev Biochem 1974; 43: 89-121

44. Bessler WG, Resch K, Hancock E, Hantke K. Induction of lymphocyte proliferation and membrane changes by lipoprotein derivatives of the lipoprotein from the outer membrane of *E. coli*. Z Immunitaetsforsch 1977; 153:11-19

45. Zhang H, Niesel DW, Peterson JW, Klimpel GR. Lipoprotein release by bacteria: Potential factor in bacterial pathogenesis. Infect Immun 1994; 66:5196-5201

46. Zhang H, Peterson JW, Niesel DW, Klimpel GR. Bacterial lipoprotein and lipopolysaccharide act synergistically to induce lethal shock and proinflammatory cytokine production. J Immunol 1997; 159:4868-4878

47. Sparwasser T, Miethke T, Lipford G, Erdman A, Hacker H, Heeg K, Wagner H. Macrophages sense pathgens via DNA motifs: induction of tumor necrosis factor-α-mediated shock. Eur J Immunol 1997; 27:1671-1679

48. Gao JJ, Zuvanich EG, Xue Q, Horn DL, Silverstein R, Morrison DC. Cutting Edge: Bacterial DNA and LPS act in synergy in inducing nitric oxide production in RAW 264.7. J Immun 1999; 163:4095-4099

49. Gao JJ, Xue Q, Zuvanich EG, Haghi KI, Morrison DC. Commercial preparation of lipoteichoic acid contains endotoxin that contributes to activation of mouse macrophages *in vitro*. Infect Immun 2001; 69:751-757

8

THE PATHOPHYSIOLOGY OF GRAM-POSITIVE SHOCK

R. Kate Beaton
Jonathan Cohen

Several Gram-positive bacteria produce toxins that are associated with very severe clinical illnesses: these include *Bacillus anthracis* (anthrax), *Clostridium botulinum* (botulism), and *Corynebacterium diphtheriae* (diphtheria). However, we are concerned here with those Gram-positive bacteria that cause the clinical syndrome of sepsis or septic shock, most commonly *Streptococcus pneumoniae*, *Staphylococcus aureus*, and *Streptococcus pyogenes*. Despite the fact that Gram-positive organisms cause sepsis with approximately the same frequency as do Gram-negative bacteria, and that the case mortality is not substantially different, the pathogenetic mechanisms associated with Gram-positive sepsis are less well understood. We review here recent developments in this field, focusing both on bacterial virulence mechanisms and host factors that contribute to pathogenesis.

CLINICAL SYNDROMES OF SHOCK ASSOCIATED WITH GRAM-POSITIVE BACTERIA

Gram-positive bacteria are implicated in 45-60% of cases of severe sepsis or septic shock in both hospital inpatients and those in critical care units [1, 2, 3]. The commonest Gram-positive organisms identified in epidemiological surveys of septic shock are *Staph. aureus* and *Strep. pneumoniae* [4]. In addition there has been an increase in *Staph. epidermidis* bacteremias of 4 to 8 fold between 1975 and 1990 [5], and signs of septic shock have been documented in 15% of these patients [6]. In most septic patients, it is generally impossible to tell with certainty on clinical grounds alone if the infecting organism is Gram-positive or Gram-negative [7]. However, interestingly, there are in addition a number of distinct clinical syndromes in which Gram-positive bacteria cause septic shock. The most familiar is the staphylococcal toxic shock syndrome, initially associated with tampon use but later appreciated as being associated with TSST-1 toxin-producing strains of *Staph. aureus*. Another striking clinical syndrome that appears to be reported with increasing frequency is the toxic shock syndrome associated with *Strep. pyogenes* [8]. Other, less common associations are shown in Table 1.

Organism	Syndrome
Streptococcus mitis	Sepsis in neutropenic patients [9]
Clostridium septicum	Typhlitis and shock in those with relapsed leukemia and bowel malignancies [10]
Streptococcus pyogenes	Sepsis following *Varicella zoster* infection, related to wound infection, myositis and necrotizing fasciitis, puerperal sepsis [11]
	Sepsis following
Streptococcus pneumoniae	splenectomy

Table 1. Gram-positive organisms and sepsis syndromes

The Gram-positive Cell Wall

The Gram-positive cell wall is made up of a thick layer of peptidoglycan (PG), forming up to 40% of the cell mass (Figure 1).

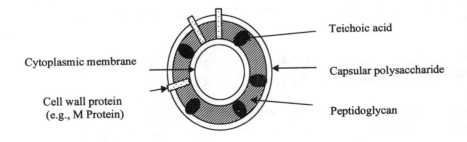

Figure 1. The Gram-positive cell wall

Gram-negative organisms contain smaller amounts of PG and this is found within the Gram-negative outer membrane. PG is a complex polymer of the hexose sugars N-acetylglucosamine and N-acetylmuramic acid which are cross linked by peptide cross bridges (Figure 2). Attached to the muramic acid residues are tetrapeptide side chains, and it is to these moieties that the cross bridging peptides bind. The tetrapeptide side chains and the cross bridges vary between species.

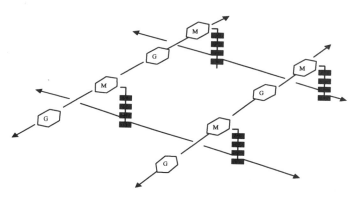

Figure 2. *Schematic representation of peptidoglycan structure. M = N-acetyl muramic acid. G = N-acetyl glucosamine*

Teichoic acids are unique to Gram-positive bacteria. There are two types of these water soluble polymers: wall teichoic acid, covalently bound to PG, and membrane teichoic acid, covalently linked to membrane glycolipid and known as lipoteichoic acid (LTA). All Gram-positive species contain membrane teichoic acids, whereas some lack the wall bound type. In some species a high molecular weight polysaccharide or hyaluronic acid capsule may surround the bacterium.

Peptidoglycan

It has been known for some time that PG is able to cause inflammation although it is a much less potent inducer of proinflammatory substances than lipopolysaccharide (LPS) [2, 12]. PG from *Staph. aureus* was 100-1000 times less potent at stimulating tumor necrosis factor (TNF)-α and interleukin (IL)-1 production by human monocytes when compared to the same weight of LPS [13]. PG has been shown to be proinflammatory in several *ex vivo* experiments. Exposure of human monocytes to PG from *Strep. pneumoniae* causes IL-1 production, but no induction of TNF-α [14]. PG from both coagulase-negative and coagulase-positive staphylococci is able to stimulate TNF-α production from human monocytes in a concentration dependent fashion [15]. TNF-α and IL-6 are produced by human monocytes stimulated with PG from a variety of Gram-positive bacteria, and the concentrations produced are greatly enhanced by the addition of serum [16].

Most of the studies that have examined the proinflammatory properties of PG have been done with relatively crude or poorly defined preparations, and little was known of the structural components of the molecule that were responsible for the biological activity. Recently however, more detailed biochemical analyses have been conducted. Digestion of *Strep. pneumoniae* cell walls with the major PG hydrolase from the organism results in a variety of products which can be separated by reverse phase high pressure chromatography. Complex branched peptides were able to stimulate TNF-α production, weight for weight, at equal levels to LPS [17]. Kengatharam et al have also attempted to characterize the moiety of PG responsible for synergism with LTA. In the presence of interferon (IFN)-γ or LTA, NAG-NAM-L-ala-D-isoglutamine caused an increase of nitric oxide (NO) formation by macrophages. This activity was abolished by hydrolysis of the NAM and L-ala bond and by the use of stereoisomers [18].

Lipoteichoic Acid

LTA is also proinflammatory and LTA from a number of species including *Staph. epidermidis*, *Strep. pneumoniae*, *Enterococcus faecalis*, *Listeria monocytogenes* and *Bacillus subtilis* can stimulate the production of TNF-α, IL-1, IL-6, and IL-10 from human monocytes [5, 12, 19]. LTA has also been shown to induce secretion of IL-8 from human peripheral blood monocytes [20]. IL-8 is chemotactic for leukocytes, predominantly neutrophils, and a feature of Gram-positive sepsis is the accumulation of neutrophils at foci of infection [2]. Several groups have noted that LTA is also able to induce NO synthase (NOS) activity from vascular smooth muscle cells [21] and macrophages [22]. Like PG, some actions seem to be CD14 and serum-dependent [2, 23]. The C substance of *Strep. pneumoniae* is a teichoic acid of special interest as it binds C-reactive protein (CRP) and can activate complement. It is a potent inducer of IL-1 production, but not of TNF-α [14], and is believed to participate in the proinflammatory events leading to shock [2, 5].

In clinical sepsis PG and LTA presumably do not exist in isolation. When LTA and PG from *Staph. aureus* were studied in a rat model, neither alone was toxic but together they caused NO production and evidence of organ failure with TNF-α and IFN-γ production [24]. However, the significance of these observations is far from clear, since the LTA of *Staph. aureus* is able to interact with PG from *Staph. aureus* or *B. subtilis* (a non pathogenic bacterium), while that of *B. subtilis* is unable to interact with either. It was proposed that the species specific structure of the LTA may therefore determine an organism's ability to go on to cause shock [18].

Evidence for Circulating Cell Wall Constituents

Recently it has been shown that PG is released by bacteria during infection and is present in the circulation [25]. The silk worm larvae test has been used to detect circulating PG in septic patients and also as a diagnostic test [26]. The literature on this area however remains small and as yet there is no evidence of correlation of plasma level of PG with patient outcome. To our knowledge, no studies have demonstrated the detection of circulating LTA in patients. Thus, while there is compelling evidence that various Gram-positive cell wall components can, in the appropriate experimental setting, demonstrate marked pro-inflammatory activity there are as yet no data comparable to those that exist for LPS that show these Gram-positive cell wall fragments play an important role in the clinical setting of sepsis.

Polysaccharide and Hyaluronic Acid Capsules

Many pathogenic Gram-positive bacteria possess a capsule that may have a number of functions. The type-specific polysaccharide capsules of group B streptococci are a major virulence factor and the presence of capsular polysaccharides increases the ability of Group B streptococci to induce macrophages to release TNF-α [27]. The hyaluronate capsule of group A streptococci (GAS) is critical for the development of tissue necrosis, bacteremia and lethal infection in mice [28]. Recent studies with human keratinocytes suggest that the capsule may act as a ligand, binding to CD44 on the cell surface, and mediating the attachment of M proteins to the cell [29]. The GAS capsule may also increase resistance to phagocytosis, a feature that has also been described in encapsulated strains of *Staph. aureus*. [30].

Soluble Factors from Gram-positive Bacteria

The ability of Gram-positive bacteria to produce soluble toxins is a well recognized pathogenic mechanism (e.g., the toxins of *B. anthracis*, *C. botulinum* and *C. diphtheriae*). The role of toxins in Gram-positive shock is less well defined.

Superantigens

Toxins produced by *Staph. aureus* and *Strep. pyogenes* have been implicated in the development of shock-like syndromes. The pyrogenic exotoxins of GAS (SPE A, C, F, G, H, J, SMEZ and SSA) and the *Staph. aureus* enterotoxins (SEA, SEB, SEC, SED, SEE, SEH) are a family of structurally related toxins sharing similar biological activities [31, 32]. TSST-1 produced by *Staph. aureus* has some differences in amino acid composition but shares similar biological activities and its overall topology is similar to the SE/SPE family of toxins [33, 34]. These toxins are able to function as superantigens. They do not require processing and presentation by antigen presenting cells in order to stimulate T cells. Superantigens interact directly with the class II major histocompatability complex (MHC) molecule on antigen presenting cells and with the β chain variable region (Vβ) portion of the T cell receptor (TCR) and induce activation, clonal expansion and deletion of a substantial proportion of T lymphocytes (Figure 3).

Structure and Relationships with MHC Class-II and the TCR

X ray crystallography studies have elucidated the structure of superantigens and also determined the interactions with MHC class II and the TCR. The SE/SPE family of superantigens are a family of soluble proteins of approximately 230 amino acids, with a central disulphide loop. TSST-1 does not possess this loop and is shorter at 194 amino acids. Mutations in various positions of the SPEA and SEB molecules inactivate biological activity and have different effects, suggesting that activity is not related to one region alone [33]. The disulfide loop is essential for mitogenic activity, although molecules with mutations in this area showed normal MHC class II binding and monocyte stimulation [35]. Variability of the sequences in the TCR binding region provides the different superantigens with specificities for different Vβ molecules. Two distinct regions of the toxins have been identified showing close sequence homology between the family of toxins, one at the C terminal side of the cysteine loop (not shared by TSST-1) and one shared by all of the SE/SPE and TSST-1 toxins [34].

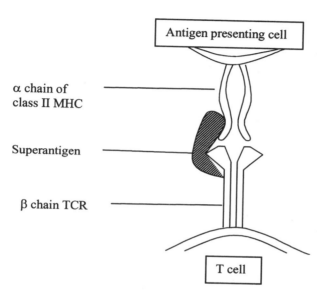

Figure 3. Schematic representation of the interaction of superantigen with TCR and MHC class II

There are two differing patterns of interaction with MHC class II. Most superantigens interact as SEB does, binding on the α-1 domain of the MHC in a readily dissociable fashion. TSST-1 binds to the β site with a strong and stable interaction, and the antigenic peptide is almost completely hidden from the TCR [36]. There is evidence that expression of MHC class-II alone is insufficient for superantigen binding [37]. Some superantigens can cause direct cross-linking of cell surface MHC class-II molecules and induce inflammatory cytokine expression. This is mediated via forming a strong bond with a distinct site on the Class II β chain, stabilized by zinc, and may allow a larger repertoire of T cells to be stimulated [36, 38, 39]. Linkage of cell surface Class II MHC molecules allows upregulation of costimulatory molecules such as B7 and may therefore precede the engagement of the TCR [40].

Superantigens show tropism for particular MHC Class II types, and modification of the MHC molecules or of the invariant chain can affect binding e.g., of TSST-1. Lavoie et al have postulated that superantigens may be preferentially presented depending on the MHC class II expressing environment, thus explaining the production of TSST-1 but not SEB by blood borne staphylococci [36]. There is evidence that non MHC class-II molecules may act as additional receptors as some superantigens still have biological activity in MHC class-II knock out mice [41].

Interaction with the TCR has been characterized recently by X ray diffraction studies. Superantigens make contact with a large interface including the CDR1, 2 and 4 loops of the TCR, with the TCR binding site falling in a groove between the two α helices. Recent studies have shown that MHC class II bound superantigens have a high affinity for the TCR, which correlates with their biological activity [42].

Evidence for Mitogenic Activity

Crosslinking of the TCR and MHC class-II via superantigens leads to a profound expansion of Vβ restricted T cells and antigen presenting cells [43, 44]. Stimulation of monocytes with SPEA and SPEC leads to production of IL-2 and IFN-γ along with IL-10 and IL-1RA [45, 46]. Stimulation of T cells with superantigens leads to a massive increase in TNF, IL-1 and IL-6 from macrophages [36]. Several studies have shown that the induction of monocyte cytokines requires the presence of T cells [47, 48] or the T cell derived cytokine IFN-γ [43]. IFN-γ also upregulates the expression of MHC class-II and therefore the number of potential superantigen receptors [36, 44]. Costimulatory molecules play an important part in response to superantigens. CD28 on T cells and its ligand on MHC class II bearing cells, B7, contribute to superantigen mitogenicity [49]. Other costimulatory molecules such as lymphocyte function-associated antigen (LFA)-1/intercellular adhesion molecule (ICAM)-1 and very late antigen (VLA)-4/vascular cell adhesion molecule (VCAM)-1 are also important [33, 45]. ICAM-1 deficient mice do not develop shock on exposure to superantigens. [50].

Knowledge of the structure and interactions of superantigenic molecules is allowing novel therapeutic approaches. Arad et al. have designed a dodecapeptide analogous to a conserved region outside the MHC and TCR binding sites. In a mouse model of toxic shock the peptide has prevented superantigen induced cytokine release and may function via blocking cosimulatory signals [51].

The Role of Superantigens in Shock

Although there is good evidence to show the interaction of superantigens with MHC and the TCR, along with evidence of clonal expansion and cytokine production, the evidence for superantigens causing shock in humans is less clear. Animals, particularly mice, are relatively resistant to superantigen-induced shock and therefore a reliable model has been difficult to produce [2]. T lymphocyte activation and expansion has been demonstrated in studies in mice [48], however large quantities of superantigen were needed and there are questions over the relationship between a model based on one large injection and that found in the clinical situation [2, 7]. There is good evidence that TSST-1 is the causative agent of the staphylococcal toxic shock syndrome. Purified toxin induces a shock-like illness in rabbits [52], and studies of patients with TSS have found markedly elevated levels of circulating Vβ2+ cells indicative of specific clonal expansion [53]. However, it is not clear whether the superantigenic properties of the toxin produce the pathology.

The increase in incidence of streptococcal shock has been associated with strains producing pyrogenic exotoxin, in particular SPEA [8] and SPEA has been detected in the serum in a small number of patients [54]. Two small clinical studies have noted selective activation [55] or deletion [56] of lymphocytes with particular Vβ chain classes and the presence of the T cell cytokine lymphotoxin α has been cited as indirect evidence of T cell activation [54]. There is also evidence that sera of patients with severe streptococcal disease are less inhibitory for streptococcal antigens acting as T cell mitogens that sera from those with less severe disease [57]. Despite this circumstantial evidence, it is still not clear if it is the superantigenic properties of SPEA (or indeed other streptococcal superantigens) that cause the tissue damage.

There is some evidence to suggest that interaction with superantigens increases susceptibility to LPS [58], however evidence for this is not universally supportive [2]. Some studies have shown a greatly increased susceptibility to endotoxin in rabbits, however anti-LPS antibodies have not proven useful in reversing superantigen-induced shock in rabbits [7, 59]. There is also evidence of synergy between TSST-1 and SE/SPE [2, 33].

Other Soluble Factors

Gram-positive organisms produce a wide variety of tissue damaging enzymes that may be involved in invasion. As Gram-positive sepsis often originates from soft tissue sites, such enzymes are important in establishing serious

Gram-positive infection. The direct evidence linking these enzymes with septic shock *per se* is less clear. Some Gram-positive organisms produce pore forming leukocidins and hemolysins. The hemolysins of *C. perfringens*, *Strep. pyogenes* and the alpha haemolysin of *Staph. aureus* in particular have been linked with the development of shock [60]. Some toxins may affect both erythrocytes and leukocytes, with others being specific for neutrophils or endothelial cells. The formation of pores leads to liberation of cellular contents, free radical release and generation of leukotrienes and other cytokines. A summary of these soluble factors putatively involved in shock is given in Table 2.

HOST FACTORS

Interaction of Cell Wall Components with Monocyte/ Macrophages

The interaction of LPS with both cell associated and soluble CD14 is reviewed elsewhere (see chapters by Morrison and Opal). The interaction of Gram-positive cell wall constituents with CD14 was shown shortly following the discovery of this mechanism in Gram-negative bacteria [67]. Anti-CD14 antibodies inhibited induction of activation of murine and human macrophage cell lines by PG [23]. Cells deficient in CD14 were unresponsive to Gram-positive cell walls, but transfection with CD14 rendered them 100 times more sensitive. PG and LPS compete for binding of CD14, however LPS binding protein (LBP) does not enhance CD14-dependent cell activation by PG [67]. Interestingly, soluble fragments of PG do not bind to CD14 [68].

The exact binding site of PG on CD14 is likely to be in the same region as that for LPS, however, certain monoclonal antibodies can block LPS binding but not PG, suggesting that the binding sites are different [68]. LTA can also bind to CD14 and induce secretion of IL-12 in human cells [23]. The exact structure responsible for activity is unknown. Both LTA and PG can bind sCD14, however unlike LPS-sCD14, these complexes do not activate endothelial and epithelial cells [69]. It is increasingly clear that CD14 can act as a pattern recognition molecule, interacting with cell surface proteins from a variety of pathogenic bacteria and discriminating between different ligands. The exact binding sites of these proteins with CD14 remain poorly understood [70]. Gram-positive organisms are also able to stimulate responses in a CD14 independent manner, the details of which are yet to be elucidated [69, 71].

Organism	Enzyme or toxin	Functions
S. aureus	Lipase, nuclease	Higher levels in bacteria causing shock [61]
	α, β, γ, δ hemolysins	Evidence for α toxin in shock strongest [33]
	leukocidin	
Streptococcus pneumoniae	neuramidase pneumolysin	Dissemination during sepsis [2] Spread and activation of local and systemic immune response [62]
Clostridium perfringens	phospholipase C α toxin	Damages cell membranes [2] Implicated in septic shock [63]
Group B Streptococci	hemolysin	Hypotension and myocardial depression [64]
Streptococcus pyogenes	SPEB cysteine protease	Multiple actions including: Cleavage of fibronectin, degradation of vitronectin, activation of matrix metalloproteinases, activation of pro IL-1β, release of bradykinin, release of M protein and C5a peptidase [2, 59, 65, 66]
	Streptolysin O and S	

Table 2. *Important enzymes, hemolysins and leucocidins of Gram-positive bacteria*

The lack of a transmembrane and cytoplasmic domain for CD14 has driven a search for a transmembrane co-receptor. Recent attention has focussed on the Toll-like receptors (TLR), in particular TLR2 and TLR4. Toll controls dorsoventral patterning during embryogenesis in *Drosophila melanogaster* and is involved in host defense to fungal infections in the adult fly [70]. TLR have been identified on mammalian cells, and the intracellular domain is similar to the mammalian IL-1 receptor. Early studies suggested that TLR 2 was involved in LPS signaling [72], but studies in C3H/HeJ mice, hyporesponsive to LPS, showed clearly that the location of the mutation giving LPS insensitivity mapped to that of TLR 4 [73]. The profound nature of LPS insensitivity in C3H/HeJ mice, despite functioning TLR 2 suggests that TLR 4 is the major component in the LPS response [74]. PG and LTA stimulate cells carrying the TLR 2 molecule, but not those lacking it, and TLR2 mutants lacking the intracellular domain do not respond to PG or LTA [75, 76]. Recently Takeuchi and colleagues have developed TLR-2 deficient mice and have compared responses to LTA, PG and LPS with TLR-4 deficient and wild type mice. As previously demonstrated TLR-4 deficient mice were hyporesponsive to LPS, but TLR-2 deficient mice responded to LPS in the same way as wild type. Macrophages from TLR-2 deficient mice were hyporesponsive to PG as well as to several Gram-positive cell walls. In contrast TLR-4 deficient macrophages lacked the response to LTA [74].

The downstream signal transduction pathway is not yet fully elucidated for Gram-positive bacteria. PG is able to stimulate the rapid and dose-dependent tyrosine phosphorylation of several cellular proteins, including *lyn* and mitogen-activated protein kinases (MAPK) along with rsk kinases [71]. There is evidence that the pattern of activation of kinases differs between LPS and PG [69]. PG induces transcription of the nuclear factor-kappa B (NF-κB), probably via TLR-2, and also activates the CREB/ATF1 (cyclic AMP responsive element binding protein/activating transcription factor-1) and activator protein (AP)-1 families of transcription factors [69].

Primary Host Response *in Vivo*

Macrophages, Neutrophils, Lymphocytes and Cytokines

In clinical Gram-positive infections, the source of the infection is often from soft tissue. In this situation accumulation of neutrophils at the site of infection is an early event, and lack of a neutrophil response at this stage has been associated with more severe disease in animal models [77]. Staphylococcal superantigens injected into mouse air pouches induce neutrophil infiltration which is dependent on the local expression of TNF-α , ICAM-1 and other cytokines, but interestingly does not require the presence of T cells [45]. A greater peripheral neutrophil leukocytosis is generally seen with Gram-positive pyogenic organisms such as *Staph. aureus* and *Strep. pyogenes* [2].

Cytokine responses to Gram-positive sepsis *in vivo* have been studied following injection and also in infection models, as well as in septic patients. Infusion of *Staph. epidermidis* into rabbits resulted in an increase of serum TNF-α and IL-1, although the inoculum size was twenty times of that of *Escherichia coli* needed to produce the same effect. A shock-like state with hypotension and organ failure resulted with both organisms [12]. Infusion of group A streptococci in a baboon sepsis model produced a rise in TNF-α and a shock-like syndrome 3 hours following the infusion. Monoclonal anti TNF-α antibodies markedly improved the outcome [78]. Rat models with injections of group B streptococci have shown sequential rises in TNF-α, IL-1, IL-6 and IFN-γ [79]. Animal models of soft tissue infection have shown a different pattern of cytokine release, with IL-6 being most prominent, and the

TNF-α response being late. Several studies suggest that the TNF-α and IL-6 responses are of a higher magnitude in Gram-negative sepsis models. Some data from clinical studies of sepsis also support this differential pattern between Gram-negative and Gram-positive sepsis [2, 7]. Studies of antiinflammatory agents in sepsis have also yielded results suggesting differences between responses in Gram-negative and Gram-positive disease. A recent review has highlighted some of the differences [7].

Nitric Oxide

NO is a critical mediator of Gram-negative induced hypotension and shock. Gram-positive cell wall components can stimulate NO production and shock in animal models [33]. A mouse model of Group A streptococcal fasciitis showed increased inducible NOS activity with increased NO levels. The levels of NO metabolites were, however, lower than those seen in similar models of Gram-negative sepsis [80]. Studies in inducible NOS (iNOS) deficient mice have demonstrated variable responses to endotoxin [81], as have studies of iNOS blockade. Inhibition of iNOS in a Gram-positive infection model made no difference to outcome [2, 81]. Mice lacking iNOS had an increased incidence of bacteremia and destructive arthritis in a staphylococcal arthritis model suggesting that NO may be important in controlling disease extent [82]. At present there are few data from clinical studies of shock on the differential role of NO in Gram-positive and Gram-negative sepsis.

Complement, Adhesion Molecules, Coagulation and Contact System.

Staph. epidermidis is capable of activating complement in a rabbit model of sepsis [12]. This has been reproduced with other Gram-positive pathogens, including Group A streptococci [78]. The role of adhesion molecules in superantigen-mediated disease in particular has been underlined by a number of studies. Mice deficient in ICAM-1 are resistant to superantigen induced shock [44], and local injection of staphylococcal superantigens resulted in increased expression of ICAM-1 on local endothelial cells. Staphylococcal superantigen related acute lung injury (ALI) also results in increased expression of ICAM-1 [83].

Disseminated intravascular coagulation (DIC) is well documented in both Gram-positive and Gram-negative shock, with no discernable differences in incidence or severity [84]. In addition to 'classical' DIC, sepsis is often complicated by activation of the contact system. Contact activation leads to the generation of bradykinin, which is implicated in local vasodilation, increased vascular permeability and generation of factor XIIa [85]. *Strep. pyogenes* cysteine protease has been shown to release kinins from precursors in *in vitro* and *ex vivo* human blood model [85]. Contact activation has been demonstrated after both experimental [86] and clinical [87] streptococcal infection. Gram-negative bacteria are also able to bind kininogen via curli and pili resulting in activation and generation of bradykinin [85]. However, although contact activation clearly occurs in severe Gram-positive sepsis, it remains unclear if this has any clinical impact.

CONCLUSION

Gram-positive sepsis is of increasing importance in clinical medicine. There is accumulating evidence that the cell wall constituents of Gram-positive organisms are crucial in stimulating the host immune response, via a CD14 dependent pathway, transduced by TLR. Superantigenic exotoxins are powerful T cell mitogens, however direct evidence that this property causes disease is elusive. There is also *in vitro* and *in vivo* evidence that the cytokine response to Gram-positive sepsis differs from that of Gram-negative sepsis, and this clearly has implications for future trials of anti inflammatory therapy.

REFERENCES

1. Bone, RC. Gram-positive organisms and sepsis. Arch Intern Med 1994; 154:26-34
2. Sriskandan S, Cohen J. Gram-positive sepsis. Mechanisms and differences from Gram-negative sepsis. Infec Dis Clin North Am 1999; 13:393-412
3. Kieft H, Hoepelman AI, Zhou W et al. The sepsis syndrome in a Dutch university hospital. Clinical observations. Arch Intern Med 1993; 153:2241-2247
4. Cohen J, Abraham E. Microbiologic findings and correlations with serum tumor necrosis factor alpha in patients with severe sepsis and septic shock. J Infect Dis 1999; 180:116-121
5. Verhoef J, Mattsson E. The role of cytokines in Gram-positive bacterial shock. Trends Microbiol 1995; 3:136-140
6. Martin MA, Pfaller MA, Wenzel RP. Coagulase-negative staphylococcal bacteremia. Mortality and hospital stay. Ann Intern Med 1989; 110:9-16
7. Opal SM, Cohen J. Clinical Gram-positive sepsis: Does it fundamentally differ from Gram-negative bacterial sepsis ? Crit Care Med 1999; 27:1608-1616
8. Eriksson BKG, Andersson J, Holm SE, et al. Epidemiological and clinical aspects of invasive group A streptococcal infections and the streptococcal toxic shock syndrome. Clin Infect Dis 1998; 27:1428-1436
9. Bochud P-Y, Calandra T, Francioli P. Bacteremia due to viridans streptococci in neutropenic patients: A review. Am J Med 1994; 97:256-264

10. Cohen J, Lynn WA. Septic Shock : From experimental models to the bedside. Rev Clin Exp Haematol 1998; 7:23-56
11. Curtis N. Invasive group A streptococcal infection. Curr Opin Infect Dis 1996; 9:191-202
12. Wakabayashi G, Gelfand J, Jung W, et al. Staphylococcus epidermidis induces complement activation, tumor necrosis factor and interleukin-1, a shock like state and tissue injury in rabbits without endotoxemia. J Clin Invest 1991; 87:1925-1935
13. Mattsson E, Verhage L, Rollof J, et al. Peptidoglycan and teichoic acid from Staphylococcus epidermidis stimulate human monocytes to release tumour necrosis factor alpha, interleukin-1 beta and interleukin-6. FEMS Immunol Med Microbiol 1993; 7:28-37
14. Reisenfeld-Orn I, Wolpe S, Garcia-Bustos JF, et al. Production of interleukin-1, but not tumor necrosis factor by human monocytes stimulated with pneumococcal cell surface components. Infect Immun. 1989; 57:1890-1893
15. Timmerman CP, Mattsson E, Martinez-Martinez L, et al. Induction of release of tumor necrosis factor from human monocytes by staphylococci and staphylococcal peptidoglycans. Infect Immun 1993; 61:4167-4172
16. Heumann D, Barras C, Severin A et al. Gram-positive cell walls stimulate synthesis of tumor necrosis factor alpha and interleukin-6 by human monocytes. Infect Immun 1994; 62:2715-2665
17. Majcherczyk PA, Langen H, Heumann D, et al. Digestion of Streptococcus pneumoniae cell walls with its major peptidoglycan hydrolase releases branch stem peptides carrying proinflammatory activity. J Biol Chem 1999; 274:12537-12543
18. Kengatharam K, De Kimpe S, Robson C, et al. Mechanism of Gram-positive Shock: Identification of peptidoglycan and lipoteichoic acid moieties essential in the induction of nitric oxide synthase, shock, and multiple organ failure. J Exp Med 1998; 188:305-315
19. Wang JE, Jørgensen, Almlöf M, et al. Peptidoglycan and lipoteichoic acid from Staphylococcus aureus induce tumor necrosis factor alpha, interleukin 6 (IL-6), and IL-10 production in both T cells and monocytes in human whole blood model. Infect Immun 2000; 68:3965-3970
20. Standiford T, Arenberg DA, Danforth JM, et al. Lipoteichoic acid induces secretion of interleukin-8 from human blood monocytes: a cellular and molecular analysis. Infect Immun 1994; 62:119-126
21. Lonchampt MO, Auguet M, Celaflotte S, et al. Lipoteichoic acid: A new inducer of nitric oxide synthase. J Cardiovasc Pharmacology 1992; 20 (Suppl 12):S146-S147
22. English BK, Patrick CC, Orlicek SL, et al. Lipoteichoic acid from viridans streptococci induces the production of tumor necrosis factor and nitric oxide by murine macrophages. J Infect Dis 1996; 174:1348-1351
23. Cleveland MG, Gorham JD, Murphy TL, et al. Lipoteichoic acid preparations of Gram-positive bacteria induce interleukin-12 through a CD14-dependent pathway. Infect Immun 1996; 64:1906-1912
24. Kimpe SJ, Kengatharam M, Thiemermann C, et al. The cell wall components peptidoglycan and lipoteichoic acid from Staphylococcus aureus act in synergy to cause shock and multiple organ failure. Proc Natl Acad Sci USA 1995; 92:10359-10363
25. Kobayashi T, Tani T, Yokota, et al. Plasma levels of peptidoglycan detected with silkworm larvae plasma in septic patient. Shock 1997; 7:139 (Abst)
26. Kobayashi T, Tani T, Yokota T, et al. Detection of peptidoglycan in human plasma using the silkworm larvae plasma test. FEMS Immunol Med Microbiol 2000; 28:49-53
27. Vallejo JG, Baker CJ, Edwards MS. Roles of the bacterial cell wall and capsule in induction of tumor necrosis factor alpha by type III group B streptococci. Infect Immun 1996; 64:5042-5046

28. Ashbaugh CD, Warren HB, Carey VJ. Molecular analysis of the role of the group A streptococcal cysteine protease, hyaluronic acid capsule and M protein in a murine model of human invasive soft-tissue infection. J Clin Invest 1998; 102: 50-560

29. Schrager HM, Rheinwald JG, Wessels MR et al. Hyaluronic acid capsule modulates M protein mediated adherence and acts as a ligand for attatchment of group A streptococci to CD44 on human lymphocytes. J Clin Invest 1998; 101:1708-1716

30. Dale JB, Washburn RG, Marques MB et al. Hyaluronate capsule and surface M protein in resistance to opsonisation of group A streptococci. Infect Immun 1996; 64:1495-1501

31. Hynes WL, Weeks CR, Iandolo JJ et al. Immunologic cross-reactivity of type A streptococcal exotoxin (erythrogenic toxin) and staphylococcal enterotoxins B and C1. Infect Immun 1987; 55:837-840

32. Dinges MM, Orwin PM, Schlievert PM. Exotoxins of Staphylococcus aureus. Clin Micro Rev 2000; 13:16-34

33. Bannan J, Visvanathan K, Zabriskie JB. Structure and function of streptococcal and staphylococcal superantigens in septic shock. Infect Dis Clin North Am 1999; 13:387-396

34. Acharya KR, Passalacqua EF, Jones EY, et al. Structural basis of superantigen action inferred from crystal structure of toxic-shock syndrome toxin-1. Nature 1994; 367:94-97

35. Grossman D, Cook RG, Sparrow JT, et al. Dissociation of the stimulatory activities of staphylococcal enterotoxins for T cells and monocytes. J Exp Med 1990; 172:1831-1841

36. Lavoie PM, Thibodeau J, Erard F, et al. Understanding the mechanisms of action of bacterial superantigens from a decade of research. Immunol Rev 1999; 168:257-269

37. Lavoie PM , Thibodeau J, Cloutier I, et al. Selective binding of bacterial toxins to major histocompatibility class II-expressing cells is controlled by invariant chain and HLA-DM. Proc Natl Acad Sci USA 1997; 94: 6892-6897

38. Roussel A, Anderson BF, Baker HM, et al. Crystal structure of the streptococcal superantigen SPE-C: dimerism and zinc binding suggest a novel mode of interaction with MHC class II molecules. Nat Struc Biol 1997; 4:635-643

39. Tiedemann RE, Frase JD. Cross-linking of MHC class II molecules by staphylococcal enterotoxin A is essential for antigen-presenting cell and T cell activation. J Immunol 1996; 157:3958-3966

40. Nabavi N, Freeman GJ, Gault A, et al. Signalling through the MHC class II cytoplasmic domain is required for antigen presentation and induces B7 expression. Nature 1992; 360:266-268

41. Avery AC, Markowitz JS, Grusby MJ, et al. Activation of T cells by superantigen in class-II-negative mice. J Immunol 1994; 153:4853-1861

42. Andersen PS, Lavoie PM, Sekaly RP et al. Role of the T-cell receptor (TCR) α chain in stabilising TCR-superantigen-MHC class II complexes. Immunity 1999; 20:473-483

43. Marrack P, Kappler J. The staphylococcal enterotoxins and their relatives. Science 1990; 248:705-711

44. Kotb M. Bacterial pyrogenic exotoxins and superantigens. Clin Micro Rev 1995; 8:411-426

45. Tessier PA, Naccache PH, Diener KR, et al. Induction of acute inflammation in vivo by staphylococcal superantigens. II. Critical role for chemokines, ICAM-1 and TNF-α. J Immunol 2998; 161:1204-1211

46. Muller-Alouf H, Alouf JE, Gerlach D, et al. Human pro- and anti-inflammatory cytokine patterns induced by Streptococcus pyogenes erythrogenic (pyrogenic) exotoxin A and C superantigens. Infect Immun 1996; 64:1450-1453

47. Muller-Alouf H, Alouf JE, Gerlach D, et al. Comparative study of cytokine release by human peripheral blood mononuclear cells stimulated with Streptococcus pyogenes superantigenic erythrogenic toxins, heat killed streptococci and lipopolysaccharide. Infect Immun 1994; 62:4915-4921

48. Marrack P, Blackman M, Kushnir E, et al. The toxicity of staphylococcal enterotoxin B in mice is mediated by T cells. J Exp Med 1990; 171:455-464

49. Blackson JN, Morse SS. The CD28/B7 pathway costimulates the response of primary murine T cells to superantigens as well as to conventional antigens. Cell Immunol 1994 ; 157 : 306-312

50. Xu H, Gonzalo JA, St. Pierre Y, et al. Leukocytosis and resistance to septic shock in intercellular adhesion molecule 1-deficient mice. J Exp Med 1994; 180:95-109

51. Arad G, Levy R, Hillman D et al. Superantigen antagonist protects against lethal shock and defines a new domain for T-cell activation. Nature Med 2000; 6:414-421

52. de Azavedo JCS, Foster TJ, Hartigan PJ. Expression of the cloned toxic shock syndrome toxin gene (tst) in vivo with a rabbit uterine model. Infect Immun 1985; 50:304-309

53. Choi Y, Lafferty JA, Clements JR, et al. Selective expansion of T cells expressing Vβ2 in toxic shock syndrome. J Exp Med 1990; 172:981-984

54. Sriskandan S, Moyes D, Cohen J. Detection of circulating bacterial superantigen and lymphotoxin alpha in patients with streptococcal toxic-shock syndrome. Lancet 1996; 348:1315-1316

55. Michie C, Scott A, Cheesbrough J, et al. Streptococcal toxic shock syndrome: evidence of superantigen activity and its toxic effects on T lymphocyte subsets in vivo. Clin Exp Immunol 1994; 98:140-144

56. Watanabe-Ohnishi R, Low DE, et al. Selective depletion of Vβ-bearing T cells in patients with severe invasive group A streptococcal infections and streptococcal toxic shock syndrome. J Infect Dis 1995; 171:74-84

57. Norrby-Teglund A, Pauksens K, Holm SE, et al. Relation between low capacity of human to inhibit streptococcal mitogens and serious manifestations of disease. J Infect Dis 1994; 170:585-591

58. Schlievert PM. Enhancement of host susceptibility to lethal endotoxin shock by staphylococcal pyrogenic exotoxin-type C. Infect Immun 1982; 36:123-128

59. Melish ME, Murata S, Fukunga C, et al. Endotoxin is not an essential mediator in toxic shock syndrome. Rev Infect Dis 1989; 11(suppl 1):S219-S228

60. Seeger W, Schutter H, Grimminger F, et al. Bacterial exotoxins and sepsis. In: Reinhart K, Eyrich K, Sprung C (eds). Sepsis. Current Perspectives in Pathophysiology and Therapy. Springer-Verlag, Berlin 1994, pp 61-85

61. Schlievert PM, Osterholm MT, Kelly JA, et al. Toxin and enzyme characterization of Staphylococcus aureus isolates from patients with and without toxic shock syndrome. Ann Intern Med 1982; 96:937-940

62. Rubins JB, Janoff EN. Pneumolysin: a multifunctional pneumococcal virulence factor. J Lab Clin Med 1998; 131:21-27

63. Stevens DL, Bryant AE. Pathogenesis of Clostridium perfringens infection: mechanisms and mediators of shock. Clin Infect Dis 1997; 25 (Suppl 2):S160-S164

64. Griffiths BB, Rhee H. Effects of hemolysins of groups A and B streptococci on cardiovascular system Microbioscience 1992; 69:17-27

65. Lukomski S, Sreevatsan S, Amberg A, et al. Inactivation of Streptococcus pyogenes extracellular cysteine protease significantly decreases mouse lethality of serotype M3 and M49 strains. J Clin Invest 1997; 99:2574-2580

66. Lukomski S, Burns EH, Wyde PR, et al. Genetic inactivation of extracellular cysteine protease (SpeB) expressed by Streptococcus pyogenes decreases resistance to phagocytosis and dissemination to organs. Infect Immun 1998; 66:771-776

67. Pugin J, Heumann D, Tomasz A, et al. CD14 is a pattern recognition receptor. Immunity 1994; 1:509-516

68. Weidemann B, Brade H, Rietschel ET, at al. Soluble peptidoglycan-induced monokine production can be blocked by anti-CD14 monoclonal antibodies and by lipid A partial structures. Infect Immun 1994; 62:4709-4715

69. Dziarski R, Ulmer AJ, Gupta D. Interactions of CD14 with components of Gram-positive bacteria. Chem Immunol 2000; 74:83-107

70. Aderem A, Ulevitch RJ. Toll-like receptors in the induction of the innate immune response. Nature 2000; 406:782-787

71. Gupta, D, Jin Y, Dziarski R. Peptidoglycan induces transcription and secretion of TNF-α and activation of lyn, extracellular signal-regulated kinase and rsk signal transduction proteins in mouse macrophages. J Immunol 1995; 155:2620-2630

72. Kirschning CJ, Wesche H, Ayres TM, et al. Human Toll-like receptor 2 confers responsiveness to bacterial lipopolysaccharide. J Exp Med 1998; 188:2091-2098

73. Poltorak A, He X, Smirnova I. Defective LPS signalling in C3H/HeJ and C57BL/10ScCr mice. Mutations in Tlr4 gene. Science 1998; 282:2085-2088

74. Takeuchi O, Hoshino K, Kawai T, et al. Differential roles of TLR2 and TLR4 in recognition of gram-negative and gram-positive bacterial cell wall components. Immunity 1999; 11:443-451

75. Schwandner R, Dziarski R, Wesche H, et al. Peptidoglycan- and lipoteichoic acid-induced cell activation is mediated by toll-like receptor 2. J Biol Chem 1999; 274:17406-17409

76. Toshimura A, Lien E, Ingalle R, et al. Recognition of Gram-positive bacterial cell wall components by the innate immune system occurs via Toll-like receptor 2. J Immunol 1999; 163:1-5

77. Schlievert PM, Assimacopoulos AP, Cleary PP. Severe invasive group A streptococcal disease: Clinical description and mechanisms of pathogenesis. J Lab Clin Med 1996; 127:13-22

78. Stevens DL, Bryant AE, Hackett SP, et al. Group A streptococcal bacteremia: The role of tumor necrosis factor in shock and organ failure. Clin Infect Dis 1996; 173:619-626

79. Teti G, Mancuso G, Tomasello F, et al. Cytokine appearance and effects of anti-tumor necrosis factor alpha antibodies in a neonatal rat model of group B streptococcal infection. Infect Immun 1993; 61:227-235

80. Sriskandan, S, Moyes D, Buttery LK, et al. The role of nitric oxide in experimental murine sepsis due to pyrogenic exotoxin A-producing Streptococcus pyogenes. Infect Immun 1997; 65:1767-1772

81. MacMiking JD, Nathan C, Hom G, et al. Altered responses to bacterial infection and endotoxic shock in mice lacking inducible Nitric oxide synthase. Cell 1995; 81:641-650

82. McInnes IB, Leung B, Wei X-Q, et al. Septic arthritis following Staphylococcus aureus infection in mice lacking inducible nitric oxide synthase. J Immunol 1998; 160:308-315

83. Neumann B, Engelhardt B, Wagner H, et al. Induction of acute inflammatory lung injury by staphylococcal enterotoxin B. J Immunol 1997; 158:1862-1871

84. Levi M, Ten Cate H. Disseminated intravascular coagulation. N Engl J Med 1999; 341:586-592

85. Herwald H, Mörgelin M, Olsen A, et al. Activation of the contact-phase system on bacterial surfaces - a clue to serious complications in infectious diseases. Nature Med 1998; 4:298-302

86. Sriskandan S, Kemball-Cook G, Moyes D, et al. Contact activation in shock caused by invasive group A Streptococcus pyogenes. Crit Care Med 2000; 28:3684-3691

87. Sriskandan S, Cohen J. Kallikrein-kinin system activation in streptococcal toxic shock syndrome. Clin Infect Dis 2000; 30:961-962

9

IMMUNOPATHOGENESIS OF GRAM-NEGATIVE SHOCK

Steven M. Opal
Christian E. Hubert

A pathogen is defined as any microorganism capable of causing disease. Microbial pathogens cause disease by one of three basic mechanisms:
1) direct invasion of tissues
2) toxin mediated tissue damage
3) induction of an injurious host inflammatory response.

Bacterial virulence connotes the capacity of a microorganism to multiply within the host at a rate faster than that of the host's antimicrobial clearance mechanisms. A concomitant measure of bacterial virulence is the intrinsic capacity of any given organism to cause disease [1].

The intrinsic virulence of bacterial organisms varies considerably. Even within a single species such as *Escherichia coli*, the virulence potentials of specific clones differ strikingly. Certain strains of *E. coli* isolated from human blood cultures (e.g., *E. coli* 018:K1) are capable of lethal infection in test animals with as little as 10 cells injected into the peritoneal space. By contrast, *E. coli* K12 requires more than 10 million cells to induce lethality under the same experimental conditions [2]. These differences exist despite the fact that the amount of bacterial endotoxin present in the cell wall of different strains of *E. coli* is essentially identical. The study of molecular pathogenesis and bacterial genomics has provided a clearer understanding of microbial virulence. A coordinated repertoire of virulence factors needs to be expressed simultaneously if a microbial pathogen is to overwhelm the formidable array of host antimicrobial defense mechanisms. While bacterial lipopolysaccharide (LPS), also known as endotoxin, is clearly a principal mediator of Gram-negative sepsis, the presence of endotoxin alone is not sufficient to explain the pathophysiology of Gram-negative septic shock.

In order for a Gram-negative bacterium to successfully induce a constellation of signs, symptoms and physiologic derangements known as septic shock, it must first gain access to the host tissues. This necessitates penetration of the physicochemical barrier of the integument and/or mucous membranes. The microorganism must then evade host antimicrobial defenses and proliferate in sufficient quantities to cause disease. This complex array of virulence properties is found in a relatively small portion of the potential bacterial pathogens that are found in abundance within the hospital environment [3-7]. Microbial flora that exists within a hospital setting are repeatedly exposed to a variety of antibacterial agents. Gram-negative bacteria are continuously selected that resist antimicrobial agents within nosocomial populations of bacterial pathogens. This feature complicates the successful management of Gram-negative infections in hospitalized patients and increases the risk of progressive infections and septic shock [8].

The essential elements of microbial pathogenesis and the host defense mechanisms that confront microbial pathogens are depicted in Table 1.

Host Defense Mechanism	Microbial Virulence Factors
Mucous barrier, ciliary action, urine flow	Adhesins, motility, host receptor binding
Intact epithelial membrane	Invasion genes, receptor-mediated endocytosis
Iron limited conditions within plasma	Siderophores, transferrin receptors, hemolysins
Complement and antibody mediated opsonic activity	K capsules, long chain O antigens on LPS, bacterial proteases
Opsonophagocytic activity by neutrophils and macrophages	K capsules, high growth potential, type III secretion systems
Pro-inflammatory cytokines	Cytokine inhibitors, use of cytokine receptors as invasion sites
Coordinated innate immunity and coagulation system	Microbial mediators of sepsis-LPS, peptidoglycan, microbial DNA

Table 1. Host-pathogen interactions in sepsis

Microbial organisms must have the capacity to bind to and penetrate host membranes, compete with the host for nutrients, and avoid clearance by the innate and adaptive, humoral and cellular, host defense mechanisms. If the organism can survive the harsh conditions found within the systemic circulation of humans, they must then proliferate and release sufficient quantities of microbial mediators to induce septic shock [1,7]. The essential microbial elements that are responsible for the immunopathogenesis of septic shock will be reviewed in this chapter.

QUORUM SENSING SYSTEMS AND COMMUNICATION BETWEEN BACTERIAL PATHOGENS

Recently, it has become apparent that many Gram-negative bacterial pathogens possess a sophisticated signaling mechanism that provides the ability for intercellular communication between bacteria [9]. This system of cell-to-cell communication permits the formation of complex microbial communities found in biofilms on medical devices and catheters. The system, known as the quorum sensing apparatus, regulates bacterial growth and gene expression in a coordinated fashion [10]. As an example, biofilms have been shown to exist as complex bacterial communities along the surfaces of medical devices. Quorum sensing mechanisms allow the bacterial pathogens to regulate their cellular density within biofilms. By this mechanism, a stable bacterial population with adequate nutrients, oxygen availability, and waste disposal is maintained. Bacteria existing in the relatively stable and quiescent growth state within biofilms are resistant to the bactericidal effects of a number of potent antimicrobial agents. Biofilm formation on vascular catheters has proven a common source of bacteremia and sepsis in intensive care units (ICUs) [9].

It has also become evident that quorum sensing systems directly contribute to microbial pathogenesis. Cell signaling among Gram-negative bacteria allows for a coordinated attack pattern against human host defense mechanisms. Bacterial biosensors in the form of N-acyl homoserine lactone (AHL) are used to signal bacterial cells among bacterial populations of the same species. AHL and other quorum sensing molecules function as autoactivators. They are secreted in the micro-environment surrounding a bacterium and diffuse into the extracellular space. If the bacterium is alone or present in small numbers, no activation occurs. However, if sufficient numbers of bacteria are present and the concentration of autoactivators reaches a critical level, the bacterial populations become activated. The activation process induces a specific set of genes including bacterial virulence genes. In this manner, a bacterial pathogen can amass sufficient numbers of bacterial cells to successfully invade a host and cause disease [9,10].

The importance of this quorum sensing apparatus to microbial pathogenesis has recently been demonstrated in a number of animal models [9-12]. *Pseudomonas aeruginosa* that have deletions in their biosensor communication systems are less capable of inducing disease in experimental animal models of bacterial pneumonia [12] or burn wound infections [9]. Cooperation between individual cells within the microbial population is an entirely new concept in microbial pathogenesis. This finding serves to emphasize the level of complexity and intricacy found in bacterial pathogens that cause disease in human populations.

PATHOGENICITY ISLANDS: CLUSTERS OF BACTERIAL VIRULENCE GENES

The detailed study of bacterial genomes over the past five years has confirmed that virulence genes are not randomly distributed in a haphazard fashion around the bacterial chromosome. Clusters of genes that mediate bacterial virulence are referred to as pathogenicity islands [5,13]. The accumulation of virulence genes closely linked to each other along the chromosome is increasingly appreciated as a genetic trait of bacterial pathogens. Pathogenicity islands contain virulence genes associated with toxin production, cell membrane adherence, Type III secretion systems, and genes associated with intracellular survival within host cells [5]. They typically occur as genetic inserts close to highly conserved, homologous gene loci found in many bacterial genomes such as the genes for tRNA synthesis. The G-C content of pathogenicity islands often differs from adjacent DNA sequences, indicating a separate evolutionary origin.

There are powerful selection forces that lead to accumulation of favorable gene products of similar or complementary virulence functions ('selfish operons') [14]. Bacterial strains appear to have inherited pathogenicity islands as a unit of genes from exogenous sources, and these gene clusters abruptly enhance the virulence potential of recipient bacterial clones [15]. Many invasive bacterial pathogens possess one or more pathogenicity island that facilitates the capacity of the organism to cause disease.

TYPE III SECRETION SYSTEMS AND MICROBIAL PATHOGENESIS

Pathogenic bacteria have evolved an eloquent and highly complex system of delivery of toxins to host cells. Gene clusters of 20 or more genes participate in the synthesis and regulation of the type III secretion system. This system specifically injects bacterial toxins into the intracellular space of host cells [16,17]. These secretion systems sense the presence of a target cell membrane and express an insertion apparatus that is structurally related to bacterial flagella. Bacterial toxins are then delivered directly into the intracellular space of target cells.

Type III secretion systems have been identified from a variety of microbial pathogens including *Yersinia* [18], *Shigella* [19], *Salmonella* [16], and *Pseudomonas* spp. [17] and numerous other bacterial genera. *P. aeruginosa* delivers exotoxin S into human cells using the type III secretion system. Exotoxin S is an ADP ribosylating toxin that disrupts actin polymerization and inhibits phagocytosis in target cells. Invasive strains of *E. coli* use Type III secretion systems to induce attachment and effacement lesions on intestinal epithelial cells. *Yersinia* spp. use the same secretion system to deliver anti-phagocytic toxins, cytokine inhibitors, and inducers of apoptosis into macrophages [16].

There is evidence that the cytotoxin system of *P. aeruginosa* contributes to pathogenesis of septic shock from localized tissue spaces such as bacterial pneumonia. Cytotoxins delivered by Type III secretion systems alter cell function and viability of epithelial membranes resulting in increased tissue permeability with systemic release of pro-inflammatory cytokines from the pulmonary tissues. This contributes to the delivery of a fatal systemic level of pro-inflammatory cytokines in experimental models of *P. aeruginosa* lung infection [20,21]. The Type III secretion system of microbial pathogens alters the balance between the host and the pathogen in favor of the invading microorganism.

THE PROCESS OF TISSUE INVASION AND DISSEMINATION BY GRAM-NEGATIVE BACTERIA

Adherence

Pathogenic bacteria express surface adhesins that allow them to bind to host cell membranes. This is an essential first step to microbial pathogenesis. Motility capacity provided by bacterial flagella often facilitates the delivery of pathogens to potential attachment sites on host cell membranes. Attachment factors recognize common surface structures on human cells such as mannose, disaccharides, and other carbohydrate structures found on the glycocalx of human cell surfaces. Other receptors for bacterial adhesins are complement receptors, integrins and cytokine receptors [5,22]. Recently, it has been shown that *P. aeruginosa* uses the cystic fibrosis transmembrane conductance regulator as its adhesin receptor in lung tissue [23]. Bacteria may also adhere directly to basement membrane structures in areas of damaged or denuded epithelial surfaces. Once attachment to host membranes has been accomplished, the critical sequence of events leading to tissue invasion commences.

Invasion

Bacterial pathogens must penetrate or bypass the epithelial barriers of the host in order to gain access to tissue sites, replicate, disseminate, and cause disease. This is accomplished by a variety of ingenious mechanisms. Many enteric pathogens have specific invasion genes that mediate the synthesis of surface proteins responsible for the uptake by human cell. These invasion genes induce receptor-mediated endocytosis by non-professional phagocytic cells (i.e., epithelial cells) [5,7,24]. These molecules induce human cells to order actin filaments in such an orientation as to initiate endocytosis of bacterial cells within the host cell. Pathogens are then carried from the luminal side of epithelial cells to the basal side where they are released into the host tissues.

Other potential pathogens insert cytotoxins into host cells and thereby induce apoptosis or disrupt cell membrane stability [16,25]. Another frequently utilized strategy by bacterial pathogens is to simply bypass the epithelial barrier to invasion through breaks in the epidermis or mucous membranes at sites of previous tissue injury.

Survival within the Host

Human plasma is a hostile environment for most bacterial populations and antibacterial properties of body fluids represent a considerable challenge to potential pathogens. The invasive organism must compete with scarce nutrients, trace elements, and oxygen supply while avoiding numerous host-derived lytic enzymes and complement-mediated lysis or opsonization [5,7]. Iron is an essential element for cell viability and is vigorously competed for by both the bacterial cells and host tissues alike [26]. Bacteria produce hemolysins, iron sequestering siderophores (aerobactins) and iron-transferrin receptors in an effort to acquire iron from host fluids [3,26]. Bacteria that are unable to acquire iron from the iron limiting conditions found in human plasma are incapable of survival or dissemination within the blood stream.

Defense against complement fixation and bacterial lysis in addition to protection against immunoglobulin binding is another essential maneuver for successful invasive microorganisms. Extracellular polysaccharide capsules are often employed along with long and bulky O specific polysaccharide side chains on LPS to prevent complement fixation to bacterial cell membranes. Extracellular proteases produced by a variety of bacterial pathogens may also degrade complement components and immunoglobulins preventing opsonization of bacteria [4-7].

Mechanisms to avoid Phagocytosis and Clearance

A critical defense mechanism against bacterial organisms is the phagocytosis and intracellular killing of bacteria by the host innate immune system. Neutrophils and macrophages recognize patterns of molecules on the cell surface of prokaryotic organisms that are not found on human cells. Complement components, mannose binding ligand, β_2 integrins (CD11/CD18) and the CD14-toll-like receptor (TLR) system [27,28], function as pattern recognition molecules to detect the presence of foreign bacterial invaders. This system is used to detect bacterial LPS and a variety of other microbial mediators (see section below).

Microorganisms express a diverse array of virulence factors in an attempt to avoid phagocytosis. These include the synthesis of large polysaccharide exocapsules to disrupt phagocytosis, release of extracellular proteases to remove opsonins, production of cytotoxins and protein inhibitors via type III secretion systems, and generation of toxins that induce apoptosis of phagocytic cells. In order to succeed as a pathogen, the microorganism must possess the ability to replicate faster than the antimicrobial clearance rate mediated by opsonophagocytosis and intracellular killing. If a pathogen has the intrinsic capacity to evade host defense mechanisms and proliferate within host tissues, the syndrome of septic shock may follow [2].

Interactions with Inflammatory Cytokines

Proinflammatory cytokines are released by macrophages, neutrophils, lymphocytes and other cells in response to microbial pathogens. These cytokines function as a defense mechanism and signaling system to promote an appropriate inflammatory response to microbial invasion. It may come as no surprise that bacterial pathogens have evolved a series of evasive maneuvers to prevent elimination by proinflammatory cytokines. Many pathogens degrade cytokines, interfere with synthesis of cytokines, or utilize cytokine receptors to invade host cells [29]. Some pathogens such as *Staph. aureus* and *P. aeruginosa* may actually utilize cytokines as a growth stimulants once phagocytized by macrophages [30]. This remarkable ability is only observed in freshly isolated clinical pathogens. This capacity is lost upon serial passage of bacteria on artificial laboratory media [30].

THE MICROBIAL MEDIATORS IMPLICATED IN THE PATHOGENESIS OF GRAM-NEGATIVE SEPSIS

While bacterial endotoxin is generally thought to be the principal mediator of Gram-negative septic shock, recent evidence indicates that LPS works in concert with a variety of other microbial mediators that contribute to systemic inflammation. Microbial mediators implicated in the pathogenesis of septic shock are listed in Table 2. These mediators work in combination with each other and probably synergize to induce systemic inflammation that contributes to the pathogenesis of septic shock.

Mediator	Host receptor/action	Relative activity
Lipopolysaccharide	LBP-CD14-TLR4-MD2	++++
Peptidoglycan	CD14-TLR2	++
Lipopeptides	CD14-TLR2	+++
Cytotoxins, type III secretion systems	Disruption of cellular activity, apoptosis	+
Unmethylated CpG motifs	TLR9	++
Bacterial flagella	TLR5	+

Table 2. Bacterial products implicated in the pathogenesis of sepsis

The most direct evidence that LPS is not essential for the induction of an inflammatory signal to host phagocytic cells is found with the LPS deficient *Neisseria meningitidis* strain [31]. Deletion of lipid A synthetic genes in this strain of *N. meningitidis* results in a viable bacterium which lacks LPS in its outer membrane. Lipid A deletion in enteric Gram-negative bacteria such as *E. coli* is a lethal mutation. The LPS-deficient strain of *N. meningitidis* is still capable of inducing inflammatory reactions via the TLR2 receptors found on macrophages. This indicates that Gram-negative bacteria have other cell wall components that induce inflammation even in the absence of bacterial LPS [32].

HOST RESPONSE TO MICROBIAL MEDIATORS THROUGH THE INNATE IMMUNE SYSTEM

The innate immune system (macrophages, neutrophils, natural killer cells and alternative complement) has evolved as an early, rapid response system to microbial invasion. Actions against invading pathogens are either direct or indirect through release of cytokines or other stimulatory molecules, which trigger the adaptive immune system by activating B and T cells.

Janeway proposed a central concept in the understanding of the innate immune system: the identification of infectious agents by means of conserved structural features through pattern-recognition receptors (PRR). The components expressed by microbial agents that trigger the immune response are termed pathogen-associated molecular patterns (PAMPs) [27]. The discovery of the Toll-like receptors (TLR) of the innate immune system is one of the great accomplishments in the understanding of molecular pathogenesis in the past decade. Comparative molecular biology has succeeded in unlocking the mystery of the cellular receptor for endotoxin. This evolutionarily conserved receptor system has allowed multicellular organisms to rapidly recognize the presence of microbial invaders. Bacterial pathogens represent an immediate threat to survival and this requires a vigorous and coordinated immune response in defense of the viability of the host [28]. The following section summarizes the major findings that defined the TLR family as the central transmembranous receptor of the innate immune system. The current knowledge about receptor structure, signaling pathways and ligand specificity is described in considerable detail.

IL-1R/TLR RECEPTOR SUPERFAMILY

The IL-1R/TLR (interleukin-1 receptor/Toll-like receptor) superfamily members (Figure 1) are found in many plants, and vertebrate and invertebrate animal species, and those with known function share the feature of being involved in host responses to injury and infection. Most notably, in humans these include not only the receptor and accessory protein for IL-1, but also the IL-18 receptor and its accessory protein, and the long-sought signaling receptor for lipopolysaccharide (LPS), TLR4. Many proteins from diverse systems show homology to the cytoplasmic domain of the type 1 interleukin-1 receptor (IL-1R1). This expanding IL-1R1-like family includes murine and human proteins, *Drosophila* (fruit fly) proteins, and a plant (tobacco) protein [28]. In *Drosophila*, Toll is involved in the rapid and transient transcriptional induction of several genes encoding potent antimicrobial peptides upon septic injury [33]. A noteworthy plant member of the IL-1R1 family is the tobacco N gene [34]. The N gene encodes a protein with an amino-terminal domain that has significant homology to Toll and the cytoplasmic domain of the IL-1R1. Introduction of the N gene into tobacco mosaic virus-sensitive strains of tobacco confers resistance to tobacco mosaic virus via the ability to mount a hypersensitive response to the virus at the site of infection within the plant. This system is fundamentally similar to the acute inflammatory response pathway stimulated by injury and mediated by IL-1 in mammals [34].

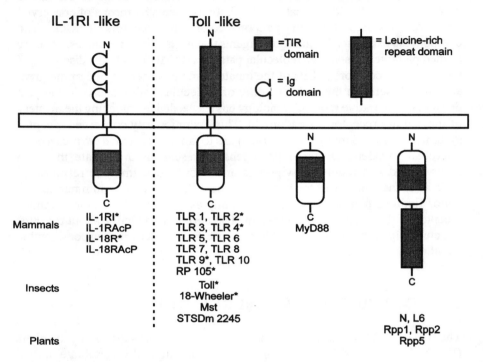

Figure 1. *The interleukin-1/Toll-like receptor family*

A growing number of mammalian homologs of IL-1R1 are being identified that contain highly conserved regions in their cytosolic domains. Homologous regions were also found in a receptor-like protein of the *Drosophila* fly called Toll. This has resulted in the defining of the IL-1R/TLR superfamily, the conserved region being termed the Toll/IL-1R (TIR) domain [33].

Drosophila Toll Members

Toll was originally described in *Drosophila* as a type I transmembrane receptor that controls the establishment of the dorsal-ventral polarity of the fly embryo [35]. Nüesslein-Volhard and Wieschaus discovered the first Toll mutants while doing genetic screens [36]. Wieschaus noted that the Toll mutant embryos failed to hatch and developed no ventral or lateral cell types. When Nüsslein-Volhard saw the particular looking embryos lacking the entire mesoderm and nervous system, she exclaimed "Toll!" (German for jazzy or cool). Thus, the new gene was given its name.

Four members of the Toll-family have been identified in *Drosophila* thus far: Toll, 18-Wheeler (18W), Mst and STSDm2245. Toll and 18W share the greatest similarity to each other and also with the cytoplasmic tail of the mammalian IL-1R1. The *Drosophila* 18W is required for morphogenesis and has many similarities to Toll. The extracellular regions of Toll and 18W contain multiple leucine rich repeats and carboxyl-terminal cysteine rich domains [37].

Drosophila Toll Signaling Pathway

Current understanding about the Toll pathway in *Drosophila* immune response comes from studies of promoters of genes induced in response to infection. Insects respond to infection with antimicrobial peptides produced by the fat body and hemocytes. All of the antimicrobial peptide genes include nuclear factor-kappa B (NF-κB) or Rel proteins in their upstream regions. The first insect protein discovered to regulate transcription through NF-κB sites was Dorsal. Subsequent genetic studies further identified Spätzle, Toll, Pelle, Tube and Cactus as necessary partners to induce Drosomycin, an antifungal *Drosophila* peptide, in response to fungal infection (Figure 2) [33].

It has been demonstrated by genetic complementation tests that Spätzle is the Toll ligand. Spätzle is endogenously secreted as an inactive precursor molecule. Protease Easter creates an active form through proteolysis into the biologically active carboxyl-terminal polypeptide fragment [38]. Binding of Spätzle to Toll activates the receptor by ligand-dependent receptor dimerization. This is of interest, because there might be an endogenous ligand for the mammalian homologs of Toll.

Activated Toll recruits of the adaptor protein Tube and the protein kinase Pelle to the intracellular part of the Toll protein [33]. As yet, no true homolog to Tube has been defined in mammals, but MyD88 appears to have a similar function.

The mammalian IRAK (IL-1R-associated kinase) appears to be homolog to *Drosophila* Pelle. Pelle interacts with another protein, the *Drosophila* homolog of mammalian tumor necrosis factor (TNF) receptor-associated factor (TRAF6) (dTRAF6). The close relationship between Toll-related signaling is also evidenced by the fact that MyD88, IRAK and TRAF6 participate not only in Toll or TLR signaling, but also in IL-1 and IL-18 signaling, leading to the activation of NF-κB [39].

The next downstream step in the signaling cascade is a direct association of dTRAF6 with the *Drosophila* homologue to ECSIT (evolutionarily conserved signaling intermediate in Toll pathways). Transfection of dECSIT in insect cells leads to production of diptericin, attacin and defensin (antimicrobial peptides) [40].

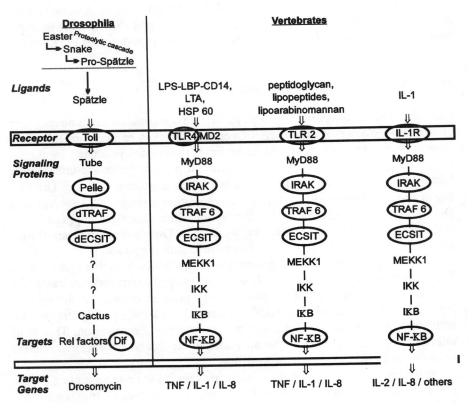

Figure 2. *Comparisons between the signaling pathways in the insect and mammalian IL-1/Toll-like receptor pathways*

The final members in signal transduction in *Drosophila* are Dorsal and Dorsal-like immunity factor (DIF) which are released from Cactus. Cactus is a cytoplasmic anchoring protein and the *Drosophila* homolog to I-κB; Dorsal and DIF are the *Drosophila* NF-κB homologs [33].

After release from Cactus, Dorsal and DIF translocate into the nucleus and induce gene transcription. There is also evidence for a *Drosophila* homolog to the mammalian I-kB kinase DLAK (*Drosophila* LPS-activated kinase), which is phosphorylating Cactus. In transfection models, DLAK-deficient cell lines fail to respond to LPS stimulation [37].

The role of the Toll receptor in the adult fly is induction of immune response in fungal infection. Toll-deficient flies fail to express Drosomycin. In infection models, Toll-mutant flies died from overwhelming growth of *Aspergillus fumigatus* [41].

The immune response of Toll deficient flies is not altered against bacteria, suggesting a different receptor and pathway. Williams et al. demonstrated recently that 18W deficient flies have an increased mortality from *E. coli* infection [42]. This might be due to a reduced expression of the antibacterial *Drosophila* protein attacin.

Another clue to the pathogen specificity is that antifungal and antibacterial signaling is also divergent further downstream: 18W deficient flies in bacterial infection have a reduced translocation of DIF into the nucleus, whereas Dorsal translocation is unaffected [43]. Toll, on the other hand, does not require DIF for intracellular signaling. This suggests that there might be a selective immune response to particular microbial pathogens.

Homologies between Drosophila Toll and the TLR Family

All members of the Toll family are membrane proteins that cross the membrane once and share similar extracellular domains [39]. Typical are 18-31 leucine-rich repeats (LRRs). The extracellular domain of TLR4 contains 22 copies of the LRR. The extracellular domains are very divergent among the different members: TLR2 and TLR4 share only 24 % of identical sequences. This makes it likely that they bind different ligands. Also the TLRs of different species are very different: mouse TLR4 and human TLR4 are only 53 % identical. Genetic studies of LRR structures among different individuals also revealed that polymorphisms are responsible for a different reaction on microbial challenge. The intracellular part contains a cytoplasmic domain of approximately 200 amino acids that is evolutionarily conserved (TIR domain).

Mammalian Toll Homologs

The mammalian homologs of *Drosophila* Toll are termed TLR proteins and have been intensively studied [39,44]. To date, six TLRs (TLR1-6) have been published [44,45]. A further four TLRs have been cloned by Schering

Corporation. These sequences will be patented and published soon (currently available on the website - http://patent.womblex.ibm.com).

TLR1-6 have been characterized by their distinctive expression patterns with mRNA detection assays. TLR1 is expressed ubiquitously and at rather high levels. TLR2 has a particularly strong expression pattern in peripheral blood mononuclear cells, but is also expressed in lymphoid tissue [46,47]. TLR3 mRNA is expressed in lung, muscle, heart, brain and intestinal cells. Alternative splicing variants have been reported from pancreas and placenta. Among peripheral blood cells, TLR3 is selectively expressed in dendritic cells. TLR4 is expressed in lymphocytes, spleen and the heart. TLR5 mRNA is detectable in peripheral blood monocytes, leukocytes, ovary and the prostate. TLR6 expression was located to spleen, thymus, ovary and lung [48]. Among these, ligands for TLR2 and TLR4, and most recently for TLR9 have been identified.

TLR Signaling Pathway

As mentioned above, the intracellular part of members of the TLR family has a high degree of homology to the IC (intracellular) domain of the IL-1R. This remarkable level of homology suggests similar intracellular signaling pathways (see Figure 2) [44,48].

Post-receptor signaling of the IL-1R is well understood. Binding of the ligand causes receptor dimerization, and with involvement of IL-1RAP, an accessory protein, the intracellular part of the receptor forms a complex of MyD88, an adapter protein, and IRAK, a kinase. IRAK then phosphorylates TRAF6, which leads to NIK (NF-κB-inducing kinase) and IKK (I-κB kinase) activation. IKK phosphorylates I-κB, which then dissociates from NF-κB [40]. NF-κB translocates to the nucleus and initiates gene transcription. When human homologs to the *Drosophila* Toll were discovered, there was great interest as to their role in innate immunity. Medzhitov et al. reported NF-κB activation as well as cytokine release through TLR4 in transfected monocytic cell lines, which were able to express TLR4 constitutively at a high level [49].

So far, TLR2 and TLR4 have been the most intensively studied members of mammalian homologs to *Drosophila* Toll. Both TLR2 and TLR4 require the adaptor protein MyD88 for signaling, and immunoprecipitation studies showed direct interaction of MyD88 and IRAK [50]. MyD88 was originally isolated and characterized as a myeloid differentiation primary response gene. MyD88 itself consists of a carboxyl-terminal TIR domain, making it a member of the TLR family. IRAK has been shown both to interact with both MyD88 and TRAF6 [48].

Further evidence for the role of TRAF6 and NIK in TLR4 signaling came from the study of TRAF6 and NIK dominant negative (DN) variants, which could not activate NF-κB [51]. Another very interesting observation came from this study. Activation of the c-Jun N-terminal kinase (JNK) pathway through TLR4 is prevented by the MyD88-DN, but not the TRAF6-DN variant. This might indicate an alternative signaling pathway divergent at the MyD88 level.

The protein ECSIT is specific for TLR/IL-1 signaling and is involved in the proteolytic cleavage and activation of the MAP-kinase MEKK-1 after TRAF6 activation [40]. ECSIT-DN inhibits NF-κB activation through MEK-1 and MEKK-1.

Recent observations by Miyake and colleagues demonstrate the necessity of another cell surface molecule for TLR4 signal transduction [52]. The protein MD-2 has no intracellular domain, but upon co-expression with TLR4 enhances LPS sensitivity in transfection models. MD-2 cotransfection with TLR2 had no effect on LPS response. MD-1 has been discovered recently as an essential partner in signaling of RP 105, another member of the TLR family that is expressed in marginal zone B cells [53].

TLR2 signaling shares many similarities with IL-1R/TLR4 signaling. TLR2 dependent NF-κB activation requires the TIR domain, which is the epitope for the TIR-MyD88-IRAK complex that induces TRAF6 [46,47].

TLR as the LPS receptor

Another exciting development in the history of TLR research has been the report that TLR4 is utilized by LPS and therefore is a candidate for the long-sought LPS-receptor [54,55]. There is still controversy about the specific ligands for members of the TLR family. It is important to stress that in receptor ligand interaction in general there are 3-10 receptors for every ligand.

Probably the most powerful microbial stimulant of innate immune responses is LPS. LPS has been known to induce signals very similar to IL-1, and also to bind to CD14 on macrophages. The best-characterized interaction is between LPS and LPS-binding protein (LBP). LPS is first bound by LBP, a plasma lipid transfer protein that moves LPS monomers from aggregates or bacterial membranes to a binding site on surface receptor CD14. Alternatively, the LBP-LPS complex can be recognized by a soluble version of CD14 that subsequently activates nonmyeloid cells [56].

CD14 is a known pattern-recognition receptor (PRR) on the surface of monocytes/macrophages. For many years it has been clear that CD14 has a major role for the effects of LPS on macrophages, monocytes, and neutrophils and that CD14 increases the sensitivity of macrophages to LPS [56]. But the precise role of CD14 in LPS signaling has remained unclear. There had to be a molecule with the ability to identify the binding partner and to discriminate LPS from host lipids and to transduce signals across the membrane. Neither LBP nor CD14 showed to have the binding specificity to discriminate LPS from host lipids. The interest in TLR biology increased greatly as evidence accumulated that these proteins participate in intracellular signaling initiated by LPS and Gram-negative bacteria.

Medzhitov et al. showed in 1997 that a constitutively active mutant of human TLR4 induces the expression of the NF-κB controlled cytokines IL-1, IL-6 and IL-8. This implicated the role of TLR4 in innate immunity [49]. Two groups of researchers demonstrated in 1998 that overexpression of TLR2 in mammalian cells renders cells responsive to LPS in a CD14 dependent manner. TLR2 was stably transfected in human kidney cell lines and activated NF-κB in the presence of CD14 and LBP and after LPS stimulation [46,47].

A second approach by Beutler and colleagues proved on a genetic level that TLR4 is involved in LPS signaling. These data were obtained in genetic analysis in two strains of mice, C3H/HeJ and C57BL/10Scr, both known for their hyporesponsiveness to LPS and their increased mortality from Gram-negative sepsis. Over the past 20 years it has been shown that hyporesponsiveness to LPS maps to a single autosomal locus (lps^d) and impaired responses can be documented both in whole animals and in cells taken from these animals.

Through extensive genetic mapping work done by Poltorak et al. and Quershi et al. the lps^d allele was shown to map to the gene encoding TLR4. The $tlr4$ locus located to the target region in chromosome 4 [54,55].

A missense mutation in the *Tlr4* gene locus was demonstrated to be responsible for the altered LPS-responsiveness in the C3H/HeJ strain. A point mutation converts a Pro residue at position 712 to His (CP712H), thus rendering the receptor inactive [57]. A further proof is that C57BL/10ScCr mice carry a large deletion mutation and do not express TLR4 mRNA.

After the initial observations with TLR2 as a physiologic LPS receptor [46,47], the relative role of TLR2 in LPS signaling has been reexamined. TLR2 exerts a cellular response to LPS, but with a lower affinity than TLR4. Therefore TLR2 does not appear to be essential for LPS signaling in native cells that also express TLR4. TLR2 could be an alternative LPS receptor in TLR4 deficient cells [58]. TLR2 has subsequently been demonstrated to be a broad spectrum PRR that interacts with a wide variety of other bacterial components including LPS itself.

Other Ligands in TLR Signaling

The concept of innate immunity demands the presence of nonclonal receptors that recognize a variety of highly conserved bacterial structures. More and more evidence has been generated that the TLR family represents this key group of innate immune response receptors. Both TLR2 and TLR4 are able to recognize more than just LPS.

While TLR2 may recognize LPS as a ligand, TLR2 has also been recognized as a signal transducer for numerous other bacterial products than LPS. So far, TLR2 has been involved in recognition of Gram-positive bacteria, mycobacteria, spirochetes, mycoplasma and yeast antigens (Table 3) [28].

Spirochetes lack LPS, but possess membrane lipoproteins in the cell wall. TLR2 antibody administered to human peripheral blood mononuclear cells prevented cytokine release after stimulation with lipoproteins and lipopeptides from *Mycoplasma fermentans, Borrelia burgdorferi and Treponema pallidum* [59]. Chinese hamster ovary cells (CHO-K1 cell lines) fail to express a functional TLR2 due to a frame-shift mutation in their TLR2 mRNA sequence. These cells were transfected with TLR2 and tested for many bacterial products. *B. burgdorferi* lipoprotein has also been shown to stimulate NF-κB through TLR2 in transfected CHO and also in TLR-2 transfected 293 cells [28].

Organism	Product
Gram-negative bacteria	LPS from various sources – possibly contaminated with peptides (*Salmonella, Shigella spp. E. coli*)
Gram-positive bacteria	*Listeria monocytogenes, Bacillus subtilis, Streptococcus spp. Staphylococcus aureus*-lipoteichoic acid, peptidoglycan, lipopeptides
Mycobacteria	Heat killed *M. tuberculosis, M. avium* lipopeptides, lipoarabinomannan
Spirochetes	*Borrelia burgdorferi Treponema. pallidum, T. maltophilum* (lipopeptides, glycolipids, Outer surface protein A)
Mycoplasma	*Mycoplasma fermentans* (R-MALP, lipopeptides)
Yeast	Zymosan

Table 3. Currently recognized ligands for TLR2

TLR4 signaling is primarily activated after lipid A/LPS challenge, but is also sensitive to lipoteichoic acid from Gram-positive bacteria and live *M.*

tuberculosis bacteria (Table 4).

Organism	Product
Gram-negative bacteria	Lipopolysaccharide, lipid A
Gram-positive bacteria	Lipoteichoic acid
Mycobacteria	Live *Mycobacteria tuberculosis*
Spirochetes	*Treponema brennaborense* glycolipids
Other ligands	Heat shock protein 60, Taxol

Table 4. Currently recognized ligands for TLR4

Purified glycolipids from *Treponema brennaborense*, a spirochete that causes an infectious disease in cattle, have been associated with TLR4-dependent signaling [60].

Ohashi et al. reported the potential first endogenous ligand for TLR4. Recent studies have shown that heat shock protein (HSP) is a danger signal to the innate immune system. Macrophages respond with a proinflammatory cytokine response to stimulation with both autologous HSP60 and microbial HSP60/65. Macrophages from C3H/HeJ responded with nitric oxide (NO) formation and TNF secretion whereas they remained unresponsive to LPS [61]. A recent publication has linked TLR4 signaling and expression in injured myocardium. Since there was no infection present in this model, these findings open the perspective that TLR4 may be responding to noninfectious and endogenous ligands in inflammation as well [62].

There now appears to be a third member of the mammalian TLR family for which ligand specificity has been defined. In a preliminary report by Akira [63], the newly recognized TLR9 appears to be a receptor for unmethylated CpG motifs found in microbial DNA. Human cells are capable of recognizing sequences of DNA that are common to bacterial genomes but rare in human DNA. These unmethylated CpG seqences in bacterial DNA induce a strong proinflammatory signal for human immune effector cells [64]. The molecular mechanism responsible for the ability to discriminate bacterial DNA from human DNA remained obscure until recent discoveries with TLR9. TLR9-DN mutants had no TNF response upon exposure to oligonucleotides containing CpG motifs found in microbial DNA [64].

Within the past few months the first ligand for TLR5 has been discovered. Bacterial flagellin from either Gram-positive or Gram-negative bacteria has been found to induce mobilization of NF6B and expression of TNF from mammalian mononuclear cells. This appears to be the means by which the innate immune system recognizes a flagellated bacterial pathogen [65].

While the precise biochemical nature of the 10 recognized human TLR proteins are being defined, there is great interest in discovering their organization and interactions in response to microbial infection. One hypothesis is that each TLR recognizes a distinct lipoprotein or glycolipid to elicit a specific response. In this manner, different PAMPs could activate different Toll family members, leading to activation of particular target genes. Results from *Drosophila* studies support this hypothesis. The 18W of the *Drosophila* system responds to bacterial stimuli and produces the antibacterial peptide gene attacin while Toll itself induces the antifungal peptide drosomycin, but no antibacterial peptides.

In humans, the same mechanism could be true, or the possibility of heterodimers with differing contributions of TLRs on their cell surface responding to different microbial mediators. There has been considerable effort to answer the question if TLR heterodimers exist on human effector cells. Underhill and coworkers constructed a mutation for TLR2 that is equivalent to the P712H mutation of TLR4 in C3H/HeJ mice. In TLR2-P681H the proline at position 681 is replaced by a histidine, thus creating a dominant-negative mutation. This group also genetically engineered the TLR4-P712H mutation [66]. These mutant TLR were transfected into RAW-TT10 murine macrophages. The cell-line with the mutant TLR2 showed impaired TNF-α production when stimulated with *Staph. aureus*, whereas there was normal reaction to LPS and *Salmonella minnesota*. Expression of the TLR4 mutant allowed normal cytokine response to *Staph. aureus*, but strong inhibition of TNF-α response to LPS and moderate inhibition to *S. minnesota*. There is no evidence to date that supports the importance of TLR2/TLR4 heterodimers in LPS signaling. Recently, it has been suggested that TLR6 may form heterodimers with TLR2 in response to bacterial peptidoglycan but not with lipopeptides where TLR2 homodimers are found [67]. Combinations of TLR signals could mediate the variable host response signals induced by a variety of different microbial pathogens and mediators.

BLOCKING TLR FUNCTION AS A POTENTIAL THERAPEUTIC OPTION?

The development of antagonists for TLR proteins may serve as a useful tool in counteracting the harmful pro-inflammatory response that complicates systemic microbial infections. There are at least three basic strategies for reducing signal transduction of TLRs with the specific goal of reducing the consequences of their biological effects.

The first strategy is the development of specific soluble TLR family members that bind and neutralize their respective microbial or mammalian ligands. Examples would be soluble TLR4 in Gram-negative sepsis or soluble TLR2 for the treatment of toxic shock syndromes caused by staphylococcal exotoxins. In the case of TLR4, this approach has been questioned recently [68].

The second strategy is the development of small molecules or antibody molecules that interfere with the extracellular domains of the TLRs. This approach could prevent interaction with distal intracellular signaling molecules before a natural ligand binds to TLR at the cell surface of effector cells. An example of this strategy would be a LPS antagonist molecule that binds to TLR4 but fails to activate an intracellular signal [68]. This strategy will be greatly facilitated once the ligand binding pockets of the TLRs are precisely characterized. X-ray crystallographic structure analysis of the TLR protein with a specific ligand has so far not been successful. This information would allow for the design of novel therapeutic agonists and antagonists that could influence the outcome of a wide range of fatal infectious states.

The third strategy is the development of small molecules that interfere with the intracellular domains of the TLRs. This approach could prevent interaction with distal intracellular signaling molecules after ligand binding to TLRs. An example of this strategy would be small molecules that might prevent recruitment of MyD88, a central intracellular member of the IL-1R/TLR family [39].

CONCLUSION

It has become evident that Gram-negative bacterial pathogens have evolved an elaborate array of virulence factors that contribute to the immunopathogenesis of systemic infection and septic shock. Microorganisms are capable of invading the human host if even subtle defects develop in the antimicrobial defense systems of the host. The human immune system is well endowed with potent detection and alarm systems to respond to the ever-present threat of microbial pathogens. The recent discovery of the TLR family now permits a detailed evaluation of the molecular pathogenesis of sepsis. The availability of human and microbial functional genomics should allow us to understand more fully the complex interactions that exist between host and pathogen in septic patients in the future.

REFERENCES

1.   Casadevall A, Pirofski L-A. Host-pathogen interactions: redefining the basic concepts of virulence and pathogenicity. Infect Immun 1999; 67:3703-3713

2. Cross AS, Opal SM, Sadoff JC, et al. Choice of bacteria in animal models of sepsis. Infect Immun 1993; 61:2741-2747
3. Opal SM, Cross AS, Gemski P, et al. Aerobactin and alpha-hemolysin as virulence determinants in *Escherichia coli* isolated from human blood, urine, and stool. J Infect Dis 1990; 161:794-796
4. Kim KS, Itabashi H, Gemski P, et al. The K1 capsule is the critical determinant in development of *Escherichia coli* meningitis in the rat. J Clin Invest 1992; 90:897-905
5. Finlay BB, Falcow S. Common themes in microbial pathogenicity revisited. Microbiol Mol Biol Rev 1997; 61:136-169
6. Johnson JR, Russo TA, Tarr PI. Molecular epidemiological and pylogenetic associations of two novel putative virulence genes, *Iha* and *iroN*$_{E. coli}$, among *Escherichia coli* isolates from patients with urosepsis. Infect Immun 2000; 68:3040-3047
7. Heumann D, Glauser MP, Calandra T. Molecular basis of host-pathogen interaction in septic shock. Curr Opin Microbiol 1998; 1:49-55
8. Opal SM, Cross AS. Clinical trials for sepsis: past failures and future hopes. Infect Dis Clin North Am 1999; 13: 285-298
9. DeKievit TR, Iglewski BH. Bacterial quorum sensing in pathogenic relationships. Infect Immun 2000; 68:4839-4849
10. Parsek MI, Greenberg EP. Acyl-homoserine lactone quorum sensing in Gram-negative bacteria: a signaling mechanism involved in associations with higher organisms. Proc Natl Acad Sci USA 2000; 97:8789-8793
11. Passador L, Cook JM, Gambello MJ. Expression of *Pseudomonas aeruginosa* virulence genes requires cell-to-cell communication. Science 1993; 260:1127-1130
12. Pearson JP, Feldman M, Iglewski BH, et al. *Pseudomonas aeruginosa* cell-to-cell signaling is required for virulence in a model of acute pulmonary infection. Infect Immun 2000; 68:4331-4334
13. Boyd EF, Hartl DL. Chromosomal regions specific to pathogenicity islands of *Escherichia coli* have a phylogenetically clustered distribution. J Bacteriol 1998; 180:1159-1165
14. Lawrence JG. Selfish operons: the evolutionary impact of gene clustering in prokaryotes and eurkaryotes. Curr Opin Genet Dev 1999; 9:642-648
15. Bloch CA, Rode CK. Pathogenicity island evaluation in *Escherichia coli* K1 by crossing with laboratory strain K-12. Infect Immun 1996; 64:3218-3223
16. Galán JE, Collmer A. Type III secretion machines: bacterial devices for protein delivery into host cells. Science 1999; 284:1322-1328
17. Hueck CJ. Type III protein secretion systems in bacterial pathogens of animals and plants. Microbiol Mol Biol Rev 1998; 62:379-433
18. Sory M-P, Boland A, Lambermont I, et al. Identification of the YopE and YopH demains required for secretion and internalization into the cytosol of macrophages, using the cyaA gene fusion approach. Proc Natl. Acad Sci USA 1995; 92:11998-12002
19. Zychlinsky, A, Prevost MC, Sansonetti PJ. *Shigella flexneri* induces apoptosis in infected macrophages. Nature 1992; 358:167-169
20. Fleiszig SM, Vallas V, Jun CH, et al. Susceptibilty of epithelial cells to *Pseudomonas aeruginosa* invasion and cytotoxicity is upregulated by hepatocyte growth factor. Infect Immun 1998; 66:3443-3446
21. Moore TA, Standiford TJ.The role of cytokines in bacterial pneumonia: an inflammatory balancing act. Proc Assoc Am Phys 1998; 110:297-305
22. Mulvey MA, Schilling JD, Martinez JJ, et al. Bad bugs and beleaguered bladders: interplay between uropathogenic *Escherichia coli* and innate host defenses. Proc Natl Acad Sci USA 2000; 97:8829-8835
23. Pier JB. Role of the cystic fibrosis transmembrane conductance regulator in innate immunity to *Pseudomonas aeruginosa* infections. Proc Natl Acad Sci USA 2000; 97:8822-8828

24. Dersch P, Isenberg RR. An immunoglobulin super family-like domain unique to the *Yersinia pseudotuberculosis* invasin protein is required for stimulation of bacterial uptake via integrin receptors. Infect Immun 2000; 68:2930-2938

25. Klapproth J-MA, Scaletsky ICA, McNamara BP, et al. A large toxin from pathogenic *Escherichia coli* strains that inhibits lymphocyte activation. Infect Immun 2000; 68:2148-2155

26. Brittigen BE, Rasmussen GT, Olokamani O, et al. Novel acquisition *Pseudomonas aeruginosa* siderophores by human phagocytes: an additional mechanism of host defense through iron sequestration? Infect Immun 2000; 568:1271-1275

27. Janeway CA Jr. The immune system evolved to discriminate infectious nonself from noninfectious self. Immunol Today. 1992; 13:11-16

28. Means TK, Golenbock DT, Fenton MJ. The biology of Toll-like receptors. Cytokine Growth Factor Rev 2000; 11:219-232

29. Wilson M, Seymour R, Henderson B. Bacterial perturbation of cytokine networks. Infect Immun 1998; 66:2401-2409

30. Kanangat S, Meduri GU, Tolley EA, et al. Effects of cytokines and endotoxin on the intracellular growth of bacteria. Infect Immun 1999; 67:2834-2840

31. Steeghs L, Kufpers B, Hendrik JH, et al. Imunogenicity of outer membrane proteins in a lipopolysaccharide-deficient mutant of *Neisseria meningitidis*: influence of adjuvants on the immune response. Infect Immun 1999; 67:4988-4993

32. Steeghs L, den Hartog R, den Boer A, et al. Meningitis bacterium is viable without endotoxin. Nature 1998; 392:449-450

33. Hoffmann JA, Reichhart JM. *Drosophila* immunity. Trends Cell Biol 1997; 7:309-316

34. Whitham S, Dinesh-Kumar SP, Choi D, et al. The product of the tobacco mosaic virus resistance gene N: similarity to toll and the interleukin-1 receptor. Cell 1994; 78:1101-1115

35. Hashimoto C, Hudson KL, Anderson KV. The Toll gene of *Drosophila*, required for dorsal-ventral embryonic polarity, appears to encode a transmembrane protein. Cell. 1988; 52:269-279

36. Stein D, Roth S, Vogelsang E, et al. The polarity of the dorsoventral axis in the *Drosophila* embryo is defined by an extracellular signal. Cell 1991; 65:725-735

37. Gay NJ, Keith FJ. *Drosophila* Toll and IL-1 receptor. Nature 1991; 351:355-356

38. DeLotto Y, DeLotto R. Proteolytic processing of the *Drosophila* Spatzle protein by Easter generates a dimeric NGF-like molecule with ventralising activity. Mech Dev 1998; 72:141-148

39. O'Neill LA, Dinarello CA. The IL-1 receptor/toll-like receptor superfamily: crucial receptors for inflammation and host defense. Immunol Today 2000; 21:206-209

40. Kopp E, Medzhitov R, Carothers J, et al. ECSIT is an evolutionarily conserved intermediate in the Toll/IL-1 signal transduction pathway. Genes Dev 1999; 13:2059-2071

41. Lemaitre B, Nicolas E, Michaut L, et al. The dorsoventral regulatory gene cassette Spatzle/Toll/Cactus controls the potent antifungal response in *Drosophila* adults. Cell 1996; 86: 973-983

42. Williams MJ, Rodriguez A, Kimbrell DA, et al. The 18-wheeler mutation reveals complex antibacterial gene regulation in *Drosophila* host defense. EMBO J 1997; 16:6120-6130

43. Wu LP, Anderson KV. Regulated nuclear import of Rel proteins in the *Drosophila* immune response. Nature 1998; 392:93-97

44. Rock FL, Hardiman G, Timans JC, et al. A family of human receptors structurally related to *Drosophila* Toll. Proc Natl Acad Sci USA 1998; 95:588-593

45. Takeuchi O, Kawai T, Sanjo H, et al. S. TLR6: A novel member of an expanding toll-like receptor family. Gene 1999; 231:59-65

46. Kirschning CJ, Wesche H, Merrill Ayres T, et al. Human toll-like receptor 2 confers responsiveness to bacterial lipopolysaccharide. J Exp Med 1998; 188:2091-2097

47. Yang RB, Mark MR, Gurney AL, et al. Signaling events induced by lipopolysaccharide-activated toll-like receptor 2. J Immunol 1999; 163:639-643
48. Bowie A, O'Neill LA. The interleukin-1 receptor/Toll-like receptor superfamily: signal generators for pro-inflammatory interleukins and microbial products. J Leukoc Biol 2000; 67:508-514
49. Medzhitov R, Preston-Hurlburt P, Janeway, CA Jr. A human homologue of the *Drosophila* Toll protein signals activation of adaptive immunity. Nature 1997; 388:394-397
50. Medzhitov R, Preston-Hurlburt P, Kopp E, et al, MyD88 is an adapter protein in the hToll/IL-1 receptor family signaling pathways. Mol Cell 1998; 2:253-258
51. Muzio M, Natoli G, Saccani S, et al. The human Toll signaling pathway: divergence of nuclear factor κB and JNK/SAPK activation upstream of tumor necrosis factor receptor-associated factor 6 (TRAF6). J Exp Med 1998;187:2097-2101
52. Shimazu R, Akashi S, Ogata H, et al. MD-2, a molecule that confers lipopolysaccharide responsiveness on Toll-like receptor 4. J Exp Med 1999; 189:1777-1782
53. Hirohashi N, Akashi S, Miyake K, et al. The expression of TLR4 and RP105 on peripheral blood mononuclear cells in systemic inflammatory response syndrome. J Endo Res 2000; 6:126 (Abst)
54. Poltorak A, He X, Smirnova I, et al. Defective LPS signaling in C3H/HeJ and C57BL/10ScCr mice: mutations in the tlr4 gene. Science 1998; 282:2085-2088
55. Qureshi ST, Lariviere L, Leveque G, et al. Endotoxin-tolerant mice have mutations in Toll-like receptor 4. J Exp Med 1999; 189: 615-625
56. Fenton MJ, Golenbock DT. LPS-binding proteins and receptors. J Leuk Biol 1998; 64:25-32
57. Poltorak A, He X, Smirnova I, et al. Defective LPS signaling in C3H/HeJ and C57BL/10ScCr mice: mutations in the tlr4 gene. Science 1998; 282:2085-2088
58. Takeuchi O, Hoshino K, Kawai T, et al. Differential roles of TLR2 and TLR4 in recognition of Gram-negative and Gram-positive bacterial cell wall components. Immunity 1999; 11:443-451
59. Lien E, Sellati TJ, Yoshimura A, et al. Toll-like receptor 2 functions as a pattern recognition receptor for diverse bacterial products. J Biol Chem 1999; 274:33419-33425
60. Schröder NWJ, Bastian O, Lamping N, et al. Involvement of lipopolysaccharide binding protein, CD14, and Toll-like receptors in the initiation of innate immune responses by *Treponema* glycolipids. J Immunol 2000; 165: 2683-2693
61. Ohashi K, Burkart V, Flohe S, et al. Heat shock protein 60 is a putative endogenous ligand of the Toll-like receptor-4 complex. J Immunol 2000; 164:558-561
62. Frantz S, Kobzik L, Kim YD, et al. Toll4 (TLR4) expression in cardiac myocytes in normal and failing myocardium. J Clin Invest 1999; 104:271-280.
63. Akira S. Roles of toll-like receptors in microbial recognition. J Endo Res 2000; 6:76 (Abst)
64. Schwartz DA, Wohlford-Henane CL, Quinn TJ, et al. Bacterial DNA or oligonucleotides containing unmethylated CpG motifs can minimize lipopolysaccharide-induced inflammation in the lower respiratory tract through a IL-12 -dependent pathway. J Immunol 1999; 163:224-231
65. Hayashi F, Smith KD,Ozinsky A, et al. The innate immune response to bacterial flagellin is mediated by Toll-like receptor 5. Nature 2001; 420:1099-1103
66. Underhill DM, Ozinsky S, Hajjar AM, et al. The Toll-like receptor 2 is recruited to macrophage phagosomes and discriminates between pathogens. Nature 1999; 401:811-815
67. Underhill D. Toll-like receptor signaling during phagocytosis. J Endo Res 2000; 6:76 (Abst)
68. Du X, Poltorak A, Silva M, et al. Analysis of TLR4-mediated LPS signal transduction in macrophages by mutational modification of the receptor. Blood Cells Mol Dis 1999; 25:328-338

10

INVOLVEMENT OF PRO- AND ANTI-INFLAMMATORY CYTOKINES IN SEPSIS

Jean-Marc Cavaillon
Minou Adib-Conquy

The appearance of detectable pro- as well as anti-inflammatory cytokines in the blood stream during sepsis is indicative of their exacerbated production. The interaction of microorganisms and their derived products with host cells rapidly leads to the production of many inflammatory mediators including cytokines. Two major features characterize the production of these factors: cascade and regulatory loops (Figure 1). This means that, once produced, a given cytokine can induce the production of others which can further induce cytokine release or on the contrary down-regulate the upper-stream synthesis. Usually absent from the plasma at homeostasis, many cytokines are produced in such large amount during sepsis that they can be detected in the circulation of the patients.

While we will not focus our review on this aspect, it should be kept in mind that the production of these inflammatory cytokines is an integral part of the processes initiated by the innate immune response to fight infection.

SEPSIS IS ASSOCIATED WITH AN EXACERBATED PRODUCTION OF ANTI-INFLAMMATORY CYTOKINES AND MEDIATORS

Interleukin-1 (IL-1α, IL-1β)

Involvement of IL-1 in Sepsis

The network of inflammatory events is mainly orchestrated by interleukin-1 (IL-1) and tumor necrosis factor (TNF). Injection of IL-1 into animals results in hypotension, increased cardiac output and heart rate, leukopenia, thrombocytopenia, hemorrhage, and pulmonary edema [1]. Cyclooxygenase inhibitors greatly prevent these different effects. IL-1 receptor antagonist (IL-1ra), a natural IL-1 inhibitor, reduces mortality from endotoxic shock [2].

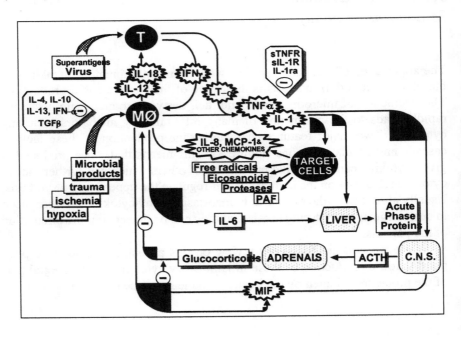

Figure 1. Cytokine loops in inflammation and sepsis

IL-1β converting enzyme (ICE) or caspase-1 is the enzyme required for the maturation of the 30 kDa biologically inactive IL-1β precursor to the mature

17 kDa active form of IL-1β. Survival to a lethal dose of endotoxin reaches 70% among ICE-deficient animals [3], while IL-1β deficient mice are normally sensitive to the lethal effect of LPS [4]. These results reflect that caspase-1 is also involved in the maturation of IL-18.

Detection of IL-1 in Sepsis

IL-1β has been regularly reported in plasma of sepsis patients whereas IL-1α has never been observed when investigated. IL-1β was found in 0 to 90% of septic patients depending on the studies, the nature of the sepsis and on the nature of the technique used to assess its presence. The highest frequency of detectable levels of IL-1β was observed among patients with meningococcal sepsis [5,6] and high levels of IL-1β correlate with the severity of meningococcemia, the presence of shock, high APACHE II scores and rapid fatal outcome [5,6,7,8]. Such correlations were not observed in other sepsis patients [9]. In a few studies, IL-1β survey was performed, and either high levels at admission followed by a decrease, or sustained levels, were reported [6,9,10].

Tumor Necrosis Factor (TNF)

Involvement of TNF in Sepsis

TNF-α toxicity includes hemodynamic instability, fever, diarrhea, metabolic acidosis, capillary leak syndrome, activation of coagulation, late hypoglycemia, induction of a catabolic state, neurotoxicity, cachexia, and renal and hematological disorders, all phenomena associated with sepsis syndrome [11]. In addition, together with IL-1, TNF induces on endothelial cells the expression of adhesion molecules involved in organ infiltration by leukocytes. A lethal effect of TNF was synergistically enhanced by IL-1 [1], interferon (IFN)-γ [12] and lipopolysaccharide (LPS) itself [13]. Anti-TNF treatments have been shown to be highly efficient in protecting animals against endotoxic shock [14] and lethal bacteremia [15]. Such treatments also protected against pulmonary microvascular injury after intestinal ischemia injury which is associated with endotoxin translocation [16]. Studies with mice rendered deficient for TNF or its receptors led to controversial results which reflected the different models - use of D-galactosamine, injection of bacteria, cecal ligation and puncture, injection of high dose LPS - and, as recently suggested by van der Meer's group in Nijmegen, differences in the bacterial origin of the LPS itself [17].

Detection of TNF in sepsis

In 1986, TNF was the first cytokine to be described in the serum of patients with septicemia [18], and later in patients with meningococcal sepsis [7,19]. While a correlation exists between poor outcome and high levels of measured circulating TNF in the case of meningococcal sepsis [7,19], in other forms of sepsis, some authors did observe such a correlation [10,20], while others did not [9,21]. Different authors have followed up the kinetics of plasma TNF and observed either an increase, a decrease, or sustained levels [9,10,20]. Indeed, as first shown by Baud et al. [21] and confirmed by Pinsky et al. [22], it seems that it is the persistence of detectable TNF rather than its peak level which is associated with the fatal outcome. When addressed, the TNF levels were found to correlate with the severity of illness and APACHE II scores [20,21]. It is worth noting that in intraperitoneal sepsis, on the contrary, high levels of circulating TNF are associated with a good prognosis while low levels correlated with fatal outcome [23,24]. Some authors reported that the TNF levels were higher in Gram-negative than in Gram-positive sepsis although this was not observed in all studies. In meningococcal sepsis, levels of TNF are higher in cerebrospinal fluids than in plasma [25] and not detected in the cerebrospinal fluid (CSF) of patients with non-bacterial meningitis [26]. Injection of LPS in human volunteers and in animal models leads to a plasma peak of TNF at 90 min, and its levels may be up-regulated by administration of ibuprofen [27] or G-CSF [28] and down-regulated by epinephrine [29].

Lymphotoxin-α (LT-α)

Lymphotoxin-α is a rare cytokine which is produced by a limited number of cells, essentially activated T-lymphocytes. It shares with TNF-α the same receptors and thus most of its activities. LT-α should be essentially expected in Gram-positive sepsis since Gram-positive bacteria release various T-cell activators known as superantigens. While the use of neutralizing antibodies could suggest that *Pseudomonas aeruginosa* infusion led to the appearance of TNF-α and LT-α in the circulation of pigs [30], LT-α has never been reported in human Gram negative sepsis [8]. On the contrary, in patients with streptococcal toxic shock syndrome, circulating LT-α was found to parallel the levels of the circulating superantigen [31].

Interleukin-2 (IL-2)

IL-2 is another cytokine which reflects T cell activation. While rarely reported in human sepsis [8,22], IL-2 was found in the circulation within two hours following injection of bacterial superantigens in mice [32] and baboons [33].

Interleukin-15 (IL-15)

IL-15 shares many functions with IL-2. The specific IL-15 receptor α-chain is associated with the IL-2 receptor β and γ-chains. While IL-2 is mainly produced by T lymphocytes, IL-15 is produced by endothelial cells and by monocytes/macrophages in response to exogenous stimuli such as bacteria and LPS. Importantly, it is expressed on the cell surface as an active molecule [34]. *In vivo*, it is induced by IL-12 [35]. In concert with other monokines (e.g. IL-12), IL-15 stimulates IFN-γ production by natural killer (NK) cells and is involved in the LPS-induced general Shwartzman reaction [36]. However, inhibition by specific antibodies of endogenous IL-15 production during *in vitro* LPS activation of murine macrophages further amplified TNF-α production [37]. The role of IL-15 during sepsis remains to be fully characterized while its presence has been reported in the plasma of septic patients [38].

Leukemia Inhibitory Factor (LIF), Oncostatin M (OSM), Ciliary Neurotrophic Factor (CNTF)

Involvement of LIF and OSM in Sepsis

LIF, CNTF, and OSM belong to the IL-6 superfamily, sharing the gp130 chain of the receptor. However, while IL-6 and IL-11 possess certain anti-inflammatory properties (see below), LIF and OSM can be considered as pro-inflammatory cytokines. Indeed, LIF is involved in the pathogenesis of inflammation and sepsis syndrome [39]. Induced by LPS and TNF, LIF can induce the release of other cytokines including IL-1, IL-6, and IL-8 by various cell types. Passive immunization against LIF in mice challenged with intraperitoneal administration of endotoxin protected them from the lethal effects and blocked increases in serum levels of IL-1 and IL-6 [40]. Subcutaneous injection of OSM in mice caused an acute inflammatory reaction [41]. OSM favored PMN adhesion to endothelial cells and transmigration via its capacity to enhance the expression of P- and E-selectin, intercellular adhesion molecule (ICAM)-1, and vascular cell adhesion molecule (VCAM)-1. Furthermore, OSM induces the release of IL-6 and ENA78 (an α-chemokine) but not that of IL-8.

Detection of LIF, CNTF, and OSM in Sepsis

First reported in 1992, detectable levels of LIF were occasionally found in plasma of 9 to 40% septic patients [39,42,43]. Levels of circulating LIF correlate with shock, temperature, creatinine and IL-6 [42]. The correlation of LIF with IL-6 has been confirmed in a baboon model of sepsis [44]. Levels of plasma CNTF and OSM are elevated in 60% and 100% septic patients, respectively [43].

Interleukin-8 (IL-8) and Chemokines

Involvement of Chemokines in Sepsis

Sepsis and SIRS are often associated with organ dysfunction that reflects the inflammatory process occurring in the tissues. One of the major features of this phenomenon is the recruitment of inflammatory leukocytes. It implies the adherence of circulating cells to the endothelium and their margination towards the tissues in response to the locally produced chemokines. Chemokines represent a family of more than 40 members. These chemokines contribute to the inflammatory cell infiltrate that participates in the disruption of tissue integrity. For example, neutralization of IL-8 profoundly inhibited neutrophil recruitment in an endotoxin-induced rabbit model of pleurisy, indicating that IL-8 is a major chemotactic factor in this model of acute inflammation [45]. During sepsis a great amount of IL-8 is detectable within the blood compartment, not only as a free cytokine [46] but also as a cell-associated form [47]. This first encounter of neutrophils with IL-8 leads to their desensitization to further signals delivered locally by IL-8. Thus, the presence of IL-8 in the vascular space may well be a mechanism that limits neutrophil accumulation at extracellular sites as illustrated by the defect in neutrophil migration capacity during sepsis or endotoxemia [48,49]. Similarly, while monocyte-chemoattractant protein-1 (MCP-1) contributes to the recruitment of inflammatory macrophages within the tissues, neutralization of MCP-1 by specific antibodies before LPS administration resulted in a striking increase in mortality and the injection of MCP-1 was protective [50]. In contrast, mice rendered deficient for the receptor of MCP-1 (CCR4-/-) which also binds macrophage inflammatory protein (MIP)-1α, regulated on activation, normal T-cell-expressed and secreted (RANTES), macrophage-derived chemokine (MDC) and thymus- and activation-regulated chemokine (TARC), exhibited significantly decreased mortality on administration of LPS [51]. These controversial results illustrate the influence of the experimental models. Furthermore, one should keep in mind that the recruitment of leukocytes by chemokines is a prerequisite to address the infectious process as elegantly shown by the deleterious effect of blocking MDC in the cecal ligation and puncture model of peritonitis in mice [52].

Detection of Chemokines in Sepsis

As first reported in 1992, a great amount of IL-8 is detectable within the blood compartment during sepsis [53,54] and in broncho-alveolar lavage (BAL) and edema fluid of acute respiratory distress syndrome (ARDS)-associated with sepsis [55]. In this study, patients with high levels of IL-8 in BAL had a high mortality rate. Similarly, high levels of plasma IL-8 correlate with the occurrence of shock [56], with the presence of infectious multiple organ failure (MOF) [46] and with poor outcome [46,53,54]. No difference in IL-8 plasma levels were found between Gram-negative and Gram positive infection [54] while in bacteremic pneumonia the type of pathogen influenced the measurable levels of IL-8 [57]. IL-8 levels also correlate with various markers including IL-6 [5,46,54], C3a, α1-anti-trypsin, lactate [54], IL-10, IL-1ra and soluble TNF receptors (sTNFR) [5]. Correlation with plasma TNF led to controversial results [5,58]. More interestingly, local levels of IL-8 often correlate with the number of recruited neutrophils [55] and plasma levels are associated with granulocyte activation as evidenced by massive release of elastase detectable in the circulation of bacteremic baboons [59] and by correlation between elastase and IL-8 in human sepsis [56].

In addition to IL-8, increased levels of various chemokines have been found in plasma of septic patients or following LPS injection in human volunteers. This is the case for MCP-1 and MCP-2 [60], MIP-1α and MIP-1β

[61] and IFN-γ-inducible protein (IP-10) [62], MCP-1 levels being higher in patients with the more severe forms of sepsis (i.e., those with shock or a lethal outcome). In a preliminary study, we found that plasma levels of RANTES were inversely correlated with APACHE II score, and lower levels of this chemokine were found in non-surviving sepsis patients (J-M. Cavaillon and D. Payen, unpublished observation).

Interleukin-12 (IL-12)

Involvement of IL-12 in Sepsis

IL-12 is a heterodimeric cytokine of p40 and p35 subunits. The measurement of p70 heterodimer is correlated with IL-12 bioactivity. IL-12 is a potent inducer of IFN-γ. Its injection in chimpanzees induces an increase in plasma concentrations of IFN-γ as well as IL-15, IL-18, α- and β-chemokines and anti-inflammatory mediators [35]. Among the adverse effects of IL-12, hepato- and splenomegaly, leukopenia, anemia, and myelodepression have been reported [63]. These phenomena were largely IFN-γ-dependent since they were not reported to occur in IFN-γ receptor deficient mice. Hepatomegaly is associated with infiltration of activated macrophages and NK cells, and single-cell necrosis. In contrast, pulmonary edema and interstitial macrophage infiltration generated by IL-12 injection were shown to be IFN-γ-independent. In a Mycobacterium bovis Bacille Calmette-Guerin (BCG)-primed model of LPS-induced shock and lethality, anti-IL-12 antibodies were associated with decreased IFN-γ and were shown to protect mice if injected before endotoxin [64]. In contrast, in a cecal ligation and puncture model, IL-12 neutralization was deleterious [65]. The later observation is in agreement with other reports which demonstrated the beneficial effects of IL-12 in the infectious process [66]

Detection of IL-12 in Sepsis

Bioactive IL-12 was detected in mouse serum at 2 to 4 h after LPS injection [67] and in baboons, surprisingly, higher levels of IL-12 were detectable in plasma of animals injected with sublethal doses of *E. coli* than in animals challenged with lethal doses [68]. In humans, an intravenous bolus injection of *E. coli* LPS in volunteers did not lead to changes in the plasma levels of IL-12 [69] and IL-12 could not be measured in most septic patients [70].

While higher levels of IL-12p40 were found in patients with severe melioidosis (infection with *Burkholderia pseudomallei*) than in healthy controls, IL-12p70, not detectable in controls, was only found in 10% of the patients [38].

Interleukin-18 (IL-18)

Involvement of IL-18 in Sepsis

IL-18 is structurally related to the IL-1 family and its maturation is under the control of caspase-1. Produced by activated macrophages and Kupffer cells, IL-18 is a potent inducer of IFN-γ [71]. While IL-18 promotes resolution of bacterial infection in mice [72], it accounts for both TNF-α and Fas ligand-mediated hepatotoxic pathways in endotoxin-induced liver injury in this model [73]. Neutralization of IL-18 protects mice against lethal *E. coli* and *S. typhimurium* endotoxemia [74] and IL-18 deficient mice showed decreased sensitivity towards LPS-induced shock [75], although this might depend upon the model since *Propionibacterium acnes*-primed IL-18-/- mice were highly susceptible to LPS [76]. It is worth noting that, in contrast, IL-18-/- mice and normal mice were similarly responsive to bacterial superantigen [75].

Detection of IL-18 in Sepsis

Plasma IL-18 is found in healthy controls and its level was enhanced in patients with melioidosis [38]; levels were higher in bacteremic patients and correlated with APACHE II score, and there was a weak correlation with IFNγ levels (r = 0.48).

Interferon-γ (IFN-γ)

Involvement of IFN-γ in Sepsis

IFN-γ is an efficient amplification cytokine produced by T-lymphocytes in response either to IL-12 and/or IL-18 produced by monocytes/macrophages activated by microbial products or by superantigens or viruses. Its synergy with the detrimental activities of LPS has been clearly established: IFN-γ enhanced LPS-induced circulating TNF-α as well as LPS- and TNF-induced mortality [12,77] and anti-IFN-γ antibodies protected against LPS- and *E. coli*-induced mortality [77,78]. As a consequence, a clinically silent viral infection may induce hypersensitivity to Gram-negative bacterial endotoxin through T cell activation and subsequent IFN-γ production, leading to a hyperproduction of TNF-α [79]. Mice lacking IFN-γ receptor have been shown to be resistant to LPS challenge after priming with BCG [80] or treatment with D-galactosamine [81]. A mouse model of endotoxemia revealed that IFN-γ was not involved in pulmonary edema [82]. Side-effects of IFN-γ include tachychardia, myalgia, malaise, leukopenia, and weakness.

Detection of IFN-γ in Sepsis

The study of circulating IFN-γ in human sepsis led to contradictory results. While in sepsis and purpura fulminans, IFN-γ was found in patients with the most severe disease [7], no correlation was reported with outcome in other studies on sepsis and septic shock [10,22]. No detectable IFN-γ was reported in meningococcal septic shock [8] and in human volunteers receiving systemic endotoxin [69]. IFN-γ was recently detected in the plasma in 71% of patients with melioidosis [38]. In a baboon septic shock model, IFN-γ levels were threefold higher in lethally challenged animals than in those receiving sublethal doses [68].

Interleukin-16 (IL-16) and IL-17

IL-16 and IL-17 are recently described cytokines with ill-defined physiologic properties. Both were discovered as T-cell products, and IL-16 can also be produced by eosinophils, mast cells, and epithelial cells. It is worth mentioning that both can stimulate the production of pro-inflammatory cytokines. IL-16 induces the secretion of IL-1β, IL-6, IL-15 and TNF-α [83] and IL-17 up-regulates the expression of IL-1β, TNF-α, IL-6, IL-12, PGE2 as well as IL-1ra and IL-10 [84]. However, their involvement during sepsis has not been addressed so far.

Colony stimulating factors (CSF)

Involvement of CSFs in Sepsis

In addition to their well known action on hematopoiesis, CSFs favor the anti-infectious process and may reduce the natural apoptosis of neutrophils. However, among these cytokines, IL-3, previously called 'multi-CSF', and granulocyte-macrophage CSF (GM-CSF) can amplify the production of IL-1 and TNF-α, and thus behave as pro-inflammatory cytokines. The deleterious effect of GM-CSF is exemplified by the response of GM-CSF-deficient mice to endotoxin: following LPS injection, hypothermia, loss in body weight, levels of circulating IFN-γ, IL-1α, and IL-6 were markedly reduced as compared to normal mice. Furthermore, the survival to one LD100 of LPS was 42% among GM-CSF-/- mice [85].

In contrast, numerous studies have reported that granulocyte-CSF (G-CSF) possesses many beneficial properties. It has been demonstrated that G-CSF reduces endotoxemia and improves survival during *E. coli* pneumonia [86], reduces bacterial translocation due to burn wound sepsis [87], and enhances the phagocytic function of neutrophils in septic animals [88]. Furthermore, in combination with antibiotics, G-CSF can prevent severe infectious complication in a peritonitis model [89] and in combination with IL-11 prevents the occurrence of lethality to a bacterial challenge in neutropenic animals [90].

Detection of CSF in Sepsis

In humans, M-CSF is present at homeostasis in the circulation and its level is increased in patients with sepsis and higher in patients with sepsis-associated hemophagocytosis [91]. G-CSF is also increased in sepsis and reaches higher levels in severe sepsis as compared to sepsis or bacteremia [92]. Enhanced levels of circulating G-CSF have been particularly associated with infection and sepsis in neonates [93]. In meningococcemia, plasma GM-CSF concentrations were briefly present in subjects with life-threatening septic shock and were strongly associated with fulminant disease [92]. GM-CSF was also markedly elevated in septic preterm infants [94].

Fas ligand (FasL)

Fas (CD95) is a member of the TNF receptor superfamily which contains a cytoplasmic death domain. Its ligation with its ligand (FasL) results in the induction of apoptosis. FasL exists as a membrane form or a soluble molecule. While sepsis is associated with a delayed apoptosis of neutrophils, an increased apoptosis in hematopoietic tissues such as thymus, Peyer's patch, spleen and bone marrow has been regularly observed. Using FasL deficient mice, it was established that the sepsis-associated apoptosis of lymphoid cells was a FasL-dependent process [95]. mRNA for Fas and FasL were highly up-regulated in BAL cells during the acute phase of human ARDS following sepsis [96] Enhanced levels of soluble FasL were measured in the BAL of these patients while soluble FasL was absent from BAL of healthy controls.

Macrophage Migration Inhibitory Factor (MIF)

MIF was first discovered in 1966 as a T-cell product released during delayed-type hypersensitivity [97] and rediscovered in 1993 as a pituitary-derived cytokine that potentiates lethal endotoxemia [98]. MIF is now recognized as a macrophage product [99] induced by the action of glucocorticoids [100]. MIF is expressed constitutively in many tissues including lung, liver, kidney, spleen, adrenal gland, and skin. MIF exists as a preformed cytokine which is rapidly released following LPS injection [101]. Bernhagen et al. [98] reported that injection of MIF together with one LD40 of LPS greatly potentiated lethality and that anti-MIF antibodies fully protected against one LD50 of LPS. Accordingly, MIF-deficient mice were more resistant to LPS induced lethality [102]. This phenomenon was associated with a reduced level of circulating TNF, an enhanced level of nitric oxide (NO) and no effect on IL-6, IL-10 and IL-12 levels. Anti-MIF antibodies also protected mice from lethal experimental peritonitis, even when treatment was started up to 8h after induction of peritonitis. [103]. While MIF is present in the plasma of healthy controls, its levels are significantly enhanced in septic patients [103].

High Mobility Group-1 (HMG-1) Protein

HMG-1 is a highly conserved nuclear protein that binds cruciform DNA. It exists as a membrane form and as an extracellular form which interacts with plasminogen and tissue type plasminogen activator (t-PA). It is produced by macrophages in response to LPS and by pituitary cell stimulated by IL-1 or TNF [104]. HMG-1 was reported to be a late mediator involved in endotoxin lethality in mice. HMG-1 has been found in plasma of septic patients, with significantly higher levels in non-survivors than in survivors [104].

Cellular Signaling Induced by Pro-inflammatory Cytokines

The Nuclear Factor-kappa B (NF-κB) and the Mitogen-activated Protein Kinase (MAPK) Pathways

During the inflammatory processes the inducible transcription factor NF-κB plays a major role in the intracellular signaling. Indeed, this is one of the main nuclear factors that regulates the transcription of numerous genes including cytokines, especially pro-inflammatory cytokines such as TNF-α, IL-1α, IL-6 and IL-8, cytokine receptors, acute phase proteins and leukocyte adhesion molecules. These components are important for the recruitment of circulating cells towards the inflammatory focus [105,106]. The NF-κB family is composed of various members, p50 (NF-κB1), p52 (NF-κB2), p65 (RelA), RelB and c-Rel, which can form homo- and heterodimers [107]. Numerous studies have shown that the transactivator form of NF-κB is the p65 unit while the p50 unit showed no or minimal activation capacities [108,109,110]. The transactivator form of NF-κB is the p65p50 heterodimer in mammalian cells, although some reports show transactivatory activities of p50p50 in cell-free *in vitro* transcription systems [111,112] or in yeast [113]. Fujita et al. [112] found that p50p50 could behave as a gene activator when complexed to the Bcl-3 protein, but another report shows that Bcl-3 facilitates the NF-κB transactivation by removing the inhibitory p50p50 from the κB-sites [114]. NF-κB is regulated by a cytoplasmic inhibitor: IκB. This protein is also a member of a large family that includes IκBα, IκBβ, IκBγ, IκBε and Bcl-3. All possess multiple regions of homology known as the ankyrin-repeat motifs, also present in the precursors of p50 and p52 (p105 and p100 respectively) which also behave as NF-κB inhibitors.

Among cytokines, TNF and IL-1 are potent activators of NF-κB, but this transcription factor is also inducible by other extracellular signals such as reactive oxygen species and complement fragments. Furthermore, endotoxin is a potent activator of NF-κB. During the past few years, many insights have been reached about the LPS signaling. These include the characterization of Toll-like receptor 4 (TLR4), the co-receptor of CD14, responsible of the signal transduction [115] and that of the MD-2 molecule which is associated to TLR4 at the cell surface [116]. In unstimulated cells, NF-κB is retained in the cytoplasm by IκB as an inactive complex. As shown in Figure 2, the binding of TNF, IL-1 or LPS to their receptors recruits adaptor molecules which leads to the activation of an NF-κB-inducing kinase (NIK) [117]. NIK seems to be the convergent point of the TNF and IL-1-mediated NF-κB activation, since mutant forms of NIK block the signaling from the receptors of both cytokines [117]. The final step of the kinase cascade leads to the activation of protein kinases that phosphorylate IκB. These IκB kinases (IKK) are associated to a high-molecular weight cytoplasmic complex [118]. In addition to NIK, MEKK-1 (a kinase implicated in the c-jun N-terminal kinase [JNK] pathway of MAPK) has been shown to phosphorylate and activate IKKα and β [119]. Recently, a new component of the IL-1RI pathway and a new intermediate in the signal transduction pathway of IL-1 and Toll have been characterized: the first molecule, called Tollip, allows the death domain of MyD88 and IL-1-receptor associated kinase (IRAK) to interact [120]; the second molecule, an adapter protein named evolutionary conserved signaling intermediate in Toll pathway (ECSIT), makes the link between TNF-receptor-associated factor (TRAF)-6 and MEKK-1 [121]. In addition, the characterization of ECSIT also supports the existence of a MEKK-1-mediated activation of NF-κB. After the activation of the IKK, IκB is phosphorylated on serines 32 and 36, leading to its subsequent ubiquitination and its degradation by the 26S proteasome pathway. Finally, after the degradation of IκB, the NF-κB dimer can translocate into the nucleus, bind to DNA and activate the transcription of target genes.

The MAPK cascades are another intracellular signaling pathway activated during the inflammatory process and they also lead to the activation of numerous transcription factors. Three MAPK cascades have been described to date, the extracellular signal-regulated kinases (ERK), the JNK/stress-activated protein kinase (SAPK) and the p38 pathways. The activation of extracellular signal-related kinase (ERK)-1 and -2, also known as p44 and p42, is triggered by mitogens and growth factors, while the two other cascades are activated by IL-1, TNF, LPS and cell stress [122,123]. c-jun is a component of the activator protein (AP)-1 transcription factor and the JNK cascade leads to its phosphorylation and an enhancement of its capacity to activate transcription.

The p38 kinase is implicated in the activation of various transcription factors and some evidence indicates that it can play a role in the activation of NF-κB. Indeed, it has been shown that the specific inhibitor of p38 (SB203580) prevented the expression of a reporter gene under the control of NF-κB [124]. However, this was not due to an inhibition of the binding of NF-κB to DNA. Thus, p38 does not seem to regulate IκB phosphorylation, but it most probably modulates the transactivation capacity of NF-κB *via* MAPK activated protein kinases (MAPKAP) that in turn phosphorylate the p65 subunit. TNF and IL-1 contribute to the activation of JNK and p38 MAPK.

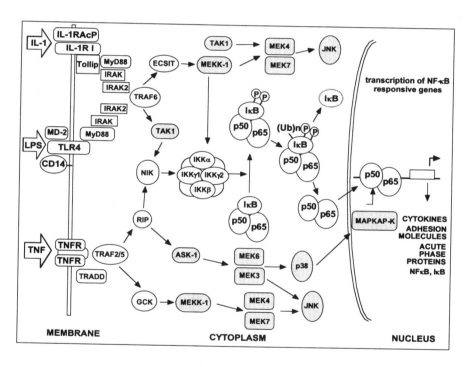

Figure 2. Cascade of NF-κB activation induced by LPS, TNF and IL-1. The binding of TNF to its receptors activates the NF-κB-inducing kinase (NIK) via its interaction with adaptor molecules: TNF receptor-associated death domain protein (TRADD), receptor interacting protein (RIP) and TNF receptor-associated factor-2 and 5 (TRAF-2/5). LPS signaling requires CD14, the Toll-like receptor 4 (TLR4) and the MD-2 surface protein. IL-1 signaling needs IL-1 receptor accessory protein (IL-1RAcP), the co-receptor of IL-1RI, MyD88 a death domain-containing protein, IL-1 receptor associated kinases (IRAK) that activate NIK via TRAF6 and TAK-1. The evolutionary conserved signaling intermediate in Toll (ECSIT) pathway is the intermediate between TRAF6 and MEKK-1 (a MAPK kinase kinase). p38 another MAPK also contributes to NF-κB activation (NB. the MAPK are represented in gray).

For TNF, it has been shown that TNF receptor-associated death domain (TRADD), TRAF2 and receptor interacting protein (RIP) are implicated in the signaling leading to JNK and p38 activation [125,126]. Furthermore, another kinase, the germinal center kinase (GCK), has been shown to interact with TRAF2 and MEKK-1 and thus could be the link between the events taking place at the receptor level and the MAPK kinase kinase (MAPKKK) [126]. For IL-1, MyD88 and IRAK are also needed for the signaling. IRAK-deficient mice showed reduced IL-1-mediated JNK and p38 activation [127]. Similarly, overexpression of MyD88 induced the activation of both JNK and NF-κB while mutant forms of MyD88 inhibited their activation [128].

NF-κB in Sepsis: A New Target for Therapy ?

NF-κB has been studied in various *in vitro* and *in vivo* models of sepsis, yet less is known about the status of this transcription factor in humans. Enhanced NF-κB activation has been reported in alveolar macrophages of patients with ARDS [129] and in the lungs and the liver of mice after experimental peritonitis [130,131]. Similarly, after hemorrhage or LPS, NF-κB was activated in lung neutrophils while it was not in circulating neutrophils [132]. The measurement of inflammatory mediators (cytokines, iNOS) also suggests that the consequence of systemic inflammation may differ in the blood and the other tissues and favors the concept of a compartmentalization of inflammation. Indeed, iNOS activity was found to be restricted to the nidus of infection in patients undergoing septic shock after cellulitis [133]. Similarly, after chest trauma, significantly higher levels of IL-1β and IL-8 were found in BAL fluid. In contrast, anti-inflammatory mediators (sTNFRI and II, IL-1ra) were present both locally and systemically [134]. Furthermore, an exacerbated production of cytokines has often been demonstrated in non-hematopoietic compartments [135,136], in contrast with the hyporeactivity of circulating cells which will be discussed later. Indeed, the analysis of NF-κB performed with cells derived from the tissues stands in contrast with the experiments performed with peripheral blood mononuclear cells (PBMC). The first reported analysis in septic patients, showed a higher *ex vivo* nuclear expression of NF-κB in the PBMC of the non-survivors [137]. We performed a similar study and confirmed that total NF-κB content is higher in the nucleus of PBMC from non-survivors as compared to survivors of severe sepsis. However, we found that the nuclear p65p50, the active form of NF-κB, was significantly reduced in all patients with severe sepsis as compared to controls and demonstrated that in the non-survivors, NF-κB was mostly composed of the inactive form p50p50 [138].

This down regulation of NF-κB in circulating mononuclear cells was also found when the systemic inflammation was not of infectious origin (major trauma).

Because of its fundamental role in acute inflammation, NF-κB has been chosen by several investigators as a target for the treatment of sepsis. Inhibitors of NF-κB, such as dithiocarbamate (PDTC) or N-acetyl-leucinyl-leucinyl-norleucinal (a potent inhibitor of the proteasome pathway) were tested in animal models of endotoxin shock, encouraged by the inhibiting effect of dithiocarbamate on human immunodeficiency virus (HIV) progression in patients [139]. Treatment with these inhibitors of NF-κB decreased NO synthase (NOS) expression within the tissues [140] and TNF and IL-6 levels in the serum [141], and reduced microvascular injury and disseminated intravascular coagulation (DIC) [142,143]. The limit of these studies is that in all but one [143], the inhibitors had to be administered before the LPS challenge in order to be effective. Furthermore, at high doses, PDTC is toxic and has non-specific effects: it can activate AP-1 another transcription factor that induces pro-inflammatory cytokines. Finally, even if NF-κB is the major transcription factor involved in the pro-inflammatory cascade, its blockade may not be sufficient as other transcription factors, such as AP-1, NF-IL6 or cAMP responsive element binding protein (CREB) can also take part in the induction of inflammatory mediators. Our observation of a dysregulation of NF-κB translocation in PBMC of patients with severe sepsis and the low presence of cytoplasmic IκBα suggest that despite the successful use of drugs in animal models of sepsis, the inhibition of NF-κB activation may not be appropriate to treat septic patients. This approach may prove to be useful if it can be delivered at the onset of inflammation or within defined compartments.

SEPSIS IS ASSOCIATED WITH AN EXACERBATED PRODUCTION OF ANTI-INFLAMMATORY CYTOKINES AND MEDIATORS

Interleukin-6 (IL-6)

Involvement of IL-6 in Sepsis

Although IL-6 is often considered as an inflammatory cytokine, most of its activities are probably associated with a negative control of inflammation thanks to its potent capacity to induce the production of acute phase proteins by the liver as well as the release of IL-1ra and sTNFR [144].

Detection of IL-6 in Sepsis

The presence of IL-6 in the plasma of sepsis patients was first reported in 1989 [8, 145]. Plasma IL-6 has been observed in 64% to 100% of studied patients. Most investigators have demonstrated that levels of circulating IL-6 correlate with severity of sepsis and may predict outcome [8,9,145,146] as illustrated by the correlation between IL-6 levels and APACHE II scores [6,147]. Numerous correlations between IL-6 levels and other markers have been reported including C3a, lactate [145], circulating endotoxin [5,148], C-reactive protein (CRP) [147] and TNF [5,8,146]. IL-6 levels are similar in Gram-positive or Gram-negative sepsis [9]. Injection of endotoxin in human volunteers revealed that the peak IL-6 level was reached 2h after injection [149,150]

Interleukin-11 (IL-11)

IL-11 belongs to the IL-6 superfamily. Although IL-11 stimulated the production of several major acute phase proteins by hepatoma cells, circulating IL-11 did not significantly participate in the production of acute-phase proteins by the liver [151]. One of the major beneficial effects of IL-11 which has been described is related to its healing activity on the intestinal tract. For example, chemotherapy and radiation both damage the small intestinal mucosa barrier and lead to the entry of gastrointestinal flora into the blood. In this lethal model, IL-11 was able to protect 80% of the animals [152]. Beneficial properties of IL-11 have also been demonstrated in a rat neonatal infectious model with group B streptococci. Prophylactic use of IL-11 enhanced the survival in this model in association with an increased number of platelets [153]. Divergent reports concern IL-11 which was detected in 67% of patients with disseminated intravascular coagulation complicated by sepsis [154] but not in patients suffering from septic shock [43].

IL-1 receptor Antagonist (IL-1ra)

Involvement of IL-1ra in Sepsis

IL-1ra is a natural IL-1 inhibitor. Produced by many cell types, including monocytes/macrophages, it is also produced by the liver as an acute phase protein [155]. Early treatment with IL-1ra reduced mortality from endotoxic shock [2], prevented *Staphylococcus epidermidis*-induced hypotension [156], and improved survival and hemodynamic performance in *E. coli* septic shock [157]. Depending on the dose of IL-1ra, it either reduced or enhanced lethality in a model of *Klebsiella pneumoniae* infection of new born rats [158]. In agreement with these observations, IL-1ra-deficient mice were more susceptible than controls to lethal endotoxemia [159].

Detection of IL-1ra in Sepsis

IL-1ra is present in plasma in healthy persons. Enhanced levels of IL-1ra have been regularly reported in critically ill patients, septic adults, and new born patients [6,160,161]. It may correlate with APACHE II score [6]. As an antagonist, its concentration has to be at least 100 fold higher than that of IL-1 to efficiently block the effects of this cytokine. Indeed 2,000 fold higher concentration have been noted in patients with septic shock [6]. In two patients who died within 3 h to 8 h after admission with a *Streptococcus* group A or *Neisseria meningitidis* septicemia we found a 3,400 and 61,000 fold higher concentration of IL-1ra than IL-1β, respectively [162,163]. These observations suggest that the balance between pro- and anti-inflammatory cytokines seems adequate to limit the effects of pro-inflammatory cytokines.

Soluble IL-1 Receptors (sIL-1R)

Both IL-1 receptors can be shed by the cells and bind to IL-1β. However, the soluble form of IL-1R type I has no discernable anti-inflammatory property following endotoxin administration in human volunteers [164]. This may reflect the fact that sIL-1RI has a similar affinity for IL-1α, IL-1β than for IL-1ra [165]. In contrast, the soluble form of the type II receptor, also known as the decoy receptor, binds IL-1β with higher affinity than IL-1ra and inhibits IL-1 activity. Plasma levels of sIL-1RII in patients with sepsis syndrome were higher than those of sIL-1RI [166].

Soluble TNF Receptors (sTNFR)

The soluble forms of the TNF receptors (sTNFRI and sTNFRII) are natural inhibitors capable of limiting TNF bioactivity. Injection into animal models of sepsis was also shown to be essentially protective [167,168]. Sepsis is associated with an enhanced plasma level of soluble TNF receptors. In children with severe meningococcemia, high levels of sTNFRI and II correlates with a poor outcome [169]. In meningococcemia as well as in sepsis, high levels of sTNFRI and II correlate with TNF-α levels [170,171]. Increased levels of sTNFR can be induced by an injection of LPS [170,171] or following injections of IL-1 [172] or TNF [173].

Interleukin-10

Involvement of IL-10 in Sepsis

IL-10 is a well known cytokine which exerts its anti-inflammatory properties particularly on monocytes/macrophages, neutrophils and T-lymphocytes. IL-10 is capable of preventing lethality in experimental endotoxemia [174] and IL-10 deficient mice were far more sensitive to LPS-induced lethality than wild-type animals [175]. In addition, neutralization of IL-10 in endotoxemia and during experimental septic peritonitis illustrated that endogenously produced IL-10 was instrumental in down-regulating the overzealous production of pro-inflammatory cytokines [176,177]. In this context, it is interesting to recall the observation by Donnelly et al. [178] that a poor prognosis in patients with ARDS was significantly associated with the lowest levels of IL-10 and IL-1ra.

Detection of IL-10 in Sepsis

Significant amounts of IL-10 are detected in the circulation of septic patients [179,180]. The highest plasma levels of this regulatory molecule are detected in the most severe cases (with shock or with poor prognosis) [178,181]. The ratio of IL-10 to TNF-α is also associated with poor outcome [181]. These observations illustrate that sepsis is not associated with a deficient anti-inflammatory response. In contrast, the exacerbated production of anti-inflammatory cytokines in sepsis cautions against a widespread use of therapeutical approaches only targeting the pro-inflammatory mediators. Indeed, the overproduction of anti-inflammatory cytokines and mediators led to the concept of the "compensatory anti-inflammatory response syndrome" (CARS) [182]. This is further suggested by the work of P. Brantzaeg et al. [183] who showed that plasma IL-10 was in part responsible for the monocyte deactivation noticed in sepsis (see below).

Interleukin-4 and Interleukin-13

In addition to IL-10, IL-4, IL-13, transforming growth factor (TGF)-β and IFN-α also possess strong anti-inflammatory activities and a potent capacity to inhibit the synthesis of the pro-inflammatory cytokines. Each individual anti-inflammatory cytokine has been demonstrated to be capable of reducing mortality in various endotoxic or septic shock models. IL-4 prevented mortality from acute but not from chronic murine peritonitis [184]. All mice pre-treated with IL-4 survived an i.p. injection of 10^7 live *E. coli* and 10^9 *Bacteroides fragilis* which killed 90% of the control animals. Using IL-4 deficient mice it was established that IL-4 can protect against TNF-mediated cachexia and death during parasitic infection [185]. However, pre-treatment with IL-4 before the induction of sepsis was protective whereas an increased mortality was reported when IL-4 was given at the time of infection [186]. This illustrates the importance of the timing and reconfirms the idea that one should be very cautious when referring to a too simplistic dichotomy between pro- and anti-inflammatory cytokines [187].

IL-13, which shares many activities with IL-4, fully protected mice from a LD90 i.p. injection of LPS [188,189]. IL-13 blockade with anti-IL-13 antibodies significantly decreased the survival rate of mice after experimental peritonitis and enhanced tissue injury which was associated with an increased expression of many chemokines [190]. This latter result suggests that, despite the absence of detectable circulating IL-4 or IL-13 in human sepsis [69,191], these cytokines may well be involved in the control of the exacerbated release of pro-inflammatory cytokines.

Interleukin-9

IL-9 is a T-cell derived cytokine, originally described as a growth factor for T cells and mast cells. Prophylactic injections of IL-9 conferred resistance of mice challenged with a lethal concentration of *Pseudomonas aeruginosa* [192]. The protective effect was correlated with a marked decrease of serum levels of TNF-α, IL-12 and IFN-γ as well as an increase of circulating IL-10 and IL-10 mRNA expression in the spleen. Interestingly, a shorter and lesser expression of IL-9 mRNA was observed in the spleen of mice after a lethal challenge than in mice after a sublethal bacterial challenge. To our knowledge, IL-9 has not yet been investigated in human sepsis.

Transforming Growth Factor-β (TGF-β)

Injection of TGF-β in mice before, or even together with, high doses of LPS was associated with a reduced mortality [193]. In a rat model of endotoxemia, TGF-β markedly reduced inducible NOS mRNA and protein levels in organs, arrested LPS-induced hypotension and decreased mortality [194]. Measurements of circulating TGF-β1 are controversial, most probably because of the difficulty to measure it and the fact that a latent and an active form already exist in normal plasma. Furthermore, since platelets are an important source of TGF-β1, measurements in plasma, platelet-poor plasma or sera may explain the discrepancies in the literature. Karres et al. [195] and Astiz et al [196] reported a reduced level in sera from septic patients. The mean levels of serum TGF-β1 in healthy controls were in the range of ng/ml in one study and pg/ml in the other, illustrating the difficulty linked to its measurement. On the other hand, we found enhanced levels in plasma and platelet-poor plasma in patients with sepsis [197]. We found a correlation (r = 0.87, p = 0.01) between levels of TGF-β1 in pleural effusion and in BAL fluid from septic patients whereas there was no correlation with plasma levels [198]. In a baboon septic model, Junger et al. [199] reported that active TGF-β levels increased while total TGF-β decreased. In a rat model of sepsis, circulating levels of TGF-β were found to be increased and to contribute to the depressed T-cell functions [200].

Interferon-α (IFN-α)

IFN-α prevented LPS-induced mortality in mice and reduced TNF mRNA expression in the spleen and liver [201]. The most fascinating observation was the capacity of IFN-α to be effective even when administered long after LPS. This contrasts with many reports in which the protective cytokine or drug had to be administered before or simultaneously with LPS. Surprisingly, very few other studies have addressed the role of IFN-α in sepsis

EX VIVO CYTOKINE PRODUCTION TO MONITOR SEPSIS-ASSOCIATED IMMUNE DEPRESSION

Sepsis syndrome is associated with an exacerbated *in vivo* production of pro- and anti-inflammatory cytokines as assessed by their increased levels in the blood stream. Paradoxically, a reduced capacity of circulating leukocytes from septic patients to produce cytokines as compared to cells from healthy controls has been regularly reported. The very first observation on the hyporeactivity of circulating cells in septic patients was demonstrated with peripheral blood lymphocytes. In the initial study, Wood et al. [202] reported a decreased IL-2 production upon phytohemaglutinin (PHA) stimulation. More recently, IFN-γ production was also reported to be affected in sepsis as well as in patients with severe injury [203]. While it is often suggested that the depressed response mainly affects the production of the Th1 cytokines (IL-2, IFN-γ), we demonstrated that the production of Th2 cytokines (IL-5, IL-10) could also be altered and that the nature of the triggering agent itself influences the observation [204]. Monocyte reactivity to LPS stimulation has been particularly studied in isolated monocytes and in whole-blood assays. Monocytes from septic patients had a diminished capacity to release TNF-α, IL-1α, IL-1β, IL-6, IL-10 and IL-12 [203,205,206,207,208] whereas this was not the case for IL-1ra [206]. Reduced cytokine production has also been observed with other stimuli such as silica, staphylococcal enterotoxin B, killed *Streptococcus* and *Staphylococcus* [196,203,209,210]. Similar hyporeactivity has been reported for the production of IL-1β, IL-1ra and IL-8 by LPS-activated neutrophils from septic patients [211,212,213].

Although the anergy of the cells observed in septic patients has been associated with endotoxin tolerance [211], this phenomenon is neither specific for endotoxin [214] nor for septic patients. Indeed, in many stressful conditions including trauma, thermal injury, hemorrhage, and severe surgery, hyporesponsiveness of circulating leukocytes and low cytokine production have been regularly reported and associated with immune depression observed in these patients.

Thus, during systemic inflammation, systemic inflammatory response syndrome (SIRS) and CARS seem to be present simultaneously; SIRS predominating within the inflamed tissues while in the blood, leukocytes show hyporeactivity (Figure 3).

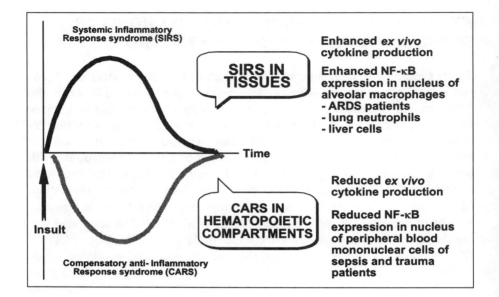

Figure 3. *Compartmentalization of the inflammatory response.*

WHICH CYTOKINE MEASUREMENTS ?

We will not discuss in detail the technical aspects linked to cytokine measurements as these have been addressed elsewhere [215]. We will just discuss the fact that cytokines assessed in any biological fluids represent the tip of the iceberg [216]. Indeed, once the specific mRNA has been translated, cytokines can be found within the cellular compartments associated with protein synthesis, and some cytokines such as IL-1α, TNF-α, IL-10, IFN-γ, and IL-15 can be found as a constitutive compound of the cell membrane. Present in the cellular environment, cytokines can be trapped by surrounding cells which possess specific receptors; finally, once bound to the receptors, cytokines are usually internalized within the cells (Figure 4). Thus, we showed that IL-1α, IL-1β and TNF-α could be found associated to monocytes of septic patients [9]. Interestingly, at the end of patient follow up, while most survivors did not have any more detectable circulating TNF, a majority still had detectable cell-associated TNF; recent studies suggest that this could be a membrane form of TNF. Indeed in patients with systemic injuries, enhanced expression of membrane TNF was reported whereas no intracellular TNF could be detected [217]. Similarly an increased expression of functionally active membrane-associated TNF has also been demonstrated on alveolar macrophages from patients with ARDS [218]. Flow cytometry analysis confirmed the presence of IL-1β positive cells among circulating leukocytes of intensive care unit patients [219]. More recently we investigated cell-associated IL-8, and found that tremendous amounts of IL-8 could be found associated to circulating neutrophils and mononuclear cells [47]. Lower, but significant amounts of IL-8 were also associated with red blood cells via their Duffy antigen. In ARDS patients, the identification of numerous IL-8 positive alveolar macrophages by immunocytochemistry has confirmed the putative detrimental role of IL-8 in the development of that syndrome [220].

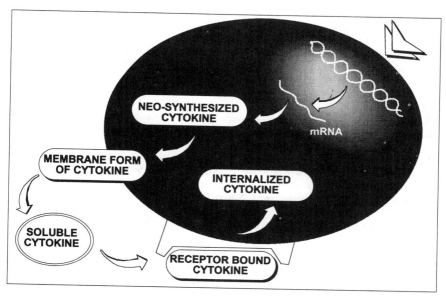

Figure 4. The source of cell-associated cytokines (adapted from [215])

REFERENCES

1. Okusawa S, Gelfand J, Ikejima T, et al. Interleukin 1 induces a shock like state in rabbit. Synergism with tumor necrosis factor and the effect of cyclooxygenase inhibition. J Clin Invest 1988; 81:1162-1172
2. Ohlsson K, Bjökk P, Bergenfield M, et al. Interleukin-1 receptor antagonist reduces mortality from endotoxin shock. Nature 1990; 348:550-552
3. Li P, Allen H, Banerjee S, et al. Mice defeficient in IL-1β converting enzyme are defective in production of mature IL-1β and resistant to endotoxic shock. Cell 1995; 80:401-411

4.   Fantuzzi G, Hui Z, Faggioni R, et al. Effect of endotoxin in IL-1β deficient mice. J. Immunol. 1996; 157:291-296
5.   Van Deuren M, Van Der Ven-Jongekrijg H, Baterlink AKN, et al. Correlation between proinflammatory cytokines and antiinflammatory mediators and the severity of disease in meningococcal infections. J Infect Dis 1995; 172:433-439
6.   Gardlund B, Sjölin J, Nilsson A, et al. Plasma levels of cytokines in primary septic shock in humans:correlation with disease severity. J Infect Dis 1995; 172:296-301
7.   Girardin E, Grau G, Dayer J, et al. Tumor necrosis factor and interleukin-1 in the serum of children with severe infectious purpura. N Engl J Med 1988; 319:397-400
8.   Waage A, Brandtzaeg P, Halstensen A, et al. The complex pattern of cytokines in serum from patients with meningococcal septic shock. Association between interleukin-6, interleukin-1, and fatal outcome. J Exp Med 1989; 169:333-338
9.   Muñoz C, Misset B, Fitting C, et al. Dissociation between plasma and monocyte-associated cytokines during sepsis. Eur J Immunol 1991; 21:2177-2184
10. Calandra T, Baumgartner JD, Grau GE, et al. Prognostic values of tumor necrosis factor/cachectin, interleukin-1, interferon-α, and interferon-γ in the serum of patients with septic shock. J Infect Dis 1990; 161:982-987
11. Van der Poll T, Romijn JA, Endert E, et al. Tumor necrosis factor mimics the metabolic response to acute infection in healthy humans. Am J Physiol 1991; 261:E457-465
12. Doherty GM, Lange JR, Langstein HN, et al. Evidence for IFN-gamma as a mediator of the lethality of endotoxin and tumor necrosis factor-alpha. J Immunol 1992; 149:1666-1670
13. Rothstein JL, Schreiber H. Synergy between tumor necrosis factor and bacterial products causes hemorrhagic necrosis and lethal shock in normal mice. Proc Natl Acad Sci USA 1988; 85:607-611
14. Beutler B, Milsark IW, Cerami AC. Passive immunization against cachectin/tumor necrosis factor protects mice from lethal effect of endotoxin. Science 1985; 229:869-871
15. Tracey KJ, Fong Y, D.G. H, et al. Anti-cachectin/TNF monoclonal antibodies prevent septic shock during lethal bacteraemia. Nature 1987; 330:662-664
16. Caty MG, Guice KS, Oldham KT, et al. Evidence for tumor necrosis factor-induced pulmonary microvascular injury after intestinal ischemia-reperfusion injury. Ann Surg 1990; 212:694-700
17. Netea MG, Kullberg BJ, Verschueren I, et al. Diferential susceptibility of cytokine knock out mice for lipopolysaccharides derived from different Gram-negative bacteria. J Endotoxin Res 2000; 6:188
18. Waage A, Espevik T, Lamvik J. Detection of tumor necrosis factor-like cytotoxicity in serum from patients with septicemia but not from untreated cancer patients. Scand. J. Immunol. 1986; 24:739-743
19. Waage A, Halstensen A, Espevik T. Association between tumor necrosis factor in serum and fatal outome in patients with meningococal disease. Lancet 1987; i:355-357
20. Offner F, Philippé J, Vogelaers D, et al. Serum tumor necrosis factor levels in patients with infectious diseases and septic shock. J Lab Clin Med 1990; 116:100-105
21. Baud L, Cadranel J, Offenstadt G, et al. Tumor necrosis factor and septic shock. Crit Care Med 1990; 18:349-350
22. Pinsky MR, Vincent JL, Deviere J, et al. Serum cytokine levels in human septic shock. Relation to multiple-system organ failure and mortality. Chest 1993; 103:565-575
23. Hamilton GH, Hofbauer S, Hamilton B. Endotoxin, TNF-alpha, interleukin-6 and parameters of the cellular immune system in patients with intraabdominal sepsis. Scand J Infect Dis 1992; 24:361-368

24. Riche F, Panis Y, Laisne MJ, et al. High tumor necrosis factor serum level is associated with increased survival in patients with abdominal septic shock:a prospective study in 59 patients. Surgery 1996; 120:801-807

25. Arditi M, Manogue KR, Caplan M, et al. Cerebrospinal fluid tumor necrosis factor-alpha and PAF concentrations and severity of bacterial meningitis in children. J Infect Dis 1990; 162:139-147

26. Dulkerian SJ, Kilpatrick L, Costarino AT, et al. Cytokine elevations in infants with bacterial and aseptic meningitis. J Pediatr 1995; 126:872-876

27. Engelhardt R, Mackensen A, Galanos C, et al. Biological response to intravenously administered endotoxin in patients with advanced cancer. J Biol Resp Mod 1990; 9:480-491

28. Pollmächer T, Korth C, Mullington J, et al. Effects of G-CSF on plasma cytokine and cytokine receptor levels and on the in vivo host response to endotoxin in healthy men. Blood 1996; 87:900-905

29. van der Poll T, Coyle SM, Barbosa K, et al. Epinephrine inhibits tumor necrosis factor-alpha and potentiates interleukin-10 production during human endotoxemia. J Clin Invest 1996; 97:713-719

30. Leeper-Woodford SK, Carey PD, Byrne K, et al. Tumor necrosis factor alpha and beta subtypes appear in circulation during onset of sepsis-induced lung injury. Am Rev Respir Dis 1991; 143:1076-1082

31. Sriskandan S, Moyes D, Cohen J. Detection of circulating bacterial superantigen and lymphotoxin-alpha in patients with streptococcal toxic-shock syndrome. Lancet 1996; 348:1315-1316

32. Wagner H, Heeg K, Miethke T. T cell mediated lethal shock induced by bacterial superantigens. Behring Inst Mitt 1992; 91:46-53

33. Tokman MG, Carey KD, Quimby FW. The pathogenesis of experimental toxic shock syndrome:the role of interleukin-2 in the induction of hypotension and release of cytokines. Shock 1995; 3:145-151

34. Musso T, Calosso L, Zucca M, et al. Human monocytes constitutively express membrane-bound, biologically active, and interferon-γ upregulated interleukin-15. Blood 1999; 93:3531-3539

35. Lauw FN, Dekkers PE, te Velde AA, et al. Interleukin-12 induces sustained activation of multiple host inflammatory mediators systems in chimpanzees. J Infect Dis 1999; 179:646-652

36. Fehniger TA, Yu H, Cooper MA, et al. IL-15 costimulates the general Shwartzman reaction and innate immune IFNγ production *in vivo*. J Immunol 2000; 164:1643-1647

37. Alleva DG, Kaser SB, Monroy MA, et al. IL-15 functions as a potent autocrine regulator of macrophage proinflammatory cytokine production. Evidence for differential receptor subunit utilization associated with stimulation or inhibition. J Immunol 1997; 159:2941-2951

38. Lauw FN, Simpson AJH, Prins JM, et al. Elevated Plasma Concentrations of Interferon (IFN) and the IFN-Inducing Cytokines Interleukin (IL)18, IL-12, and IL-15 in Severe Melioidosis. J Infect Dis 1999; 180:1878-1885

39. Waring P, Wycherley K, Cary D, et al. Leukemia inhibitory factor levels are elevated in septic shock and various inflammatory body fluids. J Clin Invest 1992; 90:2031-2037

40. Block MI, Berg M, McNamara MJ, et al. Passive immunization of mice against D factor blocks lethality and cytokine release during endotoxemia. J Exp Med 1993; 178:1085-1090

41. Modur V, Feldhaus MJ, Weyrich AS, et al. Oncostanin M is a proinflammatory mediator. In vivo effects correlates with endothelial cell expression of inflammatory cytokines and adhesion molecules. J Clin Invest 1997; 100:158-168

42. Villers D, Dao T, Nguyen JM, et al. Increased plasma levels of human interleukin for DA1a cells / leukemia inhibitory factor in sepsis correlate with shock and poor prognosis. J Infect Dis 1995; 171:232-236

43. Guillet C, Fourcin M, Chevalier S, et al. ELISA detection of circulating levels of LIF, OSM and CNTF in septic shock. Ann NY Acad Sci 1995; 762:407-412

44. Jansen PM, de Jong IW, Hart M, et al. Release of leukemia inhibitory factor in primate sepsis. Analysis of the role of TNFα. J Immunol 1996; 156:4401-4407

45. Broaddus VC, Boylan AM, Hoeffel JM, et al. Neutralization of IL-8 inhibits neutrophils influx in a rabbit model of endotoxin-induced pleurisy. J Immunol 1994; 152:2960-2967

46. Marty C, Misset B, Tamion F, et al. Circulating interleukin-8 concentrations in patients with multiple organ failure of septic and nonseptic origin. Crit. Care Med. 1994; 22:673-679

47. Marie C, Fitting C, Cheval C, et al. Presence of high levels of leukocyte-associated interleukin-8 upon cell activation and in patients with sepsis syndrome. Infect Immun 1997; 65:865-871

48. Gimbrone MA, Obin MS, Brock AF, et al. Endothelial interleukin-8:a novel inhibitor of leukocyte-endothelial interactions. Science 1989; 246:1601-1603

49. Cunha FQ, Cunha Tamashiro WMS. Tumour necrosis factor-alpha and interleukin-8 inhibit neutrophil migration in vitro and in vivo. Mediators Inflam 1992; 1:397-401

50. Zisman DA, Kunkel SL, Strieter RM, et al. MCP-1 protects mice in lethal endotoxemia. J Clin Invest 1997; 99:2832-2836

51. Chvatchko Y, Hoogewerf AJ, Meyer A, et al. A key role for CC chemokine receptor 4 in lipopolysaccharide-induced endotoxic shock. J Exp Med 2000; 191:1755-1763

52. Matsukawa A, Hogaboam CM, Lukacs NW, et al. Pivotal role of the CC chemokine, macrophage derived chemokine, in the innate immune response. J Immunol 2000; 164:5362-5368

53. Friedland J, Suputtamongkol Y, Remick D, et al. Prolonged elevation of interleukin-8 and interleukin-6 concentrations in plasma and of leukocyte interleukin-8 m-RNA levels during septicemic and localized *Pseudomonas pseudomallei* infection. Infect Immun 1992; 60:2402-2408

54. Hack C, Hart M, Strack van Schijndel R, et al. Interleukin-8 in sepsis:relation to shock and inflammatory mediators. Infect. Immun. 1992; 60:2835-2842

55. Miller EJ, Cohen AB, Nagao S, et al. Elevated levels of NAP-1/Interleukin-8 are present in the airspaces of patients with the adult respiratory distress syndrome and are associated with increased mortality. Am. J. Respir. Dis. 1992; 148:427-432

56. Endo S, Inada K, Ceska M, et al. Plasma interleukin 8 and polymorphonuclear leukocyte elastase concentrations in patients with septic shock. J Inflamm 1995; 45:136-142

57. Kragsbjerg P, Holmberg H, Vikerfors T. Dynamics of blood cytokine concentrations in patients with bacteremic infections. Scand J Infect Dis 1996; 28:391-398

58. Friedland JS, Porter JC, Daryanani S, et al. Plasma proinflammatory cytokine concentrations, acute physiology and chronic health evaluation (APACHE) III scores and survival in patients in an intensive care unit. Crit Care Med 1996; 24:1775-1781

59. Redl H, Schlag G, Bahrami S, et al. Plasma neutrophil-activating peptide-1/interleukin-8 and neutrophil elastase in a primate bacteremia model. J Infect Dis 1991; 164:383-388

60. Bossink AW, Paemen L, Jansen PM, et al. Plasma levels of the chemokines monocyte chemotactic proteins-1 and -2 are elevated in human sepsis. Blood 1995; 86:3841-3847

61. O'Grady NP, Tropea M, Preas HL, et al. Detection of macrophage inflammatory protein (MIP)-1α and MIP-1β during experimental endotoxemia and human sepsis. J Infect Dis. 1999; 179

62. Olszyna DP, Prins JM, Dekkers PEP, et al. Sequential measurements of chemokines in urosepsis and experimental endotoxemia. J Clin Immunol 1999; 19

63. Ryffel B. Interleukin-12:role of interferon-γ in IL-12 adverse effects. Clin Immunol Immunopath 1997; 83:18-20

64. Wysocka M, Kubin M, Vieira LQ, et al. Interleukin-12 is required for interferon-gamma production and lethality in lipopolysaccharide-induced shock in mice. Eur J Immunol 1995; 25:672-676

65. Steinhauser ML, Hogaboam CM, Lukacs NW, et al. Multiples roles for IL-12 in a model of acute septic peritonitis. J Immunol 1999; 162:5437-5443

66. Mancuso G, Cusumano V, Genovese E, et al. Role of interleukin-12 in experimental neonatal sepsis caused by group B streptococci. Infect Immun 1997; 65:3731-3735

67. Heinzel FP, Rerko RM, Ling P, et al. Interleukin-12 is produced in vivo during endotoxemia and stimulates synthesis of γ-interferon. Infect Immun. 1994; 62:4244-4251

68. Jansen PM, van der Pouw Kraan TCTM, de Jong IW, et al. Release of IL-12 in experimental *Escherichia coli* septic shock in baboons:relation to plasma levels to IL-10 and IFN-gamma. Blood 1996; 87:5144-5151

69. Zimmer S, Pollard V, Marshall GD, et al. The 1996 Moyer Award. Effects of endotoxin on the Th1/Th2 response in humans. J Burn Care Rehabil 1996; 17:491-496

70. Presterl E, Staudinger T, Pettermann M, et al. Cytokine Profile and Correlation to the APACHE III and MPM II Scores in Patients with Sepsis. Am. J. Respir. Crit. Care Med. 1997; 156:825-832

71. Puren AJ, Razeghi P, Fantuzzi G, et al. Interleukin-18 enhances lipopolysaccharide-induced interferon-γ production in human whole blood cultures. J Infect Dis 1998; 178:1830-1834

72. Bohn E, Sing A, Zumbihl R, et al. IL-18 regulates early cytokine production in, and promotes resolution of, bacterial infection in mice. J Immunol 1998; 160:299-307

73. Tsutsui H, Matsui K, Kawada N, et al. IL-18 accounts for both TNFα and Fas Ligand-mediated hepatotoxic pathways in endotoxin-induced liver injury in mice. J Immunol 1997; 159:3961-3967

74. Netea MG, Fantuzzi G, Kullberg BJ, et al. Neutralization of IL-18 reduces neutrophil tissue accumulation and protects mice against lethal *Escherichia coli* and *Salmonella typhimurium* endotoxemia. J Immunol 2000; 164:2644-2649

75. Hochholzer P, Lipford GB, Wagner H, et al. Role of interleukin-18 during lethal shock:decreased lipopolysaccharide sensitivity but normal surperantigen reaction in IL-18-deficient mice. Infect Immun 2000; 68:3502-3508

76. Sakao Y, Takeda K, Tsutsui H, et al. IL-18-deficient mice are resistant to endotoxin-induced liver injury but highly susceptible to endotoxic shock. Intern Immunol 1999; 11:471-480

77. Heinzel FP. The role of interferon-gamma in the pathology of experimental endotoxemia. J Immunol 1990; 145:2920-2924

78. Silva AT, Cohen J. Role of interferon-gamma in experimental Gram-negative sepsis. J Infect Dis 1992; 166:331-335

79. Nansen A, Pravsgaard Christensen J, Marker O, et al. Sensitization to lipopolysaccharide in mice with asymptomatic viral infection:role of T-cell-dependent production of interferon-γ. J Infect Dis 1997; 176:151-157

80. Kamijo R, Le J, Shapiro D, et al. Mice that lack the interferon-gamma receptor have profoundly altered responses to infection with Bacillus Calmette-Guerin and subsequent challenge with lipopolysaccharide. J Exp Med 1993; 178:1435-1440

81. Car BD, Eng VM, Schnyder B, et al. Interferon-gamma receptor deficient mice are resistant to endotoxic shock. J Exp Med 1994; 179:1437-1444

82. Heremans H, Dillen C, Groenen M, et al. Role of interferon-γ and nitric oxide in pulmonary edema and death induced by lipopolysaccharide. Am J Respir Crit Care Med 2000; 161:110-117

83. Mathy NL, Scheuer W, Lanzendörrfer M, et al. Interleukin-16 stimulates the expression and production of pro-inflammatory cytokines by human monocytes. Immunol 2000; 100:63-69

84. Jovanovic DV, Di Battista JA, Martel-Pelletier J, et al. IL-17 stimulates the production and expression of pro-inflammatory cytokines, IL-1β and TNFα by human macrophages. J Immunol 1998; 160:3513-3521

85. Basu S, Dunn AR, Marino MW, et al. Increased tolerance to endotoxin by granulocyte-macrophage colony stimulating factor deficient mice. J Immunol 1997; 159:1412-1417

86. Freeman BD, Ouezado Z, Zeni F, et al. G-CSF reduces endotoxemia and improves survival during *E.coli* pneumonia. J Appl. Physiol 1997; 83:1467-1475

87. Yalcin O, Soybir G, Koksoy F, et al. Effects of granulocyte colony-stimulating factor on bacterial translocation due to burn wound sepsis. Surgery Today 1997; 27:154-158

88. Zhang P, Bagby GJ, Stoltz DA, et al. Enhancement of peritoneal leukocyte function by granulocyte colony-stimulating factor in rats with abdominal sepsis. Crit Care Med 1998; 26:315-321

89. Villa P, Shakle CL, Meazza C, et al. Granulocyte colony stimulating factor and antibiotics in the prophylaxis of a murine model of polymicrobial peritonitis and sepsis. J Infect Dis 1998; 178:471-477

90. Opal SM, Jhung JW, Keith JC, et al. Additive effects of human recombinant interleukin-11 and granulocyte colony stimulating factor in experimental gram negative sepsis. Blood 1999; 93:3467-3472

91. Francois B, Trimoreau F, Vignon P, et al. Thrombocytopenia in the sepsis syndrome:role of hemophagocytosis and macrophage colony-stimulating factor. Am J Med 1997; 103:114-120

92. Waring PM, Presneill J, Maher DW, et al. Differential alterations in plasma colony-stimulating factor concentrations in meningococcaemia. Clin Exper Immunol 1995; 102:501-506

93. Cairo MS, Suen Y, Knoppel E, et al. Decreased G-CSF and IL-3 production and gene expression from mononuclear cells of newborn infants. Pediatric Res 1992; 31:574-578

94. Kantar M, Kultursay N, Kutukculer N, et al. Plasma concentration of granulocyte-macrophage colony stimulating factor and interleukin-6 in septic and healthy preterms. Eur J Pediat 2000; 159:156-157

95. Ayala A, Chung CS, Xu YX, et al. Increased inducible apoptosis in CD4+ T lymphocytes during polymicrobial sepsis is mediated by Fas ligand and not endotoxin. Immunol 1999; 97:45-55

96. Hashimoto S, Kobayashi A, Kooguchi K, et al. Upregulation of two death pathways of perforin/granzyme and FasL/Fas in septic acute respiratory distress syndrome. Am J Resp Crit Care Med 2000; 161:237-243

97. David JR. Delayed hypersensitivity in vitro. Its mediation by cell free substances formed by lymphoid cell-antigen interaction. Proc Natl Acad Sci USA 1966; 65:72-77

98. Bernhagen J, Calandra T, Mitchell RA, et al. MIF is a pituitary-derived cytokine that potentiates lethal endotoxaemia. Nature 1993; 365:756-759

99. Calandra T, Bernhagen J, Mitchell RA, et al. The macrophage is an important and previously unrecognized source of macrophage migration inhibitory factor. J Exp Med 1994; 179:1895-1902

100. Calandra T, Bernhagen J, Metz CN, et al. MIF as a glucocorticoid-induced modulator of cytokine production. Nature 1995; 376:68-71

101. Bacher M, Meinhardt A, Lan HY, et al. Migration inhibitory factor expression in experimentally induced endotoxemia. Am J Pathol 1997; 150:235-246

102. Bozza M, Satoskar AR, Lin G, et al. Targeted disruption of migration inhibitory factor gene reveals its critical role in sepsis. J Exp Med 1999; 189:341-346

103. Calandra T, Echtenacher B, Le Roy D, et al. Protection from septic shock by neutralization of macrophage migration inhibitory factor. Nature Med. 2000; 6:164-170

104. Wang H, Bloom O, Zhang M, et al. HMG-1 as a late mediator of endotoxin lethality in mice. Science 1999; 285:248-251

105. Wulczyn FG, Krappmann D, Scheidereit C. The NF-kB/Rel and IkB families:mediators of immune response and inflammation. J Mol Med 1996; 74:749-769

106. Baldwin AS. The NF-κB and IκB proteins:new discoveries and insights. Ann Rev Immunol 1996; 14:649-681

107. Ghosh S, May MJ, Kopp EB. NF-κB and Rel proteins:evolutionarily conserved mediators of immune responses. Ann Rev Immunol 1998; 16:225-260

108. Schmitz ML, Baeuerle PA. The p65 subunit is responsible for the strong transcription activating potential of NF-κB. EMBO J 1991; 10:3805-3817

109. Ballard DW, Dixon EP, Peffer NJ, et al. The 65-kDa subunit of human NF-κB functions as a potent transcriptional activator and target for v-Rel-mediated repression. Proc Natl Acad Sci USA 1992; 89:1875-1879

110. Bours V, Burd PR, Brown K, et al. A novel mitogen-induced gene product related to p50/p105-NF-κB participates in transactivation through a κB site. Mol Cell Biol 1992; 12:685-695

111. Kretzschmar M, Meisterernst M, Scheidereit C, et al. Transcriptinal regulation of the HIV-1 promoter by NF-κB in vitro. Genes Developement 1992; 6:761-774

112. Fujita T, Nolan GP, Liou H-C, et al. The candidate proto-oncogene *bcl-3* encodes a transcriptional coactivator that activates through NF-κB p50 homodimers. Genes Development 1993; 7:1354-1363

113. Moore PA, Ruben SM, Rosen CA. Conservation of transcriptional activation functions of the NF-κB p50 and p65 subunits in mammalian cells and *Saccharomyces cerevisiae*. Mol Cell Biol 1993; 13:1666-1674

114. Franzoso G, Bours V, Azarenko V, et al. The oncoprotein Bcl-3 can facilitate NF-κB-mediated transactivation by removing inhibiting p50 homodimers from select κB sites. The EMBO J 1993; 12:3893-3901

115. Medzhitov R, Preston-Hurlburt P, Janeway CA. A human homologue of the *Drosophila* Toll protein signals activation of adaptative immunity. Nature 1997; 388:394-397

116. Shimazu R, Akashi S, Ogata H, et al. MD-2, a molecule that confers lipopolysac-charide responsiveness on Toll-like receptor 4. J Exp Med 1999; 189:1777-1782

117. Malinin NL, Boldin MP, Kovalenko AV, et al. Map3k-related kinase involved in NK-κB induction by TNF, CD95 and IL-1. Nature 1997; 385:540-544

118. Di Donato JA, Hayakawa M, Rothwarf DM, et al. A cytokine-responsive IκB kinase that activates the transcription factor NF-κB. Nature 1997; 388:548-554

119. Hirano M, Osada S-I, Aoki T, et al. MEK kinase is involved in tumor necrosis factor α-induced NF-κB activation and degradation of IκB-α. J Biol Chem 1996; 271:13234-13238

120. Burns K, Clatworthy J, Martin L, et al. Tollip, a new componet of the IL-1RI pathway, links IRAK to the IL-1 receptor. Nature Cell Biol 2000; 2:346-351

121. Kopp E, Medzhitov R, Carothers J, et al. ECSIT is an evolutionary conserved intermediate in the Toll/IL-1 signal transduction pathway. Genes and Development 1999; 13:2059-2071

122. Westwick JK, Weitzel C, Minden A, et al. Tumor necrosis factor-α stimulates AP-1 activity through prolonged activation of the c-jun kinase. J Biol Chem 1994; 269:26396-26401

123. Raingeaud J, Gupta S, Rogers JS, et al. Pro-inflammatory cytokines and environmental stress cause p38 mitogen-activated protein kinase activation by dual phosphorylation on tyrosine and threonine. J Biol Chem 1995; 270:7420-7426

124. Wesselborg S, Bauer MKA, Vogt M, et al. Activation of transcription factor NF-κB and p38 mitogen-activated protein kinase is mediated by distinct and separed stress effector pathways. J Biol Chem 1997; 272:12422-12429

125. Liu ZG, Hsu HL, Goeddel DV, et al. Dissection of TNF receptor 1 effector functions:JNK activation is not linked to apoptosis while NF-kappa B activation prevents cell death. Cell 1996; 87:565-576

126. Yuasa T, Ohno S, Kehrl JH, et al. Tumor necrosis factor signaling to stress-activated protein kinase (SAPK)/Jun NH2-terminal kinase (JNK) and p38. J Biol Chem 1998; 273:22681-22692

127. Kanakaraj P, Schafer PH, Cavender DE, et al. Interleukin (IL)-1 receptor-associated kinase (IRAK) requirement for optimal induction of multiple IL-1 signaling pathways and IL-6 production. J Exp Med 1998; 187:2073-2079

128. Burns K, Martinon F, Esslinger C, et al. MyD88, an adapter protein involved in interleukin-1 signaling. J Biol Chem 1998; 273:12203-12209

129. Moine P, McIntyre R, Schwartz MD, et al. NF-κB regulatory mechanisms in alveolar macrophages from patients with acute respiratory distress syndrome. Shock 2000; 13:85-91

130. Williams DL, Ha T, Li C, et al. Early activation of hepatic NF-κB and NFIL6 in polymicrobial sepsis correlates with bacterremia, cytokine expression and mortality. Ann Surgery 1999; 230:95-104

131. Browder W, Ha T, Li C, et al. Early activation of pulmonary NF-κB and NFIL6 in polymicrobial sepsis. J Trauma Injury Infect Crit Care 1999; 46:590-596

132. Shenkar R, Abraham E. Mechanisms of lung neutrophil activation after hemorrhage or endotoxemia:roles of reactive oxygen intermediates, NF-κB and cyclic AMP response element binding protein. J Immunol 1999; 163:954-962

133. Annane D, Sanquer S, Sébille V, et al. Compartmentalised inducible nitric-oxide synthase activity in septic shock. The Lancet 2000; 355:1143-1148

134. Keel M, Ecknauer E, Stocker R, et al. Different pattern of local and systemic release of proinflammatory and anti-inflammatory mediators in severely injured patients with chest trauma. J Trauma 1996; 40:907-914

135. Jacobs RF, Tabor DR, Burks AW, et al. Elevated interleukin-1 release by human alveolar macrophages during adult respiratory distress syndrome. Am Rev Respir Dis 1989; 140:1686-1692

136. Fieren MWJA, Van Den Bemd GJ, Bonta IL. Endotoxin-stimulated peritoneal macrophages obtained from continuous ambulatory peritoneal dialysis patients show an increased capacity to release interleukin-1β in vitro during infectious peritonitis. Eur J Clin Invest 1990; 20:453-457

137. Böhrer H, Qiu F, Zimmermann T, et al. Role of NFκB in the mortality of sepsis. J Clin Invest 1997; 100:972-985

138. Adib-Conquy M, Adrie C, Moine P, et al. NF-κB expression in mononuclear cells of septic patients resembles that observed in LPS-tolerance. Am J Respir Crit Care Med 2000; 162:1877-1883

139. Reisinger EC, Kern P, Ernst M, et al. Inhibition of HIV progression by dithiocard. Lancet 1990; 335:679-682

140. Liu SF, Ye X, Malik AB. In vivo inhibition of nuclear factor-κB activation prevents inducible nitric oxide synthase expression and systemic hypotension in a rat model of septic shock. J Immunol. 1997; 159:3976-3983

141. Schow SR, Joly A. N-acetyl-leucinyl-leucinyl-norleucinal inhibits lipopolysaccharide-induced NF-κB activation and prevents TNF and IL-6 synthesis in vivo. Cell Immunol 1997; 175:199-202

142. Liu SF, Ye X, Malik AB. Pyrrolidine dithiocarbamate prevents I-κB degradation and reduces microvascular injury induced by lipopolysacchride in multiple organs. Mol Pharmacol 1999; 55:658-667

143. Drollinger AG, Netser JC, Rodgers GM. Dithiocarbamates ameliorate the effects of endotoxin in a rabbit model of disseminated intravascular coagulation. Sem Thromb Hemost 1999; 25:429-433

144. Tilg H, Trehu E, Atkins MB, et al. Interleukin-6 (IL-6) as an anti-inflammatory cytokine:induction of circulating IL-1 receptor antagonist and soluble tumor necrosis factor receptor p55. Blood 1994; 83:113-118

145. Hack C, de Groot E, Felt-Bersma R, et al. Increased plasma levels of interleukin-6 in sepsis. Blood 1989; 74:1704-1710

146. Calandra T, Gerain J, Heumann D, et al. High circulating levels of interleukin-6 in patients with septic shock:evolution during sepsis, prognostic value, and interplay with other cytokines. Am J Med 1991; 91:23-29

147. Damas P, Ledoux D, Nys M, et al. Cytokine serum level during severe sepsis in human IL-6 as a marker of severity. Ann Surg 1992; 215:356-362

148. Yoshimoto T, Nakanishi K, Hirose S, et al. High serum IL-6 level reflects susceptible status of the host to endotoxin and IL-1 / TNF. J Immunol 1992; 148:3596-3603

149. Fong Y, Moldawer LL, Marano M, et al. Endotoxemia elicits increased circulating beta 2-IFN/IL-6 in man. J Immunol 1989; 142:2321-2324

150. van Deventer SJH, Büller HR, ten Cate JW, et al. Experimental endotoxemia in humans:analysis of cytokine release and coagulation, fibrinolytic and complement pathways. Blood 1990; 76:2520-2526

151. Gabay C, Singwe M, Genin B, et al. Circulating levels of IL-11 and leukaemia inhibitory factor (LIF) do not significantly participate in the production of acute-phase proteins by the liver. Clin Exp Immunol 1996; 105:260-265

152. Du XX, Doerschuk CM, Orazi A, et al. A bone marrow stromal-derived growth factor, interleukin-11,, stimulates recovery of small intestinal mucosal cells after cytoablative therapy. Blood 1994; 83:33-37

153. Chang M, Williams A, Ishizawa L, et al. Endogenous interleukin-11 (IL-11) expression is increased and prophylactic use of exogenous IL-11 enhances platelet recovery and improves survival during thrombocytopenia associated with experimental group B streptococcal sepsis in neonatal rats. Blood Cells Mol & Dis 1996; 22:57-67

154. Endo S, Inada K, Arakawa N, et al. Interleukin-11 in patients with disseminated intravascular coagulation. Res Com Mol Pathol Pharmac 1996; 91:253-256

155. Gabay C, Smith MF, Eidlen D, et al. Interleukin-1 receptor antagonist is an acute phase protein. J Clin Invest 1997; 99:2930-2940

156. Aiura K, Gelgand J, Burke J, et al. Interleukin-1 receptor antagonist prevents S. epidermidis hypotension and reduces circulating levels of TNF and IL-1β in rabbits. Infect Immun 1993; 61:3342-3350

157. Fischer E, Marano MA, Van Zee KJ, et al. Interleukin-1 receptor blockade improves survival and hemodynamic performance in Escherichia coli septic shock, but fails to alter host responses to sublethal endotoxemia. J Clin Invest 1992; 89:1551-1557

158. Mancilla J, Garcia P, Dinarello CA. The interleukin-1 receptor antagonist can either reduce or enhance the lethality of *Klebsiella pneumoniae* sepsis in newborn rats. Infect Immun 1993; 61:926-932
159. Hirsch E, Irikura VM, Paul SM, et al. Functions of interleukin 1 receptor antagonist in gene knockout and overproducing mice. Proc Natl Acad Sci Usa 1996; 93:11008-11013
160. Fischer E, Van Zee KJ, Marano MA, et al. Interleukin-1 receptor antagonist circulates in experimental inflammation and in human disease. Blood 1992; 79:2196-2200
161. Rogy MA, Coyle SM, Oldenburg HS, et al. Persistently elevated soluble tumor necrosis factor receptor and interleukin-1 receptor antagonist levels in critically ill patients. J Am Coll Surg 1994; 178:132-138
162. Cavaillon JM, Müller-Alouf H, Alouf JE. Cytokines in streptococcal infections. An opening lecture. Adv Exper Med Biol 1997; 418:869-879
163. Marie C, Cavaillon JM. Negative feedback in inflammation:the role of antiinflammatory cytokines. Bull Inst Pasteur 1997; 95:41-54
164. Preas HL, Reda D, Tropea M, et al. Effects of recombinant soluble type i interleukin-1 receptor on human inflammatory responses to endotoxin. Blood 1996; 88:2465-2472
165. Giri JG, Wells J, Dower SK, et al. Elevated levels of shed type II IL-1 receptor in sepsis. Potential role for type II receptor in regulation of IL-1 responses. J Immunol 1994; 153:5802-5809
166. Pruitt JH, B WM, Edwards PD, et al. Increased soluble interleukin-1 type II receptor concentrations in postoperative patients and in patients with sepsis syndrome. Blood 1996; 87:3282-3288
167. Lesslauer W, Tabuchi H, Gentz R, et al. Recombinant soluble tumor necrosis factor receptor proteins protect mice from LPS-induced lethality. Eur. J. Immunol. 1991; 21:2883-2886
168. Ashkenazi A, Marsters S, Capon D, et al. Protection against endotoxic shock by a tumor necrosis factor receptor immunoadhesin. Proc. Natl. Acad. Sci. 1991; 88:10535-10539
169. Girardin E, Roux-Lombard P, Grau GE, et al. Imbalance between tumour necrosis factor-alpha and soluble TNF receptor concentrations in severe meningococcaemia. Immunology 1992; 76:20-23
170. Van Zee KJ, Kohno T, Fischer E, et al. Tumor necrosis factor soluble receptors circulate during experimental and clinical inflammation and can protect against excessive tumor necrosis factor alpha in vitro and in vivo. Proc Natl Acad Sci U S A 1992; 89:4845-4849
171. van der Poll T, Jansen J, van Leenen D, et al. Release of soluble receptors for tumor necrosis factor in clinical sepsis and experimental endotoxemia. J Infect Dis 1993; 168:955-960
172. van der Poll T, Fischer E, Coyle SM, et al. Interleukin-1 contributes to increased concentrations of soluble tumor necrosis factor receptor type I in sepsis. J Infect Dis 1995; 172:577-580
173. Lantz M, Malik S, Slevin ML, et al. Infusion of tumor necrosis factor (TNF) causes an increase in circulating TNF-binding protein in humans. Cytokine 1990; 2:402-406
174. Gérard C, Bruyns C, Marchant A, et al. Interleukin-10 reduces the release of tumor necrosis factor and prevents lethality in experimental endotoxemia. J. Exp. Med. 1993; 177:547-550
175. Berg D, Kühn R, Rajewsky K, et al. Interleukin-10 is a central regulator of the response to LPS in murine models of endotoxin shock and the Shwartzman reaction but not endotoxin tolerance. J. Clin. Invest. 1995; 96:2339-2347
176. Standiford TJ, Strieter RM, Lukacs NW, et al. Neutralization of IL-10 lethality in endotoxemia. J Immunol 1995; 155:2222-2229
177. van der Poll T, Marchant A, Buurman WA, et al. Endogenous IL-10 protects mice from death during septic peritonitis. J Immunol 1995; 155:5397-5401

178. Donnelly SC, Strieter RM, Reid PT, et al. The association between mortality rates and decreased concentrations of interleukin-10 and interleukin-1 receptor antagonist in the lung fluids of patients with the adult respiratory distress syndrome. Ann Intern Med 1996; 125:191-196

179. Marchant A, Devière J, Byl B, et al. Interleukin-10 production during septicaemia. Lancet 1994; 343:707-708

180. Derkx B, Marchant A, Goldman M, et al. High levels of interleukin-10 during the initial phase of fulminant meningococcal septic shock. J Infect Dis 1995; 171:229-232

181. van Dissel JT, van Langevelde P, Westendorp RGJ, et al. Anti-inflammatory cytokine profile and mortality in febrile patients. Lancet 1998; 351:950-953

182. Bone RC, Grodzin CJ, Balk RA. Sepsis:A new hypothesis for pathogenesis of the disease process. Chest 1997; 121:235-243

183. Brandtzaeg P, Osnes L, Øvstebø R, et al. Net inflammatory capacity of human septic shock plasma evaluated by a monocyte-based target cell assay:identification of interleukin-10 as a major functional deactivator of human monocytes. J Exp Med 1996; 184:51-60

184. Sawyer RG, Rosenlof LK, Pruett TL. Interleukin-4 prevents mortality from acute but not chronic murine peritonitis and induces an accelarated TNF response. Eur Surg Res 1996; 28:119-123

185. Brunet LR, Finkelman FD, Cheever AW, et al. IL-4 protects against TNF-α-mediated cachexia and death during acute shistosomiasis. J Immunol 1997; 159:777-785

186. Giampietri A, Grohmann U, Vacca C, et al. Dual effect of IL-4 on resistance to systemic gram-negative infection and production of TNFα. Cytokine 2000; 12:417-421

187. Cavaillon J-M, Adib-Conquy M. The pro-inflammatory cytokine cascade. In Immune response in the critically ill. In:Marshal, J.C., Vincent J.L. (Eds) Update in Intensive Care and Emergency Medicine, - Springer - 2000; Vol. 31:37-66

188. Muchamuel T, Menon S, Pisacane P, et al. IL-13 protects mice from lipopolysaccharide-induced lethal endotoxemia - Correlation with down-modulation of TNFα, IFN-γ, and IL-12 production. J Immunol 1997; 158:2898-2903

189. Nicoletti F, Mancuso G, Cusumano V, et al. Prevention of endotoxin-induced lethality in neonatal mice by interleukin-13. Eur J Immunol 1997; 27:1580-1583

190. Matsukawa A, Hogaboam CM, Lukacs NW, et al. Expression and contribution of endogenous IL-13 in an experimental model of sepsis. J Immunol 2000; 164:2738-2744

191. van der Poll T, de Waal Malefyt R, Coyle SM, et al. Antiinflammatory cytokine responses during clinical sepsis and experimental endotoxemia:sequential measurements of plasma soluble interleukin (IL)-1 receptor type II, IL-10, and IL-13. J Infect Dis 1997; 175:118-122

192. Grohmann U, Van Snick J, Campanile F, et al. IL-9 protects mice from Gram-negative bacterial shock:suppression of TNFα, IL-12 and IFNγ and induction of IL-10. J Immunol 2000; 164:4197-4203

193. Urbaschek R, Urbaschek B. Induction of endotoxin tolerance by endotoxin, its mediators and by monophosphoryl lipid A. In Nowotny, A. Spitzer, J.J., Ziegler, E.J. (Eds) Endotoxin Research Series, Elsevier Science Publ. 1990; 455-463

194. Perrella MA, Hsieh CM, Lee WS, et al. Arrest of endotoxin induced hypotension by transforming growth factor-β1. Proc Natl Acad Sci USA 1996; 93:2054-2059

195. Karres I, Kremer JP, Sterckholzer U, et al. Transforming growth factor-β1 inhibits synthesis of cytokines in endotoxin-stimulated human whole blood. Arch Surg 1996; 131:1310-1317

196. Astiz M, Saha D, Lustbader D, et al. Monocyte response to bacterial toxins, expression of cell surface receptors, and release of anti-inflammatory cytokines during sepsis. J Lab Clin Med 1996; 128:597-600

197. Marie C, Cavaillon J-M, Losser M-R. Elevated levels of circulating transforming growth factor-β1 in patients with the sepsis syndrome. Ann Intern Med 1996; 125:520-521

198. Marie C, Losser MR, Fitting C, et al. Cytokines and soluble cytokines receptors in pleural effusions from septic and nonseptic patients. Am J Respir Crit Care Med 1997; 156:1515-1522

199. Junger WG, Hoyt DB, Redl H, et al. Tumor necrosis factor antibody treatment of septic baboons reduces the production of sustained T-cell suppressive factors. Shock 1995; 3:173-178

200. Ahmad S, Choudhry MA, Shankar R, et al. Transforming growth factor-β negatively modulates T-cell responses in sepsis. FEBS letters 1997; 402:213-218

201. Tzung SP, Mahl TC, Lance P, et al. Interferon-alpha prevents endotoxin-induced mortality in mice. Eur J Immunol 1992; 22:3097-3101

202. Wood J, Rodrick M, O'Mahony J, et al. Inadequate interleukin 2 production. A fundamental immunological deficiency in patients with major burns. Ann. Surg. 1984; 200:311-320

203. Ertel W, Keel M, Neidhardt R, et al. Inhibition of the defense system stimulating interleukin-12 interferon-γ pathway during critical illness. Blood 1997; 89:1612-1620

204. Muret J, Marie C, Fitting C, et al. *Ex vivo* T-lymphocyte derived cytokine production in SIRS patients is influenced by experimental procedures. Shock 2000; 13:169-174

205. Muñoz C, Carlet J, Fitting C, et al. Dysregulation of in vitro cytokine production by monocytes during sepsis. J Clin Invest 1991; 88:1747-1754

206. Van Deuren M, Van Der Ven-Jongekrijg H, Demacker PNM, et al. Differential expression of proinflammatory cytokines and their inhibitors during the course of meningococcal infections. J. Infect. Dis. 1994; 169:157-161

207. Marchant A, Alegre M, Hakim A, et al. Clinical and biological significance of interleukin-10 plasma levels in patients with septic shock. J Clin Immunol 1995; 15:265-272

208. Randow F, Syrbe U, Meisel C, et al. Mechanism of endotoxin desensitization:involvement of interleukin 10 and transforming growth factor β. J. Exp. Med. 1995; 181:1887-1892

209. Luger A, Graf H, Schwarz HP, et al. Decreased serum interleukin-1 activity and monocytes interleukin-1 production in patients with fatal sepsis. Crit Care Med. 1986; 14:458-461

210. Cavaillon J-M, Muñoz C, Marty C, et al. (1993). Cytokine production by monocytes from patients with sepsis syndrome and by endotoxin-tolerant monocytes., In:Levin, J, Alving, C R, Munford, R S, Stütz, P L (Eds) Bacterial endotoxin:recognition and effector mechanisms. Elsevier Sc. Publ. 1993:275-284

211. McCall CE, Grosso-Wilmoth LM, LaRue K, et al. Tolerance to endotoxin-induced expression of the interleukin-1ß gene in blood neutrophils of humans with the sepsis syndrome. J Clin Invest 1993; 91:853-861

212. Marie C, Muret J, Fitting C, et al. Reduced ex vivo interleukin-8 production by neutrophils in septic and non-septic systemic inflammatory response syndrome. Blood 1998; 91:3439-3446

213. Marie C, Muret J, Fitting C, et al. IL-1 receptor antagonist production during infectious and noninfectious systemic inflammatory response syndrome. Crit. Care Med. 2000; 28:2277-2283

214. Cavaillon JM. The nonspecific nature of endotoxin tolerance. Trends Microbiol 1995; 3:320-324

215. Cavaillon J-M. Possibilities and problems of cytokine measurements (IN:Redl, H. and Schlag G. (Eds) . Progress in Inflammation Research. Birkäuser 1999:95-119

216. Cavaillon JM, Muñoz C, Fitting C, et al. Circulating cytokines:the tip of the iceberg ? Circ Shock 1992; 38:145-152

217. Hauser CJ, Zhou X, Joshi P, et al. The immune microenvironment of human fracture/soft-tissue hematomas and its relationship to systemic immunity. J Trauma Injury Infect Critl Care 1997; 42:895-903

218. Armstrong L, Thickett DR, Christie SJ, et al. Increased Expression of Functionally Active Membrane-Associated Tumor Necrosis Factor in Acute Respiratory Distress Syndrome. Am. J. Respir. Cell Mol. Biol. 2000; 22:68-74

219. Yentis SM, Rowbottom AW, Riches PG. Detection of cytoplasmic IL-1β in peripheral blood mononuclear cells from intensive care unit patients. Clin Exp Immunol 1995; 100:330-335

220. Donnelly S, Strieter R, Kunkel S, et al. Interleukin-8 and development of adult respiratory distress syndrom in at-risk patients groups. Lancet 1993; 341:643-647

11

PATHOPHYSIOLOGY OF IMMUNODEPRESSION IN ICU PATIENTS

Hans-Dieter Volk
Conny Höflich
Gerald Grütz
Wolf-Dietrich Döcke
Petra Reinke

Antimicrobial defense against pathogens plays a key role in the protection of the body's integrity. The first levels of defense are based on physical and biological natural barriers (e.g., skin, mucosa, pH, natural intestinal and vaginal flora) which are relatively static. If the pathogens or their toxins can pass these barriers, the inducible acute inflammatory system consisting of humoral factors (e.g., complement, interferons, defensins, proteolytic enzymes) and inflammatory cells (e.g., mast cells, macrophages) that are present in the tissue in particular at the body's surface (skin, intestine, respiratory tract) react within minutes to hours.

The resulting acute local inflammation exhibits strong antimicrobial properties. However, it is also important for tissue regeneration and wound healing which explains why inflammation is also switched on following sterile tissue trauma or hypoxic injury. In addition, local inflammation activates the endothelium and attracts further humoral and cellular components of the inflammatory system (e.g., thrombocytes, granulocytes, natural killer [NK] cells). Moreover, it activates the antigen-presenting cells in the tissue (e.g., Langerhans cells of the skin) by delivering 'danger' signals. Activated antigen-presenting cells pick up soluble (proteins, etc.), and particulate (bacteria, viruses, dead cells) antigenic material and move rapidly (within less than two hours) to the local draining lymph nodes via the lymph, or to the spleen via the venous blood. Here, the antigen-presenting cells present the processed antigenic material for a couple of days to virgin antigen-specific T cells that pass the secondary lymphoid organs during the journey through the body. Antigen-presentation, in parallel with the release of adequate co-stimulatory signals, triggers the T cells to proliferate (clonal expansion – clinically visible as lymph node swelling) and to differentiate into T-effector cells that mediate cell-mediated immunity (Th1 cells), help with B-cell derived antibody production (Th2, partially also Th1), and direct cell-mediated cytotoxicity (Th1/CTL). The activated effector T cells migrate to the site of inflammation via interaction of homing receptor pairs expressed on the cells themselves and the 'inflammation-activated' endothelial cells. Antibodies are produced by plasma cells in the lymphoid organs as well as bone marrow and circulate as plasma proteins. Inflammation-triggered changes of vascular permeability allows the immunoglobulins to migrate into tissue. This primary adaptive immune response, which starts within a few hours of the initial insult, requires, in contrast to the fast acute inflammatory response of the innate immune system, about 5-7 days but is then very efficient and long-lasting (memory).

Complex abnormalities are needed to circumvent this well balanced system resulting in severe systemic infection and inflammation as seen in septic patients. Severe trauma, major surgery, myocardial infarction etc. may result in the temporary (or irreversible) loss of essential organ functions. Modern intensive care allows patients to survive the failure of important organ functions. Over recent years, a battery of diagnostic markers have been developed to monitor various organ functions and a set of interventions introduced to substitute/reverse organ failure. However, the failure of the very important organ, the 'immune system', in the framework of multiple organ failure (MOF) was overlooked for a long time. Like other organ failures, the loss of immune competence is a negative predictor for the survival of ICU patients. Here we want to discuss the molecular mechanisms of 'immunoparalysis' – the extreme form of immune failure.

Disturbances of the natural barriers, as seen in ICU patients, dramatically increase the risk of invasive infections. In addition, many factors (stress, inflammation, pathogens by themselves, age) contribute to a depression of the innate and adaptive immune responsiveness and thus predispose severe infections. In fact, infections are one of the main clinical complications of ICU patients and they may develop into sepsis which is associated with a very high mortality.

Over the last two decades our understanding of the pathophysiology of sepsis has progressed considerably. Experimental data suggest that an overwhelming systemic inflammatory response to invasion by bacteria and fungi and/or their microbial toxins may be involved in the pathogenesis of systemic inflammatory response syndrome (SIRS), sepsis and MOF. Since tumor necrosis factor (TNF) and interleukin (IL)-1 mimic septic shock in animal models, several recent clinical trials have focused on neutralization of these inflammatory mediators. These trials, however, have had very disappointing results.

Several reasons for the failure of the anti-inflammatory approach in sepsis have been discussed [1,2]. From the immunological point of view we have had to learn that immune interventions in sepsis without immune monitoring made no sense [3]. Many ICU patients express, at least temporarily, the phenotype of a deactivated inflammatory response as well adaptive immune system, recently called 'immunoparalysis' [3].

CLINICAL AND IMMUNOLOGICAL FEATURES OF IMMUNODEPRESSION IN ICU PATIENTS

Beneficial Effects of Inflammatory Factors

During the 90s, many scientists (and companies) regarded TNF and IL-1 as the 'bad guys' in sepsis despite the fact that important experimental and clinical data contradicting this viewpoint were already available. For example TNF-targeted therapy was shown to be successful in preventing shock following a bolus application of endotoxin (lipopolysaccharide, LPS) or bacteria in many animal models even in non-human primates. However, this approach showed no benefit or was even deleterious in the cecal ligation and puncture (CLP) peritonitis model which is closer to the clinical situation [4]. Moreover, mice that are genetically deficient in the production of, or response to, TNF are relatively resistant to LPS mediated injury, but they are unable to control infection with living bacteria [5]. In case of pathogens this deficiency was associated with death even with low dose infections. Similar observations were made with LPS binding protein (LBP) knock out mice [6]. On the other hand, mice deficient in anti-inflammatory cytokines, like transforming growth factor (TGF)-β or IL-10, are very sensitive to LPS or bacterial induced shock as the result of an uncontrolled inflammatory response [7,8].

For these reasons, and from the disappointing results of the clinical trials of anti-inflammatory therapies, we learnt that most of our models were too simple. A bolus injection of LPS or bacteria does not adequately reflect the complex host-pathogen interactions that take place during sepsis. These data suggest that a well balanced inflammatory response is important to control bacterial infections. Too much inflammation in response to infection resulting in hyperinflammation, can be as lethal as too little. We now understand well the mechanisms of shock, MOF and death induced by hyperinflammation, but further studies are necessary to learn more about the pathogenesis of infection in models of 'hypoinflammation'; for example, we do not understand why LBP -/- mice die from low-dose *Salmonella* infection in the absence of any significant systemic TNF or IL-1 levels. Is the host's inflammatory system locally involved? Do the pathogens induce the inflammatory processes by direct interaction and activation with non-immune cells like endothelial cells, or do direct toxic effects by bacteria play a role?

Clinical data also challenge the simple concept of sepsis is only death 'by too much inflammation'. Most patients with septic MOF have relatively low TNF plasma levels. Moreover, septic complications are more often observed in older patients and patients with advanced tumors, most of them preoperatively express a diminished immune responsiveness (although they frequently show signs of mild systemic inflammation, e.g., elevated C-reactive protein [CRP] levels). In addition, immunosuppressed transplant patients have a strongly diminished capacity to produce proinflammatory cytokines like TNF and IL-1 but have an increased risk of developing septic complications. The course of sepsis is frequently fatal in these patients although initially typical symptoms of SIRS are less prominent suggesting that clearing of microorganism is the most important issue.

How can we Measure Immunodepression?

Several groups, including ours, have reported deactivation of monocytes and granulocytes in septic patients, particularly during the later stages of disease [3,9-11]. In contrast to the rapid and erratic fluctuations in serum cytokine concentrations, this cellular phenotype is remarkably stable. Whereas cytokines have half lives in plasma measured in minutes, monocytes and granulocytes after leaving the bone-marrow have a half-life in the peripheral blood of about 24 hrs. Monocytes migrate into the tissues where they differentiate into different subtypes of macrophages, but the granulocytes are short-lived and can only go into inflammatory tissues. These properties makes analysis of monocyte and granulocyte function suitable for daily monitoring.

In prolonged sepsis we demonstrated a state of the inflammatory system in which monocytic TNF secretion capacity (part of the innate response), HLA-DR and CD80/86 antigen expression, as well as antigen-presenting capacity (part of the adaptive immune response) are all severely depressed. However, the capacity to produce IL-1 receptor antagonist (IL-1ra) and, at least temporarily, also IL-10, is largely preserved [12]. This switch to predominant anti-inflammatory mediator release was associated with a high risk of fatal outcome from persistent, in part opportunistic, infections [3,11,12]. The high incidence of opportunistic infections in particular in long-term ICU patients is a clinical reflection of the severe immunodepression – immune organ failure. In fact, none of the > 1000 patients we have monitored survived unless their monocytes recovered proinflammatory function and HLA-DR expression. We initially observed this phenomenon in septic transplant patients and called it 'immunoparalysis' [11,13].

The main problem for the introduction of these parameters into daily clinical work is the poor standardization of flowcytometric and cytokine assays. Of course, most laboratories developed internal standardization but the values were hardly comparable between different labs. As good standardization is essential for any clinical multicenter trial, we have focused our work during the last few years on the improvement of standardization. We evaluated a semiautomatic whole blood based assay measuring the capacity of blood (monocytic) cells to produce TNF in response to low dose LPS (the kit contain standardized culture tubes, dilution medium, endotoxin, as well as a semiautomatic TNF measurement procedure). The intraassay and interassay variability was less then 5 and 20 %, respectively, even if the healthy probands were monitored over 1 year demonstrating the stability of this biological parameter if a well standardized assay (*ex vivo*-TNF; Milenia Biotec /DPC Bad Nauheim) is used. However, there is high interindividual variability: low and high responders show up to five-fold differences. Using this assay and 500 pg/ml LPS for stimulation of 100 μl heparinized 1:10 diluted whole blood, the critical level for defining 'immunoparalysis' seems to be <300 pg/ml/4hr TNF secretion (normal range 500-2500 pg/ml). For handling, less then 15 minutes/sample are necessary and the total time to obtain the result is about 5.5 hrs.

Another parameter for measurement of immunocompetence is HLA-DR expression on monocytes. Using a novel flowcytometric assay (Quantibrite HLA-DR, Becton-Dickinson, Heidelberg) it is possible to quantify exactly the number of HLA-DR molecules expressed on CD14+ monocytes. The use of a new antibody labeling technique and standard beads (Quantibrite) allows a well standardized procedure that is independent of the laboratory. The variability is less then 10 %. If the 'lysis-no wash' method is used, the total procedure time is less than 45 min. The critical level for defining 'immunoparalysis' by this method seems to be <5,000 HLA-DR molecule/monocyte (normal range: >20,000).

Thus, at least two assays for standardized measurement of monocytic function are available for multicenter trials.

Several groups have reported on disturbed T cell function as well. Faist et al. described an association between poor outcome of ICU patients and suppression of the T-cell derived interferon-gamma/IL-4 ratio. This type1/type2 cytokine shift was observed particularly in the CD8 T cell subset [14]. We observed a TH1/TH2 shift in sepsis patients too. It is not clear whether the T cell abnormalities are directly due to trauma, stress, and sepsis or indirectly to inadequate antigen-presentation.

Association between 'Immunoparalysis' induced by Exogenous Immunosuppression and Infectious Risk in Transplant Patients

Monocytes are a crucial component of resistance to infection. They phagocytose and kill pathogenic microorganisms, neutralize toxins originating from pathogens and, as antigen-presenting cells and cytokine activated effector cells, they are an important link between the innate resistance system and the highly specialized adaptive immune response. All of these functions are disturbed in monocytes from patients with 'immunoparalysis'. The question is raised whether a direct relation exists between 'immunoparalysis' and diminished antimicrobial defense/fatal outcome or whether these immunological abnormalities in the blood represent rather an epiphenomenon with prognostic value only.

The occurrence of 'immunoparalysis' is not related to the invasion by specific pathogens or toxins indicating that common host-derived regulatory processes play a role. Another indication that 'immunoparalysis' is not the direct result of pathogenic action is the fact that we and others have observed monocyte deactivation in some patients after sterile injury (burns, trauma, major surgery) or in the course of high-dose immunosuppression [11,13,15,16]. Monocyte phenotype and function are closely associated with the 'net'-immunosuppression of cell-mediated immunity, particularly of the type 1 T-cell response. The proinflammatory capacity of monocytes (secretion of TNF, IL-1, IL-12, etc.) as well their antigen-presenting capacity (expression of surface HLA-DR, HLA-DP, HLA-DQ, CD80/86) is positively regulated by immunostimulatory cytokines such as interferon-gamma (IFN-γ) or granulocyte/macrophage-colony stimulating factor (GM-CSF) and negatively influenced by several factors including IL-10, TGF-β, prostaglandins, catecholamines and apoptotic material.

Following high dose immunosuppression in transplant patients using steroid bolus, OKT 3 mAb or antithymocyte globulin (ATG), we have seen a temporary decrease both in monocytic HLA-DR expression and in the capacity to generate TNF *ex vivo*. The reason for this phenomenon may be the lack of stimulatory cytokines, such as IFN-γ, which is strongly downregulated by immunosuppression. In addition steroids directly block cytokine action on monocytes and other cells while cyclosporin up-regulates monocytic TGF-β secretion. In some patients monocyte deactivation even reaches the level of 'immunoparalysis' – a situation which is associated with an increased risk of developing infectious complications within the next few weeks. Indeed after two days of 'immunoparalysis', bacterial and/or fungal infections were seen in about 30 % of transplant patients vs. 4 % in patients without 'immunoparalysis'. The longer the 'immunoparalysis' persists the greater the incidence of infections [11,13]. In general, the immunocompetence rapidly recovers following reduction of immunosuppression which decreases the incidence of bacterial/fungal infection. Moreover, transplant patients with septic complications and 'immunoparalysis' recover from sepsis following withdraw of immunosuppression without affecting graft function. These data suggest a direct relationship between 'immunoparalysis' and insufficient control of severe infections [11,13].

Role of IL-10 in 'Immunoparalysis'

But what may be the mechanisms of 'immunoparalysis' in non-transplanted ICU patients without exogenous immunosuppression? Almost all polytrauma, burn, and major surgery patients develop a moderate, temporary, monocyte deactivation within a few hours after the traumatic event that is more evident ('immunoparalysis') and long-lasting in some than in others. The activation of the stress response plays an important role in downregulating systemic immune responsiveness following trauma. The regulatory role of the hypothalamic-pituitary-adrenal (HPA) axis resulting in corticosteroid release has long been established. Recently we have shown that activation of the catecholamine axis is also involved in a major way in monocyte deactivation following stressful events. Studies on the molecular mechanisms of this phenomenon revealed that cyclic adenosine monophosphate (cAMP) dependent processes, including the up-regulation of IL-10, turn out to play a key role [17]. Experimental studies in rats confirmed the interpretation of the clinical observations. Increase in intracranial pressure or an intraventricular release of proinflammatory cytokines simulating head trauma, were not associated with systemic release of the pro-inflammatory cytokines TNF, IL-1, or IL-6, but both protocols resulted in a rapid systemic release of the anti-inflammatory cytokine IL-10, a drop in the antigen-presenting activity, and a diminished *ex vivo* TNF secretion capacity of peripheral blood and spleen monocytes/macrophages. Parallel blocking of the β_2-adrenergic receptors could prevent IL-10 release and monocyte/macrophage deactivation by 90 and 50 %, respectively [18]. Combined blockade of both stress pathways (β_2-adrenergic and steroid receptor blockade) almost completely prevented 'immunoparalysis' in this experimental model.

In most ICU patients without further complications as well as in the rat models of acute intervention, the phenomenon appears transiently only and monocytes/macrophage function recovers spontaneously within 1-2 days following the stressful event. However, in some patients downregulation of immune responsiveness is more pronounced and long-lasting – a phenomenon that is associated with an increased risk of developing infectious complications, sepsis, and wound healing problems (including anastomosis insufficiency). The phenomenon of long-lasting 'immunoparalysis' is seen in particular in patients with sepsis / septic shock..

What is the Difference between Patients with Transient, and those with Long-lasting, Monocyte Deactivation?

Major surgery and trauma are sometimes, and sepsis is frequently, associated with endotoxemia (LPS translocation, LPS release in association with bacteremia). Following *in vitro* LPS stimulation of blood leukocytes, TNF secretion peaks about 2 hrs later, whereas peak secretion of IL-10 needs more than 14 hrs. TNF by itself can upregulate IL-10 expression [18]. A high concentration of TNF leads to hyperinflammation but at the same time induces IL-10 which counterregulates the inflammatory reaction. In fact, *in vitro* treatment of monocytes with IL-10 reduces their HLA-DR expression, antigen-presenting activity, and TNF secretion, while IL-1ra secretion is increased – a phenotype quite similar to the 'immunoparalysis' phenomenon. Moreover, neutralization of IL-10 blocks LPS desensitization, a phenomenon in which monocytic TNF release is inhibited by a prior exposure to a low dose of LPS [3,12]. These data suggest that inflammation by itself may induce its own downregulation via the nuclear factor-kappa B (NF-κB) pathway induced by TNF. The monocyte deactivation frequently observed in patients surviving septic shock (late sepsis) may be related to this phenomenon of counter-regulation, termed the compensatory anti-inflammatory response syndrome (CARS) by Roger Bone [19].

Inflammation and infection are frequently associated with apoptotic cell death. In order to prevent overwhelming inflammation during scavenging apoptotic material, uptake of apoptotic material by monocytes also downregulates TNF secretion capacity and upregulates IL-10 secretion. The molecular mechanism is not fully understood but the CD14/CD36 receptors seem to be involved [20, Doecke et al. unpublished observations]. A massive induction of apoptosis in organ failure (e.g., liver failure) may contribute to the phenomenon of 'immunoparalysis' in septic and trauma patients.

Moreover, the stress axis also seems to be involved in the regulation of IL-10 released during systemic inflammation/infection. In contrast to the situation *in vitro*, in both humans and mice, TNF and IL-10 are secreted in parallel *in vivo* within one hour following LPS challenge suggesting the involvement of TNF-independent mechanisms for IL-10 regulation. Using reverse transcriptase-polymerase chain reaction (RT-PCR) analyses we found a very high TNF and IL-10 mRNA expression in mouse or rat livers 1 hour after LPS injection while peripheral blood leukocytes expressed TNF only. Eight hours later, IL-10 mRNA was also detectable in blood leukocytes and the protein was, in contrast to TNF, still detectable in the plasma. Both late IL-10 mRNA and IL-10 protein expression were inhibited by the application of a neutralizing anti-TNF mAb in parallel with LPS. In contrast, the early IL-10 synthesis was not reduced following TNF blockade. However, when β2-adrenergic receptors were blocked, not only was early IL-10 release strongly inhibited but the early TNF release was increased (Volk et al., unpublished data).

IL-10 is not the Complete Story of 'Immunoparalysis'

Several data suggest that IL-10 is not the only mediator. Plasma samples from patients with monocyte deactivation following major surgery or from septic patients, but not those from adequate controls, inhibited the monocytic HLA-DR expression and *ex vivo* TNF secretion of indicator cells from healthy donors. In most samples elevated IL-10 levels were detectable, however, neutralizing IL-10 mAb showed variable effects in that it reversed the inhibitory plasma activity by 20 to 100 %. This suggests that, at least in some samples, additional immunosuppressive factors are present. Moreover, we recently performed a clinical trial in which IL-10 was used for treatment of psoriasis. The patients received up to 12 μg/kg body weight/day of IL-10 subcutaneously for several weeks, resulting in plasma IL-10 levels comparable with those seen in many ICU patients (20-100 pg/ml). As expected, monocytic HLA-DR expression, antigen-presenting activity, *ex vivo* TNF/IL-12 secretion capacity, and the Th1-/Th2- cytokine ratio were significantly inhibited [21]. However, we never observed such a strong downregulation of monocyte function as is seen in 'immunoparalysis'. Again, this suggests that IL-10 is an important player in monocyte deactivation - but not the only one. As long-lasting immunodepression in

ICU patients is frequently associated with endotoxemia (systemic infection, translocation), we wondered whether endotoxemia may contribute to the pathogenesis of 'immunoparalysis'. Very recently we compared the monocyte deactivation following endotoxin priming (simulation of endotoxemia) and IL-10 treatment (simulation of stress response only). Our data indicated that endotoxin mediates its suppressive effects mainly via IL-10 but provokes a more profound and longer-lasting anti-inflammatory state in monocytes than IL-10 does alone, suggesting additional co-factors which maintain the IL-10 induced monocyte deactivation in patients with endotoxemia [13].

In addition the patient's predisposition is a further factor which clearly has a major impact on the balance between inflammation and anti-inflammation. Allelic polymorphisms have been described which are associated with low or high IL-10 and TNF production, respectively [23].

CONCLUSION

- Failure of the organ, the 'immune system', that is associated with a diminished antimicrobial defense and disturbed wound healing, is a strong negative predictor for the outcome of ICU patients.
- Death by sepsis may occur not only as the result of too much inflammation (TNF, IL-1) but also by too little inflammation – in other words, TNF and IL-1 are not simply the 'bad guys'. The pathophysiology of infection-associated death under 'hypoinflammatory' conditions is, however, poorly understood.
- 'Immunoparalysis' is defined as diminished monocytic: i) HLA-DR expression, ii) antigen-presenting activity, and iii) capacity to produce proinflammatory cytokines like TNF-α.
- To make results comparable and to introduce immune monitoring into routine diagnostic programs, a well standardized procedure is essential. The development of two standardized monocyte assays (*ex vivo* TNF secretion and HLA-DR expression) is the first step in this direction.
- High-dose, exogenous immunosuppression may be associated with development of 'immunoparalysis' which predisposes to a higher incidence of bacterial/fungal infections and a poorer outcome from established infection. Recovery from 'immunoparalysis' in transplant patients by indirect immunostimulation (withdrawal of immunosuppression) improves antimicrobial defense and outcome.
- Short-term immunodepression is seen in almost all patients following trauma and major surgery. Obviously, stress mediators play a key role in the pathogenesis of temporary posttraumatic immunodepression.

However, some patients develop severe immunodepression (immunparalysis) which may persist. This situation is associated with a high incidence of infectious complications and a poor outcome.

- IL-10 is induced by different pathways (stress response, uptake of apoptotic material, and inflammation) and may play a key role in downregulating immune responsiveness. The summation of these effects in patients with LPS translocation after severe trauma/major surgery or in septic patients may explain the more long-lasting `immunoparalysis` in these patients.

- IL-10 is an important, but not the only, mediator of immunodepression in ICU patients.

The immune system should be regarded as an organ that, in ICU patients, can be driven to failure just as a liver or a kidney can. The monitoring of other system functions (kidney, liver, blood pressure, lung, coagulation, etc.) is well established on ICUs, but monitoring of the immune system is still poorly developed. However, immune responsiveness is essential for the control of infections. In this sense, the failure of immunotherapeutic approaches in sepsis introduced without immune monitoring is perhaps hardly surprising. The data from our pilot trials (IFN-γ therapy, plasmapheresis, G-CSF therapy) suggest that immunostimulation in septic patients with defined 'immunoparalysis' may provide a novel approach. Controlled multicenter trials will be necessary to test this hypothesis. The recently developed well standardized immunoassays may help to perform multicenter trials. On the one hand, immune competence can be measured by a quantitative HLA-DR flow cytometric measurement and by a semi-automatic *ex vivo* whole blood TNF secretion assay, while on the other hand inflammation and tissue injury can be detected by measurement of plasma TNF and IL-6 levels by semiautomatic systems. Moreover, it has been shown that measurement of procalcitonin plasma levels is helpful for early detection of invasive bacterial/fungal infections.

In our view, preemptive therapy of high-risk patients would be a much better approach than the treatment of established sepsis. In order to improve the cost/benefit ratio of immune interventions, measurement of immunocompetence may help to detect patients at high risk of developing infectious complications after major surgery and trauma. With the availability of standardized immune monitoring procedures we can now design appropriate clinical trials.

ACKNOWLEDGMENT

This work was supported in part by the Deutsche Forschungsgemeinschaft (DFG SFB Volk).

REFERENCES

1. Natanson C, Hoffman WD, Suffredini AF et al. Selected treatment strategies for septic shock based on proposed mechanisms of pathogenesis. Ann Intern Med 1994; 120:771-783
2. Zeni F, Freeman B, Natanson C. Anti-inflammatory therapies to treat sepsis and septic shock: a reassessment. Crit Care Med 1997; 25:1095-1100
3. Döcke WD, Randow F, Syrbe U, Krausch D, Asadullah K, Reinke P, Volk HD, Kox W . Monocyte deactivation in septic patients: restoration by IFN-γ treatment. Nature Med 1997; 3:678-681
4. Echtenacher B, Falk W, Mannel DN et al. Requirement of endogenous tumor necrosis factor/cachectin for recovery from experimental peritonitis. J Immunol 1990; 145:3762-3766
5. Pfeffer K. Mice deficient for the p55 kD tumor necrosis factor receptor are resistant to endotoxic shock, yet succumb to L. monocytogenes infection. Cell 1993; 73:457-467
6. Jack RS, Fan X, Bernheiden M et al. Lipopolysaccharide binding protein is required to combat a murine gram-negative bacterial infection. Nature 1997; 389:742-745
7. Berg DJ, Kuhn R, Rajewsky K et al. IL-10 is a central regulator of the response to LPS in murine models of endotoxic shock and the Schwartzman reaction but not endotoxin tolerance. J Clin Invest 1995; 96:2339-2347
8. Christ M, McCartney-Francis NL, Kulkarni AB et al. Immune dysregulation in TGF-beta 1 deficient mice. J Immunol 1994; 153:1936-1946
9. Rosenbloom AJ, Pinsky MR, Napolitano C et al. Suppression of cytokine-mediated beta2-integrin activation on circulating neutrophils in critically ill patients. J Leukoc Biol 1999; 66:83-89
10. Faist E, Kim C. Therapeutic immunomodulatory approaches for the control of systemic inflammatory response syndrome and the prevention of sepsis. New Horiz 1998; 6:97-102
11. Döcke WD, Reinke P, Syrbe U et al. Immunoparalysis in sepsis – from phenomenon to treatment strategies. Transplantationsmedizin 1997; 9:55-65
12. Randow F, Syrbe U, Meisel C et al. Mechanism of endotoxin desensitization – involvement of IL-10 and TGFß. J Exp Med 1995; 5:1887-1892
13. Volk HD, Reinke P, Falck P Staffa G, Briedigkeit H, von Baehr R. Diagnostic value of an immune monitoring program for the clinical management of immunosuppressed patients with septic complications. Clin Transplant 1989; 3:246-252
14. Zedler S, Bone RC, Baue AE et al. T-cell reactivity and its predictive role in immunosuppression after burns. Crit Care Med 1999; 27:66-72
15. Hershman MJ, Cheadle WG, Wellhausen SR et al. Monocyte HLA-DR antigen expression characterizes clinical outcome in the trauma patient. Br J Surg 1990; 77:204-207
16. Livingston DH, Appel SH, Wellhausen SR et al. Depressed interferon gamma production and monocyte HLA-DR expression after severe injury. Arch Surg 1988; 123:1309-1312

17. Woiciechowsky C, Asadullah K, Nestler D, Eberhardt B, Platzer C, Schöning B, Glöckner F, Lanksch WR, Volk HD, Döcke WD. Sympathetic activation triggers systemic IL-10 release in immunodepression induced by brain injury. Nature Med 1998; 4:808-813
18. Meisel C, Vogt K, Platzer C et al. Differential regulation of monocytic tumor necrosis factor-alpha and interleukin-10 expression. Eur J Immunol 1996; 26:1580-1586
19. Bone RC. Sir Isaac Newton, sepsis, SIRS, and CARS. Crit Care Med 1996; 24:1125-1128
20. Voll RE, Herrmann M, Roth EA et al. Immunosuppressive effects of apoptotic cells. Nature 1997; 390:350-351
21. Asadullah K, Stephanek K, Leupold M et al. IL-10 is a key cytokine in psoriasis. Proof of principle by IL-10 therapy: a new therapeutic approach. J Clin Invest 1998; 101:1-12
22. Wolk K, Döcke WD, von Baehr V, Volk HD, Sabat R. Impaired antigen presentation by human monocytes during endotoxin tolerance. Blood 2000; 96: 218-223.
23. Eskdale J, Gallagher G, Verweij CL et al. Interleukin 10 secretion in relation to human IL-10 locus haplotypes. Proc Natl Acad Sci USA 1998; 95:9465-9470

12

PATHOPHYSIOLOGY OF SEPSIS: THE ROLE OF NITRIC OXIDE

Simon Jonathan Finney
Timothy W Evans

In 1998, the Nobel Prize for Physiology and Medicine was awarded to Drs. Furchgott, Ignarro, and Murad in recognition of their work establishing that nitric oxide (NO) is a key signaling molecule in the cardiovascular system. Ignarro linked Murad's work on the vascular effects of exogenously applied NO to Furchgott's classic vascular ring experiments in which he demonstrated the presence of an endothelially derived relaxing factor. Subsequently, it has become apparent that this outwardly simple diatomic free radical gas modulates a wide range of biological activities including vascular homeostasis, neurotransmission and host defense; and is implicated in the pathogenesis of many disease states as diverse as arteriosclerosis and Alzheimer's disease.

BIOSYNTHESIS OF NITRIC OXIDE

Production

NO is formed stereo-specifically from the terminal guanidine nitrogen of the semi essential amino acid L-arginine, catalysed by a family of hemoproteins, the NO synthases (NOS). NOS has both oxidoreductase and oxygenase domains. The reductase domain binds flavin-adenine mononucleotide, flavin mononucleotide, and nicotinamide adenine dinucleotide phosphate (NADPH). The oxidase domain binds L-arginine, a heme moiety (iron protoporphyrin IX), and tetrahydrobiopterin. Homo-dimerization of the enzyme allows *trans* transfer of electrons from NAPDH to the oxidase domain, converting L-arginine to NO and L-citrulline, via N-hydroxy-L-arginine. The process consumes molecular oxygen.

Three isoforms of NOS, with 50-60% sequence homology, have been identified and subsequently cloned: neuronal (nNOS); endothelial (eNOS); and inducible (iNOS) or types 1, 2, and 3 respectively [1]. nNOS is encoded on chromosome 12, and is constitutively expressed in neurones, skeletal muscle, renal mesangium and pancreatic islets. eNOS is encoded on chromosome 7, and is constitutively expressed in the membrane and Golgi apparatus of endothelium, platelets, endocardium, and myocardium. iNOS is encoded on chromosome 17 and, except in the renal mesangium, is not generally expressed under physiological conditions. Immune cells, vascular smooth muscle, endothelial cells, myocardium, hepatocytes, astrocytes, renal mesangial cells, chondrocytes and fibroblasts can all be induced to express iNOS, which lacks the specific membrane targeting sequence of the other isoforms and is thus found in the cytosol. The presence of NOS in rat mitochondria (mtNOS) has been demonstrated [2], although whether this is a distinct nuclear encoded isoform or a post translational modification of type 2 NOS is unclear [3]. mtNOS has a role in the regulation of respiration, matrix pH, and transmembrane potential in mitochondria.

Regulation of NOS Activity

All three NOS isoforms have comparable specific activities in the presence of appropriate calcium levels (*vide infra*). Enzymatic output is therefore rate limited by substrate availability and the quantity of enzyme present. All three isoforms rely on the presence of calmodulin, which facilitates the transfer of electrons through the enzyme. For nNOS and eNOS, calmodulin binding occurs in response to intracellular calcium transients of the order of ~100 nM. These transients may result from activity of agonists such as bradykinin, acetylcholine, glutamate, or from changes in vascular shear stress. Constitutive NO production is rapid and short-lived and in the picomolar range. eNOS is also regulated at a transcriptional level by vascular shear stress, exercise training, chronic hypoxia, and heart failure. Calmodulin binding in iNOS unusually requires very low levels of calcium (30-70 nM); enzymatic activity is thus regulated at a transcriptional level. The promoter region of the human iNOS gene contains the appropriate response elements for shear stress and interferon-γ (IFN-γ), and a nuclear factor kappa B (NF-κB) binding consensus sequence [4]. In murine models, NF-κB activation is essential for lipopolysaccharide (LPS)-stimulated iNOS expression [5]; whereas both NF-κB and IFN-γ can cause NOS induction in humans [6, 7]. iNOS is also regulated post-transcriptionally by virtue of an 'AUUUA' motif in the 3' untranslated region of its mRNA. These motifs confer instability to mRNA, allowing the transient expression of a protein in response to a stimulus. NO production from iNOS lasts several hours, and produces levels 1000 fold higher than constitutive NOS.

Fate of Nitric Oxide

The main route of NO elimination is through combination with oxyhemoglobin which catalyses NO to nitrite and nitrate, both of which are detectable in serum and urine. The formation of S-nitrosothiols (RSNO) may act as an NO store. The manner in which S-nitrosothiols form is unclear, since NO itself is not a nitrosating agent.

NO Production in Sepsis

There are considerable *in vitro* and *in vivo* data demonstrating that NO production is increased in rodent models of sepsis [8, 9]. This is at least in part due to induction of iNOS in both immune cells and many tissues including lung, liver, kidney, muscle and spleen [10]. Induction of iNOS mRNA occurs within 20-40 minutes, is maximal at 4-6 hours, and returns to normal at 24 hours. Similarly, primary human immune and vascular cell lines stimulated *in vitro* demonstrate iNOS activity. Human *in vivo* data are more limited, NO production appearing to be less dramatic than in rodents. Nevertheless, septic and LPS-challenged humans have increased urinary and plasma levels of nitrate and nitrite [11-13] with increased iNOS mRNA and activity demonstrated in both immune cells and solid tissues [14-16]. Parenchymal cells are the dominant source of NO in human sepsis [17].

Pharmacological Manipulation of Nitric Oxide

Inhibitors of NOS

The pharmacological inhibitors of NOS are summarized in Table 1.

Considerable research has focused on the L-arginine analogs, in particular L-NMMA and L-NAME, which competitively inhibit NOS directly, but also compete for cellular substrate uptake. L-NAME is more specific for eNOS [18], whereas L-NMMA is non-selective.

Considerable efforts have been made to develop inhibitors selective to specific isoforms, particularly iNOS. Such agents include aminoguanidine, isothioureas, and 1400W. Studies using aminoguanidine are complicated by its effects on cyclooxygenase and histamine deaminase. Recently a highly specific pyrimidineimidazole based allosteric inhibitor of iNOS dimerization has been described [19]; it is still to be assessed *in vivo* or *in vitro*.

Class	Compound(s)
L-arginine derivatives	N-nitro-L-arginine methyl ester (L-NAME), N^G-monomethyl-L-arginine (L-NMMA), N-nitro-L-arginine, N-amino-L-arginine, L-cyclopropyl-arginine, L-allylarginine, L-canavanine*
Guanidines	Aminoguanidine* N-(3-(Aminomethyl)benzyl)acetamidine (1400W)*
Isothioureas	S-ethylisothiourea*, S-isopropylthiourea*
Indazoles	7-Nitroindazole
NOS dimerization inhibitors	Pyrimidineimidazoles*
Heme binders	NO, Carbon monoxide
iNOS induction inhibitors	Corticosteroids, TGF-β 1/2/3, IL-4, IL-10, PGE$_2$
BH$_4$ depletor	2,4-diamino-6-hydroxypyrimidine

Table 1. Pharmacological inhibitors of NOS (denotes relative iNOS selectivity).*

Nitric Oxide Donors

Pharmacological NO donors include the organic nitrates: nitroglycerin, isosorbide dinitrate and mononitrate. NO release is both enzymatic and non-enzymatic, possibly involving thiol groups [20]. Sodium nitroprusside, an iron-nitrosyl complex, also acts as a NO donor indirectly; requiring partial reduction by agents such as thiols to liberate the nitrosonium ion (NO^+) which acts as nitrosating species.

CELLULAR EFFECTS OF NITRIC OXIDE (FIGURE 1)

Nitric oxide acts within the interlinking network of second messenger systems [21,22]. A free radical by virtue of the unpaired electron in the outer shell of its nitrogen atom, NO has low reactivity relative to other free radicals. It interacts with transitional metals, central to cellular enzymatics; oxygen; thiols; and other free radicals. Its high lipophilicity permits easy passage across biological membranes. Mechanistically, the effects of NO may be direct or indirect. Indirect effects are mediated by virtue of the conversion of NO to peroxynitrite and dinitrogen trioxide in the presence of superoxide and oxygen. The balance between direct and indirect actions is dependent on both the rate of NO production and the prevailing redox balance. Direct effects dominate in health, whilst indirect effects occur at times of high NO flux and oxidative stress.

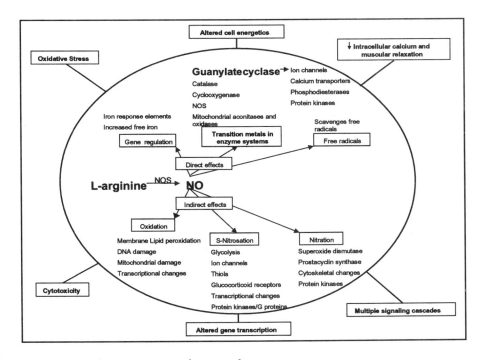

Figure 1. Cellular consequences of nitric oxide

Enzyme Systems

NO forms a nitrosyl complex with the iron of soluble guanylyl cyclase, causing it to translocate to the cell membrane where it catalyses the conversion of guanosine triphosphate to cyclic guanosine monophosphate (cGMP). The EC_{50} of NO for this reaction is relatively low (~100 nM) [23] making this the dominant signaling pathway for NO. cGMP acts on an array of other signaling pathways including the phosphodiesterases; ion channels, protein kinases, and various Ca^{2+} transporters. The net result is a fall in free intracellular calcium. The consequences are smooth muscle relaxation, inhibition of platelet aggregation, and altered cell adhesion molecule expression. Phosphodiesterase modulation provides cross talk to cAMP pathways.

NO promotes the existence of the ferric form of iron-complexes within other enzyme systems, including cyclooxygenase (COX), catalase and cytochrome oxidases as well as NOS itself [21]. Cross-talk to both constitutive and induced COX pathways modulates vasoreactivity, platelet aggregation, and leukocyte-endothelial interactions. NO-mediated inhibition of NOS activity acts as a negative feedback loop, and probably explains the decline in eNOS activity in profound sepsis.

Mitochondrial Function

NO causes reversible inhibition of cytochrome oxidase, the terminal complex of the electron transport chain, by competing with oxygen for its binding site to the a_3 heme moiety. This effectively increases the K_m for respiration, and reduces oxidative phosphorylation. Aconitases in the citric acid cycle are also inhibited by NO. Thus NO profoundly influences cellular energetics, directing them towards anaerobic glycolysis and lactate formation. Whilst this may be physiologically advantageous in areas of low oxygen flux, it may be profoundly negative and promote cytotoxicity. The function and control of mtNOS in septic humans is largely unexplored; studies are pressing.

Hemoglobin

NO is oxidized by oxyhemoglobin to nitrate and methemoglobin. This is the main route of NO elimination and provides the rationale for the use of free hemoglobin solutions as pressor agents. Addition reactions result in Fe^{2+}-nitrosyl hemoglobin and S-nitrosohemoglobin; these promote peripheral oxygen unloading and act as temporary NO stores respectively.

Redox Balance

NO is anti-oxidant reacting with highly oxidant species such as ferryl ions (Fe^{4+}) and hydroxyl ($\Box OH$) from the Fenton reaction. NO can also increase oxidative stresses by effects on catalase or intracellular free iron, a key catalyst in oxidative chemistry. Nitrosylation of catalase by high levels of NO is inhibitory, reducing the consumption of hydrogen peroxide. At lower levels NO is scavenged by hydrogen peroxide and catalase via complex I to form nitrite. NO influences intracellular iron by promoting the binding of iron binding proteins to their response elements thus modulating transcription of ferritin and transferrin receptors, and tending to increase free iron. Release of iron from ferritin is also reduced by NADPH oxidase inhibition.

Indirect Effects

Peroxynitrite

Peroxynitrite is formed from the combination of NO with superoxide, generated by the xanthine and NAPDPH oxidase systems (in inflammatory cells), or electron leak along the transport chain (exacerbated by NO inhibition of cytochrome oxidase), or even from NOS. Superoxide is usually scavenged by superoxide dismutase which is present in sufficient quantity to ensure that peroxynitrite only forms in settings of high superoxide flux or in close proximity to production; typically at endothelial cells. Peroxynitrite causes nitration (addition of NO_2) and oxidation. Oxidation of DNA results in base modifications and strand breakage (triggering poly(ADP-ribose) synthase and necrosis). Cytotoxicity is enhanced by lipid peroxidation of membranes. Thiol oxidation can alter gene transcription via nuclear zinc-thiolate centres. Nitration reactions result in the inhibition of mitochondrial superoxide dismutase, altered cytoskeletal structure, altered sarcoplasmic calcium ATPase, kinases, and inhibition of prostacyclin synthase with consequent platelet aggregation, vasodilatation, myocardial dysfunction, and altered leukocyte adhesion.

S-Nitrosation

NO may combine with oxygen to form the potent nitrosating (addition of NO) species dinitrogen trioxide. In high NO flux environments nitrosation of thiols and amines can become significant. S-nitrosation of proteins influences many other signalling pathways, and metabolic processes. S-nitrosation of glucocorticoid receptors reduces their affinity for steroids, maybe explaining the reduced efficacy of steroids in septic shock. Intracellular calcium is modulated directly via ryanodine receptors, and L-type calcium channels, but also indirectly via potassium channels thus causing vasodilatation and myocardial dysfunction.

Glyceraldehyde-3-phosphate dehydrogenase (GAPDH), creatine-kinase, enzymes of glycolysis, are inhibited: this may promote cytotoxicity in cells with already impaired oxidative phosphorylation.

S-nitrosation of signalling proteins such as protein kinase C and G-proteins, as well as transcription factors may have profound implications for catecholamine signalling, surface adhesion molecule expression, and cytokine production.

S-nitrosation of key synthetic enzymes results in reduced levels of glutathione (GSH), an important cellular defense against both nitrosative and oxidative stresses. S-nitrosation also stimulates the hexose monophosphate shunt which provides the reducing energy for GSH biosynthesis.

SYSTEMIC EFFECTS OF NITRIC OXIDE

Microcirculatory Function

Vascular Tone

Hypotension and hyporesponsiveness to vasoconstrictors are striking clinical manifestations of systemic sepsis. In rodents, LPS causes a sustained drop in blood pressure and a hyporesponsiveness to norepinephrine within 60 minutes, lasting at least 180 minutes. The blood pressure and response to norepinephrine is restored by L-NAME. Vasodilatation is primarily a consequence of NO-mediated guanylate cyclase activation, increased cGMP, and hence lower intracellular calcium levels. Dexamethasone, which prevents transcription of many genes including iNOS, abrogates hypotension at 180 minutes, but not that occurring within 60 minutes [24]. Furthermore, iNOS mRNA is not detected until at least 20 minutes after LPS administration; actual protein synthesis undoubtedly takes longer. Thus iNOS, whilst accounting for the massive increase in NO production from endothelium and vascular smooth muscle at 3 hours, cannot explain the rodent vascular response in the first 60 minutes. It is hypothesized that the early response may be due to constitutive NOS activity [25] triggered by kinins, endothelin, and platelet activating factor (PAF) [26-28], or guanylate cyclase activation by carbon monoxide produced by hemoxygenase-1 [29], hyperpolarization of smooth muscle membranes by potassium channels [30], or direct guanylate cyclase activation by LPS [31].

Despite NO-mediated vasodilatation and a global fall in systemic vascular resistance, endotoxemic models in vivo and using vascular rings demonstrate vasoconstriction in the mesenteric [32], pulmonary [33], and renal [34] circulations. This is due to the unopposed action of released vasoconstrictors such as endothelin [35], leukotrienes, and thromboxane [34]. Heterogeneity within each vascular bed is likely. In this setting, NO has a protective role, with NOS inhibition exacerbating vasoconstriction, regional hypoperfusion [36], and hence tissue oxygenation. In endotoxemic rats, low skeletal muscle tissue oxygen tensions are further reduced by non-selective NOS inhibition, with a reduced response to increases in administered oxygen [37].

In the lung, hypoxic pulmonary vasoconstriction is diminished by NO, worsening shunt [33]; NOS inhibition improves but does not normalize hypoxic pulmonary vasoconstriction, implying the presence of alternative mechanisms. Inhaled NO has been employed by some attempting to improve pulmonary hemodynamics [38].

Platelet function

NO has significant anti-aggregatory properties on platelets mediated via increased levels of cGMP, which influences phospholipase C activity and prevents diacylglycerol and inositol 1,4,5-triphosphate production; key secondary messengers in the activation of platelets via agonists [39]. cGMP also mediates a reduction in cytosolic calcium, which is central to platelet activation [40]. Thus, under physiological conditions, eNOS prevents activation of platelets within the circulation, and helps to preserve microvascular flow.

The effects of NO on the microcirculation are summarized in Figure 2.

Barrier Function

Vascular permeability increases in sepsis by mechanisms including LPS-induced caspase activation of intercellular adherent junctions with paracellular flux, and loss of endothelial cells by cytotoxicity [41]. iNOS derived NO is also important. The role of NO in modulating increased vascular permeability is complex; NO from constitutive NOS activity is seemingly protective under physiological conditions, whereas excessive iNOS-derived NO is detrimental [42]. iNOS inhibition with an isothiourea abrogates the permeability increase in response to intradermal LPS in mice [43]. Similar results have been obtained in iNOS knockout mice using both dermal and mesenteric vessels. It is hypothesised that the detrimental effect of excessive NO on permeability is mediated by cGMP stimulated phosphodiesterases reducing cAMP levels. Elevated cAMP phosphorylates myosin light chain kinase and causes the formation of tight junctional strands, modulating cytoskeletal changes and preserving vascular integrity.

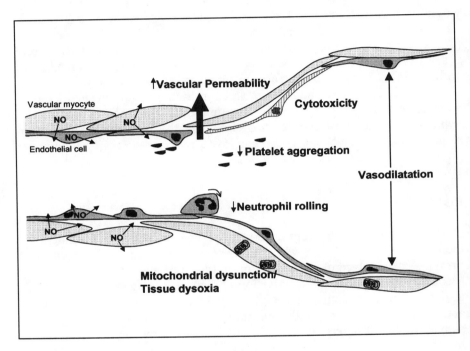

Figure 2. Microcirculatory effects of nitric oxide.

Immune Function

There is strong evidence to suggest NO has anti-microbial properties [44]. Mice unable to produce NO from iNOS, either by virtue of a genetic deletion or the presence of a specific inhibitor are more susceptible to infection by *Listeria monocytogenes* [45], *Chlamydia pneumoniae* [46], *Mycobacterium tuberculosis* [47], and *Staphylococcus aureus* [48]. The anti-microbial activity is not universal, with iNOS knockout mice being no more susceptible than wild-type mice to *Mycobacterium avium intracellulare* complex [49]. NO mediates its anti-microbial action by both direct cytotoxicity [50] and through modification of T cell responses [51]. iNOS is induced in rodent and human neutrophils and macrophages, triggered by stimuli (e.g., IFN-γ) that also stimulate phagocytic NADPH oxidase. The consequence is a diverse arsenal of reactive nitrogen and oxygen species released in the vicinity of the phagocyte, with potential to damage microbial (and host) DNA, protein, and membranes.

The anti-microbial action of NO contrasts with its ability to reduce neutrophil recruitment to tissues, which may include sites of infection. Leukocyte capture, and subsequent rolling on the endothelium are an essential prelude to firm adhesion and migration out of the circulation into tissues. This process results from interactions between endothelial selectins and intercellular adhesion molecule (ICAM)-1, with neutrophil integrins. Genetically iNOS deleted rodents demonstrate increased rolling in the microcirculation [52]; possibly since NO can influence the expression of endothelial selectins [53]. This effect may be less important at sites of infection, where local chemokines may dominate the picture up-regulating neutrophil recruitment. NO may then simply function to prevent the overspill of leukocyte adhesion to the whole circulation.

Cardiac Function

Myocardial dysfunction is typical of human septic shock, even in the setting of a hyperdynamic circulation. It is characterized by a reduced ejection fraction, biventricular dilatation, and a decreased response to catecholamines or fluid resuscitation. Studies in rodent isolated myocytes and papillary muscles suggest that myocyte dysfunction is due to a circulating factor(s), and that this is at least in part mediated via both autocrine and extra-myocytic NO loops [54], and increased cGMP production via guanylate cyclase [55]. The force of cardiac contraction is intimately linked to intracellular calcium levels: calcium activates troponin which exposes actin binding sites and allows actin-myosin cross bridge cycling. Increased cGMP reduces intracellular calcium directly and reduces agonist induced cAMP rises via stimulation of cGMP dependent phosphodiesterases [56].

Additional mechanisms have been implicated in NO mediated cardiac dysfunction. NO inhibits mitochondrial oxidative phosphorylation in rat cardiac myocytes [57], reflected by a fall from 70% to 40% in the heart's oxygen extraction ratio. Depletion of intramyocyte energy stores reduce the myocyte's ability to sustain cross-bridge cycling and normal contractile function [58].

In vivo studies in animals, confirm the decline in contractility which is prevented by L-NMMA [59]. Cardiac output, however, classically falls with non-selective blockade; the importance of changes in coronary flow or alterations in right and ventricular loading are undefined.

THE INTEGRATED RESPONSE

The role of NO in the integrated response, with other effector systems present, is provided by systemic inhibition of NOS *in vivo*, or the use of mice with targeted genetic deletions.

Nitric Oxide Synthase Inhibition

L-NMMA has been extensively studied in animal models and increases systemic vascular resistance (SVR) and arterial blood pressure in septic rodents, canines, pigs [60-62]. The rise in SVR is characteristically accompanied by a fall in cardiac index and rise in pulmonary vascular resistance. Improved global hemodynamics are not translated into a survival advantage; in most studies mortality was unchanged or increased. In one anesthetized porcine model, death was averted during the 9 hour study period [62]. This disparity may be accounted for by experimental differences in species used, the timing of interventions, use of anesthesia, and nature of the septic insult. However, the results reflect that widespread inhibition of NOS may be inappropriate either due to unfavorable effects on regional hemodynamics or other roles of NO in redox balance, immune function, or hemostasis [63].

In clinical sepsis, L-NMMA causes a sustained increase in SVR and systemic arterial blood pressure [12,64], allowing partial or complete withdrawal of concomitant norepinephrine infusions. Predictably, L-NMMA infusion is also accompanied by a fall in cardiac index and increase in pulmonary vascular resistance [64]; there are no data concerning right ventricular functional changes. Following a successful phase II trial demonstrating accelerated recovery from shock and better urine output, a phase III randomized placebo-controlled trial of L-NMMA was undertaken in septic patients for up to 14 days, with dobutamine employed to maintain the cardiac index. The trial was terminated early after enrolling 795 patients due to an excess mortality in the treatment group [65] attributed to cardiovascular events rather than multi-organ failure (MOF). It is not clear whether the failure was due to the non-selective nature of the drug or the manner of its administration. Similar results have been obtained in humans using L-NAME [66].

Subsequently interest has focused on selective iNOS blockade, using agents such as isothioureas, aminoguanidine, and L-canavanine. Whilst improving global hemodynamics, such agents may avoid deleterious effects on regional hemodynamics. In rodent endotoxemic models the drugs result in improved in liver enzymes, creatinine, and lactate [67,68], implying improved organ function if not perfusion. Moreover, some studies have demonstrated an improved short-term survival [69,70]. Isothiourea dramatically improved survival and parameters of both global and regional haemodynamics in pigs infused with streptococci [71]. However, control pigs did not show evidence of increased NO production, and the improved survival may be attributable to the additional free radical scavenging effects of the agent.

iNOS Knockout Mice

MacMicking et al [45] were some of the first to report on iNOS knockout mice. This phenotypically normal mouse had no compensatory increase in constitutive NOS expression. Anesthetized endotoxemic iNOS deleted mice survived for five hours without hypotension. Non-anaesthetized mice were only protected from higher doses of LPS, and showed similar liver dysfunction to wild type animals at lower doses of LPS. Any advantages were removed by prior activation of the immune system with autoclaved *Proprioniobacterium acnes*. Furthermore, knockout animals succumbed to ten fold lower innocula of whole bacteria *(Listeria monocytogenes)* in comparison to wild types.

Survival studies in similar models of knockout mice undergoing caecal ligation and puncture report both survival advantage and disadvantage [72,73]. These disparities once again reflect the importance of other mediators and the potential protective role of iNOS derived NO.

CONCLUSION

Nitric oxide is a key molecule in vascular regulation in health; its production is significantly increased in systemic sepsis. Clinically, sepsis is characterized by hyporeactivity to pressor agents, increased vascular permeability, myocardial dysfunction, reduced tissue oxygen consumption, and disseminated intravascular coagulation. In vitro and animal studies have implicated NO in all of these clinical observations. However, it is increasingly apparent that NO has a duplicitous role; on the one hand promoting microvascular flow and aiding bacterial killing; whilst on the other disabling metabolic processes, reducing leukocyte recruitment to tissues, and causing hypotension and cardiac dysfunction severe enough to threaten the perfusion of vital organs.

The importance of NO in the integrated host response to a septic insult is more difficult to define. Results in both animal and human clinical studies are contrasting, explained by differences in species, septic insult, timing and nature of interventions, and patient co-morbidities. Septic rodents produce considerably more NO than humans, and these models may thus unfairly favor NOS blockade; some authors even suggest that the study of higher mammals is more appropriate [74].

Nevertheless, it is evident that in both humans and animals, NO is important in hypotension and vascular dysfunction. Inhibitors universally increase systemic vascular resistance and reverse hypotension. This hypotension starts before iNOS can be both transcripted and transcribed, reflecting the role of either constitutive NOS or alternative effector pathways in this phenomenon. The clinical use of a NOS inhibitor as simple a replacement for norepinephrine would only be justified if either regional hemodynamics improve, or there are other beneficial effects; animal and human studies have not been able to consistently demonstrate this effect. Indeed many studies have shown detrimental effects of NOS inhibition.

The lack of benefit of NOS inhibition in clinical trials has been attributed in part to the non-selectivity of the drugs used. It is hypothesized, that problems encountered with NOS inhibition namely reduced cardiac index, increased pulmonary hypertension, leukocyte rolling, and platelet aggregation may be prevented by the use of selective iNOS inhibitors, and thus preservation of eNOS activity.

Selective iNOS inhibitors have only been applied in animal models to date. Several studies have demonstrated improved early survival, by averting hypotensive deaths. Early hypotensive deaths are uncommon in clinical practice, and thus the relevance of this observation is debatable. Death is usually attributable to MOF. The studies also demonstrate improved regional hemodynamics, which may help curtail the development of organ dysfunction. We suggest that regional hemodynamics should be one of the yardsticks against which selective inhibitors are measured rather than global parameters such as systemic pressure and reduction in norepinephrine dosage. Adequate organ perfusion is difficult to quantify numerically, but can be implied by surrogate markers such as urine output, gastrointestinal function and acid base balance. The effects on hemostasis, redox balance, immune function, and metabolic function are likely to be important, but goals are difficult to define. The implications of altered mitochondrial function and other cell energy pathways, have profound implications for tissue and hence organ function, especially when coupled with low tissue oxygen tensions. More basic science studies are needed in these areas to allow us to hypothesize about the potential consequences in human sepsis.

NO production therefore results in both good and bad effects in clinical and experimental sepsis. NOS inhibition should aim to restore this balance in favor of the patient, and not at total NOS inhibition. Where this balance lies in terms of NO production relative to the healthy state is not established. It is also likely that this balance will fluctuate according to insult and during the evolution of sepsis.

REFERENCES

1. Singh S,Evans TW. Nitric oxide, the biological mediator of the decade: fact or fiction? Eur Respir J 1997; 10:699-707
2. Bates TE, Loesch A, Burnstock G, et al. Immunocytochemical evidence for a mitochondrially located nitric oxide synthase in brain and liver. Biochem Biophys Res Commun 1995; 213:896-900
3. Tatoyan A,Giulivi C. Purification and characterization of a nitric-oxide synthase from rat liver mitochondria. J Biol Chem 1998; 273:11044-11048
4. Nunokawa Y, Ishida N,Tanaka S. Promoter analysis of human inducible nitric oxide synthase gene associated with cardiovascular homeostasis. Biochem Biophys Res Commun 1994; 200:802-807
5. Liu SF, Ye X,Malik AB. In vivo inhibition of nuclear factor-kappa B activation prevents inducible nitric oxide synthase expression and systemic hypotension in a rat model of septic shock. J Immunol 1997; 159:3976-3983
6. Kamijo R, Harada H, Matsuyama T, et al. Requirement for transcription factor IRF-1 in NO synthase induction in macrophages. Science 1994; 263:1612-1615
7. Spink J,Evans T. Binding of the transcription factor interferon regulatory factor-1 to the inducible nitric-oxide synthase promoter. J Biol Chem 1997; 272:24417-24425
8. Granger DL, Hibbs JB, Jr.,Broadnax LM. Urinary nitrate excretion in relation to murine macrophage activation. Influence of dietary L-arginine and oral NG-monomethyl-L-arginine. J Immunol 1991; 146:1294-1302
9. Lai CS,Komarov AM. Spin trapping of nitric oxide produced in vivo in septic-shock mice. FEBS Lett 1994; 345:120-124
10. Liu S, Adcock IM, Old RW, et al. Lipopolysaccharide treatment in vivo induces widespread tissue expression of inducible nitric oxide synthase mRNA. Biochem Biophys Res Commun 1993; 196:1208-1213
11. Ochoa JB, Udekwu AO, Billiar TR, et al. Nitrogen oxide levels in patients after trauma and during sepsis. Ann Surg 1991; 214:621-626
12. Grover R, Zaccardelli D, Colice G, et al. An open-label dose escalation study of the nitric oxide synthase inhibitor, N(G)-methyl-L-arginine hydrochloride (546C88), in patients with septic shock. Glaxo Wellcome International Septic Shock Study Group. Crit Care Med 1999; 27:913-922
13. Strand OA, Leone A, Giercksky KE, et al. Nitric oxide indices in human septic shock. Crit Care Med 2000; 28:2779-2785
14. Tsukahara Y, Morisaki T, Horita Y, et al. Expression of inducible nitric oxide synthase in

circulating neutrophils of the systemic inflammatory response syndrome and septic patients. World J Surg 1998; 22:771-777

15. Annane D, Sanquer S, Sebille V, et al. Compartmentalised inducible nitric-oxide synthase activity in septic shock. Lancet 2000; 355:1143-1148

16. Wheeler MA, Smith SD,Weiss RM. Induction of nitric oxide synthase with urinary tract infections. Adv Exp Med Biol 1999; 462:359-369

17. Wang LF, Scott JA, Weicker S, et al. Relative contribution of hemopoietic and pulmonary parenchymal Cells to lung inducible nitric oxide synthase (iNOS) activity in murine sepsis. Biochem Biophys Res Commun 2001; 283:694-699

18. Southan GJ,Szabo C. Selective pharmacological inhibition of distinct nitric oxide synthase isoforms. Biochem Pharmacol 1996; 51:383-394

19. McMillan K, Adler M, Auld DS, et al. Allosteric inhibitors of inducible nitric oxide synthase dimerization discovered via combinatorial chemistry. Proc Natl Acad Sci U S A 2000; 97:1506-1511

20. Al-Sa'doni H,Ferro A. S-Nitrosothiols: a class of nitric oxide-donor drugs. Clin Sci (Colch) 2000; 98:507-520

21. Liaudet L, Soriano FG,Szabo C. Biology of nitric oxide signaling. Crit Care Med 2000; 28 (suppl 4):N37-N52

22. Wink DA,Mitchell JB. Chemical biology of nitric oxide: insights into regulatory, cytotoxic, and cytoprotective mechanisms of nitric oxide. Free Radic Biol Med 1998; 25:434-456

23. Forstermann U, Ishii K: Measurement of cyclic GMP as an indicator of nitric oxide production. In: Feelisch M, Stamler J (eds) Methods in Nitric Oxide Research. Wiley, New York, 1996, pp 555.

24. Szabo C, Mitchell JA, Thiemermann C, et al. Nitric oxide-mediated hyporeactivity to noradrenaline precedes the induction of nitric oxide synthase in endotoxin shock. Br J Pharmacol 1993; 108:786-792

25. Salvemini D, Korbut R, Anggard E, et al. Immediate release of a nitric oxide-like factor from bovine aortic endothelial cells by Escherichia coli lipopolysaccharide. Proc Natl Acad Sci USA 1990; 87:2593-2597

26. Fleming I, Dambacher T,Busse R. Endothelium-derived kinins account for the immediate response of endothelial cells to bacterial lipopolysaccharide. J Cardiovasc Pharmacol 1992; 20 (suppl 12):S135-138

27. Paya D, Stoclet JC. Involvement of bradykinin and nitric oxide in the early hemodynamic effects of lipopolysaccharide in rats. Shock 1995; 3:376-379

28. Szabo C, Wu CC, Mitchell JA, et al. Platelet-activating factor contributes to the induction of nitric oxide synthase by bacterial lipopolysaccharide. Circ Res 1993; 73:991-999

29. Yet S-F, Pellacani A, Patterson C, et al. Induction of heme oxygenase-1 expression in vascular smooth muscle cells. A link to endotoxic shock. J Biol Chem 1997; 272:4295-4301

30. Miyoshi H,Nakaya Y. Endotoxin-induced nonendothelial nitric oxide activates the Ca(2+)-activated K+ channel in cultured vascular smooth muscle cells. J Mol Cell Cardiol 1994; 26:1487-1495

31. Wu CC, Szabo C, Chen SJ, et al. Activation of soluble guanylyl cyclase by a factor other than nitric oxide or carbon monoxide contributes to the vascular hyporeactivity to vasoconstrictor agents in the aorta of rats treated with endotoxin. Biochem Biophys Res Commun 1994; 201:436-442

32. Drazenovic R, Samsel RW, Wylam ME, et al. Regulation of perfused capillary density in canine intestinal mucosa during endotoxemia. J Appl Physiol 1992; 72:259-265

33. Griffiths MJ, Curzen NP, Mitchell JA, et al. In vivo treatment with endotoxin increases rat pulmonary vascular contractility despite NOS induction. Am J Respir Crit Care Med 1997; 156:654-658

34. Badr KF. Sepsis-associated renal vasoconstriction: potential targets for future therapy. Am J Kidney Dis 1992; 20:207-213

35. Snapper JR, Thabes JS, Lefferts PL, et al. Role of endothelin in endotoxin-induced sustained pulmonary hypertension in sheep. Am J Respir Crit Care Med 1998; 157:81-88

36. Mulder MF, van Lambalgen AA, Huisman E, et al. Protective role of NO in the regional hemodynamic changes during acute endotoxemia in rats. Am J Physiol 1994; 266:H1558-H1564

37. Anning PB, Sair M, Winlove CP, et al. Abnormal tissue oxygenation and cardiovascular changes in endotoxemia. Am J Respir Crit Care Med 1999; 159:1710-1715

38. Weitzberg E, Rudehill A, Modin A, et al. Effect of combined nitric oxide inhalation and NG-nitro-L-arginine infusion in porcine endotoxin shock. Crit Care Med 1995; 23:909-918

39. Siess W,Lapetina EG. Platelet aggregation induced by alpha 2-adrenoceptor and protein kinase C activation. A novel synergism. Biochem J 1989; 263:377-385

40. Rink TJ,Sage SO. Calcium signalling in human platelets. Annu Rev Physiol 1990; 52:431-439

41. Bannerman DD, Sathyamoorthy M,Goldblum SE. Bacterial lipopolysaccharide disrupts endothelial monolayer integrity and survival signaling events through caspase cleavage of adherens junction proteins. J Biol Chem 1998; 273:35371-35380

42. Singh S, Winlove CP, Evans TW. Microvascular permeability in experimental sepsis: mechanisms, modulation and management. In: Vincent JL (ed) Yearbook of Intensive Care and Emergency Medicine. Springer, Heidelberg, 2000, pp 80-86

43. Muraki T, Fujii E, Okada M, et al. Effect of S-ethylisothiourea, a putative inhibitor of inducible nitric oxide synthase, on mouse skin vascular permeability. Jpn J Pharmacol 1996; 70:269-271

44. Singh S, Wort SJ,Evans TW. Inducible nitric oxide and pulmonary infection. Thorax 1999; 54:959-960

45. MacMicking JD, Nathan C, Hom G, et al. Altered responses to bacterial infection and endotoxic shock in mice lacking inducible nitric oxide synthase. Cell 1995; 81:641-650

46. Rottenberg ME, Gigliotti Rothfuchs AC, Gigliotti D, et al. Role of innate and adaptive immunity in the outcome of primary infection with Chlamydia pneumoniae, as analyzed in genetically modified mice. J Immunol 1999; 162:2829-2836

47. MacMicking JD, North RJ, LaCourse R, et al. Identification of nitric oxide synthase as a protective locus against tuberculosis. Proc Natl Acad Sci USA 1997; 94:5243-5248

48. Sasaki S, Miura T, Nishikawa S, et al. Protective role of nitric oxide in Staphylococcus aureus infection in mice. Infect Immun 1998; 66:1017-1022

49. Doherty TM,Sher A. Defects in cell-mediated immunity affect chronic, but not innate, resistance of mice to Mycobacterium avium infection. J Immunol 1997; 158:4822-4831

50. Fang FC. Perspectives series: host/pathogen interactions. Mechanisms of nitric oxide-related antimicrobial activity. J Clin Invest 1997; 99:2818-2825

51. MacLean A, Wei XQ, Huang FP, et al. Mice lacking inducible nitric-oxide synthase are more susceptible to herpes simplex virus infection despite enhanced Th1 cell responses. J Gen Virol 1998; 79:825-830

52. Hickey MJ, Sharkey KA, Sihota EG, et al. Inducible nitric oxide synthase-deficient mice have enhanced leukocyte- endothelium interactions in endotoxemia. Faseb J 1997; 11:955-964

53. Davenpeck KL, Gauthier TW,Lefer AM. Inhibition of endothelial-derived nitric oxide promotes P-selectin expression and actions in the rat microcirculation. Gastroenterology 1994; 107:1050-1058

54. Finkel MS, Oddis CV, Jacob TD, et al. Negative inotropic effects of cytokines on the heart mediated by nitric oxide. Science 1992; 257:387-389

55. Finkel MS, Oddis CV, Mayer OH, et al. Nitric oxide synthase inhibitor alters papillary muscle force-frequency relationship. J Pharmacol Exp Ther 1995; 272:945-952

56. Joe EK, Schussheim AE, Longrois D, et al. Regulation of cardiac myocyte contractile function by inducible nitric oxide synthase (iNOS): mechanisms of contractile depression by nitric oxide. J Mol Cell Cardiol 1998; 30:303-315

57. Oddis CV,Finkel MS. Cytokine-stimulated nitric oxide production inhibits mitochondrial activity in cardiac myocytes. Biochem Biophys Res Commun 1995; 213:1002-1009

58. Schulz R, Dodge KL, Lopaschuk GD, et al. Peroxynitrite impairs cardiac contractile function by decreasing cardiac efficiency. Am J Physiol 1997; 272:H1212-H1219

59. Kaszaki J, Wolfard A, Bari F, et al. Effect of nitric oxide synthase inhibition on myocardial contractility in anesthetized normal and endotoxemic dogs. Shock 1996; 6:279-285

60. Hollenberg SM, Cunnion RE,Zimmerberg J. Nitric oxide synthase inhibition reverses arteriolar hyporesponsiveness to catecholamines in septic rats. Am J Physiol 1993; 264:H660-H663

61. Cobb JP, Natanson C, Quezado ZM, et al. Differential hemodynamic effects of L-NMMA in endotoxemic and normal dogs. Am J Physiol 1995; 268:H1634-H1642

62. Strand OA, Leone AM, Giercksky KE, et al. N(G)-monomethyl-L-arginine improves survival in a pig model of abdominal sepsis. Crit Care Med 1998; 26:1490-1499

63. Harbrecht BG, Billiar TR, Stadler J, et al. Inhibition of nitric oxide synthesis during endotoxemia promotes intrahepatic thrombosis and an oxygen radical-mediated hepatic injury. J Leukoc Biol 1992; 52:390-394

64. Petros A, Lamb G, Leone A, et al. Effects of a nitric oxide synthase inhibitor in humans with septic shock. Cardiovasc Res 1994; 28:34-39

65. Grover R, Lopez A, Lorente J, et al. Multi-center, randomized, placebo-controlled, double blind study of the nitric oxide synthase inhibitor 546C88: effect on survival in patients with septic shock. Crit Care Med 1999; 27:33A (Abst)

66. Avontuur JA, Tutein Nolthenius RP, van Bodegom JW, et al. Prolonged inhibition of nitric oxide synthesis in severe septic shock: a clinical study. Crit Care Med 1998; 26:660-667

67. Liaudet L, Fishman D, Markert M, et al. L-canavanine improves organ function and tissue adenosine triphosphate levels in rodent endotoxemia. Am J Respir Crit Care Med 1997; 155:1643-1648

68. Szabo C, Southan GJ,Thiemermann C. Beneficial effects and improved survival in rodent models of septic shock with S-methylisothiourea sulfate, a potent and selective inhibitor of inducible nitric oxide synthase. Proc Natl Acad Sci USA 1994; 91:12472-12476

69. Liaudet L, Rosselet A, Schaller MD, et al. Nonselective versus selective inhibition of inducible nitric oxide synthase in experimental endotoxic shock. J Infect Dis 1998; 177:127-132

70. Wu CC, Chen SJ, Szabo C, et al. Aminoguanidine attenuates the delayed circulatory failure and improves survival in rodent models of endotoxic shock. Br J Pharmacol 1995; 114:1666-1672

71. Saetre T, Höiby EA, Aspelin T, et al. Aminoehytl-isourea, a nitric oxide synthase inhibitor and free radical oxygen scavenger, imporves survival and counteracts deterioration in a porcine model of streptococcal shock. Crit Care Med 2000; 28:2697-2706

72. Cobb JP, Hotchkiss RS, Swanson PE, et al. Inducible nitric oxide synthase (iNOS) gene deficiency increasesthe mortality of sepsis in mice. Surgery 1999; 126:438-442
73. Hollenberg SM, Broussard M, Osman J, et al. Increased microvascular reactivity and imporved mortality in septic mice lacking inducible nitric oxide synthase. Circ Res 2000; 86:774-778
74. Kilbourn RG, Szabo C,Traber DL. Beneficial versus detrimental effects of nitric oxide synthase inhibitors in circulatory shock: lessons learned from experimental and clinical studies. Shock 1997; 7:235-246

13

APOPTOSIS AND THE RESOLUTION OF INFLAMMATION IN SEPSIS

Geoffrey John Bellingan

The inflammatory response is designed to protect the host. Correctly regulated it swiftly deals with pathogenic stimuli and then resolves, allowing the tissue to return to its normal structure and function. This process of resolution requires the rapid clearance of inflammatory cells in a manner that does not damage the host and for this the body employs two major mechanisms: apoptosis and cell emigration. This chapter will focus on our understanding of these two mechanisms and how they may, if not correctly regulated, contribute to the pathogenesis of severe sepsis or organ dysfunction.

Little attention has been paid so far to how leukocytes are removed after inflammation has served its purpose. This is particularly relevant, not only to harness the mechanisms governing the resolution of inflammation, but also because there is increasing evidence that the host may be just as at risk from an inadequate inflammatory reaction as it is from an overwhelming inflammatory response [1,2]. The key events in the resolution of inflammation are know to be apoptosis and emigration [3,4]. Apoptosis is fundamental in the regulation of neutrophils, monocytes, eosinophils and lymphocytes [3,5-7]. The clearance of apoptotic cells is effected through engulfment by macrophages which, along with the remaining viable lymphocytes, then emigrate from the inflamed site to the draining lymphatics [4,8-10].

Potential areas where there may be loss of normal regulation are thus; delayed apoptosis, excessive apoptosis, imperfect phagocytosis of apoptotic cells and defective leukocyte emigration. Prolonged leukocyte survival (delayed apoptosis) could increase the burden of inflammatory cells or their mediators and thus lead to an excessive inflammatory response. Apoptotic cells may progress too rapidly through to necrosis leading to release of histotoxic cellular contents (defective phagocytosis). Excessive leukocyte apoptosis could impair normal immune/inflammatory responses while parenchymal cell apoptosis could lead to organ failure [11]. Finally defective macrophage or lymphocyte emigration could lead to persisting inflammation (delayed emigration) or contribute to a hyporesponsive state (excessive/early emigration).

THE SYSTEMIC INFLAMMATORY RESPONSE SYNDROME AND IMMUNOPARESIS

Sepsis and septic shock continue to be leading causes of mortality and morbidity in critically ill patients. Historically sepsis was thought to occur when infection overwhelmed the inflammatory defenses, our beliefs on this have evolved however [12]. The realization that non-infective inflammatory states and endogenously elaborated cytokines could mimic sepsis resulted in the term systemic inflammatory response syndrome (SIRS) and the concept that SIRS may occur as a consequence of an excessive endogenous response [1,13].

Along with the abundant pro-inflammatory cascades there are numerous anti-inflammatory pathways that are stimulated as part of the normal immune/inflammatory response. These compensatory anti-inflammatory mechanisms help balance the response appropriately and are pivotal to the successful resolution of inflammation. They may, however, also contribute to inappropriate immunosuppression [12,14].

Many studies show that a profound immunosuppression occurs with severe trauma or sepsis, this is termed immunoparesis [2,15-17]. Some of the marked alterations that have been documented in the innate and acquired immune systems with severe inflammation are listed in Table 1. Sepsis tends to follow two phases, an early hyperdynamic response that can be followed by a hypodynamic response associated with depressed organ function. The immune system similarly can follow such a two-phase response although the mechanisms leading to immunoparesis are poorly understood. Many factors may contribute including endotoxin and other bacterial component(s), glucocorticoids, nitric oxide and prostaglandins, in particular prostaglandin $(PG)E_2$ as well as altered cytokine expression with a relative excess of interleukin (IL)-10 or diminished IL-12 and IL-18 which all have a immunosuppressive capacity [15,16,18-20]. Recent studies show that there is also increased apoptosis in immune and parenchymal cells in septic patients and animals [11,20-26]. This loss of immune cells may be part of the normal homeostatic response limiting inflammation and leading to resolution but it may also contribute to immunosuppression.

- Anergy to common recall antigens
- Suppression of T and B cell responsiveness
- Defective opsonization
- Diminished phagocytic function
- Suppressed neutrophil killing function
- Depressed monocyte HLA-DR expression
- Altered pro- and anti-inflammatory mediator release

Table 1. *Facets of immunosuppression associated with severe sepsis*

WHAT IS APOPTOSIS?

Kerr first coined the term apoptosis thirty years ago [27]. Apoptosis describes a series of morphologic changes in dying cells which are clearly distinct from the only previously recognized form of cell death, necrosis. Apoptosis is essential to normal growth, development and survival as the body must rid itself of cells that it no longer needs. It has thus developed the ability to eliminate specific cells in specific circumstances, hence apoptosis is also known as cell suicide or programmed cell death.

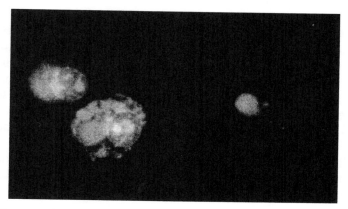

Figure 1: *Two normal macrophages on the left and one apoptotic macrophage on the right demonstrating the condensed and fragmented nucleus and loss of cytoplasmic volume typical of apoptosis in any cell type. Stained with acridine orange and viewed under fluorescent light.*

Apoptosis progresses through distinct stages with cytoplasmic membrane ruffling and formation of blebs followed by a decrease in cell volume, while in the nucleus the chromatin condenses, marginates to nuclear envelope and the nucleus eventually condenses to a dense shrunken structure [3,7,11,27] (Figure 1). The condensed apoptotic body can fragment further and eventually break apart but the usual fate is for apoptotic cells to be rapidly phagocytosed by tissue macrophages prior to loss of cell membrane integrity. The seminal studies of Metchnikoff over 100 years ago showed that intact neutrophils are phagocytosed by macrophages and Savill has clearly shown that this represents phagocytosis of apoptotic neutrophils as macrophages phagocytose only apoptotic neutrophils not live ones [8,28]. The phagocytosis of apoptotic neutrophils at sites of inflammation has now been shown for the lung, gut, joint and kidney [3,8].

Apoptosis as a Cornerstone of Inflammatory Resolution

Typically neutrophils have a life span of approximately 24 hours or less before they undergo constitutive apoptosis, eosinophils, like neutrophils undergo constitutive apoptosis although over a more prolonged time span [3,6]. Apoptosis is also an essential part of lymphocyte maturation with up to 90% of immature T cells being deleted by apoptosis during positive and negative selection, a similar fate awaits B cell precursors that do not productively rearrange their immunoglobulin genes [7,11,29]. Furthermore, Akbar et al. have shown that activation of T cells is associated with a reduction in Bcl-2 expression and propensity to undergo apoptosis although this could be suppressed by exogenous stimuli such as IL-2 [30].

Monocytes also undergo constitutive apoptosis but if exposed to pro-inflammatory stimuli such as lipopolysaccharide (LPS), tumor necrosis factor (TNF)-α or macrophage colony-stimulating factor (M-CSF) they survive and instead migrate into the site of inflammation to mature into macrophages [5]. Macrophages can also die by apoptosis but this seems to require a significant noxious stimulus [31]. The normal fate of the inflammatory macrophage in successfully resolving acute inflammation is not to die at the inflamed site by apoptosis but instead to emigrate to the draining lymph nodes [4]. Clearly it may well undergo apoptosis there or in other secondary lymphoid organs at a later stage. Finally parenchymal cells probably undergo slow but steady apoptosis as part of normal repair and regeneration mechanisms.

Regulation of Apoptosis

Studies in the worm *Caenorhabditis elegans* show that apoptosis is genetically regulated, with 131 of the 1090 somatic cells programmed to die during its development [32]. This is controlled by specific genes including CED 3 and 4 which promote apoptosis and CED 9 which inhibits it [33].

INDUCERS	SUPPRESSERS
Bad	bcl-2
bcl-X$_S$	bcl-X$_L$
Bad	al
Bak	mcl-1
e2f	bag
p53	
c-myc	
p34^{cdc2}	

Table 2. Some of the genes known to induce or suppress apoptosis in humans.

Several mammalian homologs have now been identified including the anti-apoptotic gene bcl-2, which is related to CED 9, and IL-1β converting enzyme (ICE), a member of the caspase family, which is related to CED 3. There is an increasing family of mammalian genes that have been identified as playing a role in apoptosis regulation, many of which also regulate cell proliferation (Table 2) [34,35]. In mammals the direct genetic controls of apoptosis are overlaid by many other factors. For example, it is well described that at certain stages of differentiation apoptosis occurs by default unless the cell is supported by survival factors. This is particularly apparent following removal of trophic factors from hematological cells including lymphocytes, neutrophils, eosinophils and monocytes [5,7,36]. Equally cell survival can be prolonged by the continued presence or elevated levels of certain hormones or cytokines. This is typically seen for neutrophils whose life span can be dramatically prolonged in inflammatory states [37,38]. Ceramide acts as an endogenous mediator of apoptosis and increased levels are related to the development of apoptosis [39].

TNF-α is an activator of the sphyngomyelin pathway which leads to the generation of ceramide [40]. In addition to inflammatory cytokine regulation, cell survival can be affected by a number of agents seen in sepsis including hypoxia, free radical generation, glucocorticoids and heat shock proteins [41-44]. A particularly important route through which apoptosis is initiated is by signaling through one of a family of receptors known as death receptors [45]. These factors are members of the TNF receptor super-family, and are listed in Table 3; they contain an intracellular death domain, which signals to the intracellular apoptotic machinery through adapter protein(s), which lead to apoptosis.

RECEPTOR	LIGAND
CD120a or TNFR1 (p55)	TNF-α
CD95 or Fas (Apo1)	Fas Ligand
Death Receptor 3 (Apo3)	Apo3 Ligand
TNF-related apoptosis inducing ligand [TRAIL] (Apo2)	Apo2 Ligand

Table 3. Death receptors in the TNF super-family and their ligands

Independent of whether apoptosis is induced by signaling through the death domain or through other mechanisms (steroids, cytotoxic drugs, etc.), they all lead to mitochondrial and nuclear changes. Central to both is activation of the caspases, so termed because they are cysteine proteases with an aspartate-specific cleavage site [46]. There are 13 known enzymes in this family, they exist in inactive precursor form and there are three major groupings. The initiators (caspases 2, 8, 9 and 10) are activated in response to apoptotic signals and they in turn cleave the effector caspases (3, 6 and 7) into their active forms which drive the pro-apoptotic pathways. There are a number of other caspases (1, 4, 5, 11, 12 and 13) which seem to be involved in regulation of inflammatory rather than apoptotic pathways.

There are a number of proteins that inhibit caspases and block apoptosis that, in animal models, have been shown to be effective in the treatment of stroke, myocardial ischemia/reperfusion injury, liver disease and traumatic brain injury [47, 48]. Their importance in sepsis is at present unclear but will be of great interest. Caspase 3 is the archetypal pro-apoptotic enzyme, once activated it translocates to the nucleus and drives DNA cleavage. Indeed apoptosis is characterized by DNA laddering where the nuclear DNA is cleaved by endonucleases into 180 base pair multiples. As noted the mitochondria also undergoes key changes including dissipation of the mitochondrial membrane potential because the mitochondrial permeability transition pore opens [49]. This leads to flux of Ca^{2+} and other ions and the release of mitochondrial constituents including cytochrome c. Cytochrome c binds apoptotic protease-activating factor 1 (APAF-1), a homolog of CED 4, which activates caspase 9 and thus caspase 3. This exerts a positive feedback at the mitochondria promoting pore opening which can be inhibited by bcl-2 which blocks opening of this pore.

NORMAL RESOLUTION OF INFLAMMATION

The Importance of Apoptosis

A fundamental feature of apoptosis is that the cell membrane remains intact until very late in the process thus the histotoxic intracellular contents are retained until the cell is disposed of by macrophages. This contrasts with necrotic cell death where the cell ruptures, spilling its contents into the local environment which, in the case of neutrophils for example, includes damaging enzymes such as elastase which can provoke further inflammation. Apoptotic cells are specifically recognized, through CD36, CD44 and phosphatidyl serine mechanisms, which allow macrophages to distinguish apoptotic from live cells [9,50,51]. Phagocytosis using these receptors does not invoke the macrophage to release pro-inflammatory mediators which contrasts with the phagocytosis of pathogens or opsonised particles, which elicit the release pro-inflammatory stimuli such as leukotrienes [52]. Indeed the phagocytosis of apoptotic cells leads instead to the release of TGF-β and FasL which are anti-inflammatory limiting pro-inflammatory mediator production and inducing further apoptosis in bystander cells [53,54]. The phagocytosis of apoptotic cells is extremely rapid and is mainly undertaken by macrophages but other cells for example fibroblasts can participate in this clearance response. Thus apoptotic cell death and clearance by macrophages is a powerfully anti-inflammatory mechanism and is uniquely suited to the resolution of inflammation.

Emigration and the Clearance of Inflammatory Cells

Having cleared apoptotic cells the inflammatory site will still be populated by macrophages and lymphocytes, indeed these are archetypal chronic inflammatory cells. Macrophages can undergo apoptosis but in successfully resolving acute inflammation they have been shown to be cleared not by apoptosis but by emigration, passing into the lymphatics and draining specifically to the regional lymph nodes [4] (Figure 2). This provides the macrophage with a dual life cycle, rescued from early apoptotic death as a monocyte by the presence of pro-inflammatory stimuli they migrate into the inflamed site [5]. Here they phagocytose and kill pathogens, regulate inflammation through cytokine secretion, contribute to wound healing and clear apoptotic cells [12]. They then emigrate to the draining lymph nodes where they can present antigen and thus further regulate the immune response. Macrophage emigration mimics that of dendritic cells which emigrate to regional lymph nodes very early during the inflammatory process. What is surprising about macrophage emigration is that it is regulated, resident macrophages are cleared at a very different rate to inflammatory macrophages and preliminary evidence suggests that adhesion events are critical to this regulation [55].

Figure 2: Section of a parathymic lymph node (the draining lymph node for the peritoneal cavity) from a mouse after the induction of peritonitis, viewed under fluorescent light. Inflammatory macrophages in the peritoneal cavity have been labeled with the fluorescent dye PKH26-PCL and are seen here to have emigrated in abundant numbers to the draining lymph node.

Lymphocytes, like macrophages, can be cleared by both apoptosis and emigration [7,10]. Apoptosis is an essential part of lymphocyte maturation, however, mature lymphocytes can survive for prolonged periods and participate in a complex pattern of trafficking. They drain from sites of inflammation into the lymph ducts, passing to the regional lymph nodes. Arrival of antigen arrives at a lymph node is usually accompanied by a shutdown in traffic through the node and expansion of specific cell populations. Lymphocytes do drain out of the nodes into the thoracic duct and enter the circulation, particularly in the absence of inflammation. They can then cross back from the circulation into tissue or lymph nodes under the regulation of specific vascular and lymphocyte homing receptors (Figure 3).

PROBLEMS WITH INFLAMMATORY RESOLUTION

Delayed Apoptosis and Systemic Inflammation

Neutrophil survival is significantly prolonged in inflammatory states such as sepsis, acute respiratory distress syndrome (ARDS), trauma, burns, bronchiectasis and cystic fibrosis [37,38]. Multiple pro-inflammatory signals including elevations in colony stimulating factors, and cytokines such as TNF-α and interferon (IFN)-γ or decreased levels of IL-10 may all contribute to this. These complex controls are mirrored by complex signaling mechanisms including through nuclear factor kappa-B (NF-κB), phosphoinositide 3-kinase, extracellular signal regulated kinase, reactive oxygen and bcl-2 dependant pathways [34,56-58]. Drugs can also influence survival with dopamine promoting, and glucocorticoids delaying, neutrophil apoptosis [43,59].

Delayed phagocyte apoptosis may allow a more robust inflammatory reaction and thus protect the host. It may however cause damage through increased leukocyte numbers or increased production of pro-inflammatory mediators and free radicals provoking a systemic inflammatory response. It is also clear that neutrophil apoptosis has the potential to limit inflammation as these cells have suppressed respiratory burst, are unable to degranulate and lose important activation ligands [3,60]. Moreover agents that promote neutrophil apoptosis can promote inflammatory resolution for example IL-10, which is known to augment neutrophil apoptosis, enhances resolution of pulmonary inflammation *in vivo* [61]. Although there are thus many reasons to speculate that delayed neutrophil apoptosis could exacerbate or provoke a damaging pro-inflammatory state, there is as yet no clear evidence to show that this occurs. Prolonged survival may simply be a consequence of systemic inflammation.

Excessive Apoptosis and Immunoparesis

Most attention for a pathological role for apoptosis in sepsis has focused on the potential for increased lymphocyte apoptosis to lead to an immunosuppressive state [11,17,20,62]. Lymphocytes are essential to immune and inflammatory functions and distinct lymphocyte sub-populations are associated with pro- and anti-inflammatory effects. Severe sepsis is associated with the development of a striking lymphopenia, loss of lymphocytes from thymic, splenic and other lymphoid tissue by apoptosis and increased apoptosis in circulating lymphocytes [20,23,62,63].

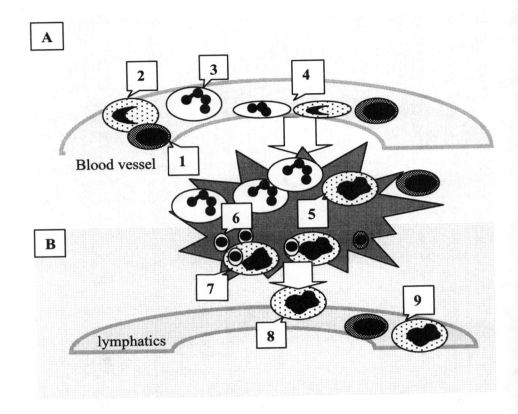

Figure 3. Overview of key events in the resolution of inflammation

A   THE NORMAL INFLAMMATORY RESPONSE
1   Mature lymphocytes enter inflammation from the circulation.
2   Monocytes die unless rescued from apoptosis by pro-inflammatory survival stimuli.
3   Neutrophils have a finite life span in the circulation.
4   Influx of leukocytes to inflamed site is under the control of adhesion molecules and
*   chemotactic signals.*
5   Monocytes mature to macrophages at the inflamed site.

B   SUCCESSFUL RESOLUTION OF INFLAMMATION
6   Neutrophils die by apoptosis not necrosis.
7   Macrophages specifically phagocytose apoptotic neutrophils.
8   Macrophage emigration into lymphatics is controlled by adhesion molecules.
9   Lymphocytes, macrophages and dendritic cells traffic to lymph nodes to present
*   antigen and regulate the immune response.*

The regulation of lymphocyte apoptosis in sepsis is complex. Some studies suggest that FasL is a key player in driving splenic CD4+ lymphocyte apoptosis in sepsis [64]. Thymocyte apoptosis however has been shown not to be regulated through FasL or endotoxin or mediated pathways, rather through the release of endogenous steroids, possibly acting through bcl-2 expression [65]. The picture is further confused as other studies suggest that sepsis induced apoptosis in spleen, thymus, lung and gut occurs through both endotoxin dependent and independent pathways [22]. Reactive oxygen species (ROS) are also implicated in driving apoptosis. One of the main antioxidant defenses is the enzyme copper/zinc SOD (Cu/Zn SOD) and mice lacking Cu/Zn SOD develop significantly more lymphocyte apoptosis after sepsis induced by cecal ligation and puncture (CLP). This confirms that oxidative stress occurs in sepsis and that this is, at least in part, regulated by Cu/Zn SOD. It also demonstrates that free radical production is a stimulus for lymphocyte apoptosis [42]. Thus the mechanisms driving lymphocyte apoptosis depend on many factors.

The importance of lymphocyte cell apoptosis as a poor prognostic indicator in sepsis is suggested by Hotchkiss et al. who prospectively studied 20 patients dying of sepsis and 16 non-septic ICU controls [24]. Apoptosis was shown in diverse organs in 50% of septic patients and was accompanied by lymphopenia, apoptosis was only seen in 1 control patient. Transgenic mice overexpressing bcl-2 in T lymphocytes have reduced T cell apoptosis and improved mortality in response to a septic challenge [66,67]. Similarly Hotchkiss also blocked apoptosis using the broad spectrum caspase inhibitor z-VAD which gave complete protection against sepsis induced T cell apoptosis and markedly increase survival [62]. These results strongly suggest that loss of lymphocytes may contribute to the mortality from sepsis.

The importance of lymphocyte apoptosis is not that clear however as other models have shown that apoptosis can be reduced without conferring a survival benefit. For example, Hotchkiss et al. showed that p53 dependent (thymus) and independent (spleen) pathways exist for sepsis-induced lymphocyte apoptosis but that p53 knockout mice had no survival benefit in sepsis [68]. Indeed in mice deficient in inducible nitric oxide synthase (NOS) lymphocyte apoptosis is reduced but mortality from sepsis is increased [69].

Severe or overwhelming sepsis may induce excessive apoptosis in other cells such as macrophages. As these cells are vital to clearing apoptotic cells their loss may be a poor prognostic indicator. Sepsis also leads to changes in the bone marrow [21]. Mixed bone marrow cells from mice show increased apoptosis at 24 hours following CLP which is accompanied by increased cell proliferation. Stem cell assays show increased colony formation by granulocyte macrophage colony stimulating factor (GM-CSF) stem cells but reduced formation by the erythroid cells, the importance of these observations to the septic process is unclear.

Sepsis-Induced Apoptosis in Parenchymal Cells

Apoptosis is seen in endothelial cells in a number of diseases and may be implicated in the pathogenesis of sepsis [25]. Endotoxin induces disseminated endothelial apoptosis which is mediated by TNF-α and requires ceramide generation. Sphymingomyelinase deficient mice, which do not lead to significant ceramide generation, have a normal TNF-α response to endotoxin but are protected from endothelial apoptosis and from death. Sepsis can also lead to parenchymal cell apoptosis which may have pathological consequences. For example endotoxin leads to time and dose dependent apoptosis in hepatocytes and pro-inflammatory cytokines cause a significant increase in apoptosis and shedding of cells from a proximal tubule monolayer, which may exacerbate acute tubular injury with tubule obstruction [70]. Apoptosis is also seen in the lung, gut, kidney and skeletal muscle but not in heart, liver or brain in a CLP model of sepsis, the relevance of this to the development of MOF is not known [22].

CONCLUSION

This review has emphasized the multiple different pathways that are involved in the resolution of inflammation including the role of cytokines, caspases, bcl-2 and other genes, free radicals, endotoxin, other bacterial components, death receptors, ceramide, endogenous glucocorticoids and adhesion molecules to portray just how complex the controls on cell emigration and death are. Just because inhibitors or promoters of one aspect of these regulatory mechanisms exist and work in one situation does not mean that these will be a universal panacea. For example G-CSF, which prolongs neutrophil survival, reduces complications from severe pneumonia while IL-10, which increases neutrophil apoptosis, also improves the resolution of pulmonary inflammation [61,71].

In summary it is clear that apoptosis is a key event in the normal resolution of inflammation. Emigration, particularly of macrophages, is another fundamental route for inflammatory cell clearance. Both clearance mechanisms are controlled by complex regulatory mechanisms. We need to understand these processes very clearly before attempting to manipulate the resolution of inflammation.

ACKNOWLEDGEMENT

This work was supported by the Medical research Council, UK.

REFERENCES

1. Bone RC. Sir Isaac Newton, sepsis, SIRS, and CARS. Crit Care Med 1996; 24:1125-1128
2. Docke WD, Randow F, Syrbe U, et al. Monocyte deactivation in septic patients: restoration by IFN-gamma treatment. Nat Med 1997; 3:678-681
3. Haslett C. Granulocyte apoptosis and its role in the resolution and control of lung inflammation. Am J Respir Crit Care Med 1999; 160: S5-S11
4. Bellingan GJ, Caldwell H, Howie SE, et al. In vivo fate of the inflammatory macrophage during the resolution of inflammation: inflammatory macrophages do not die locally, but emigrate to the draining lymph nodes. J Immunol 1996; 157:2577-2585
5. Mangan DF, Wahl SM. Differential regulation of human monocyte programmed cell death (apoptosis) by chemotactic factors and pro-inflammatory cytokines. J Immunol 1991; 147:3408-3412
6. Stern M, Savill J, Haslett C. Human monocyte-derived macrophage phagocytosis of senescent eosinophils undergoing apoptosis. Mediation by alpha v beta 3/CD36/thrombospondin recognition mechanism and lack of phlogistic response. Am J Pathol 1996;149:911-921
7. Cohen JJ. Programmed cell death and apoptosis in lymphocyte development and function. Chest 1993; 103:99S-101S
8. Savill JS, Wyllie AH, Henson JE, et al. Macrophage phagocytosis of aging neutrophils in inflammation. Programmed cell death in the neutrophil leads to its recognition by macrophages. J Clin Invest 1989; 83:865-875
9. Savill J, Hogg N, Ren Y, et al. Thrombospondin cooperates with CD36 and the vitronectin receptor in macrophage recognition of neutrophils undergoing apoptosis. J Clin Invest 1992; 90:1513-1522
10. Tsokos GC, Liossis SN. Lymphocytes, cytokines, inflammation, and immune trafficking. Curr Opin Rheumatol 1998; 10:417-425
11. Mahidhara R, Billiar TR. Apoptosis in sepsis. Crit Care Med. 2000; 28:N105-N113
12. Bellingan G. Inflammatory cell activation in sepsis. Br Med Bull 1999; 55:12-29
13. Bone RC, Balk RA, Cerra FB, et al. Definitions for sepsis and organ failure and guidelines for the use of innovative therapies in sepsis. The ACCP/SCCM Consensus Conference Committee. American College of Chest Physicians/Society of Critical Care Medicine. Chest 1992; 101:1644-1655
14. Antonelli M. Sepsis and septic shock: pro-inflammatory or anti-inflammatory state? J Chemother 1999; 11:536-540
15. Bellingan GJ. Immune dysfunction associated with critical illness. In: Webb AR, Shapiro MJ, Singer M, Suter P (Eds). Oxford textbook of critical care. Oxford University Press, Oxford, 1999, pp. 898-902
16. Mannick JA. Trauma, sepsis and immune defects In: Faist E, Meakins JL, Schildberg FW (eds) Host defense dysfunction in trauma shock and sepsis. Springer-Verlag, Berlin 1993, pp. 15-21
17. Volk HD, Reinke P, Docke WD. Clinical aspects: from systemic inflammation to 'immunoparalysis'. Chem Immunol 2000; 74:162-177
18. Albina JE, Reichner JS. Nitric oxide in inflammation and immunity. New Horiz 1995; 3:46-64

19. Ayala A, Lehman DL, Herdon CD, et al. Mechanism of enhanced susceptibility to sepsis following hemorrhage. Interleukin-10 suppression of T-cell response is mediated by eicosanoid-induced interleukin-4 release. Arch Surg 1994; 129:1172-1178

20. Ayala A, Chaudry IH. Immune dysfunction in murine polymicrobial sepsis: mediators, macrophages, lymphocytes and apoptosis. Shock 1996; 6 Suppl 1:S27-S38

21. Barthlen W, Klemens C, Rogenhofer S, et al. Critical role of nitric oxide for proliferation and apoptosis of bone-marrow cells under septic conditions. Ann Hematol 2000; 79:249-254

22. Hiramatsu M, Hotchkiss RS, Karl IE, et al. Cecal ligation and puncture (CLP) induces apoptosis in thymus, spleen, lung, and gut by an endotoxin and TNF-independent pathway. Shock 1997; 7:247-253

23. Ayala A, Xin Xu Y, Ayala CA, et al. Increased mucosal B-lymphocyte apoptosis during polymicrobial sepsis is a Fas ligand but not an endotoxin-mediated process. Blood 1998; 91:1362-1372

24. Hotchkiss RS, Swanson PE, Freeman BD, et al. Apoptotic cell death in patients with sepsis, shock, and multiple organ dysfunction. Crit Care Med 1999; 27:1230-1251

25. Stefanec T. Endothelial apoptosis: could it have a role in the pathogenesis and treatment of disease? Chest 2000; 117:841-854

26. Papathanassoglou ED, Moynihan JA, Ackerman MH. Does programmed cell death (apoptosis) play a role in the development of multiple organ dysfunction in critically ill patients? a review and a theoretical framework. Crit Care Med 2000; 28:537-549

27. Kerr JF, Wyllie AH, Currie AR. Apoptosis: a basic biological phenomenon with wide-ranging implications in tissue kinetics. Br J Cancer 1972; 26:239-257

28. Metchnikoff E Immunity to infectious diseases. Translated from French by Binnie FG 1905. Cambridge University Press, London

29. Van Parijs L, Abbas AK. Homeostasis and self-tolerance in the immune system: turning lymphocytes off. Science 1998; 280:243-248

30. Akbar AN, Borthwick N, Salmon M, et al. The significance of low bcl-2 expression by CD45RO T cells in normal individuals and patients with acute viral infections. The role of apoptosis in T cell memory. J Exp Med 1993; 178:427-438

31. Zychlinsky A, Prevost MC, Sansonetti PJ. Shigella flexneri induces apoptosis in infected macrophages. Nature 1992; 358:167-169

32. Ellis HM, Horvitz HR. Genetic control of programmed cell death in the nematode C. elegans. Cell 1986; 44:817-829

33. Hengartner MO, Horvitz HR. C. elegans cell survival gene ced-9 encodes a functional homolog of the mammalian proto-oncogene bcl-2. Cell 1994;76:665-676

34. Hannah S, Cotter TG, Wyllie AH, et al. The role of oncogene products in neutrophil apoptosis. Biochem Soc Trans 1994; 22:253S

35. Camapana D, Cleveland JL. Regulation of apoptosis in normal hemopoiesis and hematological disease In: Brenner MK, Hoffbrand AV (eds) Recent Advances in Haematology. Churchill Livingstone, New York, 1996

36. Lee A, Whyte MK, Haslett C. Inhibition of apoptosis and prolongation of neutrophil functional longevity by inflammatory mediators. J Leukoc Biol. 1993; 54:283-288

37. Jimenez MF, Watson RW, Parodo J, et al. Dysregulated expression of neutrophil apoptosis in the systemic inflammatory response syndrome. Arch Surg 1997; 132:1263-1269

38. Keel M, Ungethum U, Steckholzer U, et al. Interleukin-10 counterregulates proinflammatory cytokine-induced inhibition of neutrophil apoptosis during severe sepsis. Blood 1997 ; 90:3356-3363

39. Obeid LM, Linardic CM, Karolak LA, et al. Programmed cell death induced by ceramide. Science 1993; 259:1769-1771

40. De Nadai C, Sestili P, Cantoni O, et al. Nitric oxide inhibits tumor necrosis factor-alpha-induced apoptosis by reducing the generation of ceramide. Proc Natl Acad Sci USA 2000; 97:5480-5485

41. Hannah S, Mecklenburgh K, Rahman I, et al. Hypoxia prolongs neutrophil survival in vitro. FEBS Lett 1995; 372:233-237

42. Freeman BD, Reaume AG, Swanson PE, et al. Role of CuZn superoxide dismutase in regulating lymphocyte apoptosis during sepsis. Crit Care Med 2000; 28:1701-1708

43. Meagher LC, Cousin JM, Seckl JR, et al. Opposing effects of glucocorticoids on the rate of apoptosis in neutrophilic and eosinophilic granulocytes. J Immunol 1996; 156:4422-4428

44. Wong HR. Potential protective role of the heat shock response in sepsis. New Horiz 1998; 6:194-200

45. Ashkenazi A, Dixit VM. Death receptors: signaling and modulation. Science 1998; 281:1305-1308

46. Earnshaw WC, Martins LM, Kaufmann SH. Mammalian caspases: structure, activation, substrates, and functions during apoptosis. Annu Rev Biochem 1999; 68:383-424

47. Daemen MA, van 't Veer C, Denecker G, et al. Inhibition of apoptosis induced by ischemia-reperfusion prevents inflammation. J Clin Invest 1999; 104:541-549

48. Li H, Colbourne F, Sun P et al. Caspase inhibitors reduce neuronal injury after focal but not global cerebral ischemia in rats. Stroke 2000; 31:176-182

49. Brenner C, Kroemer G. Apoptosis. Mitochondria--the death signal integrators. Science 2000; 289:1150-1151

50. Hart SP, Dougherty GJ, Haslett C, et al. CD44 regulates phagocytosis of apoptotic neutrophil granulocytes, but not apoptotic lymphocytes, by human macrophages. J Immunol 1997; 159:919-925

51. Fadok VA, Savill JS, Haslett C, et al. Different populations of macrophages use either the vitronectin receptor or the phosphatidylserine receptor to recognize and remove apoptotic cells. J Immunol 1992; 149:4029-4035

52. Meagher LC, Savill JS, Baker A, et al. Phagocytosis of apoptotic neutrophils does not induce macrophage release of thromboxane B2. J Leukoc Biol 1992; 52:269-273

53. Brown SB, Savill J. Phagocytosis triggers macrophage release of Fas ligand and induces apoptosis of bystander leukocytes. J Immunol 1999; 162:480-485

54. McDonald PP, Fadok VA, Bratton D, et al. Transcriptional and translational regulation of inflammatory mediator production by endogenous TGF-beta in macrophages that have ingested apoptotic cells. J Immunol 1999; 163:6164-6172

55. Bellingan GJ, Chua F, Cooksley H, et al. Macrophage-mesothelial adhesion may regulate the resolution of acute peritoneal inflammation. Am J Resp Crit Care Med 2000; 161:A844 (Abst)

56. Murray J, Barbara JA, Dunkley SA, et al. Regulation of neutrophil apoptosis by tumor necrosis factor-alpha: requirement for TNFR55 and TNFR75 for induction of apoptosis in vitro. Blood. 1997; 90:2772-2783

57. Ward C, Chilvers ER, Lawson MF, et al. NF-kappaB activation is a critical regulator of human granulocyte apoptosis in vitro. J Biol Chem 1999; 274:4309-4318

58. Klein JB, Rane MJ, Scherzer JA, et al. Granulocyte-macrophage colony-stimulating factor delays neutrophil constitutive apoptosis through phosphoinositide 3-kinase and extracellular signal-regulated kinase pathways. J Immunol 2000; 164:4286-4291

59. Sookhai S, Wang JH, McCourt M, et al. Dopamine induces neutrophil apoptosis through a dopamine D-1 receptor-independent mechanism. Surgery 1999; 126:314-322

60. Dransfield I, Buckle AM, Savill J, et al. Neutrophil apoptosis is associated with a reduction in CD16 (Fc gamma RIII) expression. J Immunol 1994; 153:1254-1263

61. Cox G. IL-10 enhances resolution of pulmonary inflammation in vivo by promoting apoptosis of neutrophils. Am J Physiol 1996; 271:L566-L571

62. Hotchkiss RS, Tinsley KW, Swanson PE, et al. Prevention of lymphocyte cell death in sepsis improves survival in mice. Proc Natl Acad Sci USA 1999; 96:14541-14546
63. Hotchkiss RS, Swanson PE, Cobb JP, et al. Apoptosis in lymphoid and parenchymal cells during sepsis: findings in normal and T- and B-cell-deficient mice. Crit Care Med 1997; 25:1298-1307
64. Ayala A, Chung CS, Xu YX, et al. Increased inducible apoptosis in CD4+ T lymphocytes during polymicrobial sepsis is mediated by Fas ligand and not endotoxin. Immunology 1999; 97:45-55
65. Ayala A, Xu YX, Chung CS, et al. Does Fas ligand or endotoxin contribute to thymic apoptosis during polymicrobial sepsis? Shock 1999; 11:211-217
66. Tinsley KW, Cheng SL, Buchman TG, et al. Caspases -2, -3, -6, and -9, but not caspase-1, are activated in sepsis-induced thymocyte apoptosis. Shock 2000; 13:1-7
67. Hotchkiss RS, Swanson PE, Knudson CM, et al. Overexpression of Bcl-2 in transgenic mice decreases apoptosis and improves survival in sepsis. J Immunol 1999; 162:4148-4156
68. Hotchkiss RS, Tinsley KW, Hui JJ, et al. p53-dependent and -independent pathways of apoptotic cell death in sepsis. J Immunol 2000; 164:3675-80
69. Cobb JP, Hotchkiss RS, Swanson PE, et al. Inducible nitric oxide synthase (iNOS) gene deficiency increases the mortality of sepsis in mice. Surgery 1999;126:438-442
70. Glynne PA, Evans TJ. Inflammatory cytokines induce apoptotic and necrotic cell shedding from human proximal tubular epithelial cell monolayers. Kidney Int 1999; 55:2573-2597
71. Nelson S, Belknap SM, Carlson RW, et al. A randomized controlled trial of filgrastim as an adjunct to antibiotics for treatment of hospitalized patients with community-acquired pneumonia. CAP Study Group. J Infect Dis 1998; 178:1075-1080

14

MICROVASCULAR ALTERATIONS IN SEPSIS

Andreas W. Sielenkämper
Pete Kvietys
William J. Sibbald

THE MICROCIRCULATION

Morphology

The microvasculature unit consists of a network of blood vessels (less than 250-μm) lying between the arteries and veins. Immediately downstream of the smallest arteries are the arterioles which form a diverging network of vessels ranging from first order arterioles (from 100-μm to 150-μm in diameter) to terminal arterioles (approximately 10-μm). Arterioles contain at least one layer of smooth muscle cells and are able to actively regulate their diameter in response to a variety of stimuli. Terminal arterioles supply the capillary bed, a network of diverging and converging vascular segments (diameters from 3 to 10-μm) composed of a single layer of endothelial cells. Blood draining the capillary bed is collected by post-capillary venules (lacking smooth muscle) which converge into large venules (containing smooth muscle). Venules are typically larger in diameter than arterioles of the same branching order.

In most organs, the primary function of the microvasculature is as a site for exchange of gas, nutrients, solutes and heat. In the alveoli of the lungs the sheet like structure of the capillary bed is ideally suited to maximize surface area for blood oxygenation and the off-loading of carbon dioxide. A complex branching network exists in the villi of the gut to maximize surface area for uptake of nutrients. In the myocardium and skeletal muscle where oxygen requirements can vary greatly, a mesh like network of capillaries surrounding each muscle fiber helps to ensure adequate tissue oxygenation during period of rest and activity. Tissues with higher metabolic rates, e.g. myocardium, have a higher capillary density.

Function

The function of arterioles is primarily to regulate organ blood flow and oxygen delivery (DO_2). Within the organ, arterioles regulate the local distribution of blood flow to different regions in accordance with tissue requirements. In the lungs, hypoxic vasoconstriction to divert blood flow from poorly ventilated alveoli is one example of arteriolar redistribution of local blood flow. Arterioles also regulate microvascular pressure to limit tissue edema. A unique example of pressure regulation lies in the glomerulus of the kidney [1] where it regulates glomerular filtration.

The capillary bed is the primary site of oxygen exchange within tissues. However, oxygen transport also occurs from the blood flowing through the arteriolar tree to the surrounding tissue and neighboring capillaries resulting in a significant pre-capillary fall in hemoglobin oxygen saturation [2,3]. Re-oxygenation of red blood cells (RBCs) flowing through capillaries by diffusion from nearby arterioles helps provide homogeneous tissue oxygenation despite heterogeneous capillary blood [4].

Post-capillaries venules are the primary site of inflammatory cell trafficking, and protein and water exchange [5]. As neutrophils enter post-capillary venules, RBCs push the neutrophils to the wall of the venule thus initiating the rolling/adhesion process necessary for neutrophil emigration into the tissue. While protein and water exchange can occur independently of leukocyte trafficking, direct correlations have been noted between the extent of emigration and the degree of vascular protein leak.

Rheology

At all levels of the microvasculature (except for the smallest capillaries) there is a 'cell free' plasma sleeve along the endothelial surface where erythrocyte density is less. As a consequence, erythrocytes concentrated towards the center of the vessel travel faster, on average, than the plasma which is concentrated towards the edges of the lumen. As the diameter of the microvessels approaches that of the erythrocyte, the difference between the erythrocyte and plasma velocity increases, and hence the impact of the 'plasma' layer on hematocrit increases. The observed hematocrit within the vessel falls as compared to the systemic hematocrit (Fahreaus effect). Since viscosity depends on hematocrit, the apparent viscosity of blood also decreases (Fahreaus-Lindquist effect).

A second consequence of the particulate nature of blood further acts to reduce hematocrit within the microvasculature. Beginning in smaller arterioles (less than ~50-μm), RBCs are preferentially distributed at bifurcations into the branch with the higher blood flow [6]. The branch with the higher flow (lower downstream resistance) receives a slightly higher hematocrit while the other branch (with a higher downstream resistance) receives a slightly lower hematocrit (plasma skimming). The preferential partitioning of erythrocyte at bifurcations increases as the size of the vessels decrease and as hematocrit decreases. Thus the branching characteristics of the microvascular bed cause a cascade effect resulting in a wide heterogeneity of hematocrit within the capillary bed.

Another consequence of lower capillary hematocrit is the presence of plasma gaps between individual RBCs (RBCs travel in single file through capillaries separated by plasma). Since the RBC is the primary carrier of oxygen, the area available for oxygen exchange from capillaries is restricted to the area in the immediate neighborhood of RBCs. Capillaries with large plasma gaps have a significantly reduced area for exchange [7,8].

Regulation

Since small arterioles account for a large proportion of the microvascular resistance, it was originally assumed that these vessels were solely responsible for regulating microvascular blood flow [9]. However, it is now recognized that vasodilation of a single level of the arteriolar tree cannot increase blood flow to the level seen in heart or skeletal muscle during functional hyperemia. Blood flow regulation must be integrated from the level of the capillary bed across the entire arteriolar tree and into the arterial resistance vessels [10].

At rest, flow regulation occurs at the level of the distal arterioles which primarily regulate the distribution of flow within the tissue. As metabolic demand increases, the regulation of flow shifts to include the larger arterioles and resistance vessels which control the total blood flow into the tissue. This regulatory process involves multiple control systems responding to a range of chemical (metabolic, oxygen) and physical (pressure, shear rate) signals (Table 1) [11,12].

Shear Dependent Vasodilation
     - regulated by shear dependent NO release [13] [14].
     - dependent upon functional vascular endothelium[15].
Myogenic
     - luminal pressure increases wall tension [16].
     - increased wall tension causes smooth muscle cell membrane depolarization and
       increased intracellular Ca^{2+} concentration [17].
     - independent of vascular endothelium [18,19].
     - modulated by endothelial mediators [18,19].
Metabolic
     - involvement of metabolites (e.g. adenosine, H^+, CO_2) in blood flow regulation
     - 'spill over' of acetylcholine or NO during exercise [20].
     - vasoactive metabolites stimulate NO release

Table 1. *Regulation of microvascular blood flow*

According to the metabolic hypothesis, DO_2 to mitochondria is the regulated variable. It has been proposed that oxygen sensors either in the wall of the arteriole or in the tissue regulate DO_2 to maintain tissue oxygenation [21,22]. More recently the RBC has been proposed as the site of the sensor and effector of the local regulation of DO_2. This model proposes that as the erythrocyte enters the arteriolar tree it experiences an oxygen gradient whose magnitude is proportional to the level of metabolic activity of the nearby tissue. As oxygen is offloaded from hemoglobin, a vasodilator (low molecular weight nitrosothiol [23,24] or extracellular ATP [25]) is released from the RBC which acts directly to regulate the arterioles supplying the tissue.

MICROVASCULAR DYSFUNCTION

Sepsis originates with a focus of inflammation which initiates a cascade of inflammatory events leading to injury in remote organs and ultimately to organ failure and death. Since a number of studies have shown that the microvasculature is injured at a very early stage in the progression of sepsis [26,27], it has been proposed that the failure of the microvasculature is the key event that leads to multiple organ failure (MOF) [28].

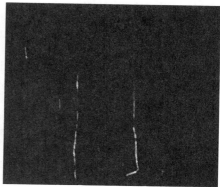

Figure 1. Loss of perfused capillaries in rat skeletal muscle (EDL muscle). Panel on left shows normal capillary density at 2.5 hours after induction of sepsis (peritonitis) and on right, significant loss of capillaries at 3.5 hours. Field of view is 350-μm wide.

Capillary Density

In sepsis, a decreased number of perfused capillaries reduces the surface area available for DO_2 while increasing the distance for oxygen diffusion (Figure 1). In a peritonitis model of sepsis in rats, intravital microscopy studies have noted a 30 % decrease in perfused capillary density and an increase in heterogeneity of flow in the remaining perfused capillaries [27].

Although there is uncertainty about the real cause of the sepsis-induced loss of capillary density, there are a number of possible explanations. For example, circulating blood cells are thought to occlude capillaries resulting in a decrease in perfused capillary density [29,30]. The activation of circulating mature leukocytes or the release of immature leukocytes from bone marrow may result in a population of less deformable cells which can be entrapped in capillaries [31,32]. The primary organs responsible for filtering these less deformable leukocytes from the circulation are the lungs, spleen, and liver. Sepsis also results in a decrease in RBC deformability which may contribute to the loss of perfused capillaries [33-35]. Disseminated intravascular coagulation (cell aggregates, DIC) has also been reported to be involved in the decrease in perfused capillary density [36]. Finally, capillary endothelial swelling and the formation of pseudopod extensions [37] are thought to reduce the capillary lumen, thus contributing to the trapping of cells.

Arteriolar Control

The loss of perfused capillaries would on its own limit the capacity of the tissue to respond to challenges to oxygen. However, impaired arteriolar vasoreactivity further compromises tissue oxygenation by limiting the ability of the microvasculature to properly distribute flow within the organs. A number of factors have been proposed for this arteriolar dysfunction, from endothelial and smooth muscle cell damage to the excess production of nitric oxide (NO). Excess NO is generated during the inflammatory process, primarily via iNOS (inducible form of NO synthase). Increased NO levels unrelated to the normal arteriolar control of microvascular blood flow may cause unregulated arteriolar vasodilation. The NO may also react with superoxide producing peroxynitrite which may cause both endothelial and smooth muscle cell injury resulting in impairing arteriolar responsiveness to circulating vasoconstrictors.

Permeability

Sepsis-induced microvascular injury is generally associated with vascular protein leakage and edema. Bacteremia or endotoxemia is associated with increases in microvascular permeability to albumin in a variety of organs. Some studies indicate that the LPS-induced increase in vascular albumin leakage into the interstitium is coupled to leukocyte emigration, i.e., prevention of leukocyte emigration also prevents albumin leakage [38,39]. However, in some cases, the macromolecular leakage is independent of leukocyte emigration [40-42]. This discrepancy may be explained by the possibility that, *in vivo*, the concentration of inflammatory mediators may achieve levels that can directly cause endothelial cell retraction of sufficient magnitude to allow protein to leak from the venules into the interstitium.

Systemic Inflammatory Response

The systemic inflammatory response associated with sepsis results in infiltration of neutrophils and endothelial barrier dysfunction (edema) in various vital organs (heart, lungs, liver, kidney, etc.), that ultimately leads to MOF. It is generally accepted that the venular end of the microcirculation is the primary locus of inflammatory events, i.e., neutrophil (PMN) adhesion and emigration, as well as, protein and water leakage (edema). In sepsis, lipopolysaccharide (LPS) and/or various cytokines (e.g., tumor necrosis factor [TNF]-α, interleukin [IL]-1, IL-8) and inflammatory mediators (e.g., platelet activating factor [PAF]) enter the circulation and activate both circulating PMN and the microvascular endothelium. Activated PMN increase their surface levels of adhesion molecules and become less deformable. Endothelial cell activation involves both synthetic (upregulation of adhesion molecules) and structural (swelling and pseudopod formation) alterations. These changes in the activation state of circulating PMN and the endothelium facilitate PMN invasion of various organ systems.

Several general concepts have emerged from experimental studies regarding the role of the microcirculation in the systemic inflammatory response that may be relevant to sepsis in humans:

Adhesion molecules involved in PMN-endothelial cell interactions

PMN infiltration of inflamed organs begins as a series of complex, yet well coordinated, interactions between adhesion glycoproteins on PMN and venular endothelium. The initial adhesive interaction induces saltatory movement or 'rolling' of PMN along the endothelium. This weak adhesive interaction is mediated by E- and P-selectins on endothelial cells and L-selectin on PMN. P-selectin, which is stored in the Weibel-Palade bodies of endothelial cells, is expressed very rapidly, reaches peak levels within 3-10 minutes, and returns to control levels within minutes thereafter [43]

Rolling PMN are maintained in close apposition to the endothelium, thereby facilitating PMN activation by locally generated inflammatory mediators. Upon activation, PMN shed their L-selectin and increase their expression/activation of β_2 integrins (CD11/CD18). The PMN integrins engage ligands on the endothelial cells to develop a strong adhesive interaction that leads to the arrest of the rolling PMN on the endothelium. The major ligand for CD18 is ICAM-1 which is constitutively expressed on endothelium and is upregulated in response to cytokine stimulation via the nuclear factor kappa B (NF-κB) pathway [44].

Adhesion molecule-dependent and -independent PMN accumulation in organs

When animals are rendered septic, their circulating PMN accumulate in a variety of organ systems [45-50]. Typically, PMN sequestration within organ systems can occur through two basic mechanisms: rolling, adhesion, and emigration in postcapillary venules utilizing the classic adhesion pathways or by simply becoming lodged in precapillary vessels (plugging). The classical adhesion mechanisms in postcapillary venules have been described above. With respect to entrapment of PMN in capillaries, this process may be facilitated by a decrease in PMN deformability either upon activation of mature circulating PMN or the recruitment of the less deformable immature PMN from the bone marrow [51,52].

The relative contribution of the classical adhesion pathways versus simple plugging in PMN accumulation may be organ specific. For example, sepsis induced leukocyte rolling and adhesion has been reported in postcapillary venules of the mesentery [48], cremaster muscle [49,53], and postsinusoidal venules of the liver [49]. By contrast, the sepsis-induced PMN accumulation in the lung is primarily due to the plugging of the less deformable PMN in precapillary vessels and PMN accumulation can occur by a CD18-independent pathway [54].

PMN diapedesis

The bulk of the evidence indicates that PMN transendothelial migration occurs via a paracellular pathway, i.e, pseudopodia being extended through the junctional complexes between endothelial cells [52,55-58]. In addition, while some early studies [59,60] suggested that PMN do not utilize endogenous proteases to traverse the endothelial barrier, more recent studies indicate that PMN-derived proteases (particularly elastase) play an important role in diapedesis [56,61].

Role of PMN in vascular dysfunction and organ failure

Interfering with PMN adhesion and infiltration provides protection against organ injury and increases survival rate. Inhibition of CD18 activity offered protection from the consequences of sepsis with respect to survival [62,63] and lung [64,65] and liver [66] injury. Mutant mice which are intercellular adhesion molecule (ICAM)-1 deficient are resistant to the lethal effects of endotoxin and have significantly less PMN infiltration of the liver [67]. These observations indicate that PMN emigration is an important step in sepsis induced tissue injury.

The means by which PMN inflict microvascular dysfunction remain somewhat controversial. Some contend that it is lytic in nature, i.e., endothelial cell death [68]. Alternatively, others have provided evidence that PMN induced microvascular dysfunction is due to the ability of PMN to induce non-lytic disruption of endothelial cell monolayers [69,70], thus creating endothelial barrier dysfunction.

Modulators of the systemic inflammatory response associated with sepsis

Sepsis is associated with an increase in circulating proinflammatory cytokines and mediators. In addition, sepsis is associated with the production of anti-inflammatory cytokines and mediators. Thus, the systemic inflammation induced by sepsis is the result of an imbalance in favor of the proinflammatory mediators.

The most frequently implicated proinflammatory cytokines in the systemic inflammatory response associated with sepsis are TNF and IL-1 [68,71]. In addition to their well recognized ability to promote PMN adhesion to endothelial cells, these two cytokines can also cause direct injury to endothelial cell monolayers and increase monolayer permeability [68].

Some interleukins can be anti-inflammatory. For example, IL-10 can be very effective in suppressing cytokine (TNF, IL-1 and IL-6) release, especially when administered prior to the onset of sepsis [38,72,73].

NO, a potent anti-adhesive molecule [74] has received a great deal of attention with respect to its modulatory role the inflammatory response induced by sepsis. *In vivo*, NOS inhibitors increased leukocyte adherence in both the liver [75] and mesentery [76]. Inhaled NO attenuates the sepsis-induced PMN migration in the lung and the associated tissue injury [77]. The endotoxemia-induced rolling and adhesion of leukocytes in the postcapillary venules of the cremaster muscle and liver were significantly elevated in iNOS-deficient animals when compared to their wild-type counterparts [49].

One mechanism by which NO may exert its anti-inflammatory effects is by inhibiting expression of adhesion molecules on endothelial cells. This effect of NO on adhesion molecule expression has been attributed to the ability of NO to increase intracellular levels of IκB, thereby inhibiting NF-κB activation [78,79].

Under certain circumstances, NO can also promote PMN-endothelial cell adhesive interactions. NO can interact with superoxide to form peroxynitrite resulting in the activation of the nuclear enzyme poly (ADP-ribose) synthase (PARS). In several models of inflammation, inhibition of PARS activity reduced leukocyte infiltration and tissue injury. Moreover, PARS inhibition has been shown to lead to diminished ICAM-1 [80,81] and P-selectin expression [80], providing evidence for the regulation of adhesion molecules by PARS. Thus, the potential interaction of NO with superoxide resulting in PARS activation should be taken into consideration when evaluating the role of NO in the sepsis-induced inflammation.

Development of LPS Tolerance

LPS tolerance refers to the adaptational phenomenon by which animals or cells that have been pretreated with LPS become more resistant to a subsequent LPS challenge. For example, intraperitoneal LPS or cecal ligation and perforation (CLP) elicits an increase in PMN sequestration in the heart, an organ remote from the challenge [45,82]. Pretreatment of animals with LPS attenuates this inflammatory response. It is assumed that the development LPS tolerance in involves modulation of NF-κB activation.

CLINICAL MANIFESTATIONS OF MICROVASCULAR INJURY IN SEPSIS

During the course of sepsis, the obvious consequence of both the inflammatory response and the abnormalities in microvascular blood flow is organ dysfunction and eventually, MOF. To understand the implications of the microvascular abnormalities for the clinical situation, it is important to view the underlying pathophysiology of sepsis, which has been detailed before, in context with the resulting alterations in organ function.

Oxygen Transport

One of the most obvious consequences of the microvascular abnormalities in sepsis is that both diffusive and convective oxygen transport are impaired in sepsis. Diffusive oxygen transport may be compromised in the lung, due to acute respiratory distress syndrome (ARDS) or pulmonary edema [83,84], or in the peripheral microcirculations, where tissue edema increases diffusion distances [85]. Convective DO_2 may be impaired because of myocardial dysfunction [86,87], blood flow maldistribution, and inadequate capillary perfusion [26,27]. The clinical significance of a possible dysfunction in mitochondrial oxygen utilization, which if present may prevent the optimal use of oxygen, remains to be defined clearly.

For long it has been postulated that because of the abnormalities in microvascular blood flow and oxygen transport, the maximal oxygen extraction capacity of the tissues is decreased in sepsis [28,88]. In animal studies, this becomes manifest as an elevation of the critical DO_2 (DO_2crit), the point where systemic oxygen uptake (VO_2) becomes dependent on oxygen supply [88,89]. However, results from numerous clinical trials on the effects of sepsis on the relationship between DO_2 and VO_2 have been conflicting, partly to be explained by methodological problems [90]. The few clinical studies that directly obtained DO_2crit data from critically ill humans observed high values for DO_2crit, at least in comparison to data from studies on anesthetized patients before or after coronary bypass graft surgery (Table 2). The only controlled trial on this issue was performed in dying patients and did not demonstrate any effect of sepsis on DO_2crit [91]. The bottom line is that for now, the exact influence of sepsis on DO_2crit – and therefore, on oxygen extraction capabilities - in humans remains unclear.

	Patients	DO₂crit ml/kg/min	Methodology
Shibutani et al. [95]	before CABG	8-10	RA
Komatsu et al. [96]	after CABG	8-10	RA
Tuchschmidt et al. [97]	sepsis	15	RA
Mohsenifar et al. [98]	ARDS	21	RA
Ronco et al. [91]	control/sepsis	4.5 ± 1.3 / 3.8 ± 1.5	RA

CABG, coronary artery bypass grafting; RA: regression analysis

Table 2. *Effects of sepsis/ARDS on critical oxygen delivery (DO₂crit) in the clinical setting*

Cardiovascular System

Myocardial failure is a common finding in sepsis. Echocardiographic studies have demonstrated that myocardial performance is usually compromised, ranging from isolated diastolic dysfunction to both diastolic and systolic ventricular failure [86,87]. Since studies in septic patients argue against an ischemic origin of sepsis-induced cardiac dysfunction [92], it is therefore believed that the dysfunctional microcirculation produces regional flow disturbances and abnormal tissue oxygenation in the heart, as reported from animal studies [93].

Sepsis is also associated with a ('hyperdynamic') high cardiac output/low vascular resistance hemodynamic profile that is thought to reflect an attempt of the organism to compensate for increased tissue oxygen needs, blood flow maldistribution (caused by disordered arteriolar reactivity) and peripheral mismatch between oxygen supply and demand [94].

Lung

If ARDS is developing in the septic patient, this is often a sign for ubiquitous microvascular injury, preceding the onset of MOF. ARDS typically leads to the development of diffuse, acute parenchymal lung injury as a result of the inflammatory response to sepsis. Important roles in this process have been attributed to complement system activation, PMN activation and sequestration and increased production of cytokines such as IL-1β, IL-6, IL 8 and TNF [99,100].

As a result of microvascular injury, microvascular permeability increases, leading to edema formation and mechanical dysfunction in the lungs [101]. Also, hypoxic pulmonary vasoconstriction is compromised, probably because of an altered vascular reactivity of pulmonary microvessels [102]. The clinical consequences of sepsis-induced lung injury are, therefore pulmonary hypertension and arterial hypoxemia.

Bowel

Gut mucosal hypoperfusion resulting in hypoxia of the mucosal layer is often named a major factor in the development of multi-organ failure following sepsis. For example, prolonged hypoperfusion to the intestinal mucosa could foster bacterial translocation and/or local production of cytokines and mediators. In humans, however, it has been difficult to confirm the presence of sepsis-related microcirculatory oxygen deprivation in the gut mucosa. In a recent study, Temmersfeld-Wolbrück et al. [103], using microlight guide reflectance spectophotometry in septic patients to assess microvascular HbO$_2$, were the first to demonstrate the occurrence of severely hypoxic microregional areas. These findings were associated with an increase in the mucosal-to-arterial PCO$_2$ gap and the Intramucosal pH (pHi), thus suggesting a link between the presence of microvascular hypoxia and intramucosal acidosis [103].

Kidney

In sepsis, renal hypoperfusion can occur because of volume depletion or intrinsic causes such as sympathetic vasoconstriction following mediator release and microthrombosis due to disseminated intravascular coagulation. However, the final common pathway leading to renal failure appears to be outer medullary ischemia and hypoxia [104].

Brain

Sepsis-associated alterations in mental function are summarized as 'septic encephalopathy'. Formerly, sepsis encephalophathy was seen primarily as a result of hypotension and MOF. Now, it is recognized that sepsis encephalopathy may also occur early in the disease, independent from failure of other organs. It is assumed that DO_2 to the brain is decreased because of cerebral hypoperfusion and reduced erythrocyte deformability [105]. Also, the blood-brain barrier function is impaired, thus allowing mediators and free radicals to cross [105]. However, in contrast to other organs such as the lung, the brain is resistant to leukocyte accumulation [106].

MARKERS OF SEPTIC MICROCIRCULATORY INJURY

The current definition of sepsis is based on characteristic changes in general markers of hemostasis which are known to be representative for a systemic inflammatory response following an infection [107]. Although these surrogate markers of sepsis (e.g., blood pressure, leukocyte count, temperature) are useful to follow up the course of sepsis, there is an ongoing search to develop more direct markers of systemic inflammation to optimize the therapy. While a large number of markers and tests have been proposed to diagnose septic microcirculatory injury to organ systems, only few were found to be sensitive enough to allow judgments about the presence and severity of sepsis on the whole body level. Among those, procalcitonin, IL 6, and lactate are probably most widely accepted to determine the severity or the clinical course of human sepsis.

Procalcitonin

The role of the hormone precursor procalcitionin in the inflammatory process underlying the sepsis syndrome has not been defined, but a close relationship to the severity of the disease has been established. While physiologic procalcitonin levels range below 0.5 ng/ml, increases by 10- to several hundred fold are found in sepsis. A recent study investigating the predictive accuracy of increased procalcitonin levels reported a sensitivity of 89% and a specifity of 94% for the diagnosis of sepsis [108]. In addition, the time course of procalcitonin levels may be a useful diagnostic criterion to determine prognosis and mortality [109,110].

IL-6

Many studies have been able to demonstrate a diagnostic or predictive value of increased levels of the cytokine, IL-6, in sepsis. However, recent studies are questioning the usefulness of IL-6 as a sepsis marker in the clinical setting, at least for the prediction of sepsis-related mortality [109,111]. Müller et al. also demonstrated that in comparison to procalcitonin, both the sensitivity and the specificity of IL-6 levels in the diagnosis of sepsis are lower (65% and 79%, respectively) [108].

Lactate

Lactate is formed from pyruvate by many tissues as the endproduct of glycolysis, and can be utilized by liver, kidney, and skeletal muscle. Under physiologic conditions most of pyruvate is metabolized by pyruvate dehydrogenase to acetyl-coA. If microcirculatory failure creates hypoxic conditions, pyruvate metabolism is depressed, and lactate levels rise [112]. The trend in arterial lactate is, therefore, often used as a surrogate marker for tissue hypoperfusion in sepsis. A problem is that because lactate levels depend on both production and utilization, abnormalities in utilization (e.g., reduced pyruvate dehydrogenase activity or liver failure) are also a potential cause of elevated plasma levels [113,114].

STRATEGIES TO MODIFY MICROVASCULAR INJURY IN SEPSIS

After more than two decades of intensive research an interim analysis results in the conclusion that at the time, only one of the numerous studied therapeutic strategies, this is activated protein C infusion, has been proven to lower the high mortality from sepsis. Researchers are still left with two major questions:

i)   What are the appropriate targets of a possible successful therapy? In addition to activated protein C infusion, candidates, for example, may include vascular reactivity, microvascular blood flow, cytokine response, or mitochondrial dysfunction.

ii)   When do we need to intervene? Most therapeutic strategies have been studied in patients with a diagnosis of sepsis. Since it has been demonstrated in different animal models that pretreatment with inflammatory mediators such as endotoxin can induce tolerance against a subsequent septic hit, the question has opened if, for example, an upregulation of tolerance pathways could be used to develop preventive strategies [115].

Target level	Strategies/Agents
Inflammatory response	Modulation of cytokine responses Modulation of neutrophil function (e.g. GCSF) NF-κB-inhibition
Vascular reactivity	α-adrenergic support (catecholamines) NO synthase inhibition/NO binding Vasopressin
Tissue oxygenation	Increase in oxygen extraction capabilities (Cell-free hemoglobin)
Coagulation	Coagulation inhibitor replacement (antithrombin III, activated protein C)
Preventive therapy	Upregulation of endotoxin tolerance

Table 3. Therapeutic strategies to modulate whole body septic microcirculatory injury

Table 3 lists a number of therapies directed at modifying the microcirculatory response to sepsis. As a result of the increasing knowledge about the complex cytokine response associated with systemic infection, numerous approaches to block individual mediators have been tested, including anti-TNF antibodies, IL-1 receptor antagonist (IL-1ra), and anti-PAF. However, so far all these strategies have failed to show a substantial benefit on outcome from sepsis, similar to approaches to block common pathways of inflammation (e.g., anti-prostaglandins and high-dose steroids) [116].

Since a ubiquitous loss of vascular resistance is a regular and almost pathognomonic finding in sepsis, it has also been appealing to develop strategies to normalize vascular reactivity. Two major class of agents have been used for such therapy, the one of which is catecholamines with α-adrenergic reactivity, while the other comprises various drugs that either inhibit the production of, or scavenge, NO. Drugs with α-adrenergic activity such as norepinephrine, epinephrine and dopamine are used routinely in septic and other shock forms to elevate vascular resistance and perfusion pressure if volume infusion alone is insufficient. While their clinical usefulness as supportive therapies to elevate blood pressure in acute shock situations is not questioned, it is still unclear if the well-documented effects on vascular reactivity and regional blood flow distribution result in improved tissue oxygenation or organ function (reviewed in [117]). NOS inhibition has been extensively studied for years, but evidence has been increasing that excessive NO blockade offers no benefit [118]. Recently, the use of NO-scavenging hemoglobin solutions has been advocated as an alternative means to support vascular reactivity in sepsis. Hemoglobin solutions are characterized by complex pharmacologic effects, but appear to offer additional benefits in sepsis because they also improve microvascular blood flow and increase oxygen extraction capabilities [119,120]. Recent work demonstrated, in different animal models, that hemoglobin solutions prevent the sepsis-induced increase in DO_2crit [89,121]. Infusion of norepinephrine, but not NO inhibition, has been shown to cause a similar effect on DO_2crit (Fig. 2) [89,122,123].

Since sepsis affects the organ microcirculations in different ways and often at different times in the disease process, it may be logical to treat individual organs separately. A good example for the potential benefits of such treatment is NO inhalation to optimize the ventilation-perfusion relationship in ARDS, a therapy which has gained clinical acceptance although no survival benefit has ever been demonstrated. Other strategies to influence regional microvascular blood flow selectively have been proposed, including epidural sympathetic blockade [124] or topical administration of vasoactive drugs [49]. The possible usefulness of such techniques in sepsis remains to be clarified.

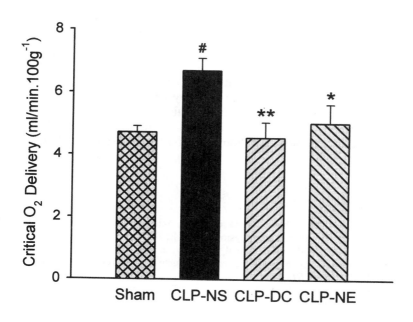

Figure 2. *DO$_2$crit after an 18 hour infusion of DCLHb or norepinephrine targeted to raise blood pressure by 10-20% in septic rats; Sham, sham controls, CLP-NS, septic controls; CLP-DC, septic rats treated with DCLHb infusion; CLP-NE, septic rats treated with norepinephrine infusion; [#]p<0.05 vs. Sham, *p < 0.05 vs. CLP-NS, **p < 0.01 vs. CLP-NS*

Currently, the most promising strategy to attenuate sepsis-related microvascular injury is the modification of activated coagulation pathways to diminish the extent of microthrombosis. In sepsis, levels of the coagulation inhibitors antithrombin III and protein C are lowered mainly as a result of complex formation and proteolytic inactivation. The endogenous control mechanism for thrombin generation are therefore impaired, resulting in activation of coagulation and inflammatory processes [125]. Experimental work demonstrated that in this situation infusion of activated protein C may have salutary effects on critical pathways of inflammation, for example, blockade of NF-κB activation [126]. The results from a recent multi-center trial using activated protein C in septic patients indicate that coagulation inhibitor replacement may improve survival from sepsis. Both experimental and clinical work is needed to explore the reasons for the therapeutic efficacy of activated protein C and to guide the development of treatment plans that include the use of coagulation inhibitors.

For long it has been known that following pretreatment with endotoxin, some degree of tolerance is developing against ischemia ('cross tolerance') and also to subsequent endotoxin exposure (endotoxin tolerance). For example, it was demonstrated that endotoxin pretreatment before LPS infusion is associated with a reduction of changes that are attributable to the inflammatory response to LPS, such as decreased neutrophil entrapment and decreased cytokine production in the microcirculation [127,128]. Recent observations also suggested that the sepsis-associated increase in microvascular permeability is ameliorated by LPS-pretreatment [129]. This information is important, since reduced microvascular permeability may translate into improved microvascular and organ function. Despite these promising results, endotoxin tolerance has not been studied beyond the experimental level.

REFERENCES

1. Ito S, Carretero OA, Abe K. Role of nitric oxide in the control of glomerular microcirculation. Clin Exp Pharm Physiol 1997; 24:578-581
2. Duling BR, Berne RM. Longitudinal gradients in periarteriolar oxygen tension. A possible mechanism for the participation of oxygen in local regulation of blood flow. Circ Res 1970; 27:669-678
3. Ellsworth ML, Ellis CG, Popel AS, Pittman RN. Role of microvessels in oxygen supply to tissue. News Physiol Sci 1994; 9:119-123
4. Ellsworth ML, Pittman RN. Arterioles supply oxygen to capillaries by diffusion as well as by convection. Am J Physiol 1990; 258:H1240-H1243
5. Lush CW, Kvietys PR. Microvascular dysfunction in sepsis. Microcirculation 2000; 7:83-101
6. Pries AR, Ley K, Claassen M, Gaethgens P. Red cell distribution at microvascular bifurcations. Microvasc Res 1989; 38:81-101
7. Federspiel WJ, Popel AS. A theoretical analysis of the effect of the particulate nature of blood on oxygen release in capillaries. Microvasc Res 1986; 32:164-189
8. Varela FE, Popel AS. Effect of intracapillary resistance to oxygen transport on the diffusional shunting between capillaries. J Biomed Eng 1998; 10:400-405
9. Pohl U, De Wit C, Gloe T. Large arterioles in the control of blood flow: role of endothelium-dependent dilatation. Acta Physiol Scand 2000; 168:505-510
10. Duling BR, Hogan RD, Langille BL, Lelkes P, Segal SS, Vatner SF, Weigelt H, Young MA. Vasomotor control: functional hyperemia and beyond. Fed Proc 1987; 46:251-263
11. Liao JC, Kuo L. Interaction between adenosine and flow-induced dilation in coronary microvascular network. Am J Physiol 1997; 272:H1571-H1581
12. Rivers RJ. Remote effects of pressure changes in arterioles. Am J Physiol 1995; 268:H1379-H1382
13. Sun D, Huang A, Koller A, Kaley G. Flow-dependent dilation and myogenic constrictionn interact to establish the resistance of skeletal muscle arterioles. Microcirculation 1995; 2:289-295
14. Ngai AC, Winn HR. Modulation of cerebral arteriolar diameter by intraluminal flow and pressure. Circ Res 1995; 77:832-840

15. Falcone JC. Endothelial cell calcium and vascular control. Med Sci Sports Exerc 1995; 27:1165-1169

16. Schubert R, Mulvany MJ. The myogenic response: established facts and attractive hypotheses. Clin Sci 1999; 96:313-326

17. Hill MA, Zou H, Davis JM, Potocnik Sj, Price S. Transient increases in diameter and [Ca(2+)](i) are not obligatory for myogenic constriction. Am J Physiol 2000; 278:H354-H352

18. Falcone JC, Meininger GA. Endothelin mediates a component of the enhanced myogenic responsiveness of arterioles from hypertensive rats. Microcirculation 1999; 6:305-313

19. Nagi MM, Ward ME. Modulation of myogenic responsiveness by CO2 in rat diaphragmatic arterioles: role of the endothelium. Am J Physiol 1997; 272:H1419-H1425

20. Welsh DG, Segal SS. Coactivation of resistance vessels and muscle fibers with acetylcholine release from motor nerves. Am J Physiol 1998; 273:H156-H163

21. Harder DR, Narayanan J, Birks EK, Liard JF, Imig JD, Lombard JH, Lange AR, Roman RJ. Identification of a putative microvascular oxygen sensor. Circ Res 1996; 79:54-61

22. Jackson WF. Arteriolar oxyge reactivity: where is the sensor? Am J Physiol 1987; 253:H1120-H1126

23. Gow AJ, Stamler JS. Reactions between nitric oxide and haemoglobin under physiological conditions. Nature 1998; 391:169-173

24. Stamler JS, Jia L, Eu JP, McMahon TJ, Demchenko IT, Bonaventura J, Gernert K, Piantadosi CA. Blood flow regulation by S-nitrosohemoglobin in the physiological oxygen gradient. Science 1997; 276:2034-2037

25. Ellsworth ML, Forrester CG, Ellis CG, Dietrich HH. The erythrocyte as a regulator of vascular tone. Am J Physiol 1995; 269:H2155-H2161

26. Farquhar I, Martin CM, Lam C, Potter R, Ellis CG, Sibbald WJ. Decreased capillary density *in vivo* in bowel mucosa of rats with normotensive sepsis. J Surg Res 1996; 61:190-196

27. Lam C, Tyml K, Martin C, Sibbald W. Microvascular perfusion is impaired in a rat model of normotensive sepsis. J Clin Invest 1994; 94:2077-2083

28. Schumacker PT, Samsel RW. Oxygen delivery and uptake by peripheral tissues: physiology and pathophysiology. Crit Care Clin 1989; 5:255-269

29. Astiz ME, DeGent GE, Lin RY, Rackow EC. Microvascular function and rheologic changes in hyperdynamic sepsis. Crit Care Med 1995; 23:265-271

30. Kirschenbaum LA, Aziz M, Astiz ME, Saha DC, Rackow EC. Influence of rheologic changes and platelet-neutrophil interactions on cell filtration in sepsis. Am J Respir Crit Care Med 2000; 161:1602-1607

31. Linderkamp O, Ruef P, Brenner B, Gulbins E, Lang F. Passive deformability of mature, immature, and active neutrophils in healthy and septicemic neonates. Pediatr Res 1998; 44:946-950

32. Yodice PC, Astiz ME, Kurian BM, Lin RY, Rackow EC. Neutrophil rheologic changes in septic shock. Am J Respir Crit Care Med 1997; 155:38-42

33. Baskurt OK, Gelmont D, Meiselman HJ. Red blood cell deformability in sepsis. Am J Respir Crit Care Med 1998; 157:421-427

34. Langenfeld JE, Machiedo GW, Lyons M, Rush BF, Dikdan G, Lysz TW. Correlation between red blood cell deformability and changes in hemodynamic function. Surgery 1994; 116:859-867

35. Machiedo GW, Powell RJ, Rush BF, Swislocki NI, Dikdan G. The incidence of decreased red blood cell deformability in sepsis and the association with oxygen free radical damage and multiple-systems organ failure. Arch Surg 1989; 124:1386-1389

36. ten Cate H. Pathophysiology of disseminated intravascular coagulation in sepsis. Crit Care Med 2000; 28:S9-S11

37. Goddard CM, Poon BY, Klut ME, Wiggs BR, Van Eeden SF, Hogg JC, Walley KR. Leukocyte activation does not mediate myocardial leukocyte retention during endotoxemia in rabbits. Am J Physiol 1998; 275:H1548-H1557
38. Schmidt H, Schmidt W, Muller T, Bohrer B, Gebhard MM, Martin E. N-acetylcysteine attenuates endotoxin-induced leukocyte-endothelial cell adhesion and macromolecular leakage in vivo. Crit Care Med 1997; 25:858-863
39. Schmidt W, Stenzel K, Gebhard MM, Martin E. C1-esterase inhibitor and its effects on endotoxin-induced leokocyte adherence and plasma extravasation in postcapillary venules. Surgery 1999; 125:280-287
40. Klabunde RE, Calvello C. Inhibition of endotoxin-induced microvascular leakage by a platelet-activating factor antagonist and 5-lipoxygenase inhibitor. Shock 1995; 4:368-372
41. Laniyonu AA, Coston AF, Klabunde RE. Endotoxin-induced mirovascular leakage is prevented by a PAF antagonist and NO synthase inhibitor. Shock 1997; 7:49-54
42. Schmidt H, Schmidt W, Muller T, Bohrer B, Bach A, Gebhard MM, Martin E. Effect of the 21-aminosteroid tirilazad mesylate on leukocyte adhesion and macromolecular leakage during endotoxemia. Surgery 1997; 121:328-334
43. Eppihimer MJ, Wolitzky B, Anderson DC, Labow MA, Granger DN. Heterogeneity of expression of E- and P-selectins in vivo. Circ Res 1996; 79:560-569
44. Haraldsen G, Kvale D, Lien B, Farstad IN, Brandtzaeg P. Cytokine-regulated expression of E-selectin, intracellular adhesion molecule-1 (ICAM-1), and vascular cell adhesion molecule-1 (VCAM-1) in human microvascular endothelial cells. J Immunol 1996; 156:2558-2565
45. Barroso-Arranda J, Schmid-Schonbien G, Sweifach BW, Mathison JC. Polymorphonuclear neutrophil contribution to induced tolerance to bacterial lipopolysaccharide. Circ Res 1991; 69:1196-1206
46. Goddard CM, Allard MF, Hogg JC, Walley KR. Myocardial morphometric changes related to decreased contractility after endotoxin. Am J Physiol 1996; 270:H1446-H1452
47. Neviere RR, Pitt-Hyde ML, Piper RD, Sibbald WJ, Potter RF. Microvascular perfusion deficits are not a prerequisite for mucosal injury in septic rats. Am J Physiol 1999; 276:G933-G940
48. Davenpeck KL, Zagorski J, Schleimer RP, Bochner BS. Lipopolysaccharide-induced leukocyte rolling and adhesion in the rat mesenteric microcirculation: regulation by glucocorticoids and role of cytokines. J Immunol 1998; 161:6861-6870
49. Hersch M, Madorin WS, Sibbald WJ, Martin CM. Selective gut microcirculatory control (SGMC) in septic rats: a novel approach with a locally applied vasoactive drug. Shock 1998; 10:292-297
50. Makita H, Nishimura N, Miyamoto K, Nakano T, Tanino Y, Hirokawa J, Nishihara J, Kawakamy Y. Effect of anti-macrophage migration inhibitory factor antibody on lipopolysaccharide-induced pulmonary neutrophil accumulation. Am J Respir Crit Care Med 1998; 158:573-579
51. Kvietys PR, Granger DN. The vascular endothelium in GI inflammation. In: Wallace J, (ed) Immunopharmacology of the gastrointestinal system. Academic Press Ltd., London, 1993 pp:69-103
52. Panes J, Granger DN. Leukocyte-endothelial cell interactions: molecular mechanisms and implications in gastrointestinal disease. Gastroenterology 1998; 114:1066-1090
53. Sundrani R, Easington CR, Mattoo A, Parillo JE, Hollenberg SM. Nitric oxide synthase inhibition increases venular leukocyte rolling and adhesion in septic rats. Crit Care Med 2000; 28:2898-2903
54. Hogg JC, Doerschuk CM. Leukocyte traffic in the lung. Ann Rev Physiol 1995; 57:97-114

55. Burns AR, Walker DC, Brown ES, Thurmon LT, Bowden RA, Keese CR, Simon SI, Entman ML, Smith CW. Neutrophil transendothelial migration is independent of tight junctions and occurs preferentially at tricellular corners. J Immunol 1997; 159:2893-2903
56. Cepinskas G, Sandig M, Kvietys PR. PAF-induced elastase-dependent neutrophil transendothelial migration is associated with the mobilization of elastase to the neutrophil surface and localization to the migrating front. J Cell Sci 1999; 112:1937-1945
57. Granger HJ, Yuan Y, Zawieja DC. Ultrastructural basis of leukocyte migration through the microvascular membrane. In: Granger DN, Schmid-Schonbein GW (eds) Physiology and pathophysiology of leukocyte adhesion. Oxford University Press, Oxford, 1995, pp:185-195
58. Kishimoto TK, Anderson DC. The role of integrins in inflammation. In: Gallin JL, Goldstein IM, Snyderman R, eds. Inflammation. Basic principles and clinical correlates. Raven Press Ltd., New York, 1992 pp:353-495
59. Furie MB, Naprstek BL, Silverstein SC. Migration of neutrophils across monolayers of cultured microvascular endothelial cells. J Cell Sci 1987; 88:161-175
60. Huber AR, Weiss SJ. Disruption of the subendothelial basement membrane during neutrophil diapedesis in an in vitro construct of a blood vessel wall. J Clin Invest 1995; 83:1122-1136
61. Cepinskas G, Noseworthy R, Kvietys PR. Transendothelial neutrophil migration. Role of neutrophil-derived proteases and relationship to transendothelial protein movement. Circ Res 1997; 81:618-626
62. Thomas JR, Harlan JM, Rice JL, Winn RK. Role of leukocyte CD11/CD18 complex in endotoxic and septic shock in rabbits. J Appl Physiol 1992; 73:1510-1516
63. Bandel JW, Goldberg RN, Suguihara C, Nagoshi R, Martinez O, Rothlein R, Ruiz P, Bancalari E. Effects of anti-CD18 monoclonal antibody, R17.7, on the cardiopulmonary manifestations of group B streptococcal sepsis in piglets. Biol Neonate 2000; 78:121-128
64. Walsh CJ, Carey PD, Cook DJ, Bechard DE, Fowler AA, Sugerman HJ. Anti-CD18 antibody attenuates neutropenia and alveolar capillary-membrane injury during gram-negative sepsis. Surgery 1991; 110:205-211
65. Xu N, Rahman A, Mishall RD, Tiruppathi C, Malik AB. Beta(2)-integrin blockade driven by E-selectin promotor prevents neutrophil sequestration and lung injury in mice. Circ Res 2000; 87:254-260
66. Jaeschke H, Farhood A, Smith CW. Neutrophil-induced liver cell injury in endotoxin shock is a CD11b/CD18-dependent mechanism. Am J Physiol 1991; 261:G1051-G1056
67. Xu H, Gonzalo JA, St.Pierre Y, et al. Leukocytosis and resistance to septic shock in intercellular adhesion molecule 1-deficient mice. J Exp Med 1994; 180:95-109
68. Lentsch AB, Ward PA. Regulation of inflammatory vascular damage. J Pathol 2000; 190:343-348
69. Kvietys PR, Granger DN. Endothelial cell monolayers as a tool for studying microvascular pathophysiology. Am J Physiol 1997; 273:G1189-G1199
70. Yoshida N, Cepinskas G, Granger DN, Anderson DC, Wolf RE, Kvietys PR. Aspirin-induced, neutrophil-mediated injury to vascular endothelium. Inflammation 1995; 19:297-312
71. Lehr HA, Fernando B, Kirkpatrick C, James J. Microcirculatory dysfunction in sepsis: a pathogenetic basis for therapy? J Pathol 2000; 190:373-386
72. Gerard C, Bruyns C, Marchant A, et al. Interleukin 10 reduces the release of tumor necrosis factor and prevents lethality in experimental endotoxemia. J Exp Med 1993; 177:547-550
73. Van der Poll T, Jansen PM, Montegut WJ, et al. Effects of IL-10 on systemic inflammatory responses during sublethal primate endotoxemia. J Immunol 1997; 158:1971-1975

74. Kanwar S, Kubes P. Nitric oxide is an antiadhesive molecule for leukocytes. New Horiz 1995; 3:93-104
75. Nishida J, McCuskey RS, McDonnell D, Fox ES. Protective role of NO in hepatic microcirculatory dysfunction during endotoxemia. Am J Physiol 1994; 267:G1135-G1141
76. Kubes P, Suzuki M, Granger DN. Nitric oxide: an endogenous modulator of leukocyte adhesion. Proc Natl Acad Sci USA 1991; 88:4651-4655
77. Bloomfield GL, Holloway S, Ridings PC, et al. Pretreatment with inhaled nitric oxide inhibits neutrophil migration and oxidative activity resulting in attenuated sepsis-induced acute lung injury. Crit Care Med 1997; 25:584-593
78. Spieker M, Darius H, Kaboth K, Hubner F, Liao JK. Differential regulation of endothelial cell adhesion molecule expression by nitric oxide donors and antioxidants. J Leukoc Biol 1998; 63:732-739
79. Spieker M, Peng HB, Liao JK. Inhibition of endothelial vascular cell adhesion molecule-1 expression by nitric oxide involves the induction and nuclear translocation of IkappaBalpha. J Biol Chem 1997; 272:30969-30974
80. Zingarelli B, Salzman AL, Szabo C. Genetic disruption of poly (ADP ribose) synthetase inhibits the expression of P-selectin and intercellular adhesion molecule-1 in myoardial ischemia/reperfusion injury. Circ Res 1998; 83:85-94
81. Zingarelli B, Szabo C, Salzman AL. Blockade of Poly (ADP-ribose) synthetase inhibits neutrophil recruitment, oxidant generation, and mucosal injury in murine colitis. Gastroenterology 1999; 116:335-345
82. Neviere RR, Cepinskas G, Madorin WS, et al. LPS pretreatment ameliorates peritonitis-induced myocardial inflammation and dysfunction: role of myocytes. Am J Physiol 1999; 277:H885-H892
83. Bone RC. Sepsis and its complications: The clinical problem. Crit Care Med 1994; 22:S8-S11
84. Kollef MH, Schuster DP. The acute respiratory distress syndrome. N Engl J Med 1995; 332:27-37
85. Hersch M, Gnidec AA, Bersten AD, Troster M, Rutledge FS, Sibbald WJ. Histologic and ultrastructural changes in nonpulmonary organs during early hyperdynamic sepsis. Surgery 1990; 107:397-410
86. Munt B, Jue J, Gin K, Fenwick J, Tweeddale M. Diastolic filling in human severe sepsis: an echocardiographic study. Crit Care Med 1998; 26:1829-1833
87. Polaert J, Declerck C, Vogelaers D, Colardyn F, Visser CA. Left ventricular systolic and diastolic function in septic shock. Intensive Care Med 1997; 23:553-560
88. Nelson DP, Samsel RW, Wood LDH, Schumacker PT. Pathological supply dependence of systemic and intestinal O_2 uptake during endotoxemia. J Appl Physiol 1988; 64:2410-2419
89. Sielenkämper AW, Yu P, Eichelbronner O, MacDonald T, Martin CM, Chin-Yee IH, Sibbald WJ. Diaspirin crosslinked hemoglobin and norepinephrine prevent the sepsis-induced increase in critical O2 delivery. Am J Physiol 2000; 279:H1922-H1930
90. Hanique G, Dugernier T, Laterre PF, Dougnac A, Roeseler J, Reynaert MS. Significance of pathologic oxygen supply dependency in critically ill patients: comparison between measured and calculated methods. Intensive Care Med 1994; 20:12-18
91. Ronco JJ, Fenwick JC, Tweeddale MG, Wiggs BR, Phang PT, Cooper DJ, Cunnungham KF, Russell JA, Walley KR. Identification of the critical oxygen delivery for anaerobic metabolism in critically ill septic and nonseptic humans. JAMA 1993; 270:1724-1730
92. Cunnion RE, Schaer GL, Parker MM, Natanson C, Parrillo JE. The coronary circulation in human septic shock. Circulation 1986; 73:637-644

93. Ince C, Sinaasappel M. Microcirculatory oxygenation and shunting in sepsis and shock. Crit Care Med 1999; 27:1369-1377

94. Sielenkämper AW, Sibbald WJ. Pathophysiology of hypotension. In: Webb A, Shapiro MJ, Singer M, Suter PM (eds). Oxford Textbook of Critical Care. Oxford University Press, Oxford, 1999 pp:215-219

95. Shibutani K, Komatsu T, Kubal K, Sanchala V, Kumar V, Bizarri DV. Critical level of oxygen delivery in anesthetized man. Crit Care Med 1983; 11:640-643

96. Komatsu T, Shibutani K, Okamoto K, Kumar V, Kubal K, Sanchala V, Lees DE. Critical level of oxygen delivery after cardiopulmonary bypass. Crit Care Med 1987; 15:194-197

97. Tuchschmidt J, Fried J, Swinney R, Sharma OP. Early hemodynamic correlates of survival in patients with septic shock. Crit Care Med 1989; 17:719-723

98. Mohsenifar Z, Goldbach P, Tashkin DP, Campisi DJ. Relationship between O2 delivery and O2 consumption in the adult respiratory distress syndrome. Chest 1983; 84:267-271

99. Meduri G, Headley S, Kohler G, Stentz F, Tolley E, Umberger R, Leeper K. Persistent elevation of inflammatory cytokines predicts a poor outcome in ARDS. Plasma IL-1 beta and IL-6 levels are consistent and efficient predictors of outcome over time. Chest 1995; 107:1062-1073

100. Schutte H, Lohmeyer J, Rosseau S, et al. Bronchoalveolar and systemic cytokine profiles in patients with ARDs, severe pneumonia and cardiogenic pulmonary edema. Eur Respir J 2000; 9:1858-1867

101. Bernard GR, Artigas A, Brigham KL, et al. The American-European Consensus Conference on ARDS. Definitions, mechanisms, relevant outcomes, and clinical trial coordination. Am J Respir Crit Care Med 1994; 149:818-824

102. Fischer SR, Deyo DJ, Bone HG, McGuire R, Traber LD, Traber DL. Nitric oxide synthase inhibition restores hypoxic pulmonary vasoconstriction in sepsis. Am J Respir Crit Care Med 1997; 156:833-839

103. Temmesfeld-Wollbruck B, Szalay A, Mayer K, Olschewski H, Seeger W, Grimminger F. Abnormalities of gastric mucosal oxygenation in septic shock: partial responsiveness to dopexamine. Am J Respir Crit Care Med 1998; 157:1586-1592

104. Heyman SN, Fuchs S, Brezis M. The role of medullary ischemia in acute renal failure. New Horizons 1995; 597-607

105. Papadopoulos MC, Davies C, Moss RF, Tighe D, Bennett ED. Pathophysiology of septic encephalopathy: A review. Crit Care Med 2000; 28:3019-3024

106. Perry VH, Andersson PB, Gordon S. Macrophages and inflammation in the central nervous system. Trends Neurosci 1993; 16:268-273

107. ACCP/SCCM Consensus Conference. Definitions for sepsis and organ failure and guidelines for the use of innovative therapies in sepsis. Chest 1992; 101:1644-1655

108. Muller B, Becker KL, Schachinger H, Rickenbacher PR, Zimmerli W, Ritz R. Calcitonin precursors are reliable markers of sepsis in a medical intensive care unit. Crit Care Med 2000; 977-983

109. Herrmann W, Ecker D, Quast S, Klieden M, Rose S, Marzi I. Comparison of procalcitonon, sCD14 and interleukin-6 values in septic patients. Clin Chem Lab Med 2000; 38:41-46

110. Hatherill M, Tibby SM, Turner C, Ratnavel N, Murdoch IA. Procalcitonin and cytokine levels: relationship to organ failure and mortality in pediatric septic shock. Crit Care Med 2000; 28:2591-2594

111. Arnalich F, Garcia-Palomero E, Lopez J, Jimenez M, Madero R, Renart J, Vazquez JJ, Montiel C. Predictive value of nuclear factor kappa B activity and plasma cytokine levels in patients with sepsis. Infect Immun 2000; 68:1942-1954

112. Vincent JL. The available clinical tools - oxygen-derived variables, lactate, and pHi. In: Sibbald WJ, Messmer K, Fink MP (eds) Tissue Oxygenation in Acute Medicine. Springer, Heidelberg, 1998 pp:193-203
113. Curtis SE, Cain SM. Regional and systemic oxygen delivery/uptake relations and lactate flux in hyperdynamic endotoxin treated dogs. Am Rev Respir Dis 1992; 145:348-354
114. Levraut J, Ciebiera JP, Chave S, Rabary O, Jambou P, Carles M, Grimaud D. Mild hyperlactatemia in stable septic patients is due to impaired lactate clearance rather than overproduction. Am J Respir Crit Care Med 1998; 157:1021-1026
115. Neviere RR, Sibbald WJ. Development of myocardial tolerance to ischemia/reperfusion and septic injury. In: Vincent JL, ed. Yearbook of intensive care and emergency medicine. Springer, Heidelberg, 1998, pp:125-132
116. Glauser MP. Pathophysiologic basis of sepsis: Considerations for future strategies of intervention. Crit Care Med 2000; 28:S4-S8
117. Treggiari-Venzi MM, Suter PM, Romand JA. Effects of catecholamine therapy on regional perfusion in septic shock. In: Vincent JL (ed) Yearbook of intensive care and emergency medicine. Springer, Heidelberg, 2000 pp:658-670
118. Kilbourn RG, Szabo C, Traber DL. Beneficial versus detrimental effects of nitric oxide synthase inhibitors in circulatory shock: Lessons learned from experimental and clinical studies. Shock 1997; 7:235-246
119. Sielenkämper AW, Eichelbrönner O, Martin CM, Madorin SW, Chin-Yee IH, Sibbald WJ. Diaspirin crosslinked hemoglobin improves mucosal perfusion in ileum of septic rats. Crit Care Med 2000; 27:782-787
120. Sielenkämper AW, Chin-Yee IH, Martin CM, Sibbald WJ. Diaspirin crosslinked hemoglobin improves systemic oxygen uptake in oxygen supply-dependent septic rats. Am J Respir Crit Care Med 1997; 156:1066-1072
121. Creteur J, Zhang H, De Backer D, Sun Q, Vincent JL. Diaspirin cross-linked hemoglobin improves oxygen extraction capabilities in endotoxic shock. J Appl Physiol 2000; 89:1437-1444
122. Zhang H, Smail N, Cabral A, Rogiers P, Vencent JL. Effects of norepinephrine on regional blood flow and oxygen extraction capabilities during endotoxic shock. Am J Respir Crit Care Med 1997; 155:1965-1971
123. Zhang H, Rogiers P, Smail N, Cabral A, Presier JC, Peny MO, Vincent JL. Effects of nitric oxide on blood flow distribution and O2 extraction capabilities during endotoxic shock. J Appl Physiol 1997; 83:1164-1173
124. Sielenkämper AW, Eicker K, Van Aken H. Thoracic epidural anesthesia increases mucosal perfusion in ileum of rats. Anesthesiology 2000; 93:844-851
125. Thijs LG. Coagulation inhibitor replacement in sepsis is a potentially useful clinical approach. Crit Care Med 2000; 28 (Suppl 9):S68-S73
126. White B, Schmidt M, Murphy C, et al. Activated protein C inhibits lipopolysaccharide-induced nuclear translocation of nuclear factoor kappaB (NF-kappaB) and tumor necrosis factor alpha (TNF-alpha) production in the THP-1 monocytic cell line. Br J Haematol 2000; 110:130-134
127. Ziegler-Heitbrock HW. Molecular mechanisms in tolerance to lipopolysaccharide. J Inflamm 1995; 45:13-26
128. Barroso-Aranda J, Schmid-Schonbein GW, Zweifach BW. Polymorphonuclear neutrophil contribution to induced tolerance to bacterial lipopolysaccharide. Circ Res 1991; 69:1196-1206
129. Fujii E, Yoshioka T, Ishida H, Irie K, Muraki T. Evaluation of iNOS-dependent and independent mechanisms of the microvascular permeability change induced by lipopolysaccharide. Br J Pharmacol 2000; 130:90-94

15

CYTOPATHIC HYPOXIA

Mitchell P. Fink

Adenosine triphosphate (ATP) is the energy currency of the cell. Virtually all cellular processes are driven by the energy released when ATP undergoes hydrolysis to form adenosine diphosphate (ADP) and inorganic phosphate (Pi).

ATP is normally generated in cells as a result of both anaerobic and aerobic processes. Anaerobic generation of ATP (or the biochemically equivalent high-energy phosphate compound, guanosine triphosphate), occurs in both the cytosol and mitochondria during three *substrate level phosphorylation* reactions. Aerobic generation of ATP occurs in mitochondria by means of a process called *oxidative phosphorylation*, wherein two compounds that are produced during glycolysis and the tricarboxylic acid (TCA) cycle, namely the reduced forms of nicotine adenine dinucleotide (NADH) and flavin adenine dinucleotide (FADH$_2$), are oxidized by O$_2$.

The reaction of a strong reducing agent, like NADH, with a powerful oxidizing agent, like O$_2$, releases a large amount of energy. In order to take optimal advantage of this highly exothermic (energy-releasing) reaction and capture as much of the energy released as possible in a usable form (i.e., the high-energy terminal pyrophosphate bond in ATP), mitochondria 'step-down' the reducing potential of NADH (and FADH$_2$) in stages. Thus, four electrons are not transferred from two moles of NADH to one mole of O$_2$ all at once, but rather are transferred through a series of intermediate compounds that have progressively lower reducing potentials.

Several of the electron carriers involved in the respiratory chain are organized as enzyme complexes located within the inner mitochondrial membrane. These complexes (called complexes I, II, III, and IV) couple the energy released during electron transfer (from moieties with greater to lesser reducing potential) to the active extrusion of protons from the mitochondrial matrix into the intermembrane space. These reactions, therefore, generate an electrochemical gradient for hydrogen ions across the inner mitochondrial membrane. The presence of this electrochemical gradient drives hydrogen ions through another mitochondrial enzyme, the $F_0F_1ATPase$, that catalyzes the formation of ATP from ADP and Pi.

For each mole of glucose metabolized to carbon dioxide (CO_2) and water (H_2O), the net yield of ATP from substrate level (anaerobic) phosphorylation reactions is four moles. In contrast, the net yield of ATP from oxidative-phosphorylation is 32 moles. Thus, oxidative metabolism in normally functioning mitochondria is far more efficient at producing ATP than is anaerobic metabolism, and a steady supply of O_2 is needed to generate most of the energy that is required to support vital cellular functions. If the delivery of O_2 is markedly impaired for any reason, cells become relatively hypoxic and the aerobic production of ATP is compromised. Classically, cellular energy production can be impaired as a result of *hypoxic hypoxia* (i.e., when the PO_2 in arterial blood is too low), *anemic hypoxia* (i.e., when the concentration of hemoglobin, the protein responsible for transporting O_2 in blood, is too low), and/or *stagnant hypoxia* (i.e., when the rate of blood flow through the microvasculature is too low).

EVIDENCE FOR CYTOPATHIC HYPOXIA IN SEPSIS

Inadequate O_2 delivery is not the only way that ATP production can be impaired in cells under pathological conditions. Even when intracellular PO_2 is within the normal range, ATP production can be inadequate to meet normal metabolic demands, if the cell's metabolic machinery for producing high-energy phosphate bonds is deranged. Intrinsic alterations in the cell's capacity for generating ATP can occur for a variety of other reasons, including: inadequate flow of substrates through the glycolytic and/or TCA pathways; depletion of reducing equivalents, like NADH; diminished flow of electrons through the mitochondrial redox chain; or dissipation of the electrochemical gradient across the inner mitochondrial membrane (by opening of 'shunt' pathways for the movement of protons down their electrochemical gradient by means other than flow through the $F_0F_1ATPase$). Collectively, mechanisms such as these that lead to impaired aerobic ATP production despite adequate O_2 availability have been termed *cytopathic hypoxia* [1], although this term is potentially misleading (since the proper use of O_2 is the problem, rather than hypoxia *per se*).

Tissue PO₂ Measurements

Tissue hypoxia is an expected correlate of any of the classical causes of impaired cellular aerobic metabolism. If the delivery of O_2 decreases on the basis of low arterial PO_2, anemia, and/or hypoperfusion, cells extract a greater fraction of the available O_2 in an effort to defend aerobic ATP production. As a consequence, the distribution of tissue PO_2 values shifts to the left (i.e., to values closer to zero). In contrast, when ATP production is impaired as a result of an intrinsic derangement in cellular respiration, then cells extract less O_2 per unit time from the available supply, leading to a rightward shift of the tissue PO_2 distribution. Accordingly, measurements of tissue PO_2 should be informative with respect to the question of what happens to cellular respiration in sepsis. Unfortunately, the results from a number of studies have yielded conflicting data, so no clear picture has emerged regarding the effects of sepsis on tissue PO_2.

Several well done studies showed that intestinal mucosal PO_2 decreased when experimental animals were infused with lipopolysaccharide (LPS) to induce a sepsis-like state [2-4]. Similarly, Sair and colleagues reported that skeletal muscle PO_2 decreased markedly in a rat model of endotoxemia [5]. Interestingly, in this study, there was no difference between endotoxemic animals and controls with respect to skeletal muscle perfusion as assessed by measuring inert gas washout curves. Therefore, the development of tissue hypoxia following the injection of LPS was attributed to impaired microvascular control of nutritive flow.

In another study, Astiz et al. studied three groups of animals: rats rendered septic by cecal ligation and puncture (CLP); rats made septic and resuscitated with intravenous albumin solution; and control rats subjected to a sham procedure [6]. Similar to the observations obtained in some large animal models of endotoxemia, bacterial peritonitis in rats was associated with a significant decrease in both systemic O_2 delivery and mean skeletal muscle PO_2. However, if albumin was infused to expand intravascular volume, both of these parameters were restored to values not different from those observed in nonseptic controls. Similar data were reported by Anning et al. [7]. These studies suggest that sepsis is *not* associated with tissue hypoxia.

Other studies support this view as well. For example, Hotchkiss et al. used a novel approach to determine whether tissue hypoxia occurs following the induction of sepsis in rats [8]. Tissue PO_2 was not measured directly, but rather was estimated by measuring the retention of [18F]-fluoroisonidazole, a lipophilic 2-nitroimidazole derivative that is irreversibly bound to intracellular macromolecules under hypoxic, but not normoxic, conditions. As a positive control, these investigators showed that retention of [18F]-fluoroisonidazole was increased in the ipsilateral gastrocnemius muscle of rats subjected to reversible hind limb ischemia by application of a rubber tourniquet. However, retention of $[^{18}F]$-fluoroisonidazole in skeletal muscle, cardiac muscle, liver, and kidney was similar in septic rats and nonseptic controls; i.e., sepsis was not associated with the development of tissue hypoxia.

Remarkably, the results from some studies seem to go even further, suggesting that tissue PO_2 values are actually supranormal in animals or patients with sepsis or septic shock. For example, VanderMeer et al. investigated the effects of resuscitated endotoxemia on intestinal mucosal PO_2 in pigs [9]. In these studies, mean mucosal PO_2 increased significantly following infusion of LPS. Although endotoxemia was not associated with mucosal hypoxia, mucosal hydrogen ion concentration increased significantly, suggesting that the development of tissue acidosis in this model was not the result of tissue hypoxia. These findings are entirely consistent with data obtained by Rosser et al., who found that bladder mucosal PO_2 increased in rats challenged with LPS [10]. Moreover, Boekstegers et al. documented that PO_2 distribution in skeletal muscle was left-shifted (i.e. to values less than normal) in patients with cardiogenic shock, as expected, but was shifted to the right (i.e., to supranormal values) in patients with septic shock [11].

Rather than measure tissue PO_2, Simonsen et al. used a different tactic to assess the effect of sepsis on mitochondrial function [12]. These investigators used near-infrared spectroscopy to monitor the redox state of the terminal element of the mitochondrial respiratory chain, cytochrome a,a$_3$, in skeletal muscle cells of baboons rendered septic by an infusion of viable *Escherichia coli*. The functional status of cytochrome a,a$_3$ was monitored by periodically causing temporary skeletal muscle ischemia by briefly occluding arterial inflow using a proximally placed tourniquet. Inflating the tourniquet caused a decrease in the signal from oxidized cytochrome a,a$_3$, whereas deflating the tourniquet resulted in an increase in the spectroscopic signal from the reoxidized enzyme. Six hours after the induction of bacteremia, the rate of cytochrome a,a$_3$ reduction following tourniquet ischemia was the same as at baseline, although the rate of reoxidation following the release of ischemia was slowed. These data suggest that mitochondrial function was normal in skeletal muscle at this time point, but the delivery of O_2 to the tissue was impaired. However, 18 hours after the induction of bacteremia, the rate of cytochrome a,a$_3$ reduction during tourniquet ischemia was markedly slowed. This finding is consistent with either of two possibilities. Sepsis might have altered the function of cytochrome a,a$_3$, such that the enzyme's ability to accept electrons from O_2 was impaired. Alternatively, sepsis might have resulted in a limitation in the availability of reducing equivalents (i.e., NADH and FADH$_2$).

Indirect Assessment of Mitochondrial Function

A dye, 3-(4,5-dimethylthiazol-2-yl)-2,5-diphenyl tetrazolium bromide (MTT), can be used to indirectly assess mitochondrial function. MTT itself is a colorless compound, but it is reduced by functioning mitochondria to a blue product (MTT-formazan) that can be detected spectrophotometrically. Bankey et al. used the reduction of MTT to MTT-formazan to assess mitochondrial function in co-cultures of rat hepatoctyes and rat liver macrophages [13]. Sequential stimulation of the cultures with a cytokine, interleukin-6 (IL-6), and then LPS decreased mitochondrial respiration by about 50%. Similar results were reported more recently by Szabo et al., who showed that MTT reduction was decreased in cultured macrophages and vascular smooth muscle cells following incubation with a pro-inflammatory cytokine, interferon-γ (IFN-γ), plus LPS [14].

More recently, Unno et al. used the MTT method in an *in vivo* study of the effects of LPS on intestinal epithelial barrier and mitochondrial function [15]. Rats were injected with saline or LPS. Twenty-four hours later, the lumen of the intestine was loaded with a solution of MTT. After a 30 min incubation period, the epithelial layer was scraped off the intestine and the concentration of MTT-formazan in enterocytes was determined, the results being normalized to DNA content. MTT reduction was significantly lower in enterocytes from endotoxemic rats as compared to enterocytes from nonendotoxemic controls, suggesting that LPS caused mitochondrial dysfunction in the epithelial cells lining the lumen of the gut.

Direct Assessment of Cellular or Mitochondrial Respiration

The MTT assay reflects the activity of a number of different dehydrogenases, particularly succinate dehydrogenase, and therefore is only an indirect measure of mitochondrial respiration [16]. Hence, it is pertinent that several studies have obtained more direct evidence that cellular or mitochondrial respiration is impaired in animals with sepsis or endotoxemia. For example, Kantrow et al. studied a rat model of sepsis induced by CLP [17]. Sixteen hours after subjecting rats to CLP or a sham operation, livers were removed and hepatocytes isolated. Hepatocytes from septic rats consumed significantly less O_2 than did hepatocytes from control rats. By permeabilizing the hepatocytes with the detergent, digitonin, and using substrates which donate electrons at specific sites along the mitochondrial electron transport chain, Kantrow et al. [17] were able to isolate the biochemical lesion induced by sepsis. Their results suggest that Complexes I and IV function normally following the induction of sepsis, whereas O_2

consumption by substrates dependent on Complex II is impaired.

In another study, King et al. sought to determine whether ileal mucosal O_2 consumption is impaired in endotoxemic rats [18]. Rats were injected intravenously with either LPS or a similar volume of saline. A segment of ileum was excised eight hours later, and strips of mucosa were mounted in a polaragraphic apparatus to determine the *ex vivo* rate of O_2 consumption by the tissue. As depicted in Figure 1, the rate of O_2 consumption was significantly lower for mucosal samples from endotoxemic as compared to control rats. Thus, the findings from this study are consistent with the results described above using the MTT assay to assess ileal epithelial mitochondrial function, and support the view that endotoxemia is associated with an acquired defect in gut mucosal respiration that is intrinsic to the cells themselves and not a result of perturbed O_2 delivery. Recently, King et al. extended these earlier findings by showing that injection of rats with LPS also inhibits *ex vivo* O_2 consumption by slices of hepatic tissue (unpublished observations). Thus, LPS-induced defects in the intrinsic capacity of cells to utilize O_2 are observable in at least two different tissues (gut mucosa and hepatic parenchyma). Further studies are needed to determine if this phenomenon is generalized or occurs in a only few specific types of cells.

BIOCHEMICAL MECHANISMS

A number of different, but mutually compatible mechanisms, might foster the development of cytopathic hypoxia under pathological conditions. These mechanisms include: diminished delivery of pyruvate into the mitochondrial TCA cycle; inhibition of key mitochondrial enzymes involved in either the TCA cycle (*cis*-aconitase) or the electron transport chain; activation of the enzyme, poly-(ADP)-ribose polymerase (PARP); or collapse of the protonic gradient across the inner mitochondrial membrane leading to uncoupling of oxidation (of NADH or $FADH_2$) from phosphorylation (of ADP to form ATP).

Inactivation of Pyruvate Dehydrogenase

The end product of glycolysis is pyruvate. This compound can either be reduced to lactate, or enter the mitochondrial TCA cycle to be oxidized to water and carbon dioxide. Pyruvate dehydrogenase (PDH) is the enzyme complex that catalyzes the first irreversible step in the oxidation of pyruvate. PDH catalyzes the conversion of pyruvate, in the presence of NAD^+ and co-enzyme A, into acetyl-CoA. Because of its pivotal role in the regulation of intermediary metabolism, the activity of PDH is tightly regulated via both end-product inhibition and reversible phosphorylation. A group of isoenzymes, the PDH kinase (PDK) family, catalyzes the phosphorylation of PDH to its inactive form (PDH$_i$). A PDH phosphatase catalyzes the dephosphorylation of PDH$_i$ to the active form of the enzyme complex (PDH$_a$). Vary et al. documented that the PHH$_i$:PHA$_a$ ratio in skeletal muscle tissue increases during chronic sepsis in rats [19,20]. The mechanism responsible for this effect is increased PDK activity [21,22]. Because flux through the TCA cycle is inhibited (and because glucose uptake by cells is stimulated), excess pyruvate accumulates in cells, leading to increased production of lactate. Thus, according to the data obtained by Vary's laboratory, hyperlactatemia in sepsis is not evidence of impaired oxygen delivery to cells, but rather the combined effects of PDH inhibition and accelerated glucose transport into cells [20].

Inhibition of Mitochondrial Respiration by Nitric Oxide

Nitric oxide (NO) is an important signaling and effector molecule produced by a wide variety of mammalian cell types [23]. NO is formed from the amino acid, L-arginine in a reaction catalyzed by a family of enzymes called nitric oxide synthase (NOS). Whereas two isoforms of this enzyme (nNOS and eNOS) tend to be constitutively expressed, a third isoform, iNOS, is expressed primarily in cells stimulated by various pro-inflammatory cytokines and/or LPS. Sepsis is associated with increased production of NO as a result of iNOS induction. Increased production of NO seems to be at least partly responsible for impaired cellular respiration in sepsis.

At physiologically relevant concentrations (~1 μM), NO rapidly but reversibly inhibits cytochrome a,a_3 (cytochrome oxidase), the terminal complex of the mitochondrial electron transport chain [24-26]. NO-mediated inhibition of mitochondrial oxygen consumption and ATP generation via this mechanism occurs as result of competition between oxygen and NO for the same binding site on the enzyme complex [27,28]. Thus, the inhibitory effect of NO tends to be more pronounced when PO$_2$ is relatively low [25,26].

Several recent studies emphasize the potential importance of NO, whether as a direct mitochondrial inhibitor or as a precursor for the formation of peroxynitrite (ONOO$^-$) (see below), in the development of cytopathic hypoxia in sepsis. As noted above, Unno et al. showed that injecting rats with LPS inhibited the reduction of MTT by ileal enterocytes, suggesting that endotoxemia leads to impaired mitochondrial function in this cell type [15]. In this same report, Unno et al. also showed that if endotoxemic rats were treated with aminoguanidine (AG), a relatively isoform-selective iNOS inhibitor, then normal mitochondrial function was preserved. Similarly, King et al. showed that treating rats with AG ameliorated the depressed *ex vivo* ileal mucosal oxygen utilization that is induced by injecting rats with LPS (Figure 1). More recently, King et al. have extended these findings by showing that treatment of endotoxemic rats with AG also partially prevented the decrease in *ex vivo* oxygen consumption by hepatic slices (unpublished observations).

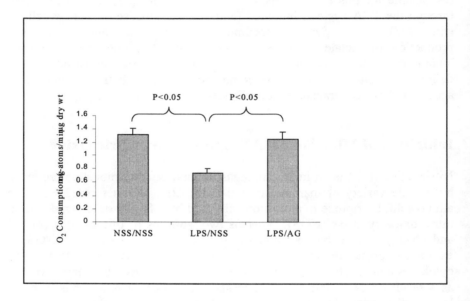

Figure 1. *Effect of LPS on ileal mucosal O_2 consumption. Rats in the NSS/NSS group were injected at $T=0$ h with normal saline (NS) and treated with NS. Rats in the LPS/NSS group were injected with LPS at $T=0$ h and treated with NS. Rats in the LPS/AG group were challenged with LPS and treated with aminoguanidine. Ex vivo O_2 consumption was measured at $T=8$ h. Adapted from [18] with permission*

The Role of Peroxynitrite and Other Oxidants

When NO , which is a free radical, is formed in the presence of another free radical, superoxide (O_2^-), the two compounds react at near diffusion-limited rates to form the potent oxidizing agent, $ONOO^-$. Whereas NO is derived from the partial oxidation of L-arginine, O_2^- is produced as a result of the partial reduction of molecular oxygen. O_2^- is one of the 'reactive oxygen species' (ROS) that are produced by the enzymes xanthine oxidase (XO) and

NADPH oxidase during a variety of acute inflammatory conditions, including sepsis. Increased NO production, secondary to iNOS induction, is also a feature of these conditions. Thus, conditions are ripe during sepsis for the production of ONOO⁻. In addition, as a result of a process called 'electron leakage', small quantities of O_2^- are continually produced by mitochondria at the level of the three enzymatic complexes that interact with co-enzyme Q_{10}. Under certain conditions, such as when cytochrome oxidase is inhibited by NO, mitochondria can generate increased quantities of O_2^- [29]. Moreover, a novel mitochondria-specific NOS isoform, mtNOS, was recently described [30,31]. Thus, within the confines of the organelle itself, mitochondria are capable of generating both NO and O_2 and, hence, under appropriate conditions, large quantities of the potentially toxic moiety, ONOO⁻ [32].

Exogenous ONOO⁻ causes irreversible inhibition of mitochondrial respiration via several mechanisms, including: inhibition of the F_0F_1ATPase [33]; inhibition of complex II [33]; inhibition of complex I [33]; and inhibition of mitochondrial aconitase (the enzyme in the TCA cycle that converts citrate into isocitrate) [34]. Endogenous production of ONOO⁻ secondary to iNOS induction plus O_2^- generation has been implicated as the major factor leading to impaired mitochondrial respiration in some tissues, such as rat diaphragm, following *in vivo* challenge with LPS [35]. Unno et al. have obtained indirect evidence that endogenous production of ONOO⁻ is responsible for ATP depletion in cultured enterocytes incubated with the pro-inflammatory cytokine, IFN-γ [36].

ONOO⁻ and other oxidants (e.g., hydroxyl radical and hydrogen peroxide) are capable of damaging many cellular constituents, including membrane lipids and nuclear DNA. In the latter case, oxidants typically causes single-strand disruptions in the integrity of DNA. Single-strand breaks in nuclear DNA are capable of activating the enzyme, PARP [37,38]. This enzyme catalyzes the cleavage of NAD^+ into ADP-ribose and nicotinamide and the polymerization of the resultant ADP-ribose units into branching poly-ADP-ribose homopolymers [39]. Intense activation of PARP can lead to massive depletion of its substrate, NAD^+/NADH. Since NADH is the main reducing equivalent used to support oxidative phosphorylation, activation of PARP can lead to a marked impairment in aerobic respiration. PARP activation has been implicated as a major factor contributing to the development of cytopathic hypoxia in sepsis. For example, studies in animal models of sepsis or endotoxemia have shown that using pharmacological agents to block PARP can prevent mitochondrial dysfunction in a variety of cell types [40,41] as well as vascular contractile dysfunction [42,43]. Moreover, in comparison to wild-type controls, mice with a genetic defect in the PARP enzyme (i.e., PARP knock-out mice) are relatively resistant to the lethal effects of LPS [44,45].

The importance of oxidant stress as a factor contributing to the development of cytopathic hypoxia was illustrated in a series of *in vitro* experiments carried out by Motterlini et al. [46]. These authors showed that exposing porcine endothelial or vascular smooth muscle cells to LPS significantly decreased oxygen utilization. Pretreatment of the cells with N-acetyl-L-cysteine (NAC), a potent antioxidant, prevented the deleterious effect of LPS exposure on oxygen utilization.

Uncoupling of Oxidative Phosphorylation

The term *mitochondrial uncoupling* implies that the utilization of oxygen (as the final electron acceptor for the oxidation of NADH and $FADH_2$) is not tightly linked to the phosphorylation of ADP to form ATP. Uncoupled respiration is manifested by an increase in the ratio of oxygen consumption under *State 4* conditions (excess substrate, ADP absent) to oxygen consumption under *State 3* conditions (excess substrate, ADP present). In experimental studies, uncoupling of oxidative phosphorylation can be induced by injecting animals or incubating isolated mitochondria with agents, such as dinitrophenol (DNP). These *uncoupling agents* dissipate the electrochemical gradient that normally supports the movement of protons through the $F_0F_1ATPase$ leading to the formation of ATP. Uncoupling of mitochondrial oxidative phosphorylation also can occur under physiological and pathophysiological conditions in the absence of added chemicals like DNP. For example, the tightness of coupling is regulated physiologically by various uncoupling proteins (UCP1, UCP2, and UCP), probably to control thermogenesis and body mass [47,48].

Even more pertinent to the present discussion is a phenomenon called the 'mitochondrial permeability transition' or MPT, which is caused by the opening of a nonspecific pore in the inner mitochondrial membrane. Whereas the inner mitochondrial membrane is normally impermeable to everything except for a few metabolites and ions, opening of the MPT pore permits the diffusion of any molecule with a molecular mass less than about 1500 Da [49]. Thus, opening of the MPT pore dissipates the mitochondrial protonic gradient, leading to the uncoupling of oxidation from phosphorylation. The MPT can be triggered by a number of conditions that might occur in the context of sepsis, including oxidative stress [50-52] and exposure of cells to pro-inflammatory cytokines, such as tumor necrosis factor (TNF) [53].

Data regarding the adequacy of mitochondrial coupling in sepsis or endotoxemia are conflicting. In one early study, Decker et al. evaluated hepatic mitochondrial function in rats with peritonitis caused by *Klebsiella pneumoniae* [54]. Although ATP levels were decreased in samples of liver tissue obtained 18 hours after the induction of sepsis, the function of isolated mitochondria, as assessed by measuring oxygen utilization following addition of appropriate substrates in the presence (*State 3*) or absence (*State 4*) of ADP, was entirely normal. Similar findings were reported by other groups of investigators [55,56]. In contrast, Mela et al. reported that hepatic mitochondrial respiration is uncoupled from ADP phosphorylation in endotoxemic rats [57]. Similarly, Tavakoli and Mela [58] showed that although oxygen utilization by isolated muscle and liver mitochondria from septic rats was normal under *State 3* conditions, oxygen consumption under *State 4* conditions was markedly increased, a finding that suggests a loss of the normal coupling between substrate oxidation and phosphorylation of ADP. Partial uncoupling of oxidative phosphorylation also has been observed in *in vitro* studies, wherein hepatocytes are incubated with LPS and various pro-inflammatory cytokines [59].

CONCLUSION

Several lines of evidence support the notion that cellular energetics are deranged in sepsis, not (just) on the basis of inadequate tissue perfusion, but rather because of impaired mitochondrial respiration and/or coupling. These findings suggest the possibility that organ dysfunction in sepsis may occur on the basis of cytopathic hypoxia. If this concept is correct, then the therapeutic implications are enormous. Efforts to improve outcome in septic patients by monitoring and manipulating cardiac output, systemic oxygen delivery, and regional blood flow would seem unlikely to have a major impact on outcome. Instead, our focus should be on developing pharmacological strategies to restore normal mitochondrial function and cellular energetics.

REFERENCES

1. Fink MP. Cytopathic hypoxia in sepsis. Acta Anaesthesiol Scand 1997 (Suppl 100); 41:87-95
2. Vallet B, Lund N, Curtis SE, et al. Gut and muscle tissue PO_2 in endotoxemic dogs during shock and resuscitation. J Appl Physiol 1994; 76:793-800
3. Hasibeder W, Germann R, Wolf HJ, et al. Effects of short-term endotoxemia and dopamine on mucosal oxygenation in porcine jejunum. Am J Physiol 1996; 270:G667-G675
4. Noldge-Schomberg GF, Priebe HJ, Armbruster K, et al. Different effects of early endotoxemia on hepatic and small intestinal oxygenation in pigs. Intensive Care Med 1996; 22:795-804

5. Sair M, Etherington PJ, Curzen NP, et al. Tissue oxygenation and perfusion in endotoxemia. Am J Physiol 1996; 271:H1620-H1625

6. Astiz M, Rackow EC, Weil MH, et al. Early impairment of oxidative metabolism and energy production in severe sepsis. Circ Shock 1988; 26:311-320

7. Anning PB, Sair M, Winlove CP, et al. Abnormal tissue oxygenation and cardiovascular changes in endotoxemia. Am J Resp Crit Care Med 1999; 159:1710-1715

8. Hotchkiss RS, Rust RS, Dence CS, et al. Evaluation of the role of cellular hypoxia in sepsis by the hypoxic marker [18F]fluoroisonidazole. Am J Physiol 1991; 261:R965-R972

9. VanderMeer TJ, Wang H, Fink MP. Endotoxemia causes ileal mucosal acidosis in the absence of mucosal hypoxia in a normodynamic porcine model of septic shock. Crit Care Med 1995; 23:1217-1226

10. Rosser DM, Stidwill RP, Jacobson D, et al. Oxygen tension in the bladder epithelium rises in both high and low cardiac output endotoxemic sepsis. J Appl Physiol 1995; 79:1878-1882

11. Boekstegers P, Weidenhofer S, Kapsner T, et al. Skeletal muscle partial pressure of oxygen in patients with sepsis. Crit Care Med 1994; 22:640-650

12. Simonson SG, Welty-Wolf K, Huang Y-CT, et al. Altered mitochondrial redox responses in Gram negative septic shock in primates. Circ Shock 1994; 43:34-43

13. Bankey PE, Hill S, Geldon D. Sequential insult enhances liver macrophage-signaled hepatocyte dysfunction. J Surg Res 1994; 57:185-191

14. Zingarelli B, Day BJ, Crapo JD, et al. The potential role of peroxynitrite in the vascular contractile and cellular energetic failure in endotoxic shock. Br J Pharmacol 1997; 120:259-267

15. Unno N, Wang H, Menconi MJ, et al. Inhibition of inducible nitric oxide synthase ameliorates lipopolysaccharide-induced gut mucosal barrier dysfunction in rats. Gastroenterology 1997; 113:1246-1257

16. Gross SS, Levi R. Tetrahydrobiopterin synthesis. An absolute requirement for cytokine-induced nitric oxide generation by vascular smooth muscle. J Biol Chem 1992; 267:25722-25729

17. Premarante S, Masuda E, Nishida S, et al. Does intravenous glutamine prevent bacterial translocation in hemorrhagic shock? Shock 1994; 2:262-266

18. King CJ, Tytgat SHAJ, Delude RL, Fink MP. Ileal mucosal oxygen consumption is decreased in endotoxemic rats but is restored toward normal by treatment with aminoguanidine. Crit Care Med 1999; 27:2518-2524

19. Vary TC, Siegel JH, Nakatani T, et al. Effect of sepsis on activity of pyruvate dehydrogenase complex in skeletal muscle and liver. Am J Physiol 1986; 250:E634-E640

20. Vary TC. Sepsis-induced alterations in pyruvate dehydrogenase complex activity in rat skeletal muscle: effects on plasma lactate. Shock 1996; 6:89-94

21. Vary TC, Hazen S. Sepsis alters pyruvate dehydrogenase kinase activity in skeletal muscle. Mol Cell Biochem 1999; 198:113-118

22. Vary TC. Increased pyruvate dehydrogenase kinase activity in response to sepsis. Am J Physiol 1991; 250:E669-E674

23. Fink MP, Payen D. The role of nitric oxide in sepsis and ARDS: synopsis of a roundtable conference held in Brussels on 18-20 March 1995. Intensive Care Med 1996; 22:158-165

24. Borutaité V, Brown GC. Rapid reduction of nitric oxide by mitochondria, and reversible inhibition of mitochondrial respiration by nitric oxide. Biochem J 1996; 315:295-299

25. Cassina A, Radi R. Differential inhibitory action of nitric oxide and peroxynitrite on mitochondrial electron transport. Arch Biochem Biophys 1996; 328:309-316

26. Nishikawa M, Sato EF, Kuroki T, Inoue M. Role of glutathione and nitric oxide in the energy metabolism of rat liver mitochondria. FEBS Lett 1997; 415:341-345

27. Torres J, Darley-Usmer V, Wilson MT. Inhibition of cytochrome c oxidase in turnover by nitric oxide: mechanism and implications for control of respiration. Biochem J 1995; 312:169-173

28. Giuffre A, Sarti P, D'Itri E, et al. On the mechanism of inhibition of cytochrome c oxidase by nitric oxide. J Biol Chem 2000; 271:33404-33408

29. Poderoso JJ, Carreras MC, Lisdero C, et al. Nitric oxide inhibits electron transfer and increases superoxide radical production in rat heart mitochondria and submitochondrial particles. Arch Biochem Biophys 1996; 328:85-92

30. Ghafourifar P, Richter C. Nitric oxide synthase activity in mitochondria. FEBS Lett 1997; 418:291-296

31. Ghafourifar P, Schenk U, Klein SD, et al. Mitochondrial nitric-oxide synthase stimulation causes cytochrome c release from isolated mitochondria. Evidence for intramitochondrial peroxynitrite formation. J Biol Chem 1999; 27:31185-31188

32. Packer MA, Porteous CM, Murphy MP. Superoxide production by mitochondria in the presence of nitric oxide forms peroxynitrite. Biochem Mol Biol Int 1996;40:527-534

33. Radi R, Rodriguez M, Castro L, et al. Inhibition of mitochondrial electron transport by peroxynitrite. Arch Biochem Biophys 1994; 308:96-102

34. Castro L, Rodriguez M, Radi R. Aconitase is readily inactivated by peroxynitrite, but not its precursor, nitric oxide. J Biol Chem 1994; 269:29409-29415

35. Boczkowski J, Lisdero C, Lanone S, et al. Endogenous peroxynitrite mediates mitochondrial dysfunction in rat diaphragm during endotoxemia. FASEB J 1999; 13:1637-1646

36. Unno N, Menconi MJ, Smith M, et al. Acidic conditions ameliorate both ATP depletion and the development of hyperpermeability in cultured Caco-2 enterocytic monolayers subjected to metabolic inhibition. Surgery 1997; 121:668-680

37. Durkacz BW, Omidiji O, Gray DA, et al. (ADP-ribose)n participates in DNA excision repair. Nature 1980; 283:593-596

38. Saitoh MS, Poirier GG, Lindahl T. Dual function for poly(ADP-ribose) synthesis in response to DNA strand breakage. Biochemistry 1994; 33:7099-7106

39. Lautier D, Lageux J, Thibodeau J, et al. Molecular and biochemical features of poly (ADP-ribose) metabolism. Mol Cell Biochem 1993; 122:171-193

40. Szabó C, Zingarelli B, Salzman AL. Role of poly-ADP ribosyltransferase activation in the vascular contractile and energetic failure elicited by exogenous and endogenous nitric oxide and peroxynitrite. Circ Res 1996; 78:1051-1063

41. Szabo C, Cuzzocrea S, Zingarelli B, et al. Endothelial dysfunction in a rat model of endotoxic shock. Importance of the activation of poly (ADP-ribose) synthetase by peroxynitrite. J Clin Invest 1997; 100:723-735

42. Pulido EJ, Shames BD, Selzman CH, et al. Inhibition of PARS attenuates endotoxin-induced dysfunction of pulmonary vasorelaxation. Am J Physiol 1999; 277:L769-L776

43. Szabo A, Salzman AL, Szabo C. Poly (ADP-ribose) synthetase activation mediates pulmonary microvascular and intestinal mucosal dysfunction in endotoxin shock. Life Sci 1998; 63:2133-2139

44. Kuhnle S, Nicotera P, Wendel A, et al. Prevention of endotoxin-induced lethality, but not of liver apoptosis in poly(ADP-ribose) polymerase-deficient mice. Biochem Biophys Res Comm 1999; 263:433-438

45. Oliver FJ, Menissier-de Murcia J, Nacci C, et al. Resistance to endotoxic shock as a consequence of defective NF-kappaB activation in poly (ADP-ribose) polymerase-1 deficient mice. EMBO J 1999; 18:4446-54

46. Motterlini R, Kerger H, Green CJ, et al. Depression of endothelial and smooth muscle cell oxygen consumption by endotoxin. Am J Physiol 1998; 275:H776-H782

47. Stuart JA, Brindle KM, Harper JA, et al. Mitochondrial proton leak and the uncoupling proteins. J Bioenerg Biomembr 1999; 31:517-525

48. Ricquier D, Bouillaud F. The uncoupling protein homologues: UCP1, UCP2, UCP3, StUCP and AtUCP. Biochem J 2000; 345:161-179

49. Zoratti M, Szabo I. The mitochondrial permeability transition. Bioch Biophys Acta 1995; 1241:139-176

50. Connern CP, Halestrap AP. Recruitment of mitochondrial cyclophilin to the mitochondrial inner membrane under conditions of oxidative stress that enhance the opening of a calcium-sensitive non-specific channel. Biochem J 1994; 302:321-324

51. Griffiths EJ, Halestrap AP. Mitochondrial non-specific pores remain closed during cardiac ischaemia, but open upon reperfusion. Biochem J 1995; 307:93-98

52. Nieminen AL, Saylor AK, Tesfai SA, et al. Contribution of the mitochondrial permeability transition to lethal injury after exposure of hepatocytes to t-butylhydroperoxide. Biochem J 1995; 307:99-106

53. Bradham CA, Qian T, Streetz K, et al. The mitochondrial permeability transition is required for tumor necrosis factor alpha-mediated apoptosis and cytochrome c release. Mol Cell Biochem 1998; 18:6353-6364

54. Greer GG, Milazzo FH. *Pseudomonas aeruginosa* lipopolysaccharide: an uncouple of mitochondrial oxidative phosphorylation. Can J Microbiol 1975; 21:877-883

55. Geller ER, Jankauskas S, Kirkpatrick J. Mitochondrial death in sepsis: a failed concept. J Surg Res 1986; 40:514-517

56. Fry DE, Silva BB, Rink RD, et al. Hepatic cellular hypoxia in murine peritonitis. Surgery 1979; 85:652-661

57. Mela L, Bacalco LV, Jr., Miller LD. Defective oxidative metabolism of rat liver mitochondria in hemorrhagic and endotoxin shock. Am J Physiol 1971; 220:571-577

58. Tavakoli H, Mela L. Alterations of mitochondrial metabolism and protein concentrations in subacute septicemia. Infect Immun 1982; 38:536-541

59. Stadler J, Billiar TR, Curran RD, et al. Effect of exogenous and endogenous nitric oxide on mitochondrial respiration in rat hepatocytes. Am J Physiol 1991; 260:C910-C916

16

INVASIVE HEMODYNAMIC MONITORING

Egbert Huettemann
Samir G. Sakka
Konrad Reinhart

The complex array of cardiovascular abnormalities encountered in sepsis and septic shock are – often in combination - hypovolemia, peripheral arterial vasodilatation, myocardial dysfunction (depressed cardiac systolic and diastolic function, pulmonary hypertension, right ventricular dysfunction) and alterations in regional blood flow distribution leading to an abnormal tissue perfusion.

These hemodynamic alterations provide the rationale for an advanced hemodynamic monitoring in patients with sepsis and septic shock. Moreover, the cardiovascular system is an important determinant of outcome [1]. Hemodynamic monitoring in septic patients has to address diagnostic, therapeutic and prognostic issues. It should always be tailored according to the individual patient, taking into account sepsis-induced organ dysfunctions as well as cardiovascular comorbidities. Cardiovascular abnormalities and the corresponding hemodynamic parameters that an 'ideal' monitoring in patients with septic shock could assess are depicted in Figure 1.

Nowadays several devices for advanced hemodynamic monitoring are commercially available: the pulmonary artery catheter (PAC), systems based on the double indicator dilution technique, and (transesophageal) echocardiography. The array of hemodynamic parameters obtainable by invasive hemodynamic monitoring includes the arterial blood pressure, systolic pressure variation (SPV) (arterial line), central venous pressure (CVP), pulmonary artery pressure (PAP), pulmonary artery occlusion pressure (PAOP), right ventricular end-systolic and end-diastolic volumes

(RVESV and RVEDV) and ejection fraction (RVEF), cardiac output (CO) (pulmonary artery catheter); intrathoracic blood volume (ITBV), extravascular lung water (EVLW), cardiac output (double indicator dilution technique), and left and right heart volumes, systolic and diastolic function, wall motion abnormalities, valvular function, cardiac output and systolic pulmonary artery pressure (echocardiography) (Table 1).

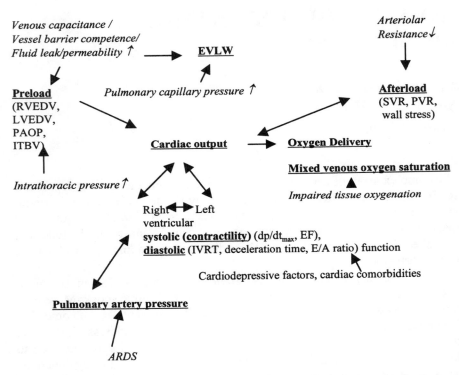

dp/dt$_{max}$ maximal pressure acceleration velocity; EF ejection fraction; IVRT isovolumetric relaxation time; E/A ratio Early filling phase / atrial filling phase velocity gradient; EVLW Extravascular lung water; RVEDV Right ventricular end-diastolic volume; LVEDV Left ventricular end-diastolic volume; PAOP pulmonary artery occlusion pressure; ITBV intrathoracic blood volume;SVR/PVR systemic/pulmonary vascular resistance

Figure 1. Hemodynamic parameters (__underlined__) that an 'ideal' monitoring in patients with septic shock would allow to assess. Pathophysiological factors affecting these parameters are set in italics.

	Arterial line	PAC	Double indicator dilution technique (COLD® /PICCO)	Echocardiography
Parameters	MAP SPV (ventilated patients)	CVP PAOP PAP SVR PVR LVSW RVSW RVEDV RVEF CO / CCO SvO_2	ITBV EVLW CO SVR LVSW CFI PDR	LV- and RV-Volumes LV- and RV- systolic function (EF) Diastolic function (relaxation, compliance) CO Wall stress Regional wall motion abnormalies Valvular function PAP_{syst}.
Advantage	Superior preload assessment compared to filling pressures	Continuous (CCO, SvO2, RVEDV) hemodynamic monitoring PAP (pulmonary hypertension) Pacing capabilities	Continuous hemodynamic monitoring (CO) ITBV better preload parameter than filling pressures EVLW may aid management of ARDS	Bedside, comprehensive evaluation of cardiac function (see above), Inexpensive (TTE)
Disadvantage	SPV only applicable to ventilated patients No information on cardiac performance and output (*exception*: pulse contour analysis)	Invasive Filling Pressures (CVP, PAOP) are poor preload parameters Beneficial effect on clinical outcome not documented	Invasive None information on PAP Beneficial effect on clinical outcome not documented	Technically limited images in majority of patients (TTE) Semi-invavise (TEE) Repeated studies longer than several hours are impractical Requires training
Evidence based medicine: Beneficial effect on outcome uncertain!				

Table 1. Invasive hemodynamic monitoring: Commercially available devices and their advantages and disadevantages

ARTERIAL BLOOD PRESSURE

One of the most prominent changes in cardiovascular function encountered in sepsis is a decrease in systemic vascular resistance (SVR) leading to a low blood pressure. The direct continuous measurement of arterial blood pressure by an arterial line, commonly inserted into the radial, femoral or axillary artery, constitutes an essential part of the hemodynamic monitoring of septic shock. Invasively monitored pressures may differ considerably from pressures recorded with a sphygmomanometer [2]. In severe hyperdynamic shock, intraarterial blood pressure may be lower than the cuff pressure due to an increased pulse wave reflection following inflation of the cuff [3]. Under these conditions, the former technique may then better approximate the true arterial blood pressure than the latter [4].

Although blood pressure *per se* does not provide information on cardiac output or cardiac preload of septic patients, changes in the arterial pressure waveform during mechanical ventilation are a very useful tool for preload assessment as has been shown recently. The SPV, i.e., the difference between the maximal and minimal values of the systolic blood pressure (SBP) during a mechanical breath [5], has been shown to be a sensitive indicator of preload experimentally and clinically. In normotensive anesthetized patients, the SPV, which is approximately 8-10 mm Hg, is normally composed of two different segments. The delta down component (Δdown) a decrease of approximately 5-6 mm Hg in the SBP relative to the SBP during a short apnea, reflects the normally occurring transient inspiratory decrease in venous return. The delta up component (Δup), an early inspiratory augmentation in the SBP of approximately 2-4 mm Hg reflects the augmentation of the stroke volume mainly due to an increase in left ventricular preload. Although the SPV cannot be interpreted in the presence of irregular arrhythmias or spontaneous breathing, it has been shown very recently in septic patients, that SPV is a useful parameter for a wide range of systemic vascular resistances and drug therapy to assess the volume status and, even more important, to predict the response to volume loading [6]. While the PAOP was of little value for predicting fluid responsiveness, a SPV value of > 10 mm Hg or a Δdown value of > 5 mm Hg were associated with a high rate of responders (increase in stroke volume 15 %) to volume expansion. It should be noted, however, that the meaning of a given SPV value might vary considerably depending on the height of the systolic pressure. Thus, the percentage of variation (SPV expressed as percentage of systolic blood pressure) rather than the absolute value in mm Hg might be more informative. A different approach for the assessment of fluid responsiveness, that has been proposed very recently, is the analysis of the respiratory changes in pulse pressure in mechanically ventilated patients. The respiratory changes in pulse pressure (ΔPP) (systolic BP – diastolic BP) were calculated as the difference between the maximal (PPmax) and the minimal (PPmin) value of pulse pressure over a single respiratory cycle, divided by the average of the two values, and expressed as a percentage:

$$\Delta PP\ (\%) = (PPmax - PPmin) / [(PPmax + PPmin) / 2] \times 100$$

In 17 ventilated patients with septic shock, a very close relationsship ($r^2=0.87$) between ΔPP before volume expansion and the percent increase in cardiac index (CI) in response to volume expansion was demonstrated [7]. In this study, the relationship between the respiratory changes in systolic pressure (calculated as ΔPP) before volume expansion and the increase in CI was weaker ($r^2= 0.66$), suggesting that ΔPP may be a better indicator of fluid responsiveness than SPV. A ΔPP value of < 15 % predicted an increase in cardiac index < 15 % with a sensitivity and a specificity of 100 %. These studies suggest that the calculation of SPV or ΔPP are the easiest and the best means to predict fluid responsiveness in mechanically ventilated patients with hypotension related to sepsis. In summary, the presence of large respiratory changes in PP, reflecting a biventricular preload-dependence, would indicate volume expansion dependency of cardiac output. On the other hand, the absence of respiratory changes in PP, indicating that at least one ventricle is preload independent, would mean that cardiac output cannot be expected to increase with fluid administration. Such a constellation might occur in sepsis-induced right ventricular dysfunction, when LV preload might be assumed to be low by PAOP and RV dilatation causing preload-independence offsets any hemodynamically beneficial effect of volume expansion.

THE PULMONARY ARTERY CATHETER (PAC)

The development of the PAC as a diagnostic tool largely contributed to the understanding of the pathophysiology of septic shock and myocardial dysfunction in septic shock. In the clinical setting, the PAC has been and is still widely used to define hemodynamic profiles in critically ill patients, especially those with septic shock. A large number of studies have documented the inability of even experienced critical care physicians to predict hemodynamic parameters accurately in a significant proportion of critically ill patients [8]. Furthermore, studies further demonstrate that the therapeutic plan is frequently changed based on the information obtained from a PAC. However, the question still remains whether the changes in therapy that are made based on hemodynamic measurements do actually influence patient outcome.

The following hemodynamic variables, that can be measured by the PAC and may be relevant to the management of septic patients, will be discussed in this chapter: CVP, PAP, PAOP, cardiac output, systemic vascular resistance (SVR), pulmonary vascular resistance (PVR), left ventricular stroke work (LVSW), right ventricular stroke work (RVSW).

Central Venous Pressure (CVP)

The CVP, a pressure related estimate of RVEDV, is the most commonly used parameter for the assessment of preload in the critical care setting. The relative ease by which this parameter is available is counter-balanced by the general limitation that pressures do not necessarily correlate with volumes. CVP is modulated by venous capacity (i.e., venous return, intravascular volume, vascular tone) and right heart function. In the normal heart the left ventricular filling pressure (i.e., end-diastolic pressure) is usually only a few mm Hg higher than the right ventricular filling pressure, so that CVP may indeed reflect cardiac preload. In the setting of sepsis, however, changes in CVP do not predict changes in PAOP [9]. Furthermore, no correlation between right atrial pressure and RVEDV was found in patients with septic shock [10]. In these patients, CVP did not allow differentiation of diminished from normal RVEF [10]. Moreover, CVP is of no predictive value regarding survival [11]. In summary, in the presence of septic shock, sepsis induced pulmonary hypertension, or biventricular dysfunction, CVP may not accurately reflect RVEDV, and left ventricular filling pressures or changes thereof.

Pulmonary Artery Pressure (PAP)

The PAP is related directly to pulmonary blood flow and inversely to PVR. In sepsis, PAP is often mildly elevated reflecting an increase in cardiac output and/or in PVR. In patients with a sepsis-related acute respiratory distress syndrome (ARDS), PAP may provide additional information and aid patient management. While there are conflicting data on the predictive value of pulmonary hypertension *per se* in septic patients [11-14], increased PVR, as evidenced by an abnormal PAP_{diast} (diastolic PAP)-PAOP gradient, has been shown to be associated with an increased mortality [13].

Pulmonary Capillary Pressure (P_{cap})

The PAOP is often used as a substitute for the intravascular hydrostatic pressure, one determinant of fluid leakage from the pulmonary capillaries. This applies only to individuals with normal cariac output and PVR and in whom the driving pressure (PAP − PAOP) across the pulmonary bed is small and P_{cap} will only be a few mm Hg above PAOP. However, in septic patients (as in all inflammatory disorders) a significant gradient between pulmonary capillary pressure and PAOP may be present, so that the PAOP will underestimate the tendency for pulmonary edema [15]. The relationship between P_{cap} and PAOP, actually being a rather complex function of cardiac output, PAP, PAOP, precapillary arterial resistance (R_a), postcapillary venous resistance (R_v) and total PVR, has been expressed by the Gaar equation [16]:

$$P_{cap} = PAOP + 0.4 (PAP-PAOP)$$

This equation is based upon the observation that, on average, 60 % of total PVR is due to R_a and 40 % is due to R_v [16,17]. However, cytokines, histamine, serotonin, vasopressors and endotoxin may change the distribution of PVR into its R_a and R_v components, resulting in increased resistance within the pulmonary venous bed between the capillaries and the left atrium. Thus, in these situations, P_{cap} is not accurately predicted by the Gaar equation [18].

In patients with sepsis versus congestive heart failure, a significant difference in the P_{cap} / PAOP gradient, 4.4 ± 4.4 vs. 1.0 ± 1.1 mm Hg (mean ± SD, respectively), was demonstrated [19]. It is impossible to directly measure pulmonary capillary hydrostatic pressure in the intact lung and, therefore, only indirect measurements are clinically possible. For bedside measurement, identification of the rapid and slow component of the capillary occlusion wedge tracing by superimposing an unwedged tracing on a wedge tracing has been proposed [20]. However, this approach is limited by a certain degree of subjectivity and the presence of artifacts in about 70% of pressure waveforms. In summary, believing, mistakenly, the PAOP to be equivalent to the pressure responsible for pulmonary capillary filtration in septic patients, raises a potential for inaccurate therapeutic interventions eventually leading to further deterioration of cardiovascular function and oxygen transport.

Pulmonary Artery Occlusion Pressure (PAOP)

Before the advent of new monitoring techniques like transpulmonary indicator dilution and echocardiography (see below) allowing bedside measurement of volume related preload parameters like intrathoracic blood volume (ITBV) and end-diastolic area (EDA), preload assessment relied solely on pressure related preload variables like CVP and PAOP. Pressure related indices like the PAOP, formerly regarded as a 'gold standard' as an indirect indicator of left ventricular end-diastolic pressure and volume, has been challenged by volume related preload indices. The physiologic correlate of ventricular preload is the end-diastolic stretch of the muscle fiber which, in the intact ventricle, is reflected by the end-diastolic volume. Although initial fiber length and end-diastolic pressure or PAOP are usually related, the relation may vary considerably because of changes in ventricular compliance or changes within the pericardium or thorax. The relationship between end-diastolic pressure and volume is curvilinear and, particularly in septic patients, subject to profound changes. Multiple studies have shown the LV pressure-volume relationsship to be abnormal in septic patients [21,22]. Furthermore, patients presenting with cardiac comorbidities (coronary heart disease, LV hypertrophy) and ventilation with positive end-expiratory pressure (PEEP) are very likely to have abnormal compliance. Moreover, RV failure and a leftward septal shift, which may be enountered in patients with sepsis, ARDS and pulmonary hypertension, may invalidate PAOP as measure of LV preload. Other pitfalls of PAOP as an indicator of preload include mitral valve disease, and aortic regurgitation.

LV end-diastolic pressure may exceed LV transmural pressure in the setting of increased pericardial or intrathoracic pressure [23]. However, most studies studying hemodynamics in septic patients use PAOP and not transmural pressures.

In the setting of sepsis, particularly if associated with sepsis related ARDS, the correct placement of the PAC within West's functional zone 3 is a prerequisite for an accurate recording of the PAOP, if pressures measured are not to be affected by alveolar pressures. Positive pressure ventilation and PEEP may increase West zone 1 and 2 of the lung at the expense of West zone 3 areas rendering a correct placement of the PAC more difficult. In ARDS, which is characterized by heterogenous disease, the region of the pulmonary vascular tree sampled by the PAC may not reflect the average pressures in the lungs.

There are several sources of error in recording the PAOP: One relates to the pressure monitoring system (improper calibration, balancing, or transducer positioning). Another is based on breathing or ventilation induced related changes in intrathoracic pressure and the presence of PEEP. The latter necessitates pressure measurements at end-expiration. In order to ensure correct recording and reading of the PAOP some criteria have been suggested: A tracing consistent with an atrial waveform, a mean PAOP substantially lower than mean PAP, and the ability to aspirate blood through the catheter tip. Ideally the PAOP should be obtained from a hard copy 'strip' or a frozen screen recorded at end-expiration. Digital estimates (by monitoring devices) may be highly erroneous.

In summary, in septic patients, absolute values (and changes) of PAOP may not accurately predict LVEDV or changes thereof due to differences (and changes) in LV distensibility [9,24]. In patients with RV dysfunction, fluid infusion may even lead to a decrease in LVEDV accompanied by an rise in PAOP [9]. Thus solely relying on filling pressures (with administration of volume) can be misleading and may result in incorrect therapeutic decisions.

One option to overcome - at least in part - these shortcomings of PAOP, are graded fluid challenges with repeated measurements of PAOP and cardiac output yielding a LV function curve thus enabling optimization of ventricular preload. Since changes in myocardial compliance have to be expected following changes in catecholamine treatment or respirator settings, this would necessitate the determination of new ventricular function curves after each adjustment of therapy in order to determine the PAOP associated with the highest cardiac output. However, this procedure is time consuming and may result in unnecessary and possibly harmful fluid loading. When guiding hemodynamic management on PAOP one should be aware that patients with septic shock may have a greatly diminished response of fluid administration. In critically ill septic patients, a marked rightward and downward shift of their Frank-Starling ventricular performance relationship was found while critically ill non-septic controls and septic patients without shock demonstrated normal responses to fluid administration with parallel increases in LVEDVI and LVSWI [25]. Due to normal fluctuations in PAP and PAOP (up to 4 mm Hg in 60 % of patients) only changes of PAOP of 3 mm Hg or more should be considered clinically meaningful [26].

Due to the limitations of the PAOP discussed above, the focus in the clinical setting should not be to achieve a given PAOP *per se*, but rather to assess how PAOP correlates with clinically meaningful parameters such as cardiac output, urine output and gas exchange.

In a study on patients with hypovolemic and septic shock, Packhan and Rackow titrated PAOP to maximize cardiac output and found values of 12 to 16 mm Hg to be optimal [27]. Most authors recommend initially achieving a PAOP of 12 mm Hg and then noting the effect of further increases in PAOP on cardiac index (CI). Especially in patients with cardiac disease an even higher PAOP (16 – 20 mm Hg) may be necessary. In such instances an echocardiographic assessment of left and right ventricular function is strongly advocated before further fluid administration.

Right Ventricular Function

The rationale for the monitoring of RV function in patients with septic shock are pulmonary hypertension and increased RV afterload, which, particularly in presence of arterial hypotension and low right coronary perfusion pressure, may adversely affect RV function. RV dysfunction and distension may in turn adversely affect LV preload, distensibility and function through septal displacement, pericardial restraint and encroachment upon the LV. Although RV dysfunction does not necessarily cause a low cardiac output, it constitutes one reason for volume-unresponsiveness in septic patients (no rise in cardiac output during volume loading).

Reduced RVEF has been demonstrated using radionuclide techniques in 52 % of patients with septic shock [10,22]. There was no correlation between RVEF and mean PAP, suggesting that primary myocardial depression or dilation, but not an increased afterload, is the causative mechanism.

Modified PAC equipped with a fast-response thermistor allows measurement of RVEF and RVEDV. The values obtained from these PAC correlate well with those obtained from radionuclide and angiographic studies [28,29]. Volumetric PACs have been assessed ino septic patients. In a study of 56 patients with sepsis, RVEF was found to decrease at the onset of shock and to improve with recovery from shock [28]. Compared to MAP, mean PAP and cardiac output, RVEF proved to the best predictor of survival. Thus, RVEF may be of prognostic value. When compared to trauma patients, hemodynamic profiles of patients with sepsis were similar to those with trauma with the exception that septic patients demonstrated greater RVEDV and lower RVEF [30]. In an investigation in 13 surgical patients with sepsis, the additional information derived from RVEDV did not alter the PAOP guided management in 43 of 46 instances with the exception of patients with increased intra-abdominal pressure [31].

New catheters allowing continuous cardiac output and RVEDV measurement have recently been introduced into clinical practice and are currently being evaluated.

Cardiac Output

The measurement of cardiac output is most commonly performed by the thermodilution technique [32], either pulmonary (PAC) or aortic (PiCCO®/COLD®). It is based on the dye indicator principle with cold solution as the indicator. Thermodilution cardiac output measurements are still regarded as gold standard. Modified PACs allow continuous measurement of cardiac output. Acceptable determinations should vary by 10 % or less for repeated measurements. Measurements in patients with tricuspid regurgitation originating from pulmonary hypertension or septic cardiomyopathy may yield variable underestimation of cardiac output of up to 15 % [33]. Further sources of error are cardiac shunting (patent foramen ovale, etc.). As to the issue of the optimal signal-to-noise ratio the use of room temperature indicator solutions is usually adequate in septic patients [34]. Given the reduced SVR of septic patients, 'normal' cardiac output values nevertheless indicate a diminished cardiac performance. Because of the inverse relationship of SVR and cardiac output, a sufficient compensation of the decreased SVR in septic shock would require an increase in cardiac output by 100 – 200 %, which is rarely seen, constituting further indirect evidence of myocardial dysfunction.

Derived Parameters (SV, SVR, PVR, LVSWI, RVSWI, DO₂, VO₂)

Based on the measurements of pressures and cardiac output, monitoring with a PAC allows calculation of several hemodynamic indices (stroke volume; RVSWI, LVSWI, SVR, PVR, shunt fraction; oxygen delivery [DO_2] and consumption [VO_2]). Mixed venous oxygen saturation (SvO_2) is discussed in a separate chapter.

Afterload-related Indices

When assessing ventricular afterload by SVR and PVR in the clinical setting, one should keep in mind that they are only approximates of LV and RV afterload. SVR has been shown to be an unreliable index of LV afterload [35]. This is explained by the fact that calculation of SVR and PVR as estimates of afterload is based on the simplifying assumption of a constant pressure and flow in the circulation (SVR = MAP-CVP/cardiac output and

PVR = PAPm-PAOP/cardiac output respectively). Actually, blood is pumped into the circulation by the heart in a pulsatile manner. Physiologically, afterload is defined as the force opposing ventricular fiber shortening during contraction or the impedance to ejection. Although it is influenced to a high degree by the arterial pressure, it is not synonymous with peripheral arterial pressure, peripheral vascular tone or SVR. Instead, afterload is determined by peripheral loading conditions as reflected by the SVR as well as intrinsic cardiac properties such as ventricular dimensions and wall thickness. (End-systolic)-wall stress ($\sigma = 1.35 \times P \times ESD/4$ h (1 + h / ESD, where P is LV end-systolic pressure; ESD is LV end-systolic diameter, and h end-systolic LV wall thickness), which can be measured by echocardiography, reflects all these factors and is a better index of afterload than SVR alone. Laplace's law states that LV wall stress is directly proportional to chamber radius and pressure and inversely proportional to wall thickness. While SVR is a function of cardiac output and arterial pressure, afterload is a function of ventricular size and arterial pressure. This explains why in a septic patient wall stress may be elevated due to a dilated ventricle while SVR may be significantly reduced. This differentiation is important, since afterload, besides the heart rate (often increased in septic patients) and contractile state, is a major determinant of myocardial oxygen consumption.

Stroke Work Indices

Stroke work is a parameter of ventricular performance representing the amount of work the ventricle performs during ejection [36]. Physiologically speaking it represents the area under the curve of the pressure volume ventricular function curve. A simplified formula applied in the clinical setting calculates LVSW from the mean arterial pressure and stroke volume. LVSW is a parameter of LV systolic function. It may underestimate true LV systolic function in the presence of hypotension for its mathematical coupling to the arterial blood pressure.

Oxygen Transport-Related Indices

Based on the knowledge of cardiac output and SvO_2 obtained by pulmonary artery catheterization, DO_2 (cardiac output x arterial oxygen content) and VO_2 (DO_2 − (cardiac output x mixed venous oxygen content) can be calculated. The issues pertaining to oxygen transport and the relationship between DO_2 and VO_2 are comprehensively covered in another chapter.

Infectious Complications

PAC use is associated with potential life-threatening iatrogenic complications of which the most frequent life-threatening complication is bloodstream infection with a median incidence of 1.1% or a median of 3.0 bloodstream infections per 1000 catheter days [37,38], carrying an attributable mortality of 14 to 28 % [39]. Most prospective studies of PAC have shown an association of the risk of infection with the duration of catheterization. The actuarial risk of PAC related bloodstream infection is very low during the first four days, but rises sharply thereafter [39]. In two prospective studies of central venous catheterization and PAC, no difference in the incidence of catheter colonization and bloodstream infection was found between patients with regular scheduled replacement at 3 days [40] or 7 days [41] versus no routine replacement. Exchange of PA catheters over a guide wire placed at an old site increased the incidence of catheter related bloodstream infection by nearly twofold [40]. Difficult catheter insertion requiring three or more punctures has been associated with a 15-fold increased risk of central venous and PA catheter infection [39].

TRANSPULMONARY INDICATOR DILUTION TECHNIQUE

The first transpulmonary indicator dilution technique clinically introduced was the double indicator dilution approach which is based on the use of two indicators with different properties. The thermo-dye dilution is the approach most commonly used, in which a freely diffusible indicator ('cold') and a plasma-bound indicator (indocyanine green, ICG) are injected simultaneously into the central circulation. In contrast to the cold, ICG remains in the intravascular space and does not equilibrate with the interstitium. Since ICG strictly remains in the intravascular space it allows measurement of the ITBV, which is the distribution volume between the right atrial injection and aortic (i.e., transpulmonary) detection site. In addition to the ITBV, the aortic thermodilution curve allows the calculation of the distribution volume of the cold and by the difference between the two distribution volumes of the two indicators, extravascular lung water (EVLW) can be calculated (Figure 2). While ITBV can be used as myocardial preload variable, EVLW may be useful for an early and accurate assessment of pulmonary edema. Since the double indicator dilution technique is relatively time consuming and expensive due to the need for a fiberoptic catheter, single transpulmonary thermodilution has been evaluated. Sufficient accuracy of this approach for the estimation of ITBV and EVLW has been shown in animal experiments [42] and clinical studies [43]. The accuracy of cardiac output by the analysis of the aortic thermodilution curve has been demonstrated in experimental and clinical studies [44-51] as long as the amount of indicator is appropriately high.

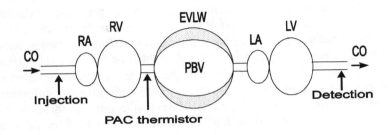

Figure 2. *The transpulmonary indicator dilution technique. RA= Right atrium, RV= right ventricle, PBV= Pulmonary blood volume, LA= Left atrium, LV= Left ventricle, ITBV= Intrathoracic blood volume, EVLW= Extravascular lung water, CO= Cardiac output, PAC= Pulmonary artery catheter. The grey shaded area represents EVLW.*

In contrast to the monitoring of pressures, the transpulmonary thermo-dye dilution technique allows direct measurement of circulatory blood volumes. In particular, ITBV is considered as an indicator of myocardial preload which is less influenced by changes in intrathoracic pressures and myocardial compliance. Animal experimental data showed that ITBV is a better indicator of myocardial preload than the RVEDV, as assessed by a fast response thermistor tipped PAC [52]. In this study, influences of changes in cardiac output on measurement of ITBV and mathematical coupling between cardiac output and ITBV could be excluded. In a clinical study, ITBV was found to correlate well with other clinical tools of preload assessment, i.e., SPV [53].

Recently, ITBV has been shown to be a more reliable indicator of myocardial preload than the cardiac filling pressures in various clinical settings. A study on the effects of varying levels of PEEP on preload parameters in patients with acute respiratory failure found that only changes in ITBV correlated well with changes in CI ($r= 0.71$) while the filling pressures did not (CVP: $r= 0.069$; PAOP: $r= 0.018$), respectively [54]. Similar results were published by Borelli who studied lung injury patients undergoing different ventilation modes [55]. In the early postoperative setting of patients after coronary revascularization, i.e., when myocardial compliance is typically changing, only ITBV ($r= 0.74$), but not the cardiac filling pressures, correlated with stroke volume index [56]. In critically ill patients, Hoeft [57] confirmed that ITBV is a better indicator of myocardial preload than the cardiac filling pressures. While changes in ITBV correlated with changes in stroke volume index according to the underlying Frank-Starling mechanism, no such correlation was observed for changes in PAOP. These findings suggest that factors other than central filling, such as the compliance of the central circulation, mean airway pressure and functional residual capacity, particularly in ventilated patients, have a major impact on the central pressure readings.

In principle, these studies determined the value of each preload variable in a controlled way and studied the influence of one factor while keeping the others unchanged. Consequently, a new Frank-Starling curve would be needed each time that intrathoracic pressure or myocardial compliance changes, for example following changes in respirator adjustments or catecholamine treatment. Thus, individual Frank-Starling curves would be necessary in short time intervals, which is time consuming and unrealistic in the clinical setting of hemodynamic stabilisation of critically ill patients.

In patients with sepsis or septic shock, we compared each preload variable in the early phase of hemodynamic stabilization during which respirator adjustments and catecholamine treatment were changed according to the clinical course [58]. In the analysis of the first hemodynamic profiles after admission to the ICU, changes in ITBV correlated best with changes in stroke volume index when compared with PAOP or CVP (Figure 3). These findings may be in part explainded by changes in dosages of vasoactive drug and/ or respirator adjustments, especially since correct determination of transmural cardiac filling pressures by PAOP may be difficult in ventilated patients with large respiratory excursions in intrathoracic pressure [59]. In summary, clinical studies in critically ill patients including patients with sepsis demonstrated that ITBV may be a more reliable indicator of myocardial preload than the cardiac filling pressures in critically ill patients with mechanical ventilation.

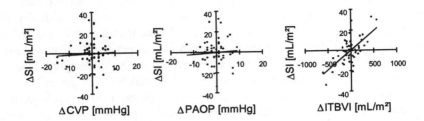

Figure 3. *Correlation between changes in central venous pressure (CVP), pulmonary artery occlusion pressure (PAOP) or intrathoracic blood volume (ITBV) and changes in stroke index (SI) in 57 critically ill patients with sepsis or septic shock. (From [57], with permission).*

Measurement of EVLW by the transpulmonary thermo-dye dilution technique has been shown to reflect EVLW when compared to gravimetry [47,60]. Especially in non-cardiac pulmonary edema, i.e., ARDS, measurement of EVLW has been found to be more reliable than chest X-ray [61] or estimation from PAOP as surrogate for hydrostatic capillary pressure [62]. PEEP and low tidal volumes have been shown to be helpful in reducing EVLW when permeability is increased [63]. ELVW has been shown to be valuable when deciding on the type of mechanical ventilation, i.e. controlled vs. pressure support [64]. Increased EVLW is strongly related to mortality and outcome may be improved by a strategy to lower EVLW [65] or limit hypervolemia.

Similar to other indices of preload, when guiding fluid therapy by ITBV, variables of organ function, i.e., lactate levels, urine output or gastric mucosal CO_2-tension should be taken into consideration.

ECHOCARDIOGRAPHY

In respect of the wide range of abnormalities in cardiac function that may be encountered in sepsis (LV systolic and diastolic dysfunction, RV dysfunction, pulmonary hypertension, hypovolemia, ARDS) and an aging population with (more) concurrent cardiac comorbidities, echocardiography is unique as it offers an instantaneous, bedside, comprehensive assessment of cardiac function in septic patients. The advent of transesophageal (TEE) approach has made this technique applicable as well to those patients in whom the transthoracic (TTE) approach does not allow satisfactory imaging for various reasons (intra-operatively, subcutaneous air or subcutaneous fat, dressings, emphysema, mechanical ventilation). Echocardiography allows qualitative and quantitative assessment of global and regional left and right ventricular systolic function, diastolic function, left and right ventricular preload, regional wall motion abnormalities, and cardiac output [66].

Quantitative estimation of preload can be done in different ways using two-dimensional echocardiography. The LV end-diastolic area (LVEDA) correlates well with volumetric analogs [67]. In particular, the LVEDA as imaged in the transgastric short axis view at the level of papillary muscles, has been shown to directly reflect changes in LVEDV [68,69]. In cardiosurgical patients with normal and abnormal LV function a linear decline in LVEDA of 0.3 cm²/% blood loss was described during graded blood loss [69]. An indexed LVEDA measured at the midpapillary level of the LV of smaller than 5.5 cm²/m² body surface area is very suggestive for a low filling status of the LV. However, if fluid management is to be guided by LVEDA, several shortcomings and limitations must be appreciated. The presence of regional wall motion abnormalities may limit the correct use of LVEDA as a preload parameter. Single data seldom provide conclusive information about the filling status, especially in septic patients with increased LVEDA. Another shortcoming is the fact that the apical region of the LV is more prone to regional wall motion abnormalities than the base of the heart. In patients with RV dysfunction, bulging of the interventricular septum towards the left decreases LVEDA. Guiding fluid management by LVEDA in these patients will lead to inappropiate therapeutic interventions. In septic patients, the superiority of volume related preload parameters like LVEDV or LVEDA over pressure related parameters like CVP or PAOP has been demonstrated by various studies (figure 4)[24,70].

The issue of the assessment of afterload by echocardiography has been addressed in a previous chapter. Using a Doppler technique cardiac output is computed by multiplying flow velocity time integral over mitral, aortic or pulmonary valve, valve opening area and heart frequency [71,72]. Compared with standard thermodilution technique for cardiac output estimation, Doppler echocardiography offers adequate assessment of cardiac output to allow monitoring of hemodynamics during initial therapeutic interventions [71,72].

In septic patients, reversible global and regional wall motion abnormalities have been described as echocardiographic evidence of septic cardiomyopathy [66]. When LV function is evaluated by echocardiography in septic patients, the degree of left ventricular dysfunction (septic cardiomyopathy), as measured by fractional shortening or ejection fraction, may be underestimated due to the decrease in afterload. New approaches like pressure-area loops by simultaneous measurement of arterial blood pressure and LV area in an automatical manner (automatical border detection) or new parameters like maximal preload recruitable stroke work, contractility can be assessed in a pre- and afterload independent manner. Up to now, however, these techniques have not gained broad application, and their use is confined to the research area.

The question of diastolic dysfunction in septic shock remains less clearly defined. In vasopressor-dependent septic shock, Poelaert et al. demonstrated a continuum of LV pathophysiology ranging from isolated diastolic dysfunction to combined systolic and diastolic abnormalities [73]. In a prospective observational study deceleration time – an index of relaxation – was (besides the APACHE II score) shown to be the only independent predictor of mortality in a multivariate analysis. Nonsurvivors had a more abnormal pattern of LV relaxation [74].

In summary, echocardiography offers a unique way for a comprehensive assessment of cardiac function. TTE/TEE should be routinely used for assessment of cardiac function, but cannot simply replace several other already established technologies in the ICU. Echocardiography provides different information than the PAC, and the methods are therefore not competitive but rather complementary. In our ICU, we advocate a combined noninvasive and invasive approach for the assessment of cardiac function. Initially – following clinical evaluation – TTE or TEE is performed for rapid morphologic diagnosis and assessment of hemodynamic state. After diagnostic evaluation, treatment can be started and its effects assessed by repeated TTE or short-term TEE monitoring. When prolonged continuous monitoring of cardiac function becomes mandatory due to persistent hemodynamic instability or treatment failure, invasive monitoring with a PAC or double indicator dilution technique system is necessary.

INVASIVE HEMODYNAMIC MONITORING IN THE MIRROR OF EVIDENCE BASED MEDICINE

Although many critical care physicians recommend the use of the PAC to optimize LV preload and monitor the effect of pharmacotherapy on CI in patients with septic shock, a recent non-randomized study intimated a possible negative effect of PAC in critically ill patients [75] and confirmatory studies of a positive effect on clinical outcome have not been published [76]. The Society of Critical Care Medicine (SCCM) PAC Consensus conference concluded that it is uncertain whether PAC improves outcome in patients with sepsis and septic shock [76]. However, the lack of outcome improvement applies as well to other monitoring techniques like arterial blood pressure measurement, transpulmonary indicator dilution technique or echocardiography. The experts felt that PAC use may be appropiate in patients with septic shock unresponsive to early resuscitative measures [76]. A fact that cannot be emphasized enough is, that to infer a positive impact on the management of septic patients, the use of the PAC (and certainly of any other monitoring technique as well) requires proper training, knowledge and thoughtful interpretation of the data obtained [77,78]. Indirect evidence that invasive monitoring has a positive impact on outcome is provided by a study from Brazil demonstrating that technology availability (besides staffing) on ICUs was inversely correlated with mortality [79].

REFERENCES

1. Parker MM, Shelhamer JH, Natanson C, et al. Serial cardiovascular variables in survivors and nonsurvivors of human septic shock: heart rate as an early predictor of prognosis. Crit Care Med 1987; 15:923-929
2. Houston MC, Thompson WL, Robertson D. Shock. Diagnosis and management. Arch Intern Med 1984; 144:1433-1439
3. Groeneveld AB, Thijs LG. Pulmonary artery catheterization in septic shock. Indications, thearpeutic and prognostic implications. Clin Intens Care 1990; 1:111-115
4. Groeneveld AB, Thijs LG. Haemodynamic monitoring in septic shock. In: Dhainaut JF, Payen D (eds) Strategy in Bedside Haemodynamic Monitoring. Update in Intensive Care and Emergency Medicine, volume 11. Springer Verlag, Berlin 1991:pp 179-197
5. Perel A, Pizov R, Cotev S. Systolic blood pressure variation is a sensitive indicator of hypovolemia in ventilated dogs subjected to graded hemorrhage. Anesthesiology 1987; 67:498-502
6. Tavernier B, Makhotine O, Lebuffe G, et al. Systolic pressure variation as a guide to fluid therapy in patients with sepsis-induced hypotension. Anesthesiology 1998; 89:1313-1321
7. Michard F, Chemla D, Richard C, et al. Clinical use of respiratory changes in arterial pulse pressure to monitor the hemodynamic effects of PEEP. Am J Respir Crit Care Med 1999; 159:935-939
8. Connors AF Jr, McCaffree DR, Gray BA. Evaluation of right-heart catheterization in the critically ill patient without acute myocardial infarction. N Engl J Med 1983; 308:263-267
9. Schneider AJ, Teule GJ, Groeneveld AB, et al. Biventricular performance during volume loading in patients with early septic shock, with emphasis on the right ventricle: a combined hemodynamic and radionuclide study. Am Heart J 1988; 116:103-112

10. Kimchi A, Ellrodt AG, Berman DS, et al. Right ventricular performance in septic shock: a combined radionuclide and hemodynamic study. J Am Coll Cardiol 1984; 4:945-951

11. D'Orio V, Mendes P, Saad G, et al. Accuracy in early prediction of prognosis of patients with septic shock by analysis of simple indices: prospective study. Crit Care Med 1990; 18:1339-1345

12. Vincent JL, Reuse C, Frank N, et al. Right ventricular dysfunction in septic shock: assessment by measurements of right ventricular ejection fraction using the thermodilution technique. Acta Anaesthesiol Scand 1989; 33:34-38

13. Sibbald WJ, Paterson NA, Holliday RL, et al. Pulmonary hypertension in sepsis: measurement by the pulmonary arterial diastolic-pulmonary wedge pressure gradient and the influence of passive and active factors. Chest 1978; 73:583-591

14. Marland AM, Glauser FL. Significance of the pulmonary artery diastolic-pulmonary wedge pressure gradient in sepsis. Crit Care Med 1982; 10:658-661

15. Taylor AE, Cope DK, Allison RC, et al. Capillary pressure measurement in human lungs. In: Zapol WM, Lemaire F (eds). Adult Respiratory Distress Syndrome. New York: Marcel Dekker, 1990

16. Gaar KA Jr, Taylor AE, Owens LJ, et al. Pulmonary capillary pressure and filtration coefficient in the isolated perfused lung. Am J Physiol 1967; 213:910-914

17. Cope DK, Allison RC, Parmentier JL, et al. Measurement of effective pulmonary capillary pressure using the pressure profile after pulmonary artery occlusion. Crit Care Med 1986; 14:16-22

18. Cope DK, Parker JC, Allison RC, et al. Gaar equation is not a reliable predictor of pulmonary capillary pressure. Crit Care Med 1989; 17:300-301

19. Levy MM. Pulmonary capillary pressure and tissue perfusion: clinical implications during resuscitation from shock. New Horiz 1996; 4:504-518

20. Collee GG, Lynch KE, Hill RD, et al. Bedside measurement of pulmonary capillary pressure in patients with acute respiratory failure. Anesthesiology 1987; 66:614-620

21. Parker MM, Shelhamer JH, Bacharach SL, et al. Profound but reversible myocardial depression in patients with septic shock. Ann Intern Med 1984; 100:483-490

22. Parker MM, McCarthy KE, Ognibene FP, et al. Right ventricular dysfunction and dilatation, similar to left ventricular changes, characterize the cardiac depression of septic shock in humans. Chest 1990; 97:126-131

23. Tyberg JV, Taichman GC, Smith ER, et al. The relationship between pericardial pressure and right atrial pressure: an intraoperative study. Circulation 1986; 73:428-432

24. Jardin F, Valtier B, Beauchet A, et al. Invasive monitoring combined with two-dimensional echocardiographic study in septic shock. Intensive Care Med 1994; 20:550-554

25. Ognibene FP, Parker MM, Natanson C, et al. Depressed left ventricular performance. Response to volume infusion in patients with sepsis and septic shock. Chest 1988; 93:903-910

26. Nemens EJ, Woods SL. Normal fluctuations in pulmonary artery and pulmonary capillary wedge pressures in acutely ill patients. Heart Lung 1982; 11:393-398

27. Packman MI, Rackow EC. Optimum left heart filling pressure during fluid resuscitation of patients with hypovolemic and septic shock. Crit Care Med 1983; 11:165-169

28. Vincent JL, Thirion M, Brimioulle S, et al. Thermodilution measurement of right ventricular ejection fraction with a modified pulmonary artery catheter. Intensive Care Med 1986; 12:33-38

29. Dhainaut JF, Brunet F, Monsallier JF, et al. Bedside evaluation of right ventricular performance using a rapid computerized thermodilution method. Crit Care Med 1987; 15:148-152

30. Mitsuo T, Shimazaki S, Matsuda H. Right ventricular dysfunction in septic patients. Crit Care Med 1992; 20:630-634

31. Yu M, Takiguchi S, Takanishi D, et al. Evaluation of the clinical usefulness of thermodilution volumetric catheters. Crit Care Med 1995; 23:681-686

32. Weisel RD, Berger RL, Hechtman HB. Current concepts measurement of cardiac output by thermodilution. N Engl J Med 1975; 292:682-684

33. Cigarroa RG, Lange RA, Williams RH, et al. Underestimation of cardiac output by thermodilution in patients with tricuspid regurgitation. Am J Med 1989; 86:417-420

34. Renner LE, Morton MJ, Sakuma GY. Indicator amount, temperature, and intrinsic cardiac output affect thermodilution cardiac output accuracy and reproducibility. Crit Care Med 1993; 21:586-597

35. Lang RM, Borow KM, Neumann A, et al. Systemic vascular resistance: an unreliable index of left ventricular afterload. Circulation 1986; 74:1114-1123

36. Glower DD, Spratt JA, Snow ND, et al. Linearity of the Frank-Starling relationship in the intact heart: the concept of preload recruitable stroke work. Circulation 1985; 71:994-1009

37. Smith RL, Meixler SM, Simberkoff MS. Excess mortality in critically ill patients with nosocomial bloodstream infections. Chest 1991; 100:164-167

38. Pittet D, Tarara D, Wenzel RP. Nosocomial bloodstream infection in critically ill patients. Excess length of stay, extra costs, and attributable mortality. JAMA 1994 25; 271:1598-1601

39. Mermel LA, Maki DG. Infectious complications of Swan Ganz Pulmonary Artery Catheters and Peripheral Arterial Catheters. In: Seifert H, Jansen B, Farr BM (eds) Catheter-Related Infections, Dekker, New York, 1997

40. Cobb DK, High KP, Sawyer RG, et al. A controlled trial of scheduled replacement of central venous and pulmonary-artery catheters. N Engl J Med 1992; 327:1062-1068

41. Eyer S, Brummitt C, Crossley K, et al. Catheter-related sepsis: prospective, randomized study of three methods of long-term catheter maintenance. Crit Care Med 1990; 18:1073-1079

42. Neumann P. Extravascular lung water and intrathoracic blood volume: double versus single indicator dilution technique. Intensive Care Med 1999; 25:216-219

43. Sakka SG, Rühl CC, Pfeiffer UJ, et al. Assessment of cardiac preload and extravascular lung water by single transpulmonary thermodilution. Intensive Care Med 2000; 26:180-187

44. Pavek K, Lindquist O, Arfors K-E. Validity of thermodilution method for measurement of cardiac output in pulmonary oedema. Cardiovasc Res 1973; 7:419-422

45. Wickerts C-J, Jakobsson J, Frostell C, et al. Measurement of extravascular lung water by thermal-dye technique: mechanisms of cardiac output dependence. Intensive Care Med 1990; 16:115-120

46. Böck JC, Barker BC, Mackersie RC, et al. Cardiac output measurements using femoral artery thermodilution in patients. J Crit Care 1989; 4:106-111

47. Lewis FR, Elings VB, Hill SL, et al. The measurement of extravascular lung water by thermal-green dye indicator dilution. Ann N Y Acad Sci 1982, 384:394-410

48. von Spiegel T, Wietasch G, Bürsch J, et al. HZV-Bestimmung mittels transpulmonaler Thermodilution. Eine Alternative zum Pulmonaliskatheter? Anaesthesist 1996; 45:1045-1050

49. Gödje O, Peyerl M, Seebauer T, et al. Reproducibility of double indicator dilution measurements of intrathoracic blood volume compartments, extravascular lung water, and liver function. Chest 1998; 113:1070-1077

50. Murdoch IA, Marsh MJ, Morrison G. Measurement of cardiac output in children. In: Vincent J-L (ed). Yearbook of Intensive Care and Emergency Medicine 1995. Berlin-Heidelberg-New York: Springer-Verlag, 1995; pp. 606-614
51. Sakka SG, Reinhart K, Meier-Hellmann A. Comparison of pulmonary artery and arterial thermodilution cardiac output in critically ill patients. Intensive Care Med 1999; 25:843-846
52. Lichtwarck-Aschoff M, Beale R, Pfeiffer UJ. Central venous pressure, pulmonary artery occlusion pressure, intrathoracic blood volume, and right ventricular end-diastolic volume as indicators of cardiac preload. J Crit Care 1996; 11:180-188
53. Preisman S, Pfeiffer U, Lieberman N, et al. New monitors of intravascular volume: a comparison of arterial pressure waveform analysis and the intrathoracic blood volume. Intensive Care Med 1997; 23:651-657
54. Lichtwarck-Aschoff M, Zeravik J, Pfeiffer UJ. Intrathoracic blood volume accurately reflects circulatory volume status in critically ill patients with mechanical ventilation. Intensive Care Med 1992; 18:142-147
55. Borelli M, Benini A, Denkewitz T, et al. Effects of continuous negative extrathoracic pressure versus positive end-expiratory pressure in acute lung injury patients. Crit Care Med 1998; 26:1025-1031
56. Hoeft A, Schorn B, Weyland A, et al. Bedside assessment of intravascular volume status in patients undergoing coronary bypass surgery. Anesthesiology 1994; 81:76-86
57. Hoeft A. Transpulmonary indicator dilution: an alternative approach for hemodynamic monitoring. In: Vincent J-L (ed). Yearbook of Intensive Care and Emergency Medicine 1995. Springer-Verlag, Heidelberg 1995; pp. 593-605
58. Sakka SG, Bredle DL, Reinhart K, et al. Comparison between intrathoracic blood volume and cardiac filling pressures in the early phase of hemodynamic instability of patients with sepsis or septic shock. J Crit Care 1999; 14:78-83
59. Hoyt JD, Leatherman JW. Interpretation of the pulmonary artery occlusion pressure in mechanically ventilated patients with large respiratory excursions in intrathoracic pressure. Intensive Care Med 1997; 23:1125-1131
60. Oppenheimer L, Elings VB, Lewis FR. Thermal-dye lung water measurements: effects of edema and embolization. J Surg Res 1979; 26:504-512
61. Sibbald WJ, Warshawski FJ, Short AK, et al. Clinical studies of measuring extravascular lung water by the thermal dye technique in critically ill patients. Chest 1983; 83:725-731
62. Sibbald WJ, Short AK, Warshawski FJ, et al. Thermal dye measurements of extravascular lung water in critically ill patients. Intravascular Starling forces and extravascular lung water in the adult respiratory distress syndrome. Chest 1985; 87:585-592
63. Colmenero-Ruiz M, Fernández-Mondéjar E, Fernández-Sacristán MA, et al. PEEP and low tidal volume ventilation reduce lung water in porcine pulmonary edema. Am J Respir Crit Care Med 1997; 155:964-970
64. Zeravik J, Borg U, Pfeiffer UJ. Efficacy of pressure support ventilation dependent on extravascular lung water. Chest 1990; 97:1412-1419
65. Mitchell JP, Schuller D, Calandrino FS, et al. Improved outcome based on fluid management in critically ill patients requiring pulmonary artery catheterization. Am Rev Respir Dis 1992; 145:990-998
66. Ellrodt AG, Riedinger MS, Kimchi A, et al. Left ventricular performance in septic shock: reversible segmental and global abnormalities. Am Heart J 1985; 110:402-409
67. Appleyard RF, Glantz SA. Two dimensions describe left ventricular volume change during hemodynamic transients. Am J Physiol 1990; 258:H277-284

68. Reich DL, Konstadt SN, Nejat M, et al. Intraoperative transesophageal echocardiography for the detection of cardiac preload changes induced by transfusion and phlebotomy in pediatric patients. Anesthesiology 1993; 79:10-15

69. Cheung AT, Savino JS, Weiss SJ, et al. Echocardiographic and hemodynamic indexes of left ventricular preload in patients with normal and abnormal ventricular function. Anesthesiology 1994; 81:376-387

70. Hüttemann E Intrathoracic blood volume versus echocardiographic parameters. Clin Intensive Care 1996; 7:S20 (Abst)

71. Savino JS, Troianos CA, Aukburg S, et al. Measurement of pulmonary blood flow with transesophageal two-dimensional and Doppler echocardiography. Anesthesiology 1991; 75:445-451

72. Darmon PL, Hillel Z, Mogtader A, et al. Cardiac output by transesophageal echocardiography using continuous-wave Doppler across the aortic valve. Anesthesiology 1994; 80:796-805

73. Poelaert J, Declerck C, Vogelaers D, et al. Left ventricular systolic and diastolic function in septic shock. Intensive Care Med 1997; 23:553-560

74. Munt B, Jue J, Gin K, et al. Diastolic filling in human severe sepsis: an echocardiographic study. Crit Care Med 1998; 26:1829-1833

75. Connors AF Jr, Speroff T, Dawson NV, et al. The effectiveness of right heart catheterization in the initial care of critically ill patients. SUPPORT Investigators. JAMA 1996 18; 276:889-897

76. Parker MM, Peruzzi W. Pulmonary artery catheters in sepsis/ septic shock. New Horiz 1997; 5:228-232

77. Gnaegi A, Feihl F, Perret C. Intensive care physicians' insufficient knowledge of right-heart catheterization at the bedside: time to act? Crit Care Med 1997; 25:213-220

78. Vincent JL, Dhainaut JF, Perret C, et al. Is the pulmonary artery catheter misused? A European view. Crit Care Med 1998; 26:1283-1287

79. Bastos PG, Knaus WA, Zimmerman JE, et al. The importance of technology for achieving superior outcomes from intensive care. Brazil APACHE III Study Group. Intensive Care Med 1996; 22:664-669

17

VALUE OF SvO₂ IN SEPSIS

Thierry Boulain
Jean-Louis Teboul

Mixed venous oxygen saturation (SvO₂) has been known for a long time to be a meaningful physiological parameter that would reflect the global balance between arterial oxygen delivery (DO₂) and oxygen consumption (VO₂) provided that arterial blood oxygen saturation (SaO₂) is well-maintained. Shock states are characterized by imbalance between oxygen supply to the tissues and tissue oxygen demand. Because monitoring of SvO₂ is now easy to perform with fiberoptic pulmonary artery catheters (PACs), it is often used to assess global oxygen balance in shock states, in particular in septic shock. In this chapter, we will see that the interpretation of SvO₂ and its changes must be particularly careful in this setting for at least two major reasons: first, in shock states, by definition, oxygen demand exceeds VO₂ and second, the capacity of the tissues to utilize oxygen is often impaired in sepsis so that VO₂ may decrease relatively to oxygen demand, even if DO₂ is normal or high. Thus, although SvO₂ monitoring has been shown to be useful in the care of cardiac patients for instance [1], its value in sepsis and septic shock may be questioned [2,3].

DETERMINANTS OF SvO₂

The blood flowing through the pulmonary artery comes from the superior and inferior vena cavae, and from the coronary sinus and is thus the mixture of all the venous returns of the body. The amount of oxygen present in mixed venous blood (the mixed venous oxygen content: CvO₂) depends upon the amount of oxygen carried from the lungs toward the peripheral tissues by the cardiovascular system, and the whole-body VO₂. In the vast majority of clinical situations, CvO₂ is well and linearly correlated with SvO₂, which represents the oxygen saturation (expressed in %) of hemoglobin contained by the red blood cells (RBC) of the mixed venous blood.

CvO$_2$ is the sum of oxygen bound to hemoglobin and of dissolved oxygen in the mixed venous blood:

$$CvO_2 \text{ (ml/100ml)} = (SvO_2 \text{ x Hb x } 1.34) + (0.003 \text{ x } PvO_2) \qquad \text{(Eqn 1)}$$

where Hb (g/dl) is the hemoglobin concentration, 1.34 is the oxygen combining capacity of hemoglobin, 0.003 is the oxygen dissolving coefficient in blood, and PvO$_2$ (mm Hg) is the partial pressure of oxygen in mixed venous blood. In most clinical cases, dissolved oxygen (PvO$_2$ x 0.003) does not contribute significantly to CvO$_2$. Thus:

$$CvO_2 = (1.34 \text{ x Hb}) \text{ x } SvO_2 \qquad \text{(Eqn 2)}$$

Similarly, the arterial oxygen content can be calculated as follows:

$$CaO_2 = (1.34 \text{ x Hb}) \text{ x } SaO_2 \qquad \text{(Eqn 3)}$$

where SaO$_2$ is the arterial blood oxygen saturation.

The Fick equation that states that:

$$VO_2 = \text{cardiac output x } (CaO_2 - CvO_2) \qquad \text{(Eqn 4)}$$

where VO$_2$ is expressed in ml/min, and cardiac output expressed in dl/min, becomes:

$$VO_2 = \text{cardiac output x } (SaO_2 - SvO_2) \text{ x } 1.34 \text{ x Hb} \qquad \text{(Eqn 5)}$$

and SvO$_2$ can be expressed as:

$$SvO_2 = SaO_2 - [VO_2/(\text{cardiac output x Hb x } 1.34)] \qquad \text{(Eqn 6)}$$

Thus, SaO$_2$, Hb, cardiac output, and VO$_2$ are the four major physiological variables which determine the value of. SvO$_2$.

In healthy subjects at rest with normal SaO$_2$ and Hb, the value of SvO$_2$ ranges from 70 to 75%. During exercise, oxygen demand is increased especially in skeletal muscles. As a consequence, VO$_2$ will increase because of the increase in cardiac output and of the increase in oxygen extraction of the tissues that occurs especially in the skeletal muscles by redistribution of the intra-organ blood flow. For this reason, values as low as 45% for SvO$_2$ can be observed in healthy subjects during exercise [4]. However, when SvO$_2$

reaches such a low value, anaerobic metabolism often appears. This point underlines the fact that oxygen extraction has physiological limits.

In pathological conditions, SvO_2 is the result of complex interactions between its four major determinants, each of which can be altered, potentially, by both the disease process and the therapeutic agents used. Moreover, these determinants are not independent since compensatory mechanisms may occur when one of them is altered. For instance, cardiac output may increase in face of a fall in SaO_2 or in Hb and may decrease after normalization of these latter variables. Thus, it must be kept in mind that SvO_2 changes are rarely linearly correlated to changes in one of its determinants.

MEASUREMENT OF SvO_2

Measurement by Transmission Spectrophotometry

A sample of mixed venous blood, drawn from a PAC, is placed between a light source and photodetectors to measure its relative light absorbance at different wavelengths. As oxyhemoglobin, deoxyhemoglobin, carboxyhemoglobin, methemoglobin, have different absorbance profiles for each of the wavelengths used that cross RBCs, it is possible to accurately determine the fractional oxygen saturation of hemoglobin (SvO_2) for the mixed venous blood. However, numerous pitfalls (reviewed elsewhere [5]) must be avoided when pulmonary artery blood is drawn through a PAC. Therefore, strict rules must be observed to avoid the sampling of oxygenated ('arterialized') capillary blood instead of pure mixed venous blood, and, in particular, the proper position of the PAC tip in a large branch of the pulmonary artery must be ensured.

The measurement of SvO_2 by cooximetry is time consuming and exposed to frequent errors. It can also cause complications such as blood wasting (especially in pediatric patients) and infections due to frequent but necessary manipulation of the PAC. For these reasons, in clinical practice, SvO_2 measurement by cooximetry is not always performed as frequently as needed.

Continuous *in Vivo* Measurement of SvO_2

For several decades now, it has been possible to measure SvO_2 through modified fiberoptic PACs by reflectance spectrophotometry, avoiding most of the pitfalls associated with mixed venous blood withdrawal, and allowing the continuous monitoring of SvO_2. The accuracy and reliability of continuous SvO_2 measurement has improved with the use of the three-wavelength, instead of the two-wavelength, systems [5].

A source of red and infrared light sends three different wavelengths (ranging from 600 to 1000 nanometers) through a fiberoptic bundle of the PAC and illuminates the blood flowing through the pulmonary artery. The intensity of light reflected by the RBCs is then transmitted back to a photodetector through another channel of optic fibers. Each reflected wavelength intensity is integrated by a computer which calculates SvO_2.

To ensure a correct measurement of reflectance SvO_2, an *in vitro* calibration must be performed prior to insertion of the PAC, in accordance with the manufacturer's instructions, with the help of a disposable optical reference. *In vivo* recalibration, that first consists of comparing the reflectance SvO_2 value with the SvO_2 measured on a blood sample, and then in correcting the SvO_2 value displayed by the computer and correcting the hemoglobin concentration initially set at insertion, should be performed every time continuous SvO_2 is suspected to be erroneous. It is not yet clear whether this recalibration is needed daily or not. Cautious care must be taken to ensure the proper position of the PAC tip (not too distal), for the accurate measurement of SvO_2. The accuracy of SvO_2 measurements given by the manufacturers of continuous SvO_2 devices is within ±2%. However, the mean precision of SvO_2 systems when compared to cooximetry is only 9% *in vitro* [6] while in the clinical setting the best limits of agreement reported between the two techniques are wide, ranging from about -9 to +9% [7]. However, discrepancies between laboratory and *in vivo* SvO_2 values are generally due to imperfect use rather than to poor quality of the SvO_2 system [8]. Therefore, misinterpretations of SvO_2 should be minimized by repositioning the PAC and by recalibrating the SvO_2 system.

INTERPRETATION OF SvO_2 IN SEPSIS

SvO_2 as an Index of Global Oxygen Extraction

The whole-body oxygen extraction ratio (O_2ER) is defined as the ratio of the whole-body VO_2 to the whole-body DO_2:

$$O_2ER = VO_2/DO_2 \qquad \text{(Eqn 7)}$$

As DO_2 = cardiac output x CaO_2, equation 6 can be transformed to:

$$SvO_2 = SaO_2 - (VO_2/DO_2) \qquad \text{(Eqn 8)}$$

When SaO_2 is close to 1 (100%), SvO_2 can thus be used to estimate O_2ER:

$$SvO_2 = 1 - O_2ER \qquad \text{(Eqn 9)}$$

In the majority of critically ill patients who are placed on mechanical ventilation and in whom arterial oxygenation is controlled by a high inspired fraction of oxygen (FiO_2) and/or positive end-expiratory pressure (PEEP), equation 9 can be reasonably applied. By contrast, in septic patients with initial severe hypoxemia, changes in SvO_2 can hardly reflect O_2ER, particularly when large changes in SaO_2 occur.

By considering that SvO_2 reflects O_2ER, SvO_2 changes can be interpreted as follows:

- a decrease in SvO_2 would mean that O_2ER has increased to match the whole-body VO_2 with the whole-body oxygen demand. This change in O_2ER can be triggered by either a drop in DO_2, or an increase in oxygen demand, or both. When, despite this normal adaptation, VO_2 does not equal oxygen demand, tissue dysoxia and anaerobic metabolism appear [9]. However, no precise value for O_2ER, and consequently for SvO_2, can be proposed as the 'critical' SvO_2 below which dysoxia occurs [9].
- inversely, an increase in SvO_2 would mean that O_2ER has decreased as a consequence of either an increase in DO_2 with VO_2 maintained or a decrease in VO_2 with DO_2 maintained or increased. We will see below that this latter situation is often encountered in hyperdynamic septic shock where the decrease in actual VO_2 (despite high whole-body oxygen demand) is not explained by reduced DO_2, but rather by oxygen extraction impairment [10].

These points underline the fact that:

- O_2ER (and thus SvO_2), which is by definition the VO_2/DO_2 ratio, cannot be a reliable marker of the adequacy between DO_2 and global oxygen demand in shock states where VO_2 is less than oxygen demand and
- interpretation of O_2ER (and thus of SvO_2) can be particularly misleading under conditions of hyperdynamic sepsis.

Clinical Use of SvO_2 Measurement in Septic Shock

Sepsis results in a complex form of shock. Some patients have reductions in systemic blood flow which eventually result in limited oxidative metabolism. In these cases, the low cardiac output is mostly related to sepsis-induced hypovolemia. However, in most patients, in whom early correction of volume depletion by aggressive fluid therapy has resulted in a hyperdynamic circulatory state, the impaired oxidative metabolism is related to the inability of tissues to extract sufficient oxygen from the blood [10,11]. Distributive abnormalities of macrocirculatory and microcirculatory blood flow mainly explain the impairment in oxygen extraction that occurs in sepsis [10,11]. As a consequence, the most frequent hemodynamic profile in human septic shock is characterized by high cardiac output and vasodilation [10,11,13], although some clinical studies reported relatively low values of cardiac output [14,15] either because of insufficient fluid resuscitation and/or presence of a patent sepsis-induced myocardial depression [11].

As we mentioned above, in septic as in non-septic shock, SvO_2 cannot serve as a reliable marker of the adequacy between DO_2 and global oxygen demand and thus as a marker of tissue hypoxia. However, SvO_2 could be helpful at the bedside to assess the adequacy of DO_2 relative to global VO_2. Therefore, SvO_2 might take a place in the cardiovascular monitoring of septic shock, by identifying patients in whom cardiac output could be further raised and then by guiding therapy aimed at increasing cardiac output. This point is of particular importance since systematic maximalization of cardiac output is not recommended in every patient with septic shock [16].

Interpretation of Absolute Values of SvO_2

Because the usual hemodynamic profile of human septic shock is characterized by high systemic blood flow, high values of SvO_2 are most often observed [3,17]. However, numerous studies have reported values less than 65 % [2,14,18,19] that would indicate that systemic blood flow is insufficiently high [3] and hence that a therapy increasing cardiac output could be selected. However, the beneficial effect of this approach on outcome remains to be proved.

When SvO_2 is within the range of 65 to 77% (i.e., the normal range in healthy subjects), it is difficult to know, from one isolated value of SvO_2, whether a further rise in DO_2 (or cardiac output) can improve significantly global tissue oxygenation. To clarify this point, we reviewed some of the most recent studies in which changes in DO_2 and whole-body VO_2 were observed in populations of resuscitated septic patients [20-31]. Some of these studies focused on splanchnic blood flow or gastric tonometry [20-25]. These studies reported mean baseline values of O_2ERs, that range from 18 to 36% that grossly correspond to SvO_2 values ranged between 64 and 82%. If these patients are classified as responders (VO_2 increase in response to DO_2 increase), non-responders with cardiac reserve (no change in VO_2 when DO_2 increases), or non-responders (no change in DO_2), initial O_2ER (or SvO_2) values do not help in discriminating responders from non-responders. Some of the populations studied had included patients with confirmed dysoxia (high lactate levels or low intramucosal gastric pH [pHi] or both), in whom it could be hoped that increasing DO_2 would compensate, at least in part the global O_2 deficit [27]. However, no O_2ER (or SvO_2) cutoff value can be found to differentiate patients with dysoxia who may further benefit (at least in part) from an increase in DO_2, from patients with dysoxia in whom raising DO_2 will fail to raise VO_2. However, a detailed analysis of these studies indicates that values of O_2ER which ranged from 30 to 35 % (or SvO_2 slightly below the range 65-70%) are most often observed in populations of patients who were not optimally resuscitated before entering the study: some had not yet received any vasoconstrictor to compensate for the non-responsiveness of blood pressure to fluids [28], some had not yet received clinically optimal fluid therapy [27], while others initially disclosed unusual high VO_2 due to high oxygen demand [30]. Thus, values of SvO_2 below 70% in septic patients would mean that initial therapy has not been sufficient [32] and/or that sedation or antipyretic drugs would be used to reduce oxygen demand. Accordingly, targeting a SvO_2 value of at least 70% might be a reasonable goal of treatment in septic shock [28]. Nevertheless, the interpretation of initial SvO_2 values between 70 and 77% remains unclear without dynamic data recorded during therapeutic interventions.

Interpretation of Changes in SvO_2

• In patients with relatively low initial values of SvO_2, following the course of SvO_2 may be helpful to assess effects on global tissue oxygenation of a therapy given for increasing cardiac output. Under conditions of oxygen supply dependence, increase in cardiac output should be accompanied by increases in VO_2 so that SvO_2 is expected to increase less than in the case of oxygen supply independence [2,33]. Consequently, relatively unchanged SvO_2 with therapy would not mean that the therapy has failed. In this case, the therapeutic agent would be rather maintained and its dose even augmented until a frank decrease in SvO_2 is obtained that would indicate that the critical level of DO_2 has been actually passed. Otherwise, SvO_2 monitoring may also be helpful to choose the appropriate dose of a therapeutic agent known to have thermogenic effects [34]. For instance, catecholamines by their β stimulation are able to increase oxygen demand and VO_2 [35]. In septic patients without evidence of shock, dobutamine was demonstrated to increase VO_2 at doses higher than 5 µg/kg/min [36]. However, if SvO_2 is actually stable despite increased DO_2, differentiating an increase in VO_2 that unmasks an oxygen debt from the thermogenic effects of inotropic drugs could be difficult and could need assessment of other metabolic variables such as lactates levels [37] and/or changes in arteriovenous PCO$_2$ gradients [38].

- In patients with SvO$_2$ higher than 70%, as we mentioned above few arguments suggest that raising further DO$_2$ would improve tissue oxygenation [32]. In this regard, Gattinoni et al. [39] did not observe any reduction in mortality, when therapy was targeted at an increase in SvO$_2$ above 70 % in a large population of critically ill patients, including septic patients. Nevertheless, monitoring of SvO$_2$ may be still useful to detect short-term decreases in SvO$_2$ that may have prognostic significance by alerting the clinician before obvious clinical aggravation such as hypotension or oliguria occur [17]. However, to better interpret SvO$_2$ changes in that high range of SvO$_2$ values, the nonlinearity of the relation between SvO$_2$ and cardiac output (equation 6) must be underlined: according to the modified Fick equation, for a constant VO$_2$, SvO$_2$ is linearly related to cardiac output in the low values of cardiac output, whereas there is a flattening of the SvO$_2$/cardiac output relationship curve in the high values of cardiac output [40]. It must be kept in mind that the SvO$_2$/cardiac output relationship will depend also on the level of VO$_2$, so that a family of hyperbolic SvO$_2$/cardiac output relationship curves for various levels of VO$_2$ (VO$_2$ isopleths) can be drawn [40] (Figure 1).

As a consequence, one must be particularly cautious in the interpretation of SvO$_2$ changes (or of absence of marked changes) under conditions of very high systemic blood flow. This point is illustrated by the analysis of data from studies in patients with hyperdynamic sepsis in whom changes in SvO$_2$ within the range of 70 to 80% were observed [26,36,41,42]. For example, in the studies of De Backer et al. [36], and Ronco et al. [41], the mean DO$_2$ in subgroups of supply independent patients increased by 36 and 49 % while SvO$_2$ increased by only 9% (from 70 to 76 % and 69 to 75 %, respectively) after dobutamine infusion. By comparison, dobutamine-induced increase in cardiac output of 33 % resulted in a 19 % increase in SvO$_2$ in supply independent patients with baseline low cardiac output and low SvO$_2$ [34] (Figure 1). In addition to the nonlinearity of equation 6, if the increase in DO$_2$ is associated with a VO$_2$ increase in supply dependent patients, SvO$_2$ can be almost unchanged as illustrated in some studies [26,43]. However, before definitive interpretation of small changes in SvO$_2$ one must take into account the relatively weak precision of reflectance spectrophotometry since a change in SvO$_2$ of at least 5 % is necessary to affirm that SvO$_2$ has actually changed [7].

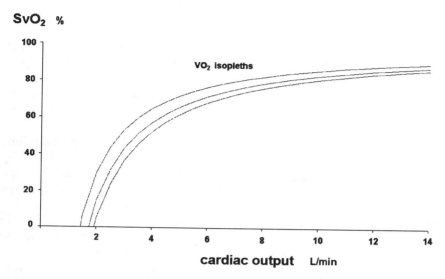

Figure 1. *SvO₂ /cardiac output relationships. According to the modified Fick equation, the SvO₂ /cardiac output relationship is curvilinear. Therefore, for a constant VO_2, changes in cardiac output result in large changes in SvO₂ in the low values of cardiac output, whereas changes in cardiac output will not result in significant changes in SvO₂ in the high values of cardiac output. These relationships are further complicated when changes in cardiac output are accompanied by changes in VO₂ and thereby by a transfer from one VO₂ isopleth to another (on the figure VO₂ increases from the left to the right).*

Thus, the two following consequences can be reasonably drawn for the clinical practice:

1) the fact that monitoring does not detect changes in SvO_2 does not rule out onset or worsening of global hypoxia. Obviously, this does not support a common idea that SvO_2 monitoring acts as an sensitive warning system in hyperdynamic septic shock. In this regard, benefits may be drawn from the use of recently available modified PACs allowing for continuous measurement of cardiac output and SvO_2 [44].

2) a decrease in SvO_2 of at least 5 % within the 'normal' range (from 77 to 65%) should be considered as clinically significant because it indicates a dramatic fall in DO_2 and/or increase in oxygen demand. This should prompt the checking of Hb, SaO_2, cardiac output, and potential causes of increased oxygen demand, and lead to appropriate treatment. However, whether application of these latter rules is superior to simple monitoring of clinical signs (blood pressure and diuresis) and could influence mortality has never be demonstrated.

SvO₂ and Regional Oxygenation

SvO₂ is the flow-weighted average of the venous saturation values from all perfused organs of the body. Organs with high blood flow and low oxygen extraction, such as the kidneys, have a greater influence on SvO₂ than do organs with low blood flow and high oxygen extraction, such as the myocardium. In sepsis the interpretation of SvO₂ is further complicated by the fact that regional and local distribution of blood flow is disturbed.

In this regard, there is now strong evidence that the hepato-splanchnic region may suffer from such unbalanced flows during septic shock [45]. Moreover, the oxygen demand of the splanchnic region is increased during sepsis [46]. This may result in splanchnic dysoxia that may be in part, the motor of multiple organ failure (MOF) [47]. Interestingly, 'normal' values of SvO₂ were observed in septic patients who exhibit very low values of hepatic vein oxygen saturation values [25, 48] and VO₂ supply dependence in the hepato-splanchnic region [48]. Furthermore, SvO₂ may remain unchanged while hepatic vein oxygen saturation and hepato-splanchnic blood flow vary by 20-30 % under drug therapy used to maintain blood pressure [25]. Therefore, SvO₂ cannot be a reliable parameter to monitor regional VO₂/DO₂.

CONCLUSION

SvO₂ can be considered as a marker of the global balance between DO₂ and actual VO₂. A decreased SvO₂ (<65 %) may be an argument that would incite the clinician to raise DO₂ in the view of preventing or reducing global hypoxia in patients with sepsis or septic shock. However, systemic blood flow is frequently high in septic shock so that SvO₂ is most often in the normal range, even in the presence of profound global and/or regional hypoxia. Furthermore, in such hyperdynamic states, interpretation of SvO₂ changes (or of absence of changes) must be particularly careful and can be improved by the concomitant assessment of cardiac output, now possible by using the recent, modified PACs.

REFERENCES

1. O'Connor JP, Townsend GE. Perioperative continuous monitoring of mixed venous oxygen saturation should be routine during high-risk cardiac surgery. J Cardiothorac Anesth 1990; 4:647-650
2. Astiz ME, Rackow EC, Falk JL, et al. Oxygen delivery and consumption in patients with hyperdynamic septic shock. Crit Care Med 1987; 15:26-28

3. Task force of the American College of Critical Care Medicine, Society of Critical Care Medicine. Practice parameters for hemodynamic support of sepsis in adult patients in sepsis. Crit Care Med 1999; 27:639-660

4. Weber KT, Andrews V, Janicki JS, et al. Amrinone and exercice paerformance in patients with chronic heart failure. Am J Cardiol 1981; 48:164-169

5. Cernaianu AC, Nelson LD. The significance of mixed venous oxygen saturation and technical aspects of continuous measurement. In: Edwards JD, Shoemaker WC, Vincent JL (eds) Oxygen transport: Principles and Practice. WB Saunders Company, London, 1993, pp 99-124

6. Janvier G, Guenard H, Lomenech AM. In vitro accuracy of three blood O_2 saturation optic catheter systems. Intensive Care Med 1994 20:480-483

7. Scuderi PE, Bowton DL, Meredith JW, et al. A comparison of three pulmonary artery oximetry catheters in Intensive Care Unit patients. Chest 1992; 102:896-905

8. Nelson LD. Mixed venous oximetry. In: Snyder JV, Pinsky MR (eds) Oxygen transport in the critically ill, Year Book Medical Publishers, Chicago,1987, pp 235-248

9. Kasnitz P, Druger GI, Yorra F, et al. Mixed venous oxygen tension and hyperlactatemia. JAMA 1976; 236:570-574

10. Astiz ME, Rackow EC. Septic shock. Lancet 1998; 351:1501-1505

11. Parillo JE. Pathogenetic mechanisms of septic shock. N Engl J Med 1993; 328:1471-1477

12. Moriyama S, Okamoto K, Tabira Y, et al. Evaluation of oxygen consumption and resting energy expenditure in critically ill patients with systemic inflammatory response syndrome. Crit Care Med 1999; 27:2133-2136

13. Groeneveld ABJ, Bronsveld W, Thijs LG. Hemodynamuic determinants of mortality in human septic shock. Surgery 1986;99:140-153

14. Astiz ME, Rackow EC, Kaufman B, et al. Relationship of oxygen delivery and mixed venous oxygenation to lactic acidosis in patients with sepsis and acute myocardial infarction. Crit Care Med 1988; 16:655-658

15. Bakker J, Vincent JL, Gris P, et al. Veno-arterial carbon dioxide gradient in human septic shock. Chest 1992; 101:509-515

16. Russell JA. Adding fuel to the fire- The supranormal oxygen delivery trial controversy. Crit Care Med 1998; 26:981-983

17. Kraft P, Steltzer H, Hiesmayr M, et al. Mixed venous oxygen saturation in critically ill septic shock patients. The role of defined events. Chest 1993; 103:900-906

18. Vincent JL, Roman A, Kahn RJ. Dobutamine administration in septic shock: addition to a standard protocol. Crit Care Med 1990; 18:689-693

19. Bakker J, Coffernis M, Leon M, et al. Blood lactate levels are superior to oxygen derived variables in predicting outcome in human septic shock. Chest 1991; 99:956-962

20. Meier-Hellmann A, Bredle DL, Specht M, et al. Dopexamine increases splanchnic blood flow but decreases gastric mucosal pH in severe septic patients treated with dobutamine. Crit Care Med 1999; 27:2166-2171

21. Levy B, Bollaert P-E, Lucchelli J-P, et al. Dobutamine improves the adequacy of gastric mucosal perfusion in epinephrine-treated septic shock. Crit Care Med 1997; 25:1649-1654

22. Levy B, Bollaert P-E, Charpentier C, et al. Comparison of norepinephrine and dobutamine to epinephrine for hemodynamics, lactate metabolism, and gastric tonometic variables in septic shock: a prospective, randomized study. Intensive Care Med 1997; 23:282-287

23. Duranteau J, Sitbon P, Teboul JL, et al. Effects of epinephrine, norepinephrine, or the combination of norepinephrine and dobutamine on gastric mucosa in septic shock. Crit Care Med 1999; 27:893-900

24. Oud L, Haupt MT. Persistant gastric intramucosal ischemia in patients with sepsis following resuscitation from shock. Chest 1999; 115:1390-1396

25. Reinelt H, Radermacher P, Kiefer P, et al. Impact of exogenous b-adrenergic receptor stimulation on hepatosplanchnic oxygen kinetics and metabolic activity in septic shock. Crit Care Med 1999; 27:325-331
26. Hayes MA, Timmins AC, Yau EHS, et al. Oxygen transport patterns in patients with sepsis syndrome or septic shock: Influence of treatment and relationship to outcome. Crit Care Med 1997; 25:926-936
27. Friedman G, De Backer D, Shahla M, et al. Oxygen supply dependency can characterize septic shock. Intensive Care Med 1998; 24:118-123
28. Yu M, Burchell S, Hasaniya NWMA, et al. Relationship of mortality to increasing oxygen delivery in patients > 50 years of age: A prospective, randomized trial. Crit Care Med 1998; 26:1011-1019
29. Bacher A, Mayer N, Limscha W, et al. Effects of pentoxifylline on hemodynamics and oxygenation in septic and non septic patients. Crit Care Med 1997; 25:795-800
30. Martin C, Viviand X, Arnaud S, et al. Effects of norepinephrine plus dobutamine or norepinephrine alone on left ventricular performance of septic shock patients. Crit Care Med 1999; 27:1708-1713
31. Rhodes A, Lamb FJ, Malagon I, et al. A prospective study of the use of a dobutamine stress test to identify outcome in patients with sepsis, severe sepsis, or septic shock. Crit Care Med 1999, 27:2361-2366
32. Alia I, Esteban A, Gordo F, et al. A randomized controlled trial of the effect of treatment aimed at maximizing oxygen delivery in patients with sever sepsis or septic shock. Chest 1999; 115: 453-461
33. Bihari D, Smithies M, Gimson A, et al. The effects of vasodilation on oxygen delivery and uptake in critically ill patients. N Engl J Med 1987; 317: 397-403
34. Teboul JL, Boujdaria R, Graini L, et al. Cardiac index vs oxygen-derived parameters for rational use of dobutamine in patients with congestive heart failure. Chest 1993; 103:81-85
35. Chiolero R, Flatt JP, Revelly JP, et al. Effects of catecholamines on oxygen consumption and oxygen delivery in critically ill patients. Chest 1991; 100:1676-1684
36. De Backer D, Moraine JJ, Berré J, et al. Effects of dobutamine on oxygen consumption in septic patients. Direct versus indirect determinations. Am J Respir Crit Care Med 1994; 150:95-100
37. Vincent JL, Dufaye P, Berré J, et al. Serial lactate determinations during circulatory shock. Crit Care Med 1983; 11:449-451
38. Teboul Jl, Mercat A, Lenique F, et al. Value of venous-arterial PCO₂ gradient to reflect the O₂ supply to demand in humans. Crit Care Med 1998; 26:1007-1010
39. Gattinoni L, Brazzi L, Pelosi P, et al. A trial of goal-oriented hemodynamic therapy in critically ill patients. SvO2 Collaborative Group. N Engl J Med 1995; 333:1025-1032
40. Jain A, Shroff SG, Janicki JS, et al. Relation between mixed venous oxygen saturation and cardiac index. Nonlinearity and normalization for oxygen uptake and hemoglobin. Chest 1991; 99:1403-1409
41. Ronco JJ, Fenwick JC, Wiggs BR, et al. Oxygen consumption is dependent of increases in oxygen delivery by dobutamine in septic patients who have normal or increased plasma lactate. Am Rev Respir Dis 1993; 147:25-31
42. Manthous CA, Shumacker PT, Pohlman A, et al. Absence of supply dependence of oxygen consumption in patients with septic shock. J Crit Care 1993; 8:203-211
43. Edwards JD, GCS Brown, Nightingale P, et al. Use of survivor's cardiorespiratory values as therapeutic goals in septic shock. Crit Care Med 1989; 17:1098-1103
44. Burchell SA, Yu M, Takiguchi SA, et al. Evaluation of a continuous cardiac output and mixed venous oxygen saturation catheter in critically ill surgical patients. Crit Care Med 1997; 25 388-91
45. Piepoli M, Garrard CS, Kontyannis DA, et al. Autonomic control of the heart and

peripheral vessels in human septic shock. Intensive Care Med, 1995; 21:112-119

46. Dahn MS, Lange MP, Lobdell K, et al. Splanchnic and total body oxygen consumption differences in septic and injured patients. Surgery 1987; 101:69-80

47. Carrico CJ, Meakins JL, Marshall JC, et al. Multiple organ failure syndrome: the gastrointestinal tract: the motor of MOF. Arch Surg 1986; 131:196-208

48. De Backer D, Creteur J, Noordally O, et al. Does hepato-splanchnic VO_2/DO_2 dependency exist in critically septic patients? Am J Respir Crit Care Med 1998; 157:1219-1225

18

BLOOD LACTATE CONCENTRATIONS IN SEPSIS

James A. Kruse

Numerous studies have demonstrated that blood lactate levels increase in humans with sepsis and in animal models of sepsis [1-22]. Some of the mechanisms leading to this hyperlactatemia are well understood, but there may be others that have not been fully elucidated. Regardless of the mechanisms, a strong association between outcome and the degree of lactate elevation has been documented repeatedly in patients with sepsis [2-4,7,8,10,16,17,19,23,24]. Lactate thus serves as a marker for severity of illness in these patients and identifies those who are at high risk for clinical decompensation. Lactate levels correlate better with survival than either cardiac index or oxygen transport indices, and predict the development of multiple organ system failure (MOF) [2,3,16].

NORMAL, RESTING LACTATE METABOLISM

A cell's ability to perform its requisite functions and maintain its own homeostasis requires a ready supply of chemical energy in the form of adenosine triphosphate (ATP). At rest, nearly all tissues of the body rely on aerobic metabolic pathways to produce ATP, derived predominantly from glucose that is oxidized to carbon dioxide (CO_2) and water in a series of chemical reactions that can be summarized as [25]:

$$\text{Glucose} + 6\,O_2 \longrightarrow 6\,CO_2 + 36\text{-}38\text{ ATP}$$

This overall process can be broken down into a simplified four step sequence that involves the reduced and oxidized forms of the enzyme cofactors nicotinamide adenine dinucleotide (NADH and NAD$^+$, respectively) and flavin dinucleotide (FADH$_2$ and FAD, respectively). The first 3 of these steps are summarized as:

$$\text{Glucose} \cdots\!\!\searrow\!\!\cdots 2\,\text{Pyruvate} \xrightarrow{\text{PD}}\searrow 2\,\text{Acetate} \cdots\!\!\xrightarrow{6\,O_2}\!\!\cdots 4\,CO_2$$

$$\begin{array}{ccc} 2\,\text{ATP}+ & 2\,CO_2 + & 2\,\text{GTP}+6\,\text{NADH} \\ 2\,\text{NADH} & 2\,\text{NADH} & +\,2\,\text{FADH}_2 \end{array}$$

Conversion of one 6-carbon molecule of glucose to two 3-carbon molecules of pyruvate is actually a series of individual reactions, each enzymatically catalyzed in the cytosol [25]. Two molecules of ATP are produced directly in this first step. In the next step, the pyruvate molecules are transported into the mitochondria where they are decarboxylated to acetate by the pyruvate dehydrogenase (PDH) enzyme complex. Acetate then enters the Krebs' cycle and is converted to carbon dioxide.

The fourth step, which also takes place in the mitochondria, utilizes NADH and FADH$_2$ to produce ATP by passing electrons from the cofactor molecules to oxygen, reducing the latter to water:

Tightly coupled to this electron transport process are oxidative phosphorylation reactions, depicted by the vertical arrows above, that generate ATP from adenosine diphosphate (ADP). Each intramitochondrial NADH molecule is thus convertible to 3 ATP molecules, whereas each FADH$_2$ molecule produces only 2 molecules of ATP.

For the 2 NADH molecules produced in the first step to be converted to ATP, they must first be translocated into the mitochondria. In brain and skeletal muscle cells this is accomplished by a shuttle reaction that takes place at the mitochondrial membrane and, in effect, converts the NADH into FADH$_2$ yielding 2 molecules of ATP per cytoplasmic NADH [25]. A more efficient mechanism takes place in the liver, kidney and heart, which moves NADH into the mitochondria and yields 3 molecules of ATP per NADH. Thus, the aerobic metabolism of one molecule of glucose yields either 36 or 38 molecules of ATP, depending on the tissue involved and its NADH shuttle mechanism.

The only direct source of lactate in human metabolism is from pyruvate by:

$$\text{Pyruvate} + \text{NADH} + \text{H}^+ \overset{\text{LDH}}{\rightleftharpoons} \text{Lactate} + \text{NAD}^+$$

This is a single-step reversible reaction catalyzed by lactate dehydrogenase (LDH), Under normal steady state conditions, the concentration of pyruvate determines that of lactate, with a molar concentration ratio of lactate:pyruvate (L:P) of approximately 10:1. In the liver and renal cortex, pyruvate can, under certain conditions, be converted back to glucose by way of the energy requiring gluconeogenic pathway.

At the tissue level, oxygen is delivered to cells by way of adjacent capillaries. Oxygen delivery (DO_2), the product of perfusion and arterial blood oxygen content, is applicable to individual cells, regions of the body (regional DO_2), or the body as a whole (systemic DO_2). To satisfy metabolic demands, sufficient oxygen must be delivered according to the stoichiometry of the above equations and the prevailing cellular ATP requirements. Cells take up the necessary amount of oxygen to accomplish the above chemical reactions and produce ATP as needed. Oxygen uptake (VO_2) is similarly applicable to individual cells, regions of the body (regional VO_2), or the body as a whole (systemic VO_2). The fraction of oxygen consumed to that delivered (VO_2/DO_2) is oxygen extraction, normally averaging about 0.25. At rest, small changes in DO_2 do not disturb VO_2. Instead, tissue oxygen extraction increases or decreases as required to maintain basal VO_2 despite mild to moderate change in DO_2.

LACTATE METABOLISM IN CIRCULATORY SHOCK

Shock is effectively a state of global tissue hypoxia [26]. It manifests clinically as hypotension accompanied by signs of organ hypoperfusion, such as cold skin, oliguria, and depression of the sensorium. If the tissue hypoxia and its inciting process are corrected early enough in the course, recovery is possible. However, due to irreversible injury to vital tissues, recovery from late stages may be impossible, even if hypoperfusion and tissue hypoxia are corrected. Thus, sustained shock is a common cause of the highly lethal syndrome of MOF [2,7].

LACTATE METABOLISM IN NON-SEPTIC SHOCK

In cardiogenic and hypovolemic shock, systemic DO_2 is severely depressed due to some impairment in cardiac function or inadequate cardiac filling. In both types of shock, the systemic vasculature responds by vasoconstriction, which maintains, or partially maintains, systemic blood pressure in the face of the low flow state. Systemic tissues respond to the inadequate DO_2 by increasing their level of oxygen extraction. Some tissues can increase their extraction fraction threefold in the face of a severely inadequate DO_2. The increased extraction results in a decrease in mixed venous oxygen saturation (SvO_2) in the venous effluent from affected tissues. Whereas oxygen uptake and aerobic metabolism normally are determined by metabolic demands, in these low-flow forms of shock VO_2 is limited by the availability of oxygen at the tissue level. Under these conditions, some vital tissues will not be able to meet all their needs for ATP by the usual aerobic pathways.

In an attempt to meet these needs, cells can utilize a modification of the first step of glucose metabolism, foregoing the 3 steps described previously. This modification adds one reaction, catalyzed by LDH, to convert much or all of the produced pyruvate to lactate [25,26]:

The advantage of this foreshortened pathway is that ATP production can proceed entirely anaerobically. However, because only 2 ATP molecules are produced from each glucose, it is only about 5% as efficient at producing ATP compared to the complete 4-step process that requires oxygen.

In aerobic metabolism, NADH produced by generation of pyruvate and other intermediates is converted back to NAD^+ by oxidative metabolism within the mitochondria, maintaining a normal ratio of $NADH:NAD^+$. NADH accumulates in hypoxia, which raises the $NADH:NAD^+$ ratio within the cytosol and helps drive the conversion of pyruvate to lactate. Thus, cellular hypoxia results in net lactate generation and raises the redox state of the cell, as reflected by raised $NADH:NAD^+$. Correspondingly, the L:P ratio is increased substantially above the normal 10:1 ratio [15,16].

Utilization of ATP, whether produced aerobically or anaerobically, results in the liberation of hydrogen ions by:

$$ATP \longrightarrow ADP + Phosphate + H^+$$

During aerobic metabolism and oxidative generation of ATP within the mitochondria, these hydrogen ions are, in effect, re-incorporated into ATP, thus maintaining neutral acid-base balance within the cell. The anaerobic production of ATP, on the other hand, does not utilize hydrogen ions. Widespread anaerobic metabolism therefore results in the net production of hydrogen ions as well as lactate ions, clinically detectable as metabolic acidosis and elevated blood lactate concentration.

A complete, global lack of oxygen, as occurs in sustained cardiac arrest, is incompatible with life because anaerobic ATP production alone cannot fulfill the energy needs of the body for more than a matter of minutes. In addition, the ensuing lactic acidosis quickly leads to profound acidosis that can itself have lethal effects. However, if DO_2 is low, but not zero, sufficient ATP production may be possible through a combination of limited aerobic metabolism in conjunction with a degree of anaerobic metabolism to maintain life for a period of hours to days until there is recovery from shock or progression to death from MOF.

These forms of shock are associated with oxygen supply dependency; i.e., a direct relationship between VO_2 and DO_2 when the latter changes incrementally [14,20,26-31]. In non-shock states, VO_2 is independent of DO_2 [32]. The juncture of the dependent and independent portions of the relationship is the critical point. Oxygen extraction is at a maximum and SvO_2 is at its minimum at DO_2 values to the left of this point, and further decreases in DO_2 are met by a corresponding decrease in VO_2. The slope of the supply dependent portion of the relationship corresponds to maximum fractional oxygen extraction. Blood lactate concentration begins to rise as DO_2 decreases below the critical point. These relationships between VO_2, DO_2, SvO_2, and lactate have been demonstrated in animals and in humans with non-septic shock [14,28-30].

LACTATE METABOLISM IN SEPTIC SHOCK

Increased blood lactate concentrations and an increased L:P ratio are characteristic findings in septic shock [1-6,8-22]. In some cases the mechanism is the same as with non-septic shock; i.e., critically subnormal systemic DO_2 leading to tissue hypoxia and anaerobic metabolism. This is a frequently observed response when sepsis is induced in laboratory animals. It can be due to associated hypovolemia, which is common in sepsis and septic shock. Often a hyperdynamic state ensues following volume expansion, but in many cases hypotension does not abate. Another mechanism of critically decreased DO_2 is myocardial depression caused by sepsis. Human volunteers injected with endotoxin develop impaired left ventricular function as manifest by decreased left ventricular ejection fraction [33]. There is evidence that this myocardial depression is mediated by tumor necrosis factor (TNF), various interleukins (IL), and nitric oxide (NO) [34]. Findings of abnormal cardiac contractility can occur despite increased cardiac output; the latter being a function of additional factors, including ventricular preload and afterload. Hypovolemia and impaired contractility can be severe enough to cause oxygen supply dependency in some patients with sepsis. The mechanism of increased lactate production in sepsis accompanied by these abnormalities is potentially no different than in other forms of shock [13,14,35,36].

Although systemic perfusion, VO_2, and DO_2 are low in some cases of septic shock, in many cases they are actually elevated above typical resting levels, especially after fluid loading [8,9,11,13,16,20,31,36,37]. Sepsis evokes a systemic inflammatory response that results in a hypermetabolic state. This is analogous to vigorous exercise or seizures, in which skeletal muscle requirements for oxygen greatly increase and are largely met by increased systemic DO_2 due to increased cardiac output. Hyperdynamic sepsis is similarly associated with both increased VO_2 and increased DO_2, although tissues other than skeletal muscle can be involved. However, if systemic oxygen requirements outstrip the ability of the cardiovascular and respiratory systems to supply oxygen to peripheral tissues, oxygen supply dependency can occur despite systemic DO_2 levels that are above the usual critical point [38].

Raised critical DO_2 points, associated with elevated blood lactate levels, have been demonstrated in bacteremic animal models of sepsis [31]. Systemic DO_2 at or above normal resting levels could similarly occur in association with supply dependency due to marked elevations in metabolic rate [1,8,13,20,36,39]. Thus, regardless of the level of systemic DO_2, septic shock associated with oxygen supply dependency could suffice to explain the associated lactate elevation [9]. Whether other mechanisms may also be involved in raising lactate levels is difficult to examine under these conditions, but can be studied in animal models and patients with sepsis not associated with frank clinical shock or oxygen supply dependency.

LACTATE METABOLISM IN SEPSIS WITHOUT SHOCK

The blood lactate concentration is frequently increased in patients with sepsis but without obvious clinical signs of septic shock. In a prospective, multicenter study, sepsis was shown to be the most common cause of lactic acidosis in the absence of shock [19]. Raised blood lactate levels are also observed in some animal models of sepsis without manifestations of circulatory shock. There are several potential explanations for these observations (Figure 1).

Occult Tissue Hypoxia

Clinical manifestations of shock, septic or otherwise, may not manifest immediately when perfusion is critically compromised. Thus, although hypotension is often regarded as a *sine qua non* of shock, inadequate vital organ perfusion can occur without hypotension. This can result in elevated systemic lactate concentrations that are due to anaerobic metabolism and tissue hypoxia from absolute or relative hypoperfusion or decreased DO_2.

One reason for this finding is the wide range in baseline systemic arterial blood pressures that occur. Just as some healthy adults can have a resting blood pressure of 80/60 mm Hg, some patients may have a statistically normal blood pressure in spite of a considerable decrease relative to their usual baseline pressure. Even if blood pressure is within a particular subject's acceptable range, perfusion to vital organs may still be critically impaired without hypotension. When this manifests as hyperlactatemia, the term 'incipient shock' has been used, because in many cases the situation progresses to hypotension and frank cardiovascular collapse in a matter of hours, associated with a high fatality rate [18,24,40].

A variety of factors can impair capillary blood flow in sepsis and potentially result in tissue hypoxia (Figure 1-1). Sepsis is associated with activation of the coagulation system and microvascular fibrin deposition. Interference with microvascular perfusion secondary to this phenomenon has been postulated as a mechanism by which organ dysfunction occurs in sepsis [41]. Alterations in blood cell deformability and other factors influencing blood rheology have been described in sepsis and could also impact microvascular DO$_2$ [42]. Interstitial edema due to increased vascular permeability occurs commonly in the lungs of patients with sepsis, and it can similarly occur in systemic tissues. Edema involving the pericapillary interstitium of vital tissues could sufficiently increase the diffusion distance between some cells and their nutritive capillaries to thereby limit oxygen availability to those cells.

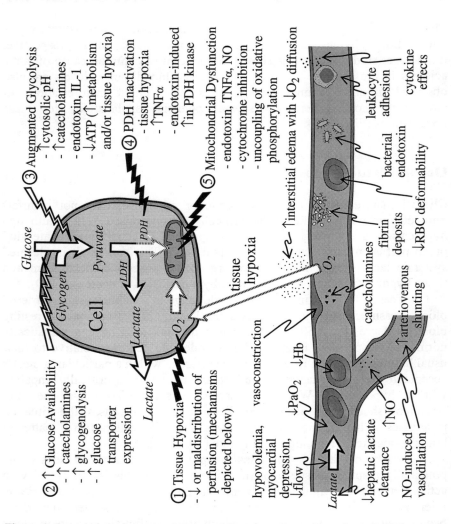

Figure 1. *Proposed mechanisms of increased lactate production in sepsis. Circled numbers are referenced in the text. Open jagged lines: stimulation; filled jagged lines: inhibition. PDH: pyruvate dehydrogenase; LDH: lactate dehydrogenase; RBC: red blood cell; Hb: hemoglobin; NO: nitric oxide*

When DO_2 is inadequate to meet tissue demands, it is most often due to inadequate perfusion. The other component of DO_2, arterial blood oxygen content, is also a potential contributory factor when there is significant anemia or hypoxemia. Perfusion that is otherwise marginally adequate can become inadequate in the face of co-existing severe anemia or hypoxemia.

Impaired Hepatic Lactate Clearance

Lactate diffusing out of lactate-producing cells enters the bloodstream where it is available to other tissues. Myocardium, e.g., preferentially takes up lactate, converts it to pyruvate, and then oxidizes it to produce ATP. Skeletal muscle can similarly utilize lactate under certain conditions. The liver and kidney can do the same, but these two organs can also utilize lactate to produce glucose via gluconeogenesis. Oxygen is required for all of these metabolic activities. Shock curtails this normal utilization of lactate, resulting in decreased lactate clearance. Because the liver is a major lactate consumer, severe hepatic dysfunction has long been considered a cause of lactic acidosis. However, patients with severe liver disease do not typically develop marked elevations of blood lactate in the absence of signs of shock [43]. Underlying hepatic disease does decrease hepatic lactate clearance, causing a higher and more prolonged level of hyperlactatemia for a given hypoxic insult [25].

Clinically, sepsis is not infrequently associated with biochemical evidence of hepatic injury. Animal models of sepsis have shown increased splanchnic lactate production in conjunction with impaired hepatic lactate extraction, without apparent reduction in splanchnic DO_2 [5]. Patients with sepsis, but without clinical signs of septic shock, have been shown to have decreased hepatic lactate clearance, but the degree of hyperlactatemia documented in these studies is quite mild [44]. Thus, while impaired lactate clearance may be a factor that contributes to increased blood lactate levels in sepsis, it is unlikely to be the major factor.

Accelerated Pyruvate Generation

Cellular mechanisms other than, or in addition to, tissue hypoxia could be involved in causing the hyperlactatemia of sepsis. One hypothesis is that pyruvate is generated at a rate that is faster than the normal ability of the cell to utilize it (Figure 1-2 and 1-3). This occurs in tissue hypoxia because decreased ATP and increased ADP levels stimulate the conversion of glucose to pyruvate, but the lack of oxygen prevents oxidation of the pyruvate. In the absence of hypoxia, some other mechanism could be proposed that enhances intracellular glucose availability and/or accelerates the rate of conversion of glucose to pyruvate at a rate beyond which the mitochondria can utilize the resulting pyruvate, even when oxygen is not rate limiting. Pyruvate can also be derived from the amino acid alanine by way of the enzyme alanine aminotransferase. Thus, increased intracellular protein catabolism could conceivably augment pyruvate production in sepsis.

Catecholamines are known to be involved in glucose metabolism, and their circulating levels are elevated in sepsis. In some tissues they may have enough of a calorigenic effect to raise regional oxygen requirements relative to available DO_2 and cause local supply dependency. Epinephrine increases glucose availability by stimulating glycogen breakdown in liver and muscle. Utilization of glucose derived from intracellular glycogen could accelerate pyruvate generation, which might not be oxidized in cells that either lack available oxygen or do not require extra ATP. If ATP is not needed, there would be no supply dependency, but lactate levels will rise due to accumulating pyruvate. In support of this, administration of epinephrine modestly increases blood lactate levels in normal subjects and causes further elevations in patients with septic shock [6,15].

In animals, endotoxin administration results in elevated lactate levels associated with increased plasma glucose concentration and augmented whole body glucose production [45]. Similarly, animals made septic by cecal ligation and puncture show increased glucose uptake and oxidation [46]. Using isotopic tracers, Gore et al. found significantly higher rates of pyruvate production and oxidation in patients with sepsis-associated lactic acidosis compared to control subjects [11]. The increased glucose uptake observed in muscle of animals with intra-abdominal sepsis is associated with increased expression of glucose transporter proteins [47]. IL-1 has been implicated as a mediator in this process, as shown by attenuation in the endotoxin-induced hyperlactatemia in rats following administration of IL-1 receptor antagonist (IL-1ra) [45].

Another potential mechanism of accelerated pyruvate generation that does not necessarily involve tissue hypoxia is respiratory alkalosis. This acid-base disturbance is common in sepsis, and the associated increases in systemic pH could lead to increased blood lactate levels. A rise in cytosolic pH is known to stimulate the activity of the rate-limiting enzyme controlling the conversion of glucose to pyruvate. Respiratory alkalosis is associated with increased blood lactate, probably by this mechanism, although the impact on blood levels is small [25,48].

Decreased PDH Activity

Another possible mechanism to explain increased lactate levels in sepsis, independent of tissue hypoxia, is an intracellular metabolic derangement that interferes with normal oxidative metabolism. In this case, DO_2 may be normal or even elevated, but some impediment to normal aerobic metabolism results in a lower VO_2 or lower fractional oxygen extraction. Diminished oxygen extraction translates to a higher than normal SvO_2 at the prevailing level of oxygen demand, which is frequently observed in patients with sepsis [38].

Decreased activity of the enzyme PDH impairs normal pyruvate oxidation and thus fits this model (Figure 1-4). There is evidence that PDH activity is decreased in hypoxia [49], but this may be immaterial if there is inadequate oxygen to allow oxidation of acetate. More relevant to sepsis without hypoxia is evidence from animal models of sepsis that PDH activity is decreased secondary to inactivation by PDH kinase [21]. TNF may be a mediator in this process since both increases in plasma lactate as well as inhibition of PDH activity were attenuated by administration of a TNF binding protein [22]. However, the findings of Gore and associates showing substantially elevated pyruvate production and oxidation rates in patients with sepsis-associated lactic acidosis suggests that PDH activity is not impaired in human sepsis [11].

Mitochondrial Dysfunction

Derangements of mitochondrial structure and function induced by endotoxin, or endogenous mediators such as cytokines or NO, have been invoked as a cause of impaired oxidative metabolism (Figure 1-5) [18,50-52]. One theory is that these or other substances inhibit mitochondrial cytochromes involved in the electron transport system, thereby stopping oxidative metabolism in a fashion analogous to cyanide poisoning. Oxygen could be amply available at the tissue level, but the affected cells unable to utilize it for oxidative metabolism. Decreased cytochrome activity has been observed in cell cultures in which NO synthase (NOS) was induced by incubation with endotoxin. This decrease in cytochrome activity was associated with increased lactate production, and prevented by the addition of methylarginine, an inhibitor of NOS [52]. Endotoxin has also been shown to impair oxidative phosphorylation *in vivo* by reducing intestinal cytochromes in a dose-related fashion [18]. Another hypothesis is that putative sepsis mediators could uncouple oxidative phosphorylation, analogous to the effects of dinitrophenol. In this case, substrate and oxygen would be utilized at an accelerated rate; however, because the process of phosphorylating ADP is uncoupled from electron transport, ATP is not produced.

Anatomic Arteriovenous Shunting

Theoretically, the development of anatomic shunts through non-nutritive vascular beds could divert arterial blood away from vital tissues and, if sufficiently widespread, deprive those tissues of needed perfusion. Regionally or systemically, the result would be a shallower than normal slope to the supply dependency portion of the VO_2 versus DO_2 curve [32], a phenomenon termed 'pathological supply dependency' [27,38]. As with the putative mechanisms involving interference with cellular aerobic metabolism, systemic SvO_2 could increase with anatomic arteriovenous shunting, even to levels higher than normal, despite the existence of hypoperfusion and increased lactate production at the level of metabolizing tissue. Although increases in SvO_2 are observed in many cases of sepsis, and anatomic shunting provides a mechanistic explanation for this observation, studies by Archie largely refuted the presence of significant systemic arteriovenous shunting in animal models of sepsis [35]. Nevertheless, some degree of anatomic shunting involving the splanchnic and renal circulation was demonstrated in these investigations.

Vasomotor Dysregulation

A final mechanism to explain the presence of increased lactate in the face of high levels of systemic DO_2, pathologic supply dependency, and lactate accumulation is a derangement of the microvasculature that interferes with normal matching of perfusion to metabolic requirements. Normally, local tissue perfusion is controlled so as to match the local requirements for VO_2 [32,38]. As a result, tissues of high metabolic demand (e.g., brain, myocardium, and exercising skeletal muscle) receive more perfusion than tissues with low oxygen requirements (e.g., skin, soft tissue, and resting skeletal muscle). This vasomotor control of the distribution of perfusion appears to be mediated at least in part by the endogenous vasodilator nitric oxide, generated locally by vascular endothelial cells just upstream of the target tissue (Figure 1-1) [12]. Endothelin, an endogenous vasoconstrictor, may similarly be involved.

Systemic vascular resistance, fractional oxygen extraction, and blood lactate levels all correlate with NO production and endothelin levels in patients with hyperdynamic sepsis and hyperlactatemia [12]. A model thus unfolds in which sepsis-induced cytokine production mediates excessive NO generation in some circulatory regions, leading to vasodilation and blood flow that is increased out of proportion to the local metabolic demands for oxygen. This vasomotor dysregulation results in physiologic shunting, leading to elevated SvO_2 from the affected site and, potentially, tissue hypoxia, pathological supply dependency and increased lactate production at other sites that are thereby deprived of perfusion [32,38]. Studies in septic rats have shown decreased functional capillary density and increased spatial heterogeneity of perfused capillaries consistent with this effect [53]. Also consistent with this model are clinical investigations in patients with sepsis demonstrating increased systemic VO_2 and/or decreased lactate levels following augmentation of DO_2 [1,8,13,14,36].

CONCLUSION

An increased blood lactate concentration is clearly a marker for circulatory failure and tissue hypoxia, including that associated with sepsis. Whether other mechanisms cause or contribute to lactate elevations in sepsis remains to be clearly elucidated. Hypermetabolism induced by a systemic inflammatory state, along with dysregulation of the microcirculatory distribution of perfusion, are likely explanations for the co-existence of hyperlactatemia, a hyperdynamic circulation, and a low oxygen extraction state as seen in many cases of clinical sepsis. High blood lactate levels in the patient with sepsis should alert the clinician to consider the possibility of inadequate tissue perfusion and oxygenation.

REFERENCES

1. Astiz ME, Rackow EC, Falk JL, et al. Oxygen delivery and consumption in patients with hyperdynamic septic shock. Crit Care Med 1987; 15:26-28
2. Bakker J, Gris P, Coffernils M, et al. Serial blood lactate levels can predict the development of multiple organ failure following septic shock. Am J Surg 1996; 171:221-226
3. Bakker J, Coffernils M, Leon M, et al. Blood lactate levels are superior to oxygen-derived variables in predicting outcome in human septic shock. Chest 1991; 99:956-962
4. Bernardin G, Pradier C, Tiger F, et al. Blood pressure and arterial lactate level are early predictors of short-term survival in human septic shock. Intensive Care Med 1996; 22:17-25
5. Chrusch C, Bands C, Bose D, et al. Impaired hepatic extraction and increased splanchnic production contribute to lactic acidosis in canine sepsis. Am J Respir Crit Care Med 2000; 161:517-526
6. Day NPJ, Phu NH, Bethell DP, et al. The effects of dopamine and adrenaline infusions

on acid-base balance and systemic haemodynamics in severe infection. Lancet 1996; 348:219-223

7. Duke TD, Butt W, South M. Predictors of mortality and multiple organ failure in children with sepsis. Intensive Care Med 1997; 23:684-692

8. Esen F, Telci L, Çakar N, et al. Evaluation of gastric intramucosal pH measurements with tissue oxygenation indices in patients with severe sepsis. Clin Intensive Care 1996; 7:180-189

9. Friedman G, De Backer D, Shahla M, et al. Oxygen supply dependency can characterize septic shock. Intensive Care Med 1998; 24:118-123

10. Friedman G, Berlot G, Kahn RJ, et al. Combined measurement of blood lactate and gastric intramucosal pH in patients with severe sepsis. Crit Care Med 1995; 23:1184-1193

11. Gore DC, Jahoor F, Hibbert JM, et al. Lactic acidosis during sepsis is related to increased pyruvate production, not deficits in tissue oxygen availability. Ann Surg 1996; 224:97-102

12. Groeneveld AB, Hartemink KJ, de Groot MC, et al. Circulating endothelin and nitrate-nitrite relate to hemodynamic and metabolic variables in human septic shock. Shock 1999; 11:1 60-166

13. Haupt MT, Gilbert EM, Carlson RW. Fluid loading increases oxygen consumption in septic patients with lactic acidosis. Am Rev Respir Dis 1985; 131:912-916

14. Kaufman BS, Rackow EC, Falk JL. The relationship between oxygen delivery and consumption during fluid resuscitation of hypovolemic and septic shock. Chest 1984; 85:336-340

15. Levy B, Bollaert P-E, Charpentier C, et al. Comparison of norepinephrine and dobutamine to epinephrine for hemodynamics, lactate metabolism, and gastric tonometric variables in septic shock: a prospective, randomized study. Intensive Care Med 1997; 23:282-287

16. Levy B, Sadoune L-O, Gelot A-M, et al. Evolution of lactate/pyruvate and arterial ketone body ratios in the early course of catecholamine-treated septic shock. Crit Care Med 2000; 28:114-119

17. Marecaux G, Pinsky MR, Dupont E, et al. Blood lactate levels are better prognostic indicators than TNF and IL-6 levels in patients with septic shock. Intensive Care Med 1996; 22:404-408

18. Schaefer CF, Lerner MR, Biber B. Dose-related reduction of intestinal cytochrome a,a3 induced by endotoxin in rats. Circ Shock 1991; 33:17-25

19. Stacpoole PW, Wright EC, Baumgartner TG, et al. Natural history and course of acquired lactic acidosis. Am J Med 1994; 97:47-54

20. Tuchschmidt J, Fried J, Swinney R, et al. Early hemodynamic correlates of survival in patients with septic shock. Crit Care Med 1989; 17:719-723

21. Vary TC. Sepsis-induced alterations in pyruvate dehydrogenase complex activity in rat skeletal muscle: effects on plasma lactate. Shock 1996; 6:89-94

22. Vary TC, Hazen SA, Maish G, et al. TNF binding protein prevents hyperlactatemia and inactivation of PDH complex in skeletal muscle during sepsis. J Surg Res 1998; 80:44-51

23. Vincent J-L, Dufaye P, Berré J, et al. Serial lactate determinations during circulatory shock. Crit Care Med 1983; 11:449-451

24. Aduen J, Bernstein WK, Khastgir T, et al. The use and clinical importance of a substrate-specific electrode for rapid determination of blood lactate concentrations. JAMA 1994; 272:1678-1685

25. Kruse JA. Lactic acidosis. In: Carlson RW, Geheb MA (eds). Principles & practice of medical intensive care. WB Saunders, Philadelphia, 1993, pp 1231-1245

26. Kruse JA. The cellular basis of conventional and experimental pharmacotherapies for circulatory shock. Anaesth Pharmacol Rev 1994; 2:115-127

27. Kruse JA, Carlson RW. The use of vasoactive drugs to support oxygen transport in sepsis. Crit Care Med 1991; 19:144-146

28. Guzman JA, Lacoma FJ, Najar A, et al. End-tidal PCO_2 as a noninvasive indicator of systemic oxygen supply-dependency during hemorrhagic shock and resuscitation. Shock 1997; 8:427-431

29. Guzman JA, Lacoma FJ, Kruse JA. Relationship between systemic oxygen supply dependency and gastric intramucosal PCO_2 during progressive hemorrhage. J Trauma 1998; 44:696-700

30. Shibutani K, Komatsu T, Kubal K, et al. Critical level of oxygen delivery in anesthetized man. Crit Care Med 1983; 11:640-643

31. Nelson DP, Beyer C, Samsel RW, et al. Pathological supply dependence of O_2 uptake during bacteremia in dogs. J Appl Physiol 1987; 63:1487-1492

32. Kruse JA. Blood lactate and oxygen transport. Intensive Care World 1987; 4:121-125

33. Suffredini AF, Fromm RE, Parker MM, et al. The cardiovascular response of normal humans to the administration of endotoxin. N Engl J Med 1989; 321:280-287

34. Cain BS, Meldrum DR, Dinarello CA, et al. Tumor necrosis factor-□ and interleukin-1□ synergistically depress human myocardial function. Crit Care Med 1999; 27:1309-1318

35. Archie JP Jr. Anatomic arterial-venous shunting in endotoxic and septic shock in dogs. Ann Surg 1977; 186:171-176

36. Bollaert PE, Bauer P, Audibert G, et al. Effects of epinephrine on hemodynamics and oxygen metabolism in dopamine-resistant septic shock. Chest 1990; 98:949-953

37. Guzman JA, Lacoma FJ, Kruse JA. Gastric and esophageal intramucosal PCO_2 ($PiCO_2$) during endotoxemia: Assessment of raw $PiCO_2$ vs PCO_2 gradients as indicators of hypoperfusion in a canine model of septic shock. Chest 1998; 113:1078-1083

38. Kruse JA. Lactic acidosis: Understanding pathogenesis and causes. J Crit Illness 1999; 14:456-466

39. Lucking SE, Williams TM, Chaten FC, et al. Dependence of oxygen consumption on oxygen delivery in children with hyperdynamic septic shock and low oxygen extraction. Crit Care Med 1990; 18:1316-1319

40. Kruse JA. Lactic acidosis: Clinical significance, diagnosis, and treatment. J Crit Illness 1999; 14:514-521

41. Hesselvik JF, Blombäck M, Brodin B, et al. Coagulation, fibrinolysis, and kallikrein systems in sepsis: relation to outcome. Crit Care Med 1989; 17:724-733

42. Astiz ME, DeGent GE, Lin RY, et al. Microvascular function and rheologic changes in hyperdynamic sepsis. Crit Care Med 1995; 23:265-271

43. Kruse JA, Zaidi SAJ, Carlson RW. Significance of blood lactate in critically ill patients with liver disease. Am J Med 1987; 83:77-82

44. Levraut J, Ciebiera J-P, Chave S, et al. Mild hyperlactatemia in stable patients is due to impaired lactate clearance rather than overproduction. Am J Respir Crit Care Med 1998; 157:1021-1026

45. Lang CH, Cooney R, Vary TC. Central interleukin-1 partially mediates endotoxin-induced changes in glucose metabolism. Am J Physiol 1996; 271:E309-E316

46. Haji-Michael PG, Ladriere L, Sener A, et al. Leukocyte glycolysis and lactate output in animal sepsis and ex vivo human blood. Metabol Clin Exp 1999; 48:779-785

47. Vary TC, Drnevich D, Jurasinski C, et al. Mechanisms regulating skele-tal muscle glucose metabolism in sepsis. Shock 1995; 3:403-410

48. Guzman JA, Kruse JA. Splanchnic hemodynamics and gut mucosal-arterial PCO_2 gradient during systemic hypocapnia. J Appl Physiol 1999; 87:1102-1106

49. Vary TC, Randle PJ. The effect of ischaemia on the activity of pyruvate dehydrogenase complex in rat heart. J Mol Cell Cardiol 1984; 16:723-733
50. Guo Y, Wu Y, Chen W, et al. Endotoxic damage to the stria vascularis:the pathogenesis of sensorineural hearing loss secondary to otitis media. J Laryngol Otol 1994; 108:310-313
51. Szabó C, Day BJ, Salzman AL. Evaluation of the relative contribution of nitric oxide and peroxynitrite to the suppression of mitochondrial respiration in immunostimulated macrophages using a manganese mesoporphyrin superoxide dismutase mimetic and peroxynitrite scavenger. FEBS Lett 1996; 381:82-86
52. Bolanos JP, Peuchen S, Heales SJ, et al. Nitric oxide-mediated inhibition of the mitochondrial respiratory chain in cultured astrocytes. J Neurochem 1994; 63:910-916
53. Lam C, Tyml K, Martin C, et al. Microvascular perfusion is impaired in a rat model of normotensive sepsis. J Clin Invest 1994; 94:2077-2083

19

VENO-ARTERIAL PCO$_2$ GRADIENT

Vincent Castelain
Jean-Louis Teboul

DEFINITIONS

The veno-arterial carbon dioxide (CO_2) tension (PCO_2) gradient (ΔPCO_2) is the difference between the PCO_2 in mixed venous blood ($PvCO_2$) and the PCO_2 in arterial blood ($PaCO_2$):

$$\Delta PCO_2 = PvCO_2 - PaCO_2 \qquad \text{(Eqn 1)}$$

$PaCO_2$ and PvO_2 are the partial pressures of the dissolved CO_2 in arterial and mixed venous blood respectively which represent only a fraction of arterial CO_2 content ($CaCO_2$) and mixed venous CO_2 content ($CvCO_2$) respectively.

CO$_2$ TRANSPORT IN THE BLOOD

CO_2 is carried in the blood in three forms [1]: dissolved, as bicarbonate, and in combination with proteins as carbamino compounds. CO_2 is about 20 times more soluble than oxygen (O_2), so that the dissolved form plays a more significant role in the normal carriage in the blood.

Bicarbonate is formed in the blood by the following sequence:

$$CO_2 + H_2O \Leftrightarrow H_2CO_3 \Leftrightarrow HCO_3^- + H^+ \qquad \text{(Eqn 2)}$$

where H_2O is water, H_2CO_3 is carbonic acid, HCO_3^- is bicarbonate ion and H^+ is hydrogen ion. The first reaction is very slow in the plasma, but fast in the red blood cell (RBC), because of the presence in this cell of carbonic anhydrase. The second reaction occurs rapidly within the RBC and does not need any enzyme. When the concentrations of HCO_3^- and H^+ in the cell rise, HCO_3^- diffuses out of the RBC into the plasma but H^+ cannot diffuse easily because the cell membrane is relatively impermeable to cations. Some of the H^+ liberated are bound to hemoglobin (Hb):

$$H^+ + HbO_2 \Leftrightarrow H\text{-}Hb + O_2 \qquad \text{(Eqn 3)}$$

This reaction occurs because reduced Hb is a better acceptor of H^+ than the oxygenated Hb. In the peripheral blood the loading of CO_2 is facilitated by the presence of reduced Hb (Haldane effect) [1]. Thus unloading oxygen in peripheral capillaries facilitates the loading of CO_2 while oxygenation enhances the unloading of CO_2 in the lung [2].

Carbamino compounds are formed by the combination of CO_2 with terminal amine groups of blood protein, especially the globin of Hb. Reduced Hb can load much more CO_2 as carbamino compounds than HbO_2.

The greater part of the CO_2 content (CCO_2) is in the form of bicarbonate. The relationship between the PCO_2 and the total CCO_2 is curvilinear although more linear than the oxygen dissociation curve [1]. Hematocrit, oxygen saturation, temperature and pH influence the PCO_2/CCO_2 relationship [1].

DETERMINANTS OF VENOARTERIAL CO₂ GRADIENT

The Fick Equation

The Fick equation applied to CO_2, indicates that the CO_2 excretion (equivalent to CO_2 production in a steady state) equals the product of cardiac output by the difference between CO_2 content in mixed venous blood ($CvCO_2$) and arterial blood ($CaCO_2$):

$$VCO_2 = \text{cardiac output} \times (CvCO_2 - CaCO_2) \qquad \text{(Eqn 4)}$$

The normal relationship between pressure and content of CO_2 is almost linear over the usual physiological range of the CO_2 contents so that PCO_2 can be taken as a measure of the CO_2 content of the blood [3,4]. Therefore, by rearranging the Fick equation and substituting PCO_2 for CCO_2, a modified Fick equation can be obtained:

$$VCO_2 = \text{cardiac output} \times k \times \Delta PCO_2 \text{ so that} \qquad \text{(Eqn 5)}$$
$$\Delta PCO_2 = k \times VCO_2 / \text{cardiac output} \qquad \text{(Eqn 6)}$$

where k is assumed to be constant.

Therefore, ΔPCO_2 would be linearly related to CO_2 production and inversely related to cardiac output.

Influence of CO_2 Production on ΔPCO_2

Aerobic CO_2 Production

At the cellular level, the aerobic CO_2 generation is a normal terminal product of oxidative metabolism. Thus, under aerobic conditions CCO_2 in the effluent venous blood must be higher than in the afferent arterial blood. Under these normal conditions, the total CO_2 production (VCO_2) is directly related to global oxygen consumption (VO_2):

$$VCO_2 = R \cdot VO_2$$

(Eqn 7)

where R is the respiratory quotient, that may vary between 0.7 and 1.0 with respect to the predominant energy source; for instance when lipids are the major fuel sources, R is close to 0.7 whereas under conditions of high carbohydrate intake R approaches 1.0.

Therefore, the aerobic CO_2 production should augment with increased oxidative metabolism or for a constant VO_2 when an equilibrated feeding regimen is replaced by a high carbohydrate intake regimen. Under both conditions, $CvCO_2$ - $CaCO_2$ and ΔPCO_2 should increase except if cardiac output increases to the same extent.

Anaerobic CO_2 Production

Under hypoxic conditions, H^+ ions are generated by two mechanisms [5]:
- excessive production of lactic acid owing to an acceleration of anaerobic glycolysis, since pyruvate is no longer cleared by the Krebs cycle;
- hydrolysis of adenosine triphosphate (ATP) and of adenosine diphosphate (ADP) that occurs in conditions of anaerobiosis.

HCO_3^- ions will then buffer H^+ ions into the cell so that CO_2 will be generated.

Anaerobic decarboxylation of some substrates produced by intermediate metabolism (α ketoglutarate or oxaloacetate) is a potential but minor source of anaerobic CO_2 production [5].

Anaerobic production of CO_2 in hypoxic organs is difficult to detect. Indeed, venous blood flow can be sufficiently high to wash out the CO_2 produced from the tissues under these circumstances of a marked fall in aerobic CO_2 production. Therefore, PCO_2 could be not augmented in the draining vein and anaerobic CO_2 production not detected. However, if afferent and efferent blood flows are artificially stopped, hypoxia will ensue within the organ and the continued anaerobic CO_2 generation would then be detected by measuring an increased PCO_2 either in the organ itself or in the stagnant efferent venous blood flow, and this despite the fall in aerobic CO_2 production. In experimental models of myocardial ischemia induced by ventricular fibrillation or prolonged coronary artery occlusion, striking elevations of PCO_2 consistent with anaerobic CO_2 production were measured in the myocardium and in the cardiac vein [6, 7].

Influence of Cardiac Output on ΔPCO₂

According to the modified Fick equation, ΔPCO_2 is inversely correlated to cardiac output. In experimental studies in which cardiac output was gradually reduced, under conditions of stable VO_2 and VCO_2 [8-11], ΔPCO_2 was observed to increase along with the decrease in cardiac output. Elevation of ΔPCO_2 following cardiac output reduction, under conditions of stable CO_2 production, can be explained by the CO_2 stagnation phenomenon. Because of the slowing of transit time a greater than normal addition of CO_2 per unit of blood traversing the peripheral efferent microvessels tends to generate hypercapnia in the venous circulation. As long as pulmonary ventilation is adequate, as cardiac output drops, a gradient will develop between $PvCO_2$ and $PaCO_2$. However, some authors [12,13] observed in animals allowed to breathe spontaneously, increases in ΔPCO_2 associated with cardiac output reduction and VO_2 stability, that had resulted from a decrease in $PaCO_2$ but an unchanged $PvCO_2$. Indeed, under spontaneous breathing conditions, hyperventilation stimulated by the reduced blood flow, may decrease $PaCO_2$ and then may limit the CO_2 stagnation-associated increase in $PvCO_2$ that would have occurred if $PaCO_2$ was not decreased. This finding underlines the usefulness of calculating ΔPCO_2 rather than simply measuring $PvCO_2$, especially under conditions of spontaneous breathing [14].

CAN ΔPCO₂ BE USED AS A MARKER OF TISSUE HYPOXIA ?

In cardiac arrest-resuscitated animal or patients, striking increases in ΔPCO_2 have been reported [15-17]. These findings were ascribed to the reduced blood flow during resuscitation manoeuvers [15,16] and to the development of anaerobic metabolism following cardiorespiratory arrest [17]. Adrogue et al. [17] also reported a venoarterial PCO_2 gradient greater in patients with circulatory failure, than in those without circulatory failure. From these observations, it was postulated that anaerobic CO_2 production may play a major role in the widening PCO_2 gradient under conditions of low flow states with tissue hypoxia. Thus, some authors have proposed to use ΔPCO_2 to detect tissue hypoxia or dysoxia in critically ill patients [8-10]. In fact, this is a much more complex issue than it appears, as confirmed by the existence of divergent reports in the recent literature that require further explanation.

Animal Studies

Tissue Hypoxia Induced by Reduced Blood Flow

Most studies that have addressed the issue of detecting tissue hypoxia by analysis of ΔPCO_2, used protocols of reducing blood flow. Zhang and Vincent [10] compared the values of ΔPCO_2 and venoarterial pH gradient with that of blood lactate in their relationship to changes in VO_2 and O_2 delivery (DO_2) during an acute reduction in blood flow induced by cardiac tamponade in dogs. As mentioned above, they observed during the oxygen supply independent period, a reduction in cardiac output from 4.1 ± 1.0 to 1.7 ± 0.6 l/min, a slight increase in ΔPCO_2 from 7.1 ± 4.6 to 17.5 ± 6.6 mm Hg ($p < 0.01$), while a constant VCO_2 was measured. Below the critical level of DO_2 (oxygen supply dependent period), the widening of ΔPCO_2 was magnified by a further increase in $PvCO_2$ and a reduction in $PaCO_2$. Interestingly, below the critical level of DO_2, VCO_2 decreased, while lactate increased. The critical values of DO_2 calculated for VO_2, ΔPCO_2 and lactate did not differ significantly. At the end of the study, ΔPCO_2 was 40.9 ± 14.3 mm Hg while cardiac output was 0.6 ± 0.3 l/min. Interestingly, VO_2 and VCO_2 have been observed to decrease dramatically during this period. Thus, the brisk increase in ΔPCO_2 measured during this phase could have been not due to an increase in production of CO_2 but rather to the major role played by the further reduction in cardiac output, through CO_2 stagnation phenomenon, for the lowest range of cardiac output.

Other authors used a biphasic model of the VO_2/DO_2 relationship in anesthetized dogs [8,9]. By producing a graded hemorrhage, they also found a brisk increase in ΔPCO_2 at the critical level of DO_2. However, the data presented in these studies also suggest that the ΔPCO_2 changes were mostly related to the reduction in cardiac output.

Groeneveld et al. [11] also found a hyperbolic response of ΔPCO_2 to reduction in cardiac output induced by application of incremental levels of positive end-expiratory pressure (PEEP) in pigs. Since the measured VCO_2

decreased with cardiac output during the oxygen supply dependent period, the authors concluded that during hypoperfusion and hypoxia, the increased ΔPCO_2 was caused by a greater reduction in tissue blood flow than in CO_2 production, so that tissue CO_2 removal was impaired [11].

Thus, from the analysis of available experimental data [8-11] it can be reasonably assumed that a sudden increase in ΔPCO_2 should not be readily ascribed to the onset or to the worsening of hypoxia but rather to a further reduction in blood flow.

At least, two mechanisms can explain the predominant role of reduction in cardiac output in ΔPCO_2 under conditions of very low flow:

1) The mathematical curvilinearity of the relationship between ΔCCO_2 and cardiac output (Fick equation), may explain the exaggerated ΔPCO_2 increase for the lowest range of cardiac output. In fact, this mathematical phenomenon is strong under conditions of maintained VCO_2, but attenuated here, because of gradual decreases in VCO_2 simultaneously with decreases in cardiac output (gradual shift from a VCO_2 isopleth to another one) (Figure 1). Therefore this can play only for one part of the marked ΔPCO_2 increase observed during this period.

2) The other reason for the striking widening of ΔPCO_2 may be the curvilinearity of the relationship between $CvCO_2$ and $PvCO_2$. Indeed, we previously assumed that the relationship between CCO_2 and PCO_2 is nearly linear and that the extrapolation of the Fick equation to the modified Fick equation is valid. In fact, this is not true in the highest range of CCO_2 where ΔPCO_2 changes are greater than ΔCCO_2 changes [4]. Reduced pH and high oxygen saturation would further exaggerate disparities between CCO_2 and PCO_2 at high levels of CCO_2 [4]. Consequently, as during low flow states, $CvCO_2$ would be increased because of CO_2 stagnation, $PvCO_2$ would be particularly high so that for a given cardiac output and VCO_2, ΔPCO_2 would be of greater magnitude than previously assumed from the modified Fick equation. This phenomenon may be exaggerated by the fall in venous pH which constantly follows the increase in $PvCO_2$ and may be of further importance if metabolic acidosis coexists.

Tissue Hypoxia with Maintained Blood Flow

We earlier pointed out that under conditions of tissue hypoxia, anaerobic CO_2 production should occur. However, the reduction in aerobic metabolism must decrease the aerobic CO_2 production. If the net resultant effect is a reduction in total CO_2 production as indicated by studies that have addressed this issue

[10,11,18], then ΔPCO_2 would not increase under conditions of normal or high blood flow. Indeed, the lesser quantity of CO_2 produced should easily be removed by a normal or elevated venous blood flow so that $CvCO_2$ and $PvCO_2$ should not increase. To confirm this simple physiological hypothesis, one needs experimental studies in which cell hypoxia would be created by another mechanism than reducing blood flow, for instance hypoxemic hypoxia. Recently, Vallet et al. [19] have addressed this issue in an experimental study. They decreased DO_2 delivery either by decreasing flow (ischemic hypoxia) or by decreasing arterial PO_2 at constant flow (hypoxic hypoxia) in an *in situ*, vascularly isolated, innervated dog hind limb perfused with a pump-membrane oxygenator system. Similar levels of critical DO_2 were obtained in both groups. While limb oxygen uptake linearly decreased in both groups below this level, ΔPCO_2 significantly increased in the ischemic hypoxia group, but never differed from baseline in the hypoxic hypoxia group. The authors concluded that absence of increased ΔPCO_2 does not preclude the presence of tissue dysoxia, and that decreased flow is a major determinant of increased ΔPCO_2 [19].

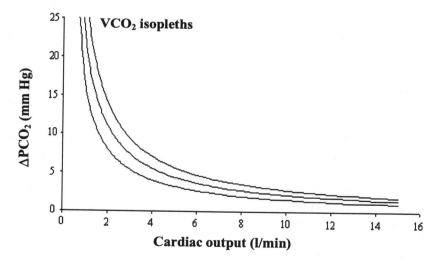

Figure 1. ΔPCO_2 /cardiac output relationships. According to the modified Fick equation, the ΔPCO_2 cardiac output relationship is curvilinear. Therefore for a constant VCO_2, changes in cardiac output result in large changes in ΔPCO_2 in the low values of cardiac output, whereas changes in cardiac output will not result in significant changes in ΔPCO_2 in the high values of cardiac output. These relationships are further complicated when changes in cardiac output are accompanied by changes in VCO_2 and thereby by a transfer from one VCO_2 isopleth to another (on the figure VCO_2 increases from the left to the right).

Clinical Studies

Clinical studies in septic patients have also suggested that reduced blood flow plays the key role in the widening of the CO_2 gradient observed under conditions of low blood flow with tissue hypoxia [20,21]. Mecher et al. [20] found that the subgroup of septic shock patients with ΔPCO_2 > 6 mm Hg (mean ± SEM = 9 ± 1 mmHg) had a mean cardiac output significantly lower than the subgroup of those with ΔPCO_2 ≤ 6 mm Hg. Interestingly, the two subgroups did not differ in terms of blood lactate (6 ± 1 vs 5.7 ± 1.1 mmol/l respectively) and blood pressure (59 ± 3 and 63 ± 4 mm Hg). In other words, many patients of this study (18/37) had a normal ΔPCO_2 despite tissue hypoxia, probably because their high blood flow had easily remove the CO_2 produced at the periphery. In the subgroup of patients with high ΔPCO_2, fluid loading had resulted in a decrease in ΔPCO_2 associated with an increase in cardiac output. The authors reasonably concluded that in patients with septic shock, an increased ΔPCO_2 is associated with a reduced systemic flow. Bakker et al. [21] also demonstrated that in patients with septic shock, ΔPCO_2 was mostly related to cardiac output. In their study including 64 patients with septic shock, only 15 patients had a ΔPCO_2 > 6 mmHg. These patients had a lower cardiac output than the patients with normal ΔPCO_2. Moreover, opposite changes in ΔPCO_2 and in cardiac output during the course of septic shock were observed [21]. Interestingly, patients with a high ΔPCO_2 had similar VO_2 and blood lactate levels than those with a normal ΔPCO_2. Although VCO_2 and VO_2 were not measured directly, these data suggest that differences in CO_2 production did not account for differences in ΔPCO_2 [21]. Clearly, the studies of Mecher et al. [20] and of Bakker et al. [21] have underlined the poor sensitivity of ΔPCO_2 to detect tissue hypoxia, since ΔPCO_2 was normal in most patients with sepsis-related circulatory shock except with those with low cardiac output.

The major role of cardiac output in the widening of ΔPCO_2 was confirmed by the study of Wendon et al. [22] including ten hypotensive patients with fulminant hepatic failure. These patients were assumed to have significant tissue hypoxia, as they demonstrated an increase in VO_2 after prostacyclin infusion. The major finding was that during baseline, ΔPCO_2 was very low (less than 3 mm Hg). This was probably explained by a low production of CO_2 – postulated in view of the low VO_2 (119 ml/min/m^2) - easily removed by the very high level of cardiac output (cardiac index = 5.4 l/min/m^2). These findings underline the fact that tissue hypoxia under conditions of high flow states should result in decreased, rather than increased, ΔPCO_2.

CLINICAL USE OF ΔPCO_2 IN SEPSIS

Interpretation of ΔPCO_2 in Sepsis

Sepsis results in a complex form of shock. Some patients have reductions in systemic blood flow which eventually result in limited oxidative metabolism. In these cases, the low cardiac output is mostly related to sepsis-induced hypovolemia. However, in most patients, in whom early correction of volume depletion by aggressive fluid therapy has resulted in hyperdynamic circulatory state, the impaired oxidative metabolism is related to the inability of tissues to extract sufficient oxygen from the blood [23]. Distributive abnormalities of macrocirculatory and microcirculatory blood flow mainly explain the oxygen extraction impairment that occurs in sepsis [24]. As a consequence, the most frequent hemodynamic profile encountered in human septic shock is characterized by high cardiac output and vasodilation [25-26], although some clinical studies reported relatively low values of cardiac output [20,21] either because of insufficient fluid resuscitation [20] and/or presence of a patent sepsis-induced myocardial depression [23]. As we will discuss below, ΔPCO_2 might take a place in the cardiovascular monitoring of septic shock, by identifying patients in whom cardiac output could be further raised.

ΔPCO_2 can be calculated after simultaneous sampling of arterial blood ($PaCO_2$) and of mixed venous blood from the distal port of a properly placed pulmonary artery catheter ($PvCO_2$). Under physiological conditions, ΔPCO_2 is assumed to be between 2 and 5 mm Hg [2]. As developed above, ΔPCO_2 cannot serve as a reliable marker of tissue hypoxia in septic, as in non septic, conditions. However, ΔPCO_2 could be helpful at the bedside to assess the adequacy of cardiac output relative to global metabolic conditions and to guide therapy aimed at increasing cardiac output. Indeed, according to the Fick equation applied to CO_2, ΔPCO_2 can be considered as a marker of adequacy of venous blood flow (i.e., cardiac output) to remove the total CO_2 produced by the peripheral tissues. The clinical implications of this concept can be summarized as follows:

- An increased ΔPCO_2, may suggest that cardiac output is not high enough with respect to the global metabolic conditions.

- under suspected hypoxic conditions (increased blood lactate levels), the existence of a high ΔPCO_2 could be one of the arguments that will incite the clinician to increase cardiac output in an attempt to reduce tissue hypoxia.
- under suspected aerobic conditions, ΔPCO_2 can be relatively high if cardiac output is low, as evidenced in septic [13] or in non septic animals [10] in which mean values of 15 mm Hg [13] and of 17.5 mm Hg [10] were found to coexist with likely aerobic conditions (oxygen supply independence period). Values as high as 10 to 12 mm Hg were also reported in patients with low cardiac output and normal blood lactates who did not exhibit any oxygen supply dependence after cardiac output was augmented by dobutamine [27]. From all these data, it may reasonably be postulated that observation of a high ΔPCO_2 in a given septic patient without evidence of global tissue hypoxia would mean that blood flow is not high enough, even if the value of cardiac output is measured in the normal range. This condition can be associated with a sepsis-induced increased oxygen demand and hence increased aerobic CO_2 production. However, whether increasing cardiac output to prevent short-term subsequent risks of onset of tissue hypoxia is actually beneficial remains to be proved.

Following the course of ΔPCO_2 can also be helpful to assess the effects on global tissue metabolism, of a therapeutic intervention aimed at increasing cardiac output in a patient with a high initial value of ΔPCO_2. Under conditions of O_2 supply dependence, increase in cardiac output must be accompanied by increases in VO_2 and hence VCO_2 so that ΔPCO_2 is expected to decrease less than in the case of O_2 supply independence. Consequently, relatively unchanged ΔPCO_2 with therapy would not mean that the therapy has failed. In this case, the therapeutic agent would be rather maintained and its dose even augmented until obtaining a frank decrease in ΔPCO_2 that would indicate that the critical level of DO_2 has been actually passed.

In additon, ΔPCO_2 can be helpful in selecting the appropriate dose of a therapeutic agent known to have thermogenic effects. For instance, catecholamines by their β stimulation may exert calorigenic effects and thus are able to increase both VO_2 and VCO_2 [28]. In septic patients without evidence of shock, dobutamine was demonstrated to increase VO_2 and VCO_2 at doses higher than 5 μg/kg/min [29]. Similarly, ΔPCO_2 - as an index of the VCO_2/cardiac output ratio - was shown to be able to detect changes in oxygen demand accompanying dobutamine-induced changes in cardiac output [27]. In this regard, ΔPCO_2 together with SvO_2 [30] may help to titrate drug therapy.

- A normal ΔPCO_2, suggests that cardiac output is high enough to wash out the CO_2 produced from the peripheral tissue. However, whether a normal ΔPCO_2 means that cardiac output has not to be further raised under hypoxic conditions, remains to be established.

Limitations in the Interpretation of ΔPCO_2

When blood flow is high, a frequent condition in sepsis [23], large changes in cardiac output will not result in significant changes in ΔPCO_2, because of the curvilinearity of the relationship between ΔPCO_2 and cardiac output (Figure 1). Indeed, according to the modified Fick equation, for a constant VCO_2, ΔPCO_2 is linearly related to cardiac output in the low values of cardiac output, whereas there is a flattening of the ΔPCO_2/cardiac output relationship curve in the high values of cardiac output [31]. This point was illustrated in a series of patients with high systemic blood flow but without evidence of tissue hypoxia and in whom significant changes in cardiac output were associated with unchanged ΔPCO_2 values [32]. It must be kept in mind that the ΔPCO_2/cardiac output relationship will depend also on the level of VCO_2, so that a family of hyperbolic ΔPCO_2/cardiac output relationship curves for various levels of VCO_2 (VCO_2 isopleths) can be drawn (Figure 1) [31]. As a consequence, interpretation of ΔPCO_2 changes (or of absence of changes) must be particularly cautious under conditions of very high systemic blood flow.

Although a normal ΔPCO_2 would suggest that global blood flow is roughly adequate to the global metabolic condition, it does not preclude inadequacy of blood flow for metabolic conditions at a regional level, for instance in the splanchnic area, as demonstrated in an experimental study [33]. In septic shock patients with high systemic blood low (and presumably low ΔPCO_2) inadequate splanchnic blood flow [34] or an increased difference between gastric mucosal and arterial PCO_2 [26] were reported. This point is of importance because gut mucosal ischemia could play a pivotal role in the pathogenesis of multiple organ failure (MOF) [35].

There are numerous additional potential causes of error in PCO_2 measurements: incorrect sample container; inadequate sample volume relative to anticoagulant volume; sample contaminated by air, venous blood, or catheter fluid; improper transport conditions; length of the delay between acquisition and analysis; technical problems of the blood gas analyzer, etc. Even if all these potential errors are prevented, there is still a proper instrument imprecision of ± 1 mm Hg, even in a laboratory with intense quality control and using the more recent models of blood gas analyzers [36].

This range of error is not so far from the usual range of ΔPCO_2. This point further emphasizes the fact that clinicians must be very careful in the interpretation of low values of ΔPCO_2 and of small changes in ΔPCO_2.

Combined Analysis of ΔPCO_2 and Oxygen-derived Parameters

Indirect evidence of anaerobic CO_2 production under conditions of tissue hypoxia have been brought by studies reporting, along with a decrease in DO_2, decreases in VO_2 and VCO_2 (calculated from expired gas analysis) but with an increased VCO_2/VO_2 ratio [11,18]. Under these conditions, an increased VCO_2/VO_2 ratio indicates that VCO_2 is less reduced than VO_2 when tissue hypoxia occurs. In others words, this probably denotes the presence of anaerobic CO_2 generation in hypoxic tissues. Therefore, the use of an increase in the respiratory quotient has been proposed to detect global tissue hypoxia through detection of anaerobic CO_2 generation [18]. This could be the useful tool that one needs to detect global tissue hypoxia. Since VO_2 is equal to the product of cardiac output and arteriovenous difference in oxygen content $(C_{A-V} O_2)$ and VCO_2 is proportional to the product of cardiac output and ΔPCO_2, the $\Delta PCO_2/C_{A-V} O_2$ ratio could be used to detect global anaerobic metabolism in patients with a pulmonary artery catheter in place. In a series of 100 critically ill patients, we recently found a close correlation between lactatemia and $\Delta PCO_2/C_{A-V} O_2$ ratio, while no correlation was found between lactatemia and ΔPCO_2 alone and between lactatemia and $C_{A-V}O_2$ alone (unpublished data). Further confirmation is obviously required before applying these concepts at the bedside.

CONCLUSION

ΔPCO_2 can be considered as a marker of adequacy of cardiac output relative to global metabolic condition. In patients with sepsis or septic shock monitored by a pulmonary artery catheter, an increased ΔPCO_2 could be an argument in favor of raising cardiac output to prevent or reduce global hypoxia. However, it must be remembered that systemic blood flow is commonly high in septic shock so that ΔPCO_2 is most often in the normal range. Furthermore, in such hyperdynamic states, interpretation of ΔPCO_2 changes (or of absence of changes) must be made with care.

REFERENCES

1. West JB. Gas transport to the periphery: how gases are moved to the peripheral tissues? In: West JB (ed) Respiratory physiology. The essentials, 4th edn. Williams & Wilkins, Baltimore,1990; pp 69-85.
2. Groeneveld ABJ. Interpreting the venous-arterial PCO_2 difference. Crit Care Med 1998; 26:979-980.
3. Giovannini I, Carlo C, Boldrini G, Castagneto M. Calculation of venoarterial CO_2 concentration difference. J Appl Physiol 1993; 74:959-964
4. McHardy GJR. The relationship between the differences in pressure and content of carbon dioxide in arterial and venous blood. Clin Sci 1967; 32:299-309
5. Randall HM, Jr., Cohen JJ. Anaerobic CO_2 production by dog kidney in vitro. Am J Physiol 1966; 211:493-505.
6. Von Planta M, Weil MH, Gazmuri RJ, et al. Myocardial acidosis associated with CO_2 production during cardiac arrest and resuscitation. Circulation 1989; 80:684-92.
7. Kette F, Weil MH, Gazmuri RJ, et al. Intramyocardial hypercarbic acidosis during cardiac arrest and resuscitation. Crit Care Med 1993; 21:901-906
8. Bowles SA, Schlichtig R, Kramer DJ, et al. Arteriovenous pH and partial pressure of carbon dioxide detect critical oxygen delivery during progressive hemorrhage in dogs. J Crit Care 1992; 7:95-105
9. Van der Linden P, Rausin I, Deltell A, et al. Detection of tissue hypoxia by arteriovenous gradient for PCO_2 and pH in anesthetized dogs during progressive hemorrhage. Anesth Analg 1995; 80:269-275
10. Zhang H, Vincent JL. Arteriovenous differences in PCO_2 and pH are good indicators of critical hypoperfusion. Am Rev Respir Dis 1993; 148:867-871
11. Groeneveld AB, Vermeij CG, Thijs LG. Arterial and mixed venous blood acid-base balance during hypoperfusion with incremental positive end-expiratory pressure in the pig. Anesth Analg 1991; 73:576-582
12. Mathias DW, Clifford PS, Klopfenstein HS. Mixed venous blood gases are superior to arterial blood gases in assessing acid-base status and oxygenation during acute cardiac tamponade in dogs. J Clin Invest 1988; 82:833-838
13. Rackow EC, Astiz ME, Mecher CE, Weil MH. Increased venous-arterial carbon dioxide tension difference during severe sepsis in rats. Crit Care Med 1994; 22:121-125
14. Benjamin E. Venous hypercarbia: a nonspecific marker of hypoperfusion. Crit Care Med 1994;22:9-10
15. Grundler W, Weil MH, Rackow EC. Arteriovenous carbon dioxide and pH gradients during cardiac arrest. Circulation 1986; 74:1071-1074
16. Weil MH, Rackow EC, Trevino R, et al. Difference in acid-base state between venous and arterial blood during cardiopulmonary resuscitation. N Engl J Med 1986; 315:153-156
17. Adrogue HJ, Rashad MN, Gorin AB, et al. Assessing acid-base status in circulatory failure. Differences between arterial and central venous blood. N Engl J Med 1989; 320:1312-1316
18. Cohen IL, Sheikh FM, Perkins RJ, et al. Effect of hemorrhagic shock and reperfusion on the respiratory quotient in swine. Crit Care Med 1995; 23:545-552
19. Vallet B, Teboul JL, Cain S, Curtis S. Veno-arterial CO_2 difference during regional ischemic or hypoxic hypoxia. J Appl Physiol 2000; 89:1317-1321
20. Mecher CE, Rackow EC, Astiz ME, et al. Venous hypercarbia associated with severe sepsis and systemic hypoperfusion. Crit Care Med 1990; 18:585-589

21. Bakker J, Vincent JL, Gris P, et al. Veno-arterial carbon dioxide gradient in human septic shock. Chest 1992; 101:509-515
22. Wendon JA, Harrison PM, Keays R, Gimson AE, Alexander G, Williams R. Arterial-venous pH differences and tissue hypoxia in patients with fulminant hepatic failure. Crit Care Med 1991; 19:1362-1364
23. Parillo JE. Pathogenetic mechanisms of septic shock. N Engl J Med 1993; 328:1471-1477
24. Astiz ME, Rackow EC. Septic shock. Lancet 1998; 351:1501-1505
25. Groeneveld ABJ, Bronsveld W, Thijs LG. Hemodynamuic determinants of mortality in human septic shock. Surgery 1986; 99:140-153
26. B Levy, PE Bollaert, C Charpentier, et al. Comparison of norepinephrine and dobutamine to epinephrine for hemodynamics, lactate metabolism and gastric tonometric variables in septic shock. A prospective, randomized study. Intensive Care Med 1997; 23:282-287
27. Teboul Jl, Mercat A, Lenique F, et al. Value of venous-arterial PCO$_2$ gradient to reflect the O$_2$ supply to demand in humans. Crit Care Med 1998; 26:1007-1010
28. Chiolero R, Flatt JP, Revelly JP, et al. Effects of catecholamines on oxygen consumption and oxygen delivery in critically ill patients. Chest 1991; 100:1676-1684
29. De Backer D, Moraine JJ, Berre J, et al. Effects of dobutamine on oxygen consumption in septic patients. Direct versus indirect determinations. Am J Respir Crit Care Med 150; 1994:95-100
30. Teboul JL, Boujdaria R, Graini L, et al. Cardiac index vs oxygen-derived parameters for rational use of dobutamine in patients with congestive heart failure. Chest 1993; 103:81-85
31. Teboul JL, Michard F, Richard C. Critical analysis of venoarterial CO$_2$ gradient as a marker of tissue hysoxia. In Vincent JL (ed) Yearbook of Intensive Care and Emergency Medicine. Springer, Heidelberg, 1996, pp 296-307
32. Bernardin G, Lucas P, Hyvernat H, et al. Influence of alveolar ventilation changes on calculated gastric intramucosal pH and gastric-arterial PCO$_2$ difference. Intensive Care Med 1999; 25:269-273
33. Heino A, Haetikainen J, Merasto ME, et al. Systemic and regional PCO$_2$ gradients as markers of intestinal ischemia. Intensive Care Med 1998; 24:599-604
34. Ruokonen E, Takala J, Kari A, et al. Regional blood flow and oxygen transport in septic shock. Crit Care Med 1993; 21:1296-1303
35. Fiddian-Green RG. Associations between intramucosal acidosis in the gut and organ failure. Crit Care Med 1993; 21: S103-S105
36. Crapo RO. Arterial blood gases: quality assessment. In Tobin M (ed) Principle and Practice of Intensive Care Monitoring, Mc Graw-Hill, New-York, 1998, pp 107-122

20

GAS TONOMETRY

Eliézer Silva
Luiz F. Poli de Figueiredo

Sepsis remains one of the most common causes of multiple organ dysfunction syndrome, in part as a consequence of sepsis-induced maldistribution of blood flow, resulting in hypoperfusion of regional vascular beds [1]. However, there is a great deal of controversy as to whether the tissue distress observed in sepsis is caused exclusively by microcirculatory hypoxia or by disturbances in cellular metabolic pathways. Several authors have shown that despite an apparently sufficient global oxygen delivery (DO_2), signs of hypoxia and/or metabolic dysfunction persist. The availability of techniques to assess regional hemodynamic and oxygen-related variables has highlighted the inadequacy of the information obtained by global measurements [2].

There are several convincing reasons to concentrate on the gut as the organ to detect occult tissue hypoxia during an apparent hemodynamic stability [3]. First, intestinal mucosal cells are normally under a low oxygen tension (PO_2), because the effective hematocrit within the villi is decreased due to a phenomenon called 'plasma skimming' [4] and the villi have a peculiar microvascular architecture, characterized by a countercurrent exchange of oxygen from arteriole to adjacent venule along their length (Figure 1). Under normal conditions, this shunting of oxygen is not harmful to the villi. However, in conditions in which blood flow to the gut becomes greatly curtailed, such as in circulatory shock, the oxygen deficit in the tips of the villi can become so severe that they can suffer ischemic death and disintegrate [4,5].

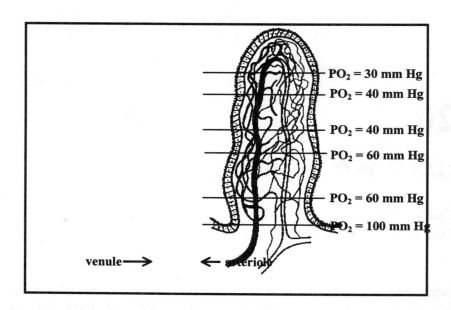

$PO_2 = 30$ mm Hg

$PO_2 = 40$ mm Hg

$PO_2 = 40$ mm Hg

$PO_2 = 60$ mm Hg

$PO_2 = 60$ mm Hg

$PO_2 = 100$ mm Hg

venule ⟶   ⟵ arteriole

Figure 1. *Intestinal villus – countercurrent exchange of oxygen between arteriole and venule*

Second, the gut is the organ with the highest critical DO_2 in the body, principally during sepsis [6]. Third, the gut is richly innervated by the sympathetic nerve system. In response to a decrease in global DO_2, intestinal vasoconstriction is greater than most vascular beds when blood is redistributed to the vital organs, and may persist when systemic hemodynamic variables have been reestablished (Figure 2). These conditions jeopardize the integrity of gut mucosal cells, predisposing to increases in gut permeability and translocation of bacteria and their toxins. Consequently, a systemic inflammatory response, incriminated in the development of multiple organ failure (MOF) [4,7], is induced by regional cytokine synthesis and several other inflammatory mediators, released by hepatic and systemic mononuclear cells [4].

Since sepsis is characterized by blood flow heterogeneity and underperfused gut mucosa can be a motor of MOF, it is reasonable to monitor its perfusion. Although several techniques have been proposed to measure the adequacy of gut perfusion [8], only gas tonometry is available for bedside clinical use. It is a minimally invasive technique that measures gut mucosal PCO_2 through a modified nasogastric tube with a CO_2-permeable balloon at its tip [9]. Because of the inverse relationship between tissue PCO_2 and local blood flow, gas tonometry has emerged as a tool for tissue perfusion assessment.

This chapter will highlight current knowledge regarding gas tonometry as a tool to better understand the pathophysiology of tissue oxygen distribution in sepsis. We will focus on the clinical applications of gas tonometry, particularly the role of gut mucosal acidosis on outcome and as an index with putative therapeutic implications.

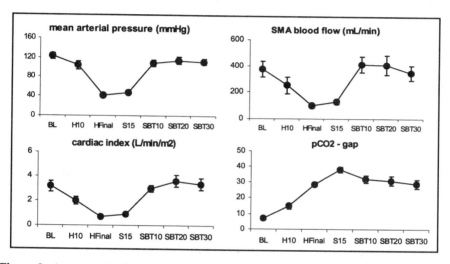

Figure 2. *A progressive hemorrhage (25 ml/min) was induced in dogs to a target mean arterial pressure of 40 mm Hg (H10-Hfinal), maintained for 15 minutes (S15) and treated by rapid total shed blood transfusion, with a 30-min follow-up. Despite immediate recovery of arterial pressure, cardiac output and mesenteric artery blood flow, PCO_2 gap remained high. This study highlights the limitation of systemic variables to predict gut mucosal perfusion and it also shows blood flow redistribution within the gut. Whether these changes were caused by the short shock state or from ischemia-reperfusion injury of mucosal cells remains to be determined (Poli de Figueiredo, et al., unpublished data).*

THE TONOMETRIC METHOD

Since the early part of this century, it has been shown that in a hollow viscus, tissue CO_2 diffuses from regional blood vessels into the lumen [10]. In 1959, Boda and Muranyi [11] published the concept of gastric tonometry. They demonstrated a close relationship between gastric PCO_2 and end-tidal CO_2 and, therefore, to arterial PCO_2, using a catheter with a balloon filled with room air into the stomach of healthy volunteers to measure PCO_2 of the gas sampled from the balloon. By introducing a saline sample into the gallbladder or urinary bladder lumen, Bergofsky [12] demonstrated that PCO_2 equilibrates with organ wall PCO_2. A more rapid equilibration between fluid PCO_2 and venous PCO_2, drained from an ileal loop mucosa, was observed by Dawson et al. [13]. More recently, the ability to measure PCO_2 by the tonometric method was clearly validated *in vitro* using solutions with known PCO_2 concentrations [14].

Fiddian-Green et al. [15] adopted the saline tonometric technique for the assessment of gut luminal PCO_2 and extended its use to the calculation of gastrointestinal intramucosal pH (pHi). They assumed that the arterial bicarbonate level, measured by an arterial blood gas analyzer, was the same as the intramucosal bicarbonate, and calculated pHi by the Henderson-Hasselbach equation as follows:

$$pHi = 6.1 + \log \frac{[HCO_3^-]}{[PCO_2] \times 0.031}$$

where $[HCO_3^-]$ is the bicarbonate concentration, calculated from arterial PCO_2 and pH, $[PCO_2]$ is the CO_2 tension, measured on saline aspirated directly from the stomach, and 0.031 is the solubility coefficient for CO_2 in plasma. Subsequently, this technique was modified to use a CO_2-permeable, silicone balloon catheter, from which aliquots of saline could be withdrawn and evaluated by routine blood gas analyzers.

The validity and reproducibility of pHi, measured by gastric tonometry, were examined in experimental models of sepsis, graded hemorrhage and mesenteric artery occlusion; compared to the pH measured by implanted microelectrodes, pHi matched closely [16-20]. It has been also shown, by several different techniques, that decreases in blood flow to the gut are paralleled by concordant decreases in pHi and increases in tissue PCO_2 determined by tonometry [19,21-28]. Also, in critically ill patients, mucosal gastric perfusion, measured by laser Doppler [29] or reflectance spectroscopy [30], was lower when an increased $PgCO_2$-$PaCO_2$ gradient or a subnormal pHi was present.

Hence, PCO_2 estimated by tonometry should correspond to that of tissue PCO_2. When fluid is instilled into the lumen of a hollow organ, gaseous CO_2 equilibrates with CO_2 in interstitial fluid and cells in the superficial layers of the organs wall [31]. However, the stomach may be an exception, because the PCO_2 of gastric juice may, in some instances, exceed the PCO_2 of the gastric wall and gastric venous blood PCO_2. PCO_2 is also generated into the gastric lumen, from neutralization of H^+ by the bicarbonate contained in the gastric juice or in the backflow of duodenal fluid. Back diffusion of CO_2 into the gastric mucosa itself increases gastric wall PCO_2, independently of gastric mucosal blood flow [32-34]. After H_2 blockade by cimetidine, H^+ production by the stomach is reduced, and the PCO_2 of gastric luminal fluid and that of the gastric venous blood approximate each other. Accordingly, the H^+ of gastric juice interferes with tonometric measurement of PCO_2, and routine H_2 blockade is therefore recommended to minimize this effect [32]. Although many critically ill patients are treated with H_2 receptor-blocking agents for the prevention of stress ulceration, their benefits are disputed. There are adverse effects of H_2 blockade in such settings, especially an increased risk of nosocomial pneumonia [35]. To avoid the short-comes (food, H_2 blockers, duodenal reflux) of the gastric tract for mucosal PCO_2 measurements, PCO_2 tonometry has been evaluated in several other tissues such as sublingual [36-38], esophageal [22], and bladder [39] mucosas. The feasibility and accuracy of these techniques remains to be validated.

There are limitations inherent to the use of saline samples, such as the time interval required for CO_2 equilibration between the saline in the tonometer's balloon and the gastric wall. Experimentally, it has been shown that the level of tissue PCO_2 has little effect on the equilibration period [24,40]. The manufacturer recommends mathematical corrections to adjust for incomplete equilibration, which is usually inversely related to the period of equilibration. However, these corrections represent average values rather than values indicating the time required for partial equilibration for an individual patient. Another source of error is that, when saline PCO_2 is measured with several blood gas analyzers, a wide variation is observed, particularly at higher PCO_2 levels, underestimating balloon PCO_2 [41]. By using other solutions instead of saline, errors in PCO_2 estimation were attenuated [41,42]. Phosphate buffer solutions have been suggested as options to improve the accuracy and reliability of PCO_2 measurement [43].

However, the use of systemic bicarbonate, assuming that it is equal to intramucosal bicarbonate concentration, is the major limitation for the use of calculated pHi in the clinical setting. Isolated regional ischemia may result in lower local bicarbonate levels when compared to systemic values. Conversely, during shock states with systemic acidosis, gastric intramucosal bicarbonate is consistently greater than that of arterial blood. Moreover, other causes of systemic hypercarbia and metabolic acidosis, without hypoperfusion, may also influence pHi calculation, despite a preserved mucosal perfusion. For all those drawbacks, calculated pHi should be replaced by the tonometer-arterial blood PCO_2 gradient, named PCO_2-gap, avoiding the confounding effects of systemic metabolic and respiratory alterations. However, Guzman et al. [44] showed that this gradient remains stable during hypoventilation, but it may increase after hyperventilation. These findings warrant cautious interpretation of the PCO_2 gap as an indicator of gastric mucosal perfusion during systemic hypocapnia. Despite this concern, PCO_2-gap remains the most reliable marker of tissue perfusion nowadays and should definitively replace pHi [45, 46].

Further advances in the tonometric method were achieved by Salzman et al. [21], who reinvestigated the concept that PCO_2 measurements could be performed on gas aspirated from the stomach. The PCO_2 of this gas correlated with that measured on saline sampled from a conventional balloon tonometer, when perfusion was decreased by pericardial tamponade. During respiratory acidosis and in the absence of shock, there was a very high correlation between the PCO_2 of stomach gas and that of the saline sampled from the balloon. This concept of air tonometry was recently expanded by Guzman and Kruse [47], who circulated gas through a gastric balloon and measured PCO_2 continuously, by an infrared capnometer. More recently, capnometry and conventional balloon tonometry have been combined and called capnometric recirculating gas tonometry (CRGT), overcoming limitations such as the long equilibration time, saline sampling and a relatively labor-intensive manipulation. Air is used in lieu of saline, and then gas is aspirated and analyzed automatically by infrared capnometry after a 10-minute equilibration, with a commercially available Tonocap (Datex-Engstrom; Tonometrics; Tewksbury, Mass). In experimental models, CRGT has been shown to be capable of detecting changes in gastric mucosal PCO_2 shortly after inducing hypoxemia and hemorrhage [48]. CRGT has been validated also in critically ill patients [14,49]. Hence, CRGT is currently the best method available, and in addition to providing semi-continuous online measurements of gastric PCO_2, can detect significant changes within minutes, and may be used during short-term interventional studies.

PCO_2 AS A MARKER OF BLOOD FLOW AND TISSUE HYPOXIA

In animal models of progressive hemorrhage or cardiac tamponade, in which DO_2 was reduced by a decreased cardiac output, an elevation in veno-arterial ΔPCO_2 was observed, while oxygen uptake (VO_2) and CO_2 production remained constant [50-52]. In this condition of oxygen supply-independency, an elevation of veno-arterial ΔPCO_2, following flow reduction, can be explained simply by CO_2 stagnation. When DO_2 was further reduced, below its critical value (DO_2crit), a decrease in VO_2 was observed, suggesting oxygen supply-dependency and consequent anaerobic metabolism. An increase in lactate concentration confirmed this assumption [51,52]. The progressive widening of veno-arterial ΔPCO_2 was magnified by a sharp increase in $PvCO_2$, when DO_2 decreased below its critical point (a veno-arterial ΔPCO_2 around 30 mm Hg). It was assumed that this steep increase in

ΔPCO_2 can be used as a reliable marker of tissue dysoxia, since the DO_2crit calculated by either using the relationship between VO_2 to DO_2, lactate to DO_2, or ΔPCO_2 to DO_2, provided similar results [51,52].

However, in a recent review, Teboul et al. [53] noted that the aerobic production of CO_2 is theoretically reduced when tissue dysoxia is present (as $VCO_2 = R \times VO_2$), and proposed that an explanation of venous and tissue hypercarbia, in low-flow states, emerges from the curvilinearity of the Fick equation. As mentioned above, if anaerobic CO_2 production occurred under conditions of tissue dysoxia, it would result from the H+ excess buffering by HCO_3^-. However, as highlighted by Teboul et al. [53], studies addressing the issue of detecting tissue dysoxia by analysis of ΔPCO_2, used experimental protocols of blood flow reduction; the associated decrease in cardiac output acts as a confounding variable, not allowing a definitive conclusion. In order to clarify this question, Vallet et al. [54], using an *in situ* isolated, innervated canine hind limb model, showed that when DO_2 was decreased, either by blood flow reduction (ischemic hypoxia) or decreasing arterial PO_2 (hypoxic hypoxia), regional veno-arterial ΔPCO_2 increased only when blood flow was reduced, even though the same oxygen deficit was observed in both protocols. The authors concluded that the absence of an increased veno-arterial ΔPCO_2 does not preclude the presence of tissue dysoxia. Hence, decreased blood flow appeared to be the major determinant of increased ΔPCO_2.

If intestinal tonometry is to be used to detect early dysoxia in low flow states, it is essential to know at which level increased tissue PCO_2 represents aerobic (stagnant flow with preserved VO_2), or anaerobic, metabolism. Some evidence has emerged from Schlichtig's group [23]. These authors observed that mucosal PCO_2, estimated by tonometry, increased to values nearly threefold higher than predicted by Dill's blood nomogram, which shows the aerobic relationship between $PvCO_2$ and mixed venous oxygen saturation (SvO_2). In this nomogram, a known $PvCO_2$ can be used to predict the SvO_2 (SvO_2^{Dill}). A SvO_2^{Dill} that agrees with a measured SvO_2 in a blood sample indicates that dissolved CO_2 appeared purely on the basis of aerobic metabolism. On the other hand, when the SvO_2^{Dill} is less than the measured SvO_2, it represents the conversion of bicarbonate to dissolved CO_2, due to anaerobic metabolism. Moreover, these authors also observed that gastric mucosal PCO_2 markedly exceeded PCO_2 values in portal venous blood, when flow was decreased below the critical DO_2. Consistency with aerobic CO_2 was only observed with a maximal mucosal-arterial ΔPCO_2 gradient, around 25-35 mm Hg, while a further increase in mucosal-arterial ΔPCO_2 was consistent with mucosal dysoxia. However, in this particular study, low blood flow remained as a confounding variable, according to Teboul's experiments [53].

To establish the exact role of a decreased blood flow on tissue PCO_2, Vallet et al. [55] evaluated the veno-arterial CO_2 gap [P(v-a)CO_2], gut mucosal-arterial CO_2 gap [P(m-a)CO_2], and gastric mucosal blood flow (laser Doppler flow probe). They showed, by using two different mechanisms of tissue hypoxia, that mucosal blood flow is not the only factor that could contribute to gastric mucosal hypercarbia. In one group, systemic hypoxia was induced by progressive reduction in the inspired oxygen fraction (FiO_2, hypoxic hypoxia [HH]) or by progressive bleeding (ischemic hypoxia, IH). While IH decreased gastric mucosal blood flow and increased both [P(v-a)CO_2] and [P(m-a)CO_2], HH increased only [P(m-a)CO_2], although gastric mucosal blood flow remained constant. As expected, IH induced a larger increase in ΔPCO_2 than HH. The peculiar microcirculatory system and its counter-current exchange of oxygen and CO_2 within the mucosal villus could explain these findings. Therefore, conditions of low tissue DO_2 may induce both tissue hypoxia and hypercarbia, by incrementing the counter-current oxygen exchange between arteriole and venule, threatening cells at the tips of the villi.

Following fluid resuscitation in sepsis, tissue DO_2 may be restored but gastric mucosal hypercarbia may not be prevented, due to disturbances in cellular metabolic pathways impairing oxygen utilization, which has been termed cytopathic hypoxia. This may explain the concomitance of high tissue PCO_2 and adequate tissue PO_2 and gastric mucosal blood flow, observed by several authors [25,56,57]. In fact, a high gastric to arterial PCO_2 gradient could be a marker of dysoxia, independent of the causes of impaired oxygen utilization.

However, a simplistic conclusion that tissue hypercarbia necessarily means hypoperfusion or anaerobic metabolism may be misleading. The rationale behind tonometry is the assumption that an increased mucosal-arterial PCO_2 gradient indicates imbalance between perfusion and metabolism. This assumes that the mucosal-arterial PCO_2 gradient is a surrogate marker of mucosal-arterial CO_2 content difference. However, when oxygen saturation, hemoglobin and/or arterial-venous pH difference change, the relationship between PCO_2 and CO_2 content is not linear. In particular, the condition in which there is an increase in blood flow, but a larger increase in CO_2 production, matching a respective change in oxygen consumption, may lead to the dissociation of PCO_2 gradients between vascular beds with different baseline oxygen extraction. Jakob et al. [58] have speculated that, particular changes in tissue oxygen extraction (Haldane effect), may explain the increasing mucosal-arterial PCO_2 gradients, despite preserved or increased mucosal tissue perfusion.

In summary, the major determinant of tissue PCO_2 is blood flow. However, because of the villus' peculiar vascular arrangement, a high gastric mucosal PCO_2 can be a marker of dysoxia and not simply a marker of disproportionately low blood flow for the tissue's metabolic status.

PATHOPHYSIOLOGY OF TISSUE HYPERCARBIA IN SEPSIS

There are many reasons for the development of gastric mucosal hypercarbia in septic patients. Metabolic needs are typically increased by the inflammatory response to infection, increasing CO_2 load. This may further enlarge veno-arterial PCO_2 and tissue-arterial PCO_2 gradients, especially when there is no compensatory increase in cardiac output or tissue blood flow. Particularly during early resuscitation, tissue blood flow can be low (stagnant flow), due to either hypovolemia and/or arterial hypotension. Gastric mucosal hypercarbia may be due also to systemic metabolic acidosis, mainly secondary to lactic acidosis, a condition in which tissue hypercarbia is universally observed, produced by bicarbonate buffering of hydrogen ions. Even in the absence of systemic acidosis, tissue CO_2 can be increased by anaerobic metabolism, due to regional blood flow maldistribution, shifting blood flow away from the mucosa. Moreover, mucosal acidosis may not be mediated by hemodynamic alterations, but may be due to direct metabolic changes induced by endotoxin [26]. Increasing mucosal blood flow by hemodynamic interventions, in this condition, may fail to reestablish normal mucosal PCO_2. Finally, a paradoxical increase in PCO_2-gap may be observed, despite an increase in mucosal blood flow and oxygen saturation. This phenomenon could be explained by the Haldane effect, which states that at any PCO_2, arterial oxygenated blood has a lower CO_2 content than reduced venous blood. Hence, for a given CO_2 content, PCO_2 will be higher at a higher hemoglobin saturation. Table 1 summarizes the main causes of elevated tissue CO_2.

Physiologic influence
- Systemic arterial PCO_2
- Low gastric mucosal blood flow (stagnant flow)
- Increased CO_2 production by aerobic metabolism*
- Increased CO_2 production by anaerobic metabolism*
- Inhibition of pyruvate dehydrogenase*
- Haldane effect

*without a proportional increase in gastric mucosal blood flow

Table 1. *Causes of increased gastric intramucosal PCO_2 in septic patients*

SPLANCHNIC BLOOD FLOW DISTRIBUTION

Although pHi and PCO_2 gap are often considered as indexes of splanchnic perfusion [59,60], this has never been shown conclusively. Some experimental and clinical studies have failed to demonstrate a linear correlation between gut mucosal PCO_2 and hepatosplanchnic blood flow. The PCO_2 gap reflects merely perfusion and/or oxygenation conditions of the gut mucosa. Therefore, we cannot generalize gut mucosal CO_2 measurements to the splanchnic area, because blood flow distribution may vary widely between and within organs, especially in sepsis.

Vallet et al. [55] demonstrated, in a canine model of resuscitated endotoxic shock, a marked redistribution of blood flow within the gut wall, from the mucosa toward the muscularis, with a simultaneous decrease in intestinal mucosal PO_2. These data contrast with Revelly et al. [57], who used microspheres to evaluate blood flow distribution within the intestinal wall during endotoxic shock in pigs. Surprisingly, they found that, whereas total mesenteric blood flow was unchanged, blood flow to the gut mucosa increased and blood flow to the muscularis decreased. Although marked blood flow redistribution was observed in both studies, their opposing findings could be explained by differences in the methods used to assess mucosal blood flow.

Lagoa et al. [61] have recently evaluated the effects of large volume infusion on splanchnic blood flow distribution, using live *E. coli* infusion in dogs. After bacteria infusion, cardiac index (CI) and mesenteric blood flow (MBF, ultrasonic flowprobe) decreased. In contrast, portal-arterial PCO_2 and gastric-arterial PCO_2 (PCO_2 gap) gradients increased. After fluid resuscitation, whereas CI and MBF increased and portal-arterial PCO_2 gradient decreased, the PCO_2 gap remained high (Figure 3). If we use CO_2 gradient as a marker of blood flow, we could analyze the behavior of CO_2 gradient in different compartments. There was no correlation between systemic venous-arterial PCO_2, portal-arterial PCO_2, and PCO_2 gap, probably reflecting a large blood flow redistribution within these compartments.

Similar findings have emerged from clinical studies. In stable septic patients, Creteur et al. [62] found no significant correlation between the PCO_2 gap and hepatosplanchnic blood flow, or between the PCO_2 gap and other regional oxygen-derived variables, such as suprahepatic venous blood oxygen saturation and mesenteric veno-arterial PCO_2 gradient. Silva et al [63] have studied the effects of norepinephrine and epinephrine infusion on systemic hemodynamic variables, hepatosplanchnic blood flow and gastric mucosal PCO_2 in septic shock patients, and no correlation between them could be demonstrated. For instance, epinephrine infusion increased CI more than norepinephrine, but fractional splanchnic blood was higher with norepinephrine. If the increase in splanchnic blood flow occurred similarly in all gut layers, ΔPCO_2 gap and $\Delta SvO_2\text{-}ShO_2$ would decrease proportionally, because $SvO_2\text{-}ShO_2$ gradient reflects the oxygenation balance in the splanchnic area. However, no correlation between ΔPCO_2 gap and $\Delta SvO_2\text{-}ShO_2$ gradient was observed (Figure 3). Our findings support the concept that there is a large blood flow redistribution inter and intra-organs in septic states.

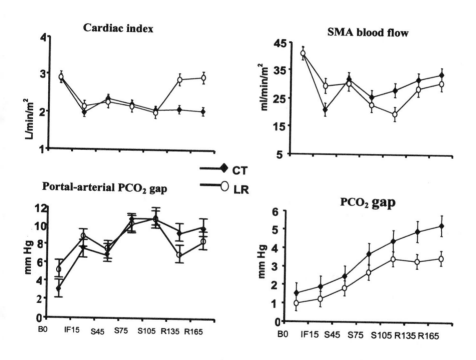

Figure 3. *Effects of live E. coli infusion during 15 min (IF15). After a 90-min period (S45, S75, S105), dogs were randomized to 2 groups: control (CT), no fluids and lactate Ringer's (LR), 32 mL/kg, over 60 min (R135, R165). Live bacterial infusion induced sustained decreases in cardiac index (CI) and SMA blood flow, while portal-arterial PCO_2 and mucosal-arterial PCO_2 gradients increased steadily. Only mucosal-arterial PCO_2 gradient was not restored after fluid infusion [adapted from **62**].*

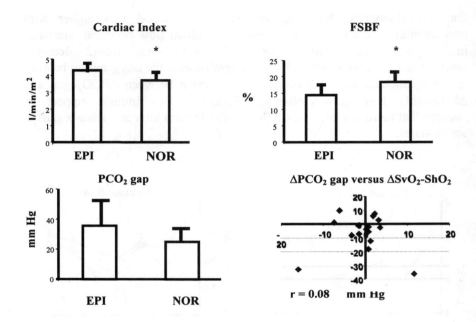

Figure 4. *The effects of epinephrine (EPI)-norepinephrine (NOR) shift on cardiac index (CI), fractional splanchnic blood flow (FSBF) and PCO$_2$ gap in 20 septic shock patients. Correlation between the PCO$_2$ gap variation (ΔPCO$_2$ gap) and the variation of mixed venous and hepatic venous O$_2$ difference (Δ SvO$_2$-ShO$_2$). *p < 0.05 [adapted from ref 63]*

In summary, gut mucosal PCO$_2$ is just a surrogate marker of local blood flow, reflecting merely the balance between CO$_2$ production and clearance within that layer of the gastrointestinal tract. Actually, we should interpret gut mucosal PCO$_2$ as a tool to better understand blood flow distribution in sepsis and its possible clinical implications.

CLINICAL USES OF GASTRIC TONOMETRY IN SEPSIS

Since gut mucosal hypoperfusion may have a pivotal role in the development of MOF in sepsis, several authors are attempting to correlate gastric tonometry with outcome. Consequently, many studies have also addressed whether gastric acidosis reversal could affect outcome and its response to potential hemodynamic interventions.

Outcome Prediction

Gastric intramucosal acidosis, detected during intensive care admission, has been related to outcome in several trials [64-68]. The predictive value of this measure, after an initial period of treatment in the intensive care unit (ICU), has been conflicting. However, these trials had several limitations. The number of patients been enrolled was not enough to exclude either a beta or an alpha error. Moreover, there was a large heterogeneity regarding inclusion criteria. Mortality has been the main endpoint, which is subject to many influences other than the ones directly related to the restoration of organ perfusion. Finally, most studies have been using calculated pHi, which incorporates systemic bicarbonate, therefore impairing comparison between the effects of systemic and regional perfusion disturbances on outcome, as previously discussed.

Preliminary results from our prospective, ongoing study in patients with severe sepsis and/or septic shock (ACCP/SCCM consensus conference definition), have been suggesting a relationship between PCO_2 gap and the development of multiple organ dysfunction, as assessed by the SOFA score [69]. We have already evaluated 44 patients with ages varying between 15-85 years. Mortality rate has been 40% and APACHE II score, 19. Patients who had a PCO_2-gap larger than 15 mm Hg, on the 3rd day following resuscitation, either had a high SOFA score (>11) or died by the 10th day. An interesting finding has been that patients with a sustained high PCO_2 gap are showing a progressive increase in relative risk for death, on days zero, 1 and 2 (Table 2).

	Day 0	Day 1	Day 2	Day 3	
PCO₂ gap	1.8	1.7	3.2	2,7	RR
(>	(0.9-3.4)	(0.9-3.1)	(1.3-7.7)	(1,2-6,3)	CI
15mmHg)	0.15	0.17	0.003	0.002	p
SOFA	1.6	1.9	4.4	3.6	RR
(> 11)	(0.8-3.4)	(0.8-4.2)	(1.5-12.9)	(1,2-10.6)	CI
	0.20	0.11	0.0008	0.006	p

RR – relative risk; CI – confidence interval.

Table 2. *Relative risk of death for septic shock patients on days zero, 1, 2, and 3 [70]*

Similarly, a high SOFA score was associated with mortality. However, caution must be exercised in interpreting these data, because gastric mucosal acidosis could be just a marker of sepsis-induced dysfunction in cellular metabolism, instead of the cause of MOF, as has been widely claimed.

Additional clinical trials are needed to confirm and better clarify this relationship.

Hemodynamic Management of Gastric Mucosal Acidosis in Septic Patients

From the preceding discussion, it seems attractive to attempt to reduce intestinal microcirculation abnormalities in sepsis. A reasonable hypothesis to be tested is that the use of vasoactive agents, which optimize intestinal perfusion, can reduce the incidence of MODS in septic patients.

Total hepatosplanchnic blood flow, measured by the indocyanine green (ICG) technique, and mucosal blood flow, measured directly by laser Doppler or indirectly by gas tonometry, have been used to assess regional oxygenation during the most commonly used hemodynamic interventions in sepsis: fluid replacement and vasoactive drug infusion.

Absolute or relative hypovolemia is commonly present in septic patients and it is responsible, in part, for tissue hypoperfusion, justifying why fluid replacement is considered an essential, early intervention in sepsis. However, the relationship between fluid resuscitation and gastric mucosal blood flow remains incompletely characterized. Current knowledge is largely based on experimental studies. In an endotoxic shock model in dogs, De Backer et al. [70] showed that fluid resuscitation increased mesenteric blood flow but did not prevent the decrease in gastric mucosal pH. Also in endotoxemic dogs, Vallet et al. [3] showed that fluid resuscitation increased cardiac output and gut serosal PO_2, and restored systemic VO_2; however, gut VO_2, mucosal PO_2 and pHi remained low, and gut lactate output high. Lagoa et al. [61] evaluated systemic and regional effects of fluid resuscitation in dogs with sepsis induced by live *E. coli* infusion. Crystalloid infusion restored both systemic and global regional variables, such as superior mesenteric artery blood flow and portal vein-arterial PCO_2.gradient. However, fluid infusion only avoided further increases in PCO_2 gap, with no improvement after 60 minutes.

Data from clinical studies are very limited. In a small group of hypovolemic septic patients, Forrest et al. [71] reported that fluid loading neither increased pHi nor decreased PCO_2 gap. Addressing the repercussions of a fluid challenge (500 ml of hetastarch over 30 minutes), on systemic hemodynamic parameters and PCO_2 gap in patients with severe sepsis or septic shock, we [72] showed a decrease in mean PCO_2 gap. However, significant individual variations in PCO_2 gap response were observed and there was no correlation between changes in cardiac index and PCO_2 gap.

These data suggest that PCO_2 gap should not be used isolated to guide fluid replacement.

When tissue oxygenation is not restored despite fluid replacement, vasoactive drugs are commonly used to increase oxygen supply and avoid hypotension. However, they induce different changes on systemic and regional blood flow. Silva et al. [72] reviewed the effects of vasoactive drugs on gastric pHi. Within the inherent limitations with the use of pHi in most studies as the gut mucosal perfusion index, we highlighted that:

a) although dopaminergic effects can increase splanchnic blood flow, low-dose dopamine usually decreases pHi, suggesting a blood flow redistribution away from gastric mucosa;

b) dobutamine most commonly increases splanchnic blood flow and tends to increase pHi in septic patients. In addition, dobutamine can disclose the presence of severe splanchnic hypoperfusion in septic patients. Creteur et al. [74] showed that, in patients with low fractional splanchnic blood flow (SBF/cardiac index), the PCO_2 gap fell significantly with increasing doses of dobutamine;

c) dopexamine has been shown to increase splanchnic oxygenation, principally in sepsis, but it can also induce undesirable hypotension;

d) data on norepinephrine are more limited, but suggest that it can increase pHi in patients with septic shock; and

e) epinephrine could impair splanchnic perfusion in patients with septic shock.

More recent data support the benefits of β-adrenergic agents on gastric mucosal perfusion [75,76]. These data can be summarized by a commonly employed statement 'β-adrenergic effects have a pivotal role in increasing gut mucosal blood flow in sepsis'.

Targeting the intestinal microcirculation with vasoactive drugs is one approach to counteract the microvascular abnormalities in the pathophysiology of sepsis. However, major individual variations are present in several studies including ours [72,74,77]. Clinicians must exercise prudence to incorporate the evidence into clinical practice and should test different doses of distinct catecholamines to achieve their physiological therapeutic aims.

Gas Tonometry Guided Therapy

In critically ill patients, a persistently high PCO_2 gap may be associated with worsening in outcome but it has not been definitively established if this finding is just an epiphenomenon or a pathophysiological event of the development of MOF. However, in this evidence-based medicine (EBM) époque, clinicians have demanded a large, multicenter, randomized clinical trial, to prove or disprove the effectiveness of PCO_2 gap-guided therapy, before actively incorporating its use in the daily practice.

To date, only five controlled studies have examined whether treatment aimed at increasing pHi improves outcome. None of these studies exclusively addressed septic patients and only two enrolled a sufficient number of patients to allow some conclusion to be drawn. Gutierrez et al. [78] performed a randomized, controlled clinical trial comparing standard therapy (not specified) to additional therapy, described as further fluid and red blood cell replacement plus dobutamine infusion, to correct low pHi in critically ill patients. They showed that the mortality rate was significantly reduced in those patients with an admission pHi of > 7.35. More recently, Gomersall et al. [79], using a more controlled resuscitation protocol, sought if additional therapy, aimed at correcting low pHi, would improve outcome in conventionally treated critically ill patients. In this study, pHi guided-therapy failed to improve outcome. However, both studies enrolled heterogeneous groups of patients. As one would expect, it is not probable that an isolated, miraculous intervention for different patients could produce outcome improvement. In the Gutierrez study, mortality in the control group was unexpectedly high, and no attempt was made to standardize treatment. In Gomersall's study, there was no difference in pHi between control and intervention groups at zero, 12, and 24 hours, when the intervention was withheld. Silva et al. demonstrated that persistent gastric mucosal acidosis, beyond 24 hours is very important to predict outcome [69]. So, a treatment protocol should be maintained until 48 or 72 hours after the start of resuscitation. Finally, as mentioned, the use of calculated pHi incorporates systemic metabolic and respiratory variables, compromising the interpretation of pHi as a regional parameter to be targeted.

Recently, Chapman et al. [80] published the state of the art on gastrointestinal tonometry. The authors emphasized that, while it may be possible to apply the principles of evidence-based medicine to the evaluation of a single intervention affecting outcome, applying them to the introduction of a new piece of monitoring is even more complex. It is the management driven by, and the therapeutic interventions taken in response to, the monitor's information which may affect outcome. Both are dependent on many other factors, not simply the numbers displayed on the monitor's screen. For example, pulse oximetry would not be used in the clinical setting based on these principles, because there is no difference in outcome or complication rate with its use. However, it was shown that it allows rapid, early and safe diagnosis, and correction of arterial hypoxemia with significantly less supplemental oxygen than with the group of patients without pulse oximetry. The same may be true for gas tonometry, which may provide information guiding interventions leading to the reversal of disturbances that may be linked to MOF.

CONCLUSION

There is evidence to support the relationship between splanchnic hypoperfusion and multiple organ dysfunction in septic patients, largely related to mucosal injury leading to increased permeability and systemic inflammatory response. As gut mucosal PCO_2 reflects the balance between flow and metabolism, gas tonometry is a valuable tool to monitor the regional effects of hemodynamic interventions and gives insight regarding blood flow heterogeneity in sepsis. The definitive role of gas tonometry to predict outcome and guide therapy for septic patients will be established by large, prospective multicenter trials.

REFERENCES

1. Schumacker P, Cain SM. The concept of a critical oxygen delivery. Intensive Care Med 1987; 13:223-229
2. Ince C, Sinaasappel M. Microcirculatory oxygenation and shunting in sepsis and shock. Crit Care Med 1999; 27:1369-1377
3. Vallet B, Lund N, Curtis SE, et al. Gut and muscle tissue PO2 in endotoxemic dogs during shock and resuscitation. J Appl Physiol 1994; 76:793-800
4. Marshall JC, Christou NV, Meakins JL. The gastrointestinal tract. The "undrained abscess" of multiple organ failure. Ann Surg 1993; 218:111-119
5. Guyton AC, Hall J. General principles of gastrointestinal function - motility, nervous control, and blood circulation. In: Guyton AC, Hall JE (eds) Textbook of Medical Physiology 9th Edition, 1996, pp793-802
6. Nelson DP, Samsel RW, Wood LD, Schumacker P. Pathological supply dependence of systemic and intestinal O2 uptake during endotoxemia. J Appl Physiol 1988; 64:2410-2419
7. Fink MP. Why the GI tract is pivotal in trauma, sepsis, and MOF. Sepsis 1991; 6:253-276
8. Mythen M, Faehnrich J. Monitoring gut perfusion. In: Rombeau JL, Takala J (eds). Gut dysfunction in critical illness. Springer-Verlag, Berlin 1996 pp 246-263
9. Fiddian-Green RG. Gastric intramucosal pH, tissue oxygenation and acid-base balance. Br J Anaesth 1995; 74:591-606
10. McIver M. Gaseous exchange between the blood and the lumen of the stomach and intestine. Am J Physiol 1926; 76:92-111

11. Boda D, Muranyi L. "Gastrotonometry": an aid to the control of ventilation during artificial respiration. Lancet 1959; 73:181-182

12. Bergofsky EH. Determinationof of tissue O2 tensions by hollow visceral tonometers: effects of breathing enriched O2 mixtures. J Clin Invest 1964; 43:193-200

13. Dawson AM, Trenchard D, Guz A. Small bowel tonometry: assessment of small gut mucosal oxygen tension in dog and man. Nature 1965; 206(987):943-944

14. Creteur J, De Backer D, Vincent JL. Monitoring gastric mucosal carbon dioxide pressure using gas tonometry: in vitro and in vivo validation studies. Anesthesiology 1997; 87:504-510

15. Fiddian-Green RG. Tonometry: theory and applications. Intensive Care World 1992; 9:60-65

16. Antonsson JB, Engstrom L, Rasmussen I, Wollert S, Haglund UH. Changes in gut intramucosal pH and gut oxygen extraction ratio in a porcine model of peritonitis and hemorrhage. Crit Care Med 1995; 23:1872-1881

17. Antonsson JB, Boyle CC, Kruithoff KL, Wang HL, Sacristan E, Rothschild HR et al.. Validation of tonometric measurement of gut intramural pH during endotoxemia and mesenteric occlusion in pigs. Am J Physiol 1990; 259:G519-G523

18. Montgomery A, Hartmann M, Jonsson K, Haglund U. Intramucosal pH measurement with tonometers for detecting gastrointestinal ischemia in porcine hemorrhagic shock. Circ Shock 1989; 29:319-327

19. Antonsson JB, Haglund UH. Gut intramucosal pH and intraluminal PO2 in a porcine model of peritonitis or haemorrhage. Gut 1995; 37:791-797

20. Schlichting E, Lyberg T. Monitoring of tissue oxygenation in shock: an experimental study in pigs. Crit Care Med 1995; 23:1703-1710

21. Salzman AL, Strong KE, Wang H, Wollert PS, Vandermeer TJ, Fink MP. Intraluminal balloonless air tonometry: a new method for determination of gastrointestinal mucosal carbon dioxide tension. Crit Care Med 1994; 22:126-134

22. Sato Y, Weil MH, Tang W, et al. Esophageal PCO2 as a monitor of perfusion failure during hemorrhagic shock. J Appl Physiol 1997; 82:558-562

23. Schlichtig R, Bowles SA. Distinguishing between aerobic and anaerobic appearance of dissolved CO2 in intestine during low flow. J Appl Physiol 1994; 76:2443-2451

24. Tang W, Weil MH, Sun SJ, et al.. Gastric intramural PCO2 as a monitor of perfusion failure during hemorrhagic and anaphylatic shock. J Appl Physiol 1994; 76:572-577

25. van der Meer JT, Wang H, Fink MP. Endotoxemia causes ileal micosal acidosis in the absence of mucosal hypoxia in a normodynamic porcine model of septic shock. Crit Care Med 1995, 23:1217-1226

26. Heino A, Hartikainen J, Merasto M, Alhava E, Takala J. Systemic and regional PCO2 gradients as markers of intestinal ischaemia. Intensive Care Med 1998; 24: 599-604

27. Knichwitz G, Rotker J, Mollhoff T, Richter KD, Brussel T. Continuous intramucosal PCO2 measurement allows the early detection of intestinal malperfusion. Crit Care Med 1998; 26:1550-1557

28. Neviere R, Chagnon JL, Vallet B, et al.. Dobutamine improves gastrointestinal mucosal blood flow in a porcine model of endotoxic shock. Crit Care Med 1997; 25: 1371-1377.

29. Neviere R, Mathieu D, Chagnon JL, Lebleu N, Wattel F. The contrasting effects of dobutamine and dopamine on gastric mucosal perfusion in septic patients. Am J Respir Crit Care Med 1996; 154:1684-1688

30. Elizalde JI, Hernandez C, Llach J, Monton C, Bordas JM, Pique JM et al.. Gastric intramucosal acidosis in mechanically ventilated patients: role of mucosal blood flow [see comments]. Crit Care Med 1998; 26:827-832

31. Fiddian-Green RG, Pittenger G, Whitehouse WM Jr. Back-diffusion of CO2 and its influence on the intramural pH in gastric mucosa. J Surg Res 1982; 33:39-48

32. Heard SO, Helmsoortel CM, Kent JC, et al.. Gastric tonometry in health volunteers:effect of ranitidine on calculated intramural pH. Crit Care Med 1991; 19:271-274

33. Kolkman JJ, Groeneveld AB, Meuwissen SG. Effect of ranitidine on basal and bicarbonate enhanced intragastric PCO_2: a tonometric study. Gut 1994; 35:737-741

34. Stevens MH, Thirlby RC, Feldman M. Mechanisms for high PCO_2 in gastric juice:roles of bicarbonate secretion and CO_2 diffusion. Am J Physiol 1987; 253:G527-G530

35. Driks MR, Graven DE, Celli BR, et al. Nosocomial pneumonia in intubated patients given sucralfate as compared with antacids or histamine type 2 blockers: the role of gastric colonization. N Engl J Med 1987; 317:1376-1382

36. Jin X, Weil MH, Sun S, Tang W, Bisera J, Mason EJ. Decreases in organ blood flows associated with increases in sublingual PCO_2 during hemorrhagic shock. J Appl Physiol 1998; 85:2360-2364

37. Weil MH, Nakagawa Y, Tang W, et al. Sublingual capnometry: a new noninvasive measurement for diagnosis and quantitation of severity of circulatory shock. Crit Care Med 1999; 27:1225-1229

38. Nakagawa Y, Weil MH, Tang W, et al. Sublingual capnometry for diagnosis and quantitation of circulatory shock. Am J Respir Crit Care Med 1998; 157:1838-1843

39. Lang JD, Evans D, Poli de Figueiredo L, Hays S, Mathru M, Kramer G. A novel approach to monitor tissue perfusion: bladder mucosal PCO_2, PO_2, and pHi during ischemia and reperfusion in pigs. J Intensive Care 1999; 14:93-98

40. Kette F, Weil MH, Gazmuri RJ, et al. Intramyocardial hyperbaric acidosis during cardiac arrest and resuscitation. Crit Care Med 1993; 21:901-906

41. Takala J, Parviainen I, Siloaho M, Ruokonen E, Hamalainen E. Saline PCO_2 is an important source of error in the assessment of gastric intramucosal pH. Crit Care Med 1994; 22:1877-1879

42. Riddington D, Venkatesh B, Clutton-Brock T, Bion J, Venkatesh KB. Measuring carbon dioxide tension in saline and alternative solutions: quantification of bias and precision in two blood gas analyzers. Crit Care Med 1994; 22:96-100

43. Knichwitz G, Kuhmann M, Brodner G, Mertes N, Goeters C, Brussel T. Gastric tonometry: precision and reliability are improved by a phosphate buffered solution. Crit Care Med 1996; 24:512-516

44. Guzman JA, Kruse JA. Gut mucosal-arterial PCO_2 gradient as an indicator of splanchnic perfusion during systemic hypo- and hypercapnia. Crit Care Med 1999; 27:2760-2765

45. Schlichtig R, Mehta N, Gayowski TJ. Tissue-arterial PCO_2 difference is a better marker of ischemia than intramural pH (pHi) or arterial pH-pHi difference. J Crit Care 1996; 11:51-56

46. Vincent JL, Creteur J. Gastric mucosal pH is definitely obsolete – please, tell us more about gastric mucosal PCO_2. Crit Care Med 1998; 26:1479-1481

47. Guzman JA, Kruse JA. Development and validation of a technique for continuous monitoring of gastric intramucosal pH. Am J Respir Crit Care Med 1996; 153:694-700

48. Guzman JA, Kruse JA. Continuous assessment of gastric intramucosal PCO_2 and pH in hemorrhagic shock using capnometric recirculating gas tonometry. Crit Care Med 1997; 25:533-537

49. Heinonen PO. Validation of air tonometric measurement of gastric regional concentration of CO_2 in critically ill septic patients. Intensive Care Med 1997; 23:524-529

50. Bowles SA, Schlichtig R, Kramer DJ, Klions HA. Arteriovenous pH and partial pressure of carbon dioxide detect critical oxygen delivery during progressive haemorrhage in dogs. J Crit Care 1992; 7:95-105

51. Van Der Linden P, Rausin I, Deltell A, et al. Detection of tissue hypoxia by arteriovenous gradient for PCO_2 and pH in anesthetized dogs during progressive hemorrhage. Anesth Analg 1995; 80:269-275

52. Zhang H, Vincent JL. Arteriovenous difference in PCO2 and pH are good indicators of critical hypoperfusion. Am Rev Respir Dis 1993; 148:867-871
53. Teboul JL, Michard F, Richard C. Critical analysis of venoarterial CO2 gradient as a marker of tissue hypoxia. In: Vincent JL (ed) Yearbook of Intensive Care and Emergency Medicine. Springer-Verlag, Berlin, 1996 pp 296-307
54. Vallet B, Teboul JL, Cain SM, Curtis SE. Veno-arterial CO2 difference during regional ischemic or hypoxic hypoxia. J Appl Physiol 2000; 89:1317-1321
55. Vallet B, Durinck JL, Chagnon JL, Neviere R. Effects of hypoxic hypoxia on veno and gut mucosal arterial PCO2 difference in pigs. Anesthesiology 1996; 85:A607 (Abst)
56. Temmesfeld-Wollbruck B, Szalay A, Mayer K, Olschewski H, Seeger W, Grimminger F. Abnormalities of gastric mucosal oxygenation in septic shock: partial responsiveness to dopexamine. Am J Respir Crit Care Med 1998; 157:1586-1592
57. Revelly JP, Ayuse A, Brienza N, et al. Endotoxic shock alters distribution of blood flow within the intestinal wall. Crit Care Med 1996; 24:1345-1351
58. Jakob SM, Kosonen P, Ruokonen E, Parviainen I, Takala J. The Haldane effect - an alternative explanation for increasing gastric mucosal PCO2 gradients? Br J Anaesth 1999; 83:740-746
59. Maynard N, Bihari D, Beale R, et al. Assessment of splanchnic oxygenation by gastric tonometry in patients with acute circulatory failure. JAMA 1993; 270:1203-1210
60. Maynard ND, Bihari DJ, Dalton RN, Smithies MN, Mason RC. Increasing splanchnic blood flow in the critically ill. Chest 1995; 108:1648-1654
61. Lagoa C, Cruz Jr R, Poli de Figueiredo L, Silva E, Rocha e Silva M. Systemic and splanchnic hemodynamics, metabolism and pCO2-gap during septic shock induced by live E. coli infusion in dogs. Crit Care Forum 2000; 4:S88 (Abst)
62. Creteur J, De Backer D, Vincent JL. Does gastric tonometry monitor splanchnic perfusion? Crit Care Med 1999; 27:2480-2484
63. Silva E, Creteur J, De Backer D, Vincent JL. Effects of norepinephrine and epinephrine on splanchnic oxygen utilization in septic shock patients. Crit Care Med 1998; 26:A63 (Abst)
64. Doglio GR, Pusajo JF, Egurrola MA, et al. Gastric mucosal pH as a prognostic index of mortality in critically ill patients. Crit Care Med 1991; 19:1037-1040
65. Mohsenifar Z. Gastric intramucosal acidosis during weaning from mechanical ventilation. Adv Exp Med Biol 1994; 361:333-343
66. Gutierrez G, Palizas F, Doglio G, et al. Gastric intramucosal pH as a therapeutic index of tissue oxygenation in critically ill patients. Lancet 1992; 339:195-199
67. Marik PE. Gastric intramucosal pH. A better predictor of multiorgan dysfunction syndrome and death than oxygen-derived variables in patients with sepsis. Chest 1993; 104:225-229
68. Joynt GM, Lipman J, Gomersall CD, Tan I, Scribante J. Gastric intramucosal pH blood lactate in severe sepsis. Anaesthesia 1997; 52:726-732
69. Silva E, Blecher S, Kai MH, et al. Gastric-arterial PCO2 gradient, but not lactate levels, is related to multiple organ dysfunction assessed by SOFA score in septic patients n septic shock. Crit Care Forum 2000; 4:S88 (Abst)
70. De Backer D, Zhang H, Manikis P, Vincent JL. Regional effects of dobutamine in endotoxic shock. J Surg Res 1996; 65:93-100
71. Forrest DM, Baigorri F, Chittock DR, Spinelli JJ, Russell JA. Volume expansion using pentastarch does not change gastric arterial CO2 gradient or gastric intramucosal pH in patients who have sepsis syndrome. Crit Care Med 2000; 28:2254-2258
72. Silva E, De Backer D, Creteur L, Vincent JL. Effects of fluid challenge on gastric-arterial CO2 gradient in septic patients. Crit Care Med 1998; 26:A136 (Abst)
73. Silva E, DeBacker D, Creteur J, Vincent JL. Effects of vasoactive drugs on gastric intramucosal pH. Crit Care Med 1998; 26:1749-1758

74. Creteur J, De Backer D, Vincent JL. A dobutamine test can disclose hepatosplanchnic hypoperfusion in septic patients. Am J Respir Crit Care Med 1999; 160:839-845

75. Duranteau J, Sitbon P, Teboul JL, et al. Effects of epinephrine, norepinephrine, or the combination of norepinephrine and dobutamine on gastric mucosa in septic shock. Crit Care Med 1999; 27:893-900

76. Levy B, Bollaert PE, Luchelli J-P, Sadoune L-D, Larcan A. Dobutamine improves the adequacy of gastric mucosal perfusion in epinephrine-treated septic shock. Crit Care Med 1997; 25:1649-1654

77. Levy B, Nace L, Bollaert PE, Dousset B, Mallie JP, Larcan A. Comparison of systemic and regional effects of dobutamine and dopexamine in norepinephrine-treated septic shock. Intensive Care Med 1999; 25:942-948

78. Gutierrez G, Palizas F, Doglio G, Wainsztein N, Gallesio A, Pacin J et al.. Gastric intramucosal pH as a therapeutic index of tissue oxygenation in critically ill patients [see comments]. Lancet 1992; 339(8787):195-199

79. Gomersall CD, Joynt GM, Freebairn RC, Hung V, Buckley TA, Oh TE. Resuscitation of critically ill patients based on the results of gastric tonometry: a prospective, randomized, controlled trial. Crit Care Med 2000; 28:607-614

80. Chapman M, Mythen MG, Webb AR, Vincent JL. Report from the meeting: gastrointestinal tonometry: state of the art. Intensive Care Med 2000; 26:613-622

21

GENERAL HEMODYNAMIC SUPPORT

Steven M. Hollenberg

Septic shock occurs when infection leads to failure of the circulatory system to maintain adequate delivery of oxygen and other nutrients to tissues, causing cellular and then organ dysfunction. In patients with septic shock, therapy has three main components. The immediate goal is to restore blood pressure and tissue perfusion before irreversible tissue damage ensues. The source of infection must be identified and eliminated. Another therapeutic goal is to interrupt the pathogenic sequence leading to septic shock. While these latter goals are being pursued, adequate organ system perfusion and function must be maintained. Thus, hemodynamic therapy in septic shock is largely supportive, aiming to restore effective tissue perfusion and to normalize cellular metabolism while allowing time for other interventions aimed at reversing the pathophysiology of sepsis to take effect.

Septic shock, the prototypical form of distributive shock, is different and more complicated than other forms of shock. In hypovolemic, cardiogenic, and extracardiac obstructive shock, hypotension results from a decrease in cardiac output, with consequent anaerobic tissue metabolism. In sepsis, tissue hypoperfusion results not only from decreased perfusion pressure attributable to hypotension but also from abnormal shunting of a normal or increased cardiac output [1]. Thus, hemodynamic support of septic patients requires consideration of both global and regional perfusion.

One practical consequence of the complexity of hemodynamics in sepsis is that it is much more difficult to define the goals of therapy with certainty than in other forms of shock in which global hypoperfusion is the dominant pathology. In cardiogenic shock, for example, the goal of therapy is to improve myocardial performance and increase cardiac output. Although different organs may be hypoperfused to variable degrees, indices of regional perfusion usually correlate well with indices of global perfusion, and both can be used to monitor the efficacy of therapy. In sepsis, maldistribution of a normal cardiac output can impair perfusion to different organs. Within the organs themselves, abnormalities of resistance vessel tone or occlusion of nutritive microvessels can result in inhomogeneity of blood flow and exacerbated organ dysfunction. To add to the complexity, cytokines and other pathogenic mediators of sepsis can perturb cellular metabolism, leading to inadequate utilization of oxygen and other nutrients despite adequate perfusion. One might not expect all of these abnormalities to be corrected by hemodynamic therapy. It is, however, possible to formulate an underlying approach to the hemodynamic support of patients with sepsis, with the understanding that the fundamental principle that therapies should be titrated to specific and definable endpoints is more important than specific recommendations.

This chapter will begin with consideration of basic principles in initial assessment of patients with septic shock. Indices of global perfusion will be discussed, followed by consideration of indices of regional perfusion. Finally, specific goals and endpoints for fluid resuscitation, vasopressor therapy, and inotropic support for patients with septic shock will be discussed. Although it is recognized that many vasoactive agents have both vasopressor and inotropic actions, distinction between the two is useful for the purpose of defining goals and endpoints of therapy.

BASIC PRINCIPLES

Patients with septic shock should be treated in an intensive care unit (ICU). Continuous electrocardiographic (EKG) monitoring should be performed for detection of rhythm disturbances, and pulse oximetry should be used to detect fluctuations in arterial oxygenation. Laboratory measurements such as arterial blood gases, serum electrolytes, complete blood counts, coagulation parameters and lactate concentrations should be done early and repeated as indicated.

In shock states, measurement of blood pressure using an arterial cannula provides the most appropriate and reproducible measurement of arterial pressure [2]. Noninvasive monitoring by auscultation or oscillometric methods is commonly inaccurate in hypotensive patients, and these methods measure arterial pressure only intermittently. Arterial cannulation allows for beat-to-beat analysis so that decisions regarding therapy can be based on immediate and reproducible blood pressure information [3]. Such monitoring facilitates the administration of large quantities of fluids and potent vasopressor and inotropic agents to critically ill patients.

Although initial therapy of patients with shock consists of rapid fluid infusion, and mild hypovolemia may be treated successfully with rapid fluid replacement, if the diagnosis remains undefined or the hemodynamic status remains unstable, consideration of right-sided heart catheterization is advisable. The limitations of clinical assessment of intravascular volume and cardiac output in critically ill patients are well recognized [4]. This is particularly true of septic patients, in whom rales on lung auscultation and pulmonary infiltrates on chest X-ray may result from either fluid overload or acute respiratory distress syndrome (ARDS).

In addition, because hemodynamics can change rapidly in sepsis, pulmonary artery catheterization is often useful for monitoring the response to therapy. Optimization of intravascular volume and cardiac output and minimization of dosages of vasoactive agents can often be achieved most rapidly with right heart catheterization.

Echocardiography is an excellent initial tool for cardiovascular evaluation in patients with shock. Echocardiography provides information on overall cardiac performance, identifies regional wall motion abnormalities suggestive of ischemia or infarction, and can rapidly diagnose other causes of shock such as tamponade and valvular disease [5]. Accurate assessment of stroke volume can be done by Doppler echocardiography [6], but serial assessment is more challenging.

Finally, it should be clear that resuscitation of patients with septic shock should be titrated to clinical end points of arterial pressure, heart rate, urine output, skin perfusion, and mental status, as well as to indices of tissue perfusion such as blood lactate concentrations and mixed venous oxygen saturation (SvO_2) [3].

INDICES OF GLOBAL PERFUSION

Bedside clinical assessment can provide a reasonably good indication of global perfusion. Shock in sepsis is usually defined as a systolic pressure below 90 mm Hg or a mean arterial pressure (MAP) below 60 mm Hg [7]. Use of MAP in this context is preferable to systolic pressure because it is a better reflection of organ perfusion pressure [1]. Any given level of arterial pressure, however, must be interpreted in light of the chronic blood pressure; thus, in patients with severe chronic hypertension, a decrease in MAP of 40 mm Hg may produce tissue hypoperfusion even if mean pressure still exceeds 60 mm Hg. Conversely, patients with chronically low blood pressures many not develop shock until the MAP drops below 50 mm Hg. Tachycardia is almost invariably present in patients with shock in the absence of chronotropic incompetence or medications which decrease heart rate.

Clinical indicators of decreased perfusion include oliguria, clouded sensorium, delayed capillary refill, and cool skin. Some caution is necessary in interpreting these signs in septic patients, however, since they are neither completely sensitive nor completely specific. In addition, it is clear that organ dysfunction in sepsis can occur in the absence of global hypoperfusion.

In most forms of shock, elevated blood lactate concentrations reflect anaerobic metabolism due to hypoperfusion, but the interpretation of blood lactate concentrations in septic patients is not as straightforward. Some studies in animal models of sepsis have found normal high-energy phosphate levels [8] but others have not [9]; the differences may relate to the severity of the septic model, with more severe sepsis being associated with depletion of adenosine triphosphate (ATP) despite maintenance of systemic oxygen delivery (DO_2) and tissue oxygenation. A number of studies have indicated that increasing either global [10] or regional DO_2 [11] fails to alter elevated lactate concentrations in patients with sepsis. Measurements of tissue PO_2 in septic patients have failed to demonstrate tissue hypoxia in the presence of lactic acidosis [12], and a number of studies have suggested that elevated lactate may result from cellular metabolic alterations rather than from global hypoperfusion in sepsis [13,14]. Accelerated glycolysis, high pyruvate production [15], and decreased clearance by the liver may contribute to elevated lactate concentrations. Nonetheless, although lactate concentrations may not always represent tissue hypoxia, the prognostic value of elevations of blood lactate has been well established in septic shock patients [16-18]. The trend of lactate concentrations is a better indicator than a single value [16,17]. It is also of interest to note that the blood lactate concentration is a better prognostic indicator than oxygen-derived variables.[19]

The saturation of oxyhemoglobin in the venous circulation is an indicator of the balance between DO_2 and oxygen consumption. For these purposes, it is important to measure saturation in a blood sample in which venous return from the superior and inferior vena cava has been adequately mixed. Thus, SvO_2 is usually measured by withdrawing a blood sample from the pulmonary artery in patients with a right heart catheter in place. Alternatively, continuous measurement of SvO_2 can be achieved using an oximetric right heart catheter. SvO_2 is dependent on cardiac output, oxygen consumption, hemoglobin concentration, and arterial oxygen saturation. In patients with a stable oxygen demand, in the absence of hypoxemia and anemia, desaturation of hemoglobin in mixed venous blood can reflect decreased cardiac output.

As is the case with measurement of blood lactate, interpretation of SvO_2 can be challenging in patients with septic shock. Normal SvO_2 is 70% in critically ill patients. In most forms of shock, hypoperfusion causes increased oxygen extraction in the periphery and decreases SvO_2. In septic patients, however, maldistribution of blood flow with shunting of blood through the tissue can elevate SvO_2. Thus, the utility of using SvO_2 as an index of global perfusion to guide therapy in patients with septic shock has not been demonstrated conclusively. Nonetheless, in septic patients, SvO_2 less than 65% usually indicates decreased perfusion.

INDICES OF REGIONAL PERFUSION

The adequacy of regional perfusion in shock is usually assessed clinically by evaluating indices of organ function. Myocardial hypoperfusion usually presents with evidence of myocardial ischemia. Renal hypoperfusion can be reflected by decreased urine output and increased blood urea nitrogen and creatinine, although acute tubular necrosis is in the differential diagnosis. Central nervous system dysfunction is indicated by an alteration in the level of consciousness or abnormal sensorium. Hepatic parenchymal injury can be manifested by increased serum concentrations of transaminases, lactic dehydrogenase, and bilirubin, and decreased concentrations of albumin and clotting factors indicate decreased hepatic synthetic capability. Splanchnic hypoperfusion can result in stress ulceration, ileus, and malabsorption. In septic shock, however, organ dysfunction can result from either perfusion failure, the effects of toxic mediators such as inflammatory cytokines, or from a combination of the two.[1]

Interest has thus focused on methods of measuring regional perfusion in septic patients more directly. The splanchnic circulation has been the focus of these investigations for several reasons: the countercurrent flow in the gut microcirculation increases the risk of mucosal hypoxia, the gut may have a higher critical DO_2 threshold than other organs, and gut ischemia increases intestinal permeability [20]. Measurements of oxygen saturation in the hepatic vein have revealed oxygen desaturation in a subset of septic patients, suggesting that hepato-splanchnic oxygen supply may be inadequate in these patients, even when more global parameters appear adequate [21].

Gastric tonometry has been proposed as a simple method to assess regional perfusion in the gut by employing a balloon in the stomach to measure intramucosal PCO_2. From this PCO_2 measurement and the arterial bicarbonate concentration, one can then calculate gastric intramucosal pH (pHi) using the Henderson-Hasselbalch equation, making the assumption that bicarbonate concentration in the gastric mucosal tissue is in equilibrium with systemic arterial bicarbonate [22]. Because this may not be the case in shock [23], and because remote systemic metabolic acidosis and alkalosis change systemic bicarbonate, use of gastric mucosal PCO_2, which is not confounded by arterial bicarbonate, has been proposed. Gastric mucosal PCO_2 is influenced directly by systemic arterial PCO_2, however, and so use of the gastric-arterial PCO_2 difference may be the most appropriate primary tonometric variable of interest, although even this parameter is not a simple measure of gastric mucosal hypoxia [23].

Despite this complexity, gastric tonometry is a good predictor for the ultimate outcome of critically ill patients [24-27]. Its usefulness in guiding therapy in patients with sepsis and septic shock, however, has not been proven. One study has shown decreased mortality with pHi-directed care in critically ill patients admitted to an ICU with initially normal pHi [26]. Interpretation of this study is complicated by the fact that mortality in the control group was high, and that therapy based on pHi was heterogeneous because decisions were made at the discretion of the clinicians and not by protocol. In addition, the degree to which the results of this trial are applicable to patients with septic shock is unclear. Gastric tonometry may prove to be a useful measure of regional perfusion in the splanchnic circulation, but randomized controlled trials with clear, reproducible treatment algorithms will be necessary to establish its utility in the management of patients with septic shock.

GOALS AND ENDPOINTS OF HEMODYNAMIC SUPPORT IN SEPTIC PATIENTS

Goals and Monitoring of Fluid Resuscitation

Because septic shock is accompanied by fever, venodilation, and diffuse capillary leakage, most septic patients present with inadequate preload [28]. In the initial phases of experimental and clinical septic shock, filling pressures are low, and a hyperdynamic state develops only after volume repletion [29, 30]. Thus, fluid resuscitation represents the best initial therapy for treatment of hypotension in sepsis. The goal of fluid resuscitation in septic shock is to restore tissue perfusion and to normalize oxidative metabolism. Increasing cardiac output and oxygen delivery is dependent on adequate expansion of blood and plasma volume [31, 32].

Fluid infusion is best initiated with predetermined boluses titrated to clinical endpoints of heart rate, urine output, and blood pressure. Patients who do not respond rapidly to initial fluid boluses, or those with insufficient physiologic reserve, should be considered for invasive hemodynamic monitoring. Filling pressures should be increased to a level associated with maximal increases in cardiac output. In most patients with septic shock, cardiac output will be optimized at pulmonary artery occlusion pressures (PAOP) between 12 mm Hg and 15 mm Hg [33]. Increases above this range usually do not significantly enhance end-diastolic volume or stroke volume and increase the risk of development of pulmonary edema.

The optimal hemoglobin and hematocrit for patients with septic shock is unclear. Hemoglobin concentrations usually range between 8 and 10 gm/dl in patients with septic shock, and a decrease in hemoglobin in the range of 1 to 3 gm/dl can be expected during resuscitation of septic shock with either crystalloids or colloids [34]. This degree of anemia is usually well tolerated in most patients, because the associated decrease in blood viscosity decreases afterload and increases venous return, thereby increasing stroke volume and cardiac output. Some patients, however, may have clinical parameters that suggest a need for increased DO_2, including excessive tachycardia, cardiac dysfunction, underlying coronary artery disease, severe mixed venous oxygen desaturation, or failure to clear lactic acidosis.

Transfusing to a predefined threshold to increase DO_2 cannot be recommended on the basis of existing data. The majority of trials have not demonstrated significant increases in systemic oxygen consumption nor shown consistent benefit in tissue perfusion when the major effect of transfusion therapy is to increase oxygen content [35-37]. A multicenter controlled trial randomizing critically ill patients to transfusion thresholds of 7 gm/dl and 10 gm/dl failed to demonstrate any improvement in clinically significant outcomes with higher hemoglobin levels [38].

Goals and Monitoring of Vasopressor Therapy

When appropriate fluid administration fails to restore adequate arterial pressure and organ perfusion, therapy with vasopressor agents should be initiated. Vasopressor therapy may be required transiently even while cardiac filling pressures are not yet adequate, in order to maintain perfusion in the face of life-threatening hypotension. Although the use of these drugs has the potential to reduce organ blood flow through arterial vasoconstriction, their final effects will depend upon the sum of the direct effects and any increase in organ perfusion pressure. In settings where organ autoregulation is lost, organ flow becomes linearly dependent on pressure [39,40] and organ perfusion pressure must be preserved to optimize flow.

All patients requiring vasopressor therapy for shock should have an arterial cannula for measurement of blood pressure, not only because these catheters are more accurate than noninvasive methods in this setting, but because they allow decisions regarding therapy to be based on immediate and reproducible blood pressure information. Such monitoring makes it possible to give optimal quantities of fluids and potent vasopressor and inotropic agents safely to critically ill patients [1].

Arterial pressure is the endpoint of vasopressor therapy, and the restoration of adequate pressure is the criterion of effectiveness. Blood pressure, however, does not always equate to blood flow, and the precise level of MAP to aim for is not necessarily the same in all patients. Animal studies suggest that below a MAP of 60 mm Hg, autoregulation in the coronary, renal, and central nervous system vascular beds blood flow is compromised, and blood flow may be reduced [39]. Thus, most authorities recommend that MAP should be maintained above 60 mm Hg in septic patients [2,3,28].

Some patients, however, may require higher blood pressures to maintain adequate perfusion. In sepsis, autoregulation curves may be shifted to the right, demanding a greater perfusion pressure to achieve adequate blood flow. There is some data from open-label clinical series to support the notion that urine output and creatinine clearance can be increased in septic patients by targeting MAP to levels as high as 75 mm Hg [41,45]. Nonetheless, a recent study of ten patients with fluid-refractory septic shock requiring vasopressor agents found no improvement in parameters of tissue perfusion when MAP was increased from 65 mm Hg to 85 mm Hg [46]. It is clear that individualization of therapy is warranted in the clinical setting; hypertensive patients, for example, may need higher pressures to maintain perfusion than normotensive patients. It is also clearly important to supplement end points such as blood pressure with assessment of regional and global perfusion using the methods outlined previously.

Goals and Monitoring of Inotropic Therapy

Inotropic therapy in septic shock is complex in that different approaches endeavor to achieve different goals. When fluid resuscitation is adequate, cardiac output is elevated in most septic patients, but myocardial contractility, as assessed by ejection fraction, is impaired [47]. Some patients, especially those with pre-existing cardiac dysfunction, may have decreased cardiac output and may require inotropic agents such as dobutamine, dopamine, and epinephrine. In septic patients with decreased cardiac output, the goal of therapy is to restore normal physiology. Because of the complexity of assessment of clinical parameters in septic patients, direct measurement of cardiac output by invasive hemodynamic monitoring is advisable, but other endpoints of global perfusion should be followed as well. When global hypoperfusion is manifested by decreased SvO_2, this measure may be used as a guide to the adequacy of inotropic therapy. Similarly, a fall in blood lactate concentrations concomitant with increased cardiac output is a good prognostic sign.

Some critically ill septic patients are hypermetabolic and may require high levels of DO_2 to maintain oxidative metabolism [9, 28]. Accordingly, it has been hypothesized that such patients would benefit from therapeutic measures to increase oxygen delivery to 'supranormal' levels. Retrospective analyses showed that achievement of cardiac index greater than 4.5 L/min/m^2, oxygen delivery greater than 600 ml/min/m^2, and oxygen consumption greater than 170 ml/min/m^2 correlated with improved survival [48]. Randomized studies to test the hypothesis that routinely increasing DO_2 to these predefined levels in all critically ill patients have produced conflicting results [49-52], and it remains unclear whether increases in cardiac index and DO_2 are the cause of increased survival or represent underlying physiologic reserve of the patient. Thus, on the basis of current data, a strategy of routinely increasing DO_2 to predetermined elevated end-points of cardiac index and DO_2 is not recommended [3, 53]. Nonetheless, some clinicians believe that this issue has not been settled definitively in those patients with septic shock, and argue that a subset of these patients may benefit from therapy aimed at supranormal DO_2. Because the trials in support of such a strategy involved titration to endpoints of cardiac output and DO_2, is seems logical that such therapy would best be guided by invasive hemodynamic monitoring to measure cardiac output and systemic and mixed venous oxygen saturation.

Despite seemingly adequate resuscitation, some patients with septic shock develop multiple organ failure (MOF), resulting in death. It has been hypothesized that even after hypotension has been corrected and global DO_2 is adequate in patients with septic shock, blood flow and tissue perfusion can remain suboptimal. Cellular perfusion is dependent on microvascular perfusion, which in turn is dependent on regional perfusion. Regional perfusion, in turn, is a function of cardiac output and its distribution, as well as of regional perfusion pressure. Thus, given the complexity of the pathogenesis of sepsis, while achievement of adequate global DO_2 is necessary for adequate cellular perfusion, it may not always be sufficient.

Although the current evidence does not support improved outcome with empiric therapy to raise cardiac output in patients with normal blood pressure, a subpopulation of patients might have regional hypoperfusion that would respond to additional therapy. Such therapy would need to be titrated to an index of regional perfusion such as gastric tonometry, although the precise endpoints are unclear. In this context, it is important to realize that different interventions to increase DO_2, such as fluid resuscitation, blood transfusion, or infusion of vasoactive agents, can have different effects on regional perfusion [54-56]. Indeed, different vasoactive agents have been shown to have divergent effects on gastric intramucosal pH. This is an area of controversy and ongoing research; randomized controlled trials, with clear, reproducible treatment algorithms and use of defined measures of regional perfusion are necessary. In the interim, clinicians should choose endpoints for inotropic therapy in septic patients and titrate therapy to these endpoints

CONCLUSION

The complexity of the pathophysiology of sepsis has led to controversy regarding optimal therapy. Nonetheless, it is possible to formulate an underlying approach to the hemodynamic support of patients with sepsis, with the understanding that the basic principles of the approach are more important than the specific recommendations. For example, as we advance our understanding of which parameters most accurately reflect the effects of therapy in septic patients, it seems clear that eventually a combination of these parameters will prove most useful. Similarly, although the particular endpoints that clinicians use may change, the notion that they should define the goals of therapy and evaluate the results of their interventions on the basis of those goals will remain. Therapies for sepsis will continue to evolve, but the notion that such therapies should be titrated to specific and definable endpoints remains a fundamental principle.

REFERENCES

1. Hollenberg SM, Parrillo JE. Shock. In: Fauci AS, Braunwald E, Isselbacher KJ, et al., eds. Harrison's Principles of Internal Medicine. New York: McGraw-Hill, 1997:214-222
2. Parrillo JE, Parker MM, Natanson C, et al. Septic shock in humans: Advances in the understanding of pathogenesis, cardiovascular dysfunction, and therapy. Ann Intern Med 1990; 113:227-242
3. Task Force of the American College of Critical Care Medicine, Hollenberg SM, Ahrens TS, et al. Practice parameters for hemodynamic support of sepsis in adult patients. Crit Care Med 1999; 27:639-660
4. Mimoz O, Rauss A, Rekei N, et al. Pulmonary artery catheterization in critically ill patients: a prospective analysis of outcome changes associated with catheter-prompted changes in therapy. Crit Care Med 1994; 22:573-579
5. Cunnion RE, Natanson C. Echocardiography, pulmonary artery catheterization, and radionuclide cineangiography in septic shock. Intensive Care Med 1994; 20:535-537
6. Hollenberg SM, Neumann AL, Schupp E, et al. Comparison of stroke volumes obtained by echocardiography and thermodilution in septic patients. Crit Care Med 1993; 22:A112 (Abst)
7. Bone RC, Fein AM, Balk RA, et al. Definitions for sepsis and organ failure and guidelines for the use of innovative therapies in sepsis. Chest 1992; 101(6):1644-1655

8. Hotchkiss RS, Karl IE. Reevaluation of the role of cellular hypoxia and bioenergetic failure in sepsis. JAMA 1992; 267:1503-1510

9. Astiz M, Rackow EC, Weil MH, et al. Early impairment of oxidative metabolism and energy production in severe sepsis. Circ. Shock 1988; 26:311-320

10. Hayes MA, Timmins AC, Yau EH, et al. Oxygen transport patterns in patients with sepsis syndrome or septic shock: influence of treatment and relationship to outcome. Crit Care Med 1997; 25:926-936

11. Steffes CP, Dahn MS, Lange MP. Oxygen transport-dependent splanchnic metabolism in the sepsis syndrome. Arch Surg 1994; 129:46-52

12. Boekstegers P, Weidenhofer S, Pilz G, et al. Peripheral oxygen availability within skeletal muscle in sepsis and septic shock: comparison to limited infection and cardiogenic shock. Infection 1991; 5:317-323

13. Bredle D, Samsel R, Schumacker P. Critical O_2 delivery to skeletal muscle at high and low PO_2 in endotoxemic dogs. J Appl Physiol 1989; 66:2553-2558

14. Rackow E, Astiz ME, Weil MH. Increases in oxygen extraction during rapidly fatal septic shock in rats. J Lab Clin Med 1987; 109:660-664

15. Gore DC, Jahoor F, Hibbert JM, et al. Lactic acidosis during sepsis is related to increased pyruvate production, not deficits in tissue oxygen availability. Ann Surg 1996; 224:97-102

16. Friedman G, Berlot G, Kahn RJ. Combined measurements of blood lactate levels and gastric intramucosal pH in patients with severe sepsis. Crit. Care Med. 1995; 23:1184-1193

17. Vincent JL, Dufaye P, Berre J. Serial lactate determinations during circulatory shock. Crit Care Med. 1983; 11:449-451

18. Weil MH, Afifi AA. Experimental and clinical studies on lactate and pyruvate as indicators of the severity of acute circulatory failure. Circulation 1970; 41:989-1001

19. Bakker J, Coffemils M, Leon M, et al. Blood lactates are superior to oxygen-derived variables in predicting outcome in human septic shock. Chest 1992; 99:956-962

20. Nelson D, Beyer C, Samsel R, et al. Pathologic supply dependence of systemic and intestinal O_2 uptake during bacteremia in the dog. J Appl Physiol 1987; 63:1487-1489

21. De Backer D, Creteur J, Noordally O, et al. Does hepato-splanchnic VO2/DO2 dependency exist in critically ill septic patients? Am J Respir Crit Care Med 1998; 157:1219-1225

22. Creteur J, De Backer D, Vincent JL. Monitoring gastric mucosal carbon dioxide pressure using gas tonometry: in vitro and in vivo validation studies. Anesthesiology 1997; 87:504-510

23. Russell JA. Gastric tonometry: does it work? Intensive Care Med. 1997; 23:3-6

24. Marik PE. Gastric intramucosal pH. A better predictor of multiorgan dysfunction syndrome and death than oxygen-derived variables in patients with sepsis. Chest 1993; 104:225-229

25. Maynard N, Bihari D, Beale R, et al. Assessment of splanchnic oxygenation by gastric tonometry in patients with acute circulatory failure. JAMA 1993; 270:1203-1210

26. Gutierrez G, Palizas F, Doglio G, et al. Gastric intramucosal pH as a therapeutic index of tissue oxygenation in critically ill patients. Lancet 1992; 339:195-199

27. Doglio GR, Pusajo JF, Egurrola MA, et al. Gastric mucosal pH as a prognostic index of mortality in critically ill patients. Crit Care Med 1991; 19:1037-1040

28. Rackow EC, Astiz ME. Mechanisms and management of septic shock. Crit Care Clin 1993; 9:219-237

29. Carroll G, Snyder J. Hyperdynamic severe intravascular sepsis depends on fluid administration in cynomolgus monkey. Am J Physiol 1982; 243:R131-R141

30. Rackow EC, Kaufman BS, Falk JL, et al. Hemodynamic response to fluid repletion in patients with septic shock: evidence for early depression of cardiac performance. Circ Shock 1987; 22:11-22

31. Astiz ME, Rackow EC, Weil MH. Pathophysiology and treatment of circulatory shock. Crit Care Clin. 1993; 9:183-203

32. Haupt MT, Gilbert EM, Carlson RW. Fluid loading increases oxygen consumption in septic patients with lactic acidosis. Am Rev Respir Dis 1985; 131:912-916

33. Packman MJ, Rackow EC. Optimum left heart filling pressure during fluid resuscitation of patients with hypovolemic and septic shock. Crit Care Med 1983; 11:165-169

34. Rackow EC, Falk JL, Fein IA. Fluid resuscitation in shock: A comparison of cardiorespiratory effects of albumin, hetastarch and saline solutions in patients with hypovolemic shock. Crit Care Med. 1983; 11:839-850

35. Conrad S, Dietch K, Hebert C. Effect of red cell transfusion on oxygen consumption following fluid resuscitation in septic shock. Circ Shock 1990; 31:419-429

36. Mink R, Pollack M. Effect of blood transfusion on oxygen consumption in pediatric septic shock. Crit. Care Med. 1990; 18:1087-1091

37. Steffes C, Bender J, Levison M. Blood transfusion and oxygen consumption in surgical sepsis. Crit Care Med. 1991; 19:512-517

38. Hebert PC, Wells G, Blajchman M, et al. A multicenter, randomized, controlled clinical trial of transfusion requirements in critical care. N Engl J Med 1999; 340:409-417

39. Bersten AD, Holt AW. Vasoactive drugs and the importance of renal perfusion pressure. New Horiz 1995; 3:650-661

40. Kirchheim HR, Ehmke H, Hackenthal E, et al. Autoregulation of renal blood flow, glomerular filtration rate and renin release in conscious dogs. Pflugers Arch 1987; 410:441-449

41. Desjars P, Pinaud M, Bugnon D, et al. Norepinephrine therapy has no deleterious renal effects in human septic shock. Crit Care Med 1989; 17:426-429

42. Fukuoka T, Nishimura M, Imanaka H, et al. Effects of norepinephrine on renal function in septic patients with normal and elevated serum lactate levels. Crit Care Med 1989; 17:1104-1107

43. Hesselvik JF, Brodin B. Low dose norepinephrine in patients with septic shock and oliguria: effects on afterload, urine flow, and oxygen transport. Crit Care Med 1989; 17:179-180

44. Martin C, Eon B, Saux P, et al. Renal effects of norepinephrine used to treat septic shock patients. Crit Care Med 1990; 18:282-285

45. Redl-Wenzl EM, Armbruster C, Edelmann G, et al. The effects of norepinephrine on hemodynamics and renal function in severe septic shock states. Intensive Care Med 1993; 19:151-154

46. LeDoux D, Astiz ME, Carpati CM, et al. Effects of perfusion pressure on tissue perfusion in septic shock. Crit Care Med 2000; 28:2729-2732

47. Parker MM, Shelhamer JH, Bacharach SL, et al. Profound but reversible myocardial depression in patients with septic shock. Ann Intern Med 1984; 100:483-490

48. Tuchschmidt J, Fried J, Astiz M, et al. Elevation of cardiac output and oxygen delivery improves outcome in septic shock. Chest 1992; 102:216-220

49. Yu M, Levy MM, Smith P, et al. Effect of maximizing oxygen delivery on morbidity and mortality rates in critically ill patients: a prospective, randomized, controlled study. Crit Care Med 1993; 21:830-838

50. Hayes MA, Timmins AC, Yau EHS, et al. Elevation of systemic oxygen delivery in the treatment of critically ill patients. N Engl J Med 1994; 330:1717-1722

51. Gattinoni L, Brazzi L, Pelosi P, et al. A trial of goal-oriented hemodynamic therapy in critically ill patients. N Engl J Med 1995; 333:1025-1032

52. Boyd O, Grounds RM, Bennett ED. A randomized clinical trial of the effect of deliberate perioperative increase of oxygen delivery on mortality in high-risk surgical patients. JAMA 1993; 270:2699-2707

53. Heyland DK, Cook DJ, King D, et al. Maximizing oxygen delivery in critically ill patients: a methodologic appraisal of the evidence. Crit. Care Med. 1996; 24:517-524

54. Levy B, Bollaert PE, Charpentier C, et al. Comparison of norepinephrine and dobutamine to epinephrine for hemodynamics, lactate metabolism, and gastric tonometric variables in septic shock: a prospective, randomized study. Intensive Care Med. 1997; 23:282-287

55. Marik PE, Mohedin M. The contrasting effects of dopamine and norepinephrine on systemic and splanchnic oxygen utilization in hyperdynamic sepsis. JAMA 1994; 272:1354-1357

56. Schreuder WO, Schneider AJ, Groeneveld ABJ, et al. Effect of dopamine vs norepinephrine on hemodynamics in septic shock. Chest 1989; 95:1282-1288

22

FLUID ADMINISTRATION

Andrew R Webb

Sepsis is the systemic response to infection and may be associated with organ dysfunction or shock. Shock in sepsis is often characterized by low peripheral resistance and, particularly after fluid resuscitation, high cardiac output [1,2]. In clinical shock inadequate tissue perfusion may be overt (with obvious clinical signs) or covert (with few clinical signs). Both may lead to organ dysfunction and failure. Recognizing covert shock requires a high degree of suspicion, early recognition of hypovolemia and tools for assessment of tissue perfusion.

Managing shock follows the basic principles of resuscitation followed by attention to the cause. Resuscitation requires a functional approach to the circulation after ensuring adequate oxygenation and appropriate hemodynamic monitoring. The circulation may be thought of as a system of conduits carrying oxygen and nutrient containing fluid (blood) to tissues and driven by a pump (the heart). Resuscitation must target the four main components of the circulation individually, i.e., the heart, the blood vessels, the blood (volume and constituents) and the tissues. This chapter will concentrate on the management of the blood volume.

Usually the circulating volume will be targeted first [3, 4]. Apart from attention to the oxygen supply, correction of volume deficit is the most critical intervention in shock and may even modulate the immune response [5]. This was realized in the 19th century [6] when it was stated that volume replacement rather than erythrocyte replacement was most critical in hemorrhage. The situation is no different in the management of hypovolemia associated with sepsis. Towards the end of World War I it was demonstrated that colloid rather than saline infusions produced more effective blood pressure correction and less edema in hemorrhagic shock [7].

Few would disagree that early administration of fluid often corrects features of shock, such as hypotension or oliguria. Indeed, approximately 50% of septic patients will have hemodynamic stability restored after adequate fluid resuscitation [8] and more than 90% will have a normal or high cardiac output [1]. Hypovolemia must be treated urgently to avoid the serious complication of organ dysfunction.

It is important that assumptions are not made about appropriate filling pressures, which may bear little relation to filling volumes. Rather, a fluid challenge approach is adopted with careful assessment of the circulatory response to small, incremental fluid aliquots. In this way subclinical hypovolemia is uncovered and treated at the same time.

ROLE OF VOLUME REPLACEMENT IN SEPSIS

The Hemodynamic Problem

The hallmarks of sepsis-induced peripheral vascular failure are vasodilatation and capillary leak. Vasodilatation increases the size of the intravascular space such that a greater than normal circulating volume is required. In this situation hypovolemia may be relative rather than absolute. Capillary leak clearly reduces the circulating volume by exudation to the interstitial space. Sepsis induced myocardial depression is associated with a reduced ejection fraction such that a normal stroke volume requires a greater than normal end-diastolic volume. End-systolic volume is also increased. Providing for an increase in cardiac filling may require a higher than normal circulating volume. In addition insensible fluid loss through sweat is often increased due to fever and, in some cases, an inappropriate polyuria contributes as a result of impaired renal concentrating capacity [9].

Thus, sepsis is associated with both absolute and relative hypovolemia [10]. Provision of an adequate circulating volume is a priority since it is associated with an improvement in survival [11].

The Problem of Capillary Leak

Because of the associated capillary leak, some choose to maintain a reduced circulating volume in an attempt to avoid edema formation while supporting the circulation with inotropes. Both inotropes and colloids used in resuscitation would be expected to increase capillary pressure and therefore increase transcapillary fluid flux. The use of inotropic agents in hypovolemic patients often leads to tachycardia with an associated increase in myocardial oxygen demand [12,13]. Inotropes also have various effects in different parts of the circulation depending on the balance of α, β and dopaminergic stimulation. However, the balance of vasodilatation versus vasoconstriction is not predictable for particular tissues [14], particularly in the critically ill and in view of the endogenous sympathetic response to hypovolemia. The result is an unpredictable maldistribution of flow.

The use of fluid to restore circulating volume overcomes many of the problems associated with inotropes in the hypovolemic patient. Increase in stroke volume is achieved without further increase in sympathetic drive, thus avoiding the problem of increasing tachycardia. Likewise, a reduction in adrenergic peripheral vasoconstriction secondary to hypovolemia will improve microcirculatory blood flow [15]. Only after the circulating volume has been restored can the use of additional circulatory support be recommended.

Notwithstanding the above, the 'dry and drive' philosophy exists because of concern over the effects of edema. This, and cost-effectiveness issues, predominate in the colloid-crystalloid controversy. Proponents of the crystalloid school accept an increase in edema formation and suggest that this does not affect outcome [16-19].

DIAGNOSING HYPOVOLAEMIA

The Gold Standard

The gold standard for the diagnosis of hypovolemia is the measurement of blood volume. Techniques available rely on the principles of indicator dilution, usually involving radio-isotopes as the indicators. Most techniques do not lend themselves to rapid, bedside estimation and, therefore, preclude rapid intervention. Furthermore, true estimation of blood volume requires an indicator that is detectable before it distributes outside the circulation. The only indicator that can currently be used in this fashion, mixing with the whole circulation before any loss from the circulation, is radio-chromium labeled red blood cells (RBCs) [20]. The development of methods based on carbon monoxide labeled red cells [21] is more promising. However, normal blood volume is a poor indicator of physiological requirement and is dependent on body composition, being lower in obese patients [22]. We therefore rely on surrogate markers of volume status.

Clinical Signs

Clinical signs of hypovolemia (reduced skin turgor, oliguria, tachycardia and hypotension) are late indicators. The presence of these signs signifies hypovolemia of a degree that requires urgent intervention. The absence of these signs does not exclude hypovolemia. Indeed paradoxical bradycardia has been described in severe hemorrhagic shock [23]. More difficult is the diagnosis of lesser degrees of hypovolemia which require treatment for maintenance of tissue perfusion and avoidance of the sequelae of organ dysfunction. Clinical assessment is dependent on patient position, there being an increase in plasma volume, and therefore a minimization of clinical signs, associated with supine positioning [24]. Where hypovolemia is suspected in a supine patient, lifting the legs and watching for an improvement in the circulation is a useful indicator.

The Central Venous Pressure

The central venous pressure (CVP) is the most popular surrogate marker of volume status. Its popularity is based on ease of measurement but there are a number of pitfalls. CVP is dependent on venous return to the heart, right ventricular compliance, peripheral venous tone [25] and posture [26]. A normal CVP does not exclude hypovolemia [22] and the CVP is particularly unreliable in pulmonary vascular disease, right ventricular disease, isolated left ventricular failure and valvular heart disease. In patients with an intact sympathetic response to hypovolemia, the CVP may fall in response to fluid [27]. Although peripheral vasodilatation is more common in sepsis it is dangerous to rely on absolute CVP measurements as the sole arbiter of volume status.

Pulmonary Artery Wedge Pressure and Cardiac Output

The pulmonary artery catheter (PAC) has become a popular technique for measurement of pulmonary artery wedge pressure (PAWP) and cardiac output. The PAWP provides similar information regarding fluid status as the CVP and, since the purpose of fluid resuscitation is to provide optimal blood flow, measurement of PAWP without assessment of cardiac output cannot be justified. As with CVP the absolute level of PAWP does not confirm or exclude hypovolemia. Although it has been suggested that cardiac filling pressures of 12-15 mmHg will produce an optimal cardiac output in most septic patients [28], using this as an absolute target does not guarantee optimal filling for the individual. Left ventricular disease may increase the level of PAWP compatible with adequate circulating volume and interpretation of PAWP requires caution in ventilated patients [29]. PAWP is a useful indicator of relative hypovolemia where CVP is high and PAWP is significantly lower, e.g., in selective right ventricular dysfunction or chronic airflow limitation where the CVP is unreliable.

Pulmonary artery catheterization is known to be associated with significant complications [30] and has even been suggested as a cause of increased mortality [31]. Cardiac output can now be measured by non-invasive techniques such as thoracic bioimpedence [32] and esophageal Doppler ultrasound [33]. Both techniques have been used to assess body fluid status [34, 35].

As with other surrogate markers of volume status knowledge of the absolute cardiac output does not confirm or refute hypovolemia. More important is the response of cardiac output to fluid therapy and whether cardiac output is adequate depends on whether tissue perfusion is adequate.

Tissue Perfusion

Irrespective of the volume status, adequate tissue perfusion does not require treatment. Global assessment of tissue perfusion is based on demonstration of the absence of anaerobic metabolism, i.e., no lactic or metabolic acidosis. The presence of lactic acidosis does not necessarily indicate an inadequate circulation, e.g. liver dysfunction, and the absence of lactic acidosis does not guarantee adequate perfusion of all tissues [36].

The gut mucosa is one of the earliest tissues to be compromised in hypovolemia [37, 38] and tonometry provides a simple, non-invasive method of assessment of the adequacy of perfusion [38, 39]. Refinement of the method of gastric tonometry has produced a semi-continuous, automated system. Although the technique may be used to monitor tissue perfusion, correction of which may be the ultimate goal of fluid resuscitation, it must be remembered that alternative treatments may be required to correct tissue perfusion. Global hemodynamic assessment in response to fluid therapy is still required, although the tonometer may help with the difficult diagnosis of otherwise covert hypovolemia [40].

The Fluid Challenge

The fluid challenge is a method of safely restoring circulating volume [41]. Rather than using fixed hemodynamic endpoints, fluid is given in small aliquots to produce a known increment in circulating volume with assessment of the dynamic hemodynamic response to each aliquot. No fixed hemodynamic endpoint is assumed and the technique provides a diagnostic test of hypovolemia (via an appropriate positive response of the circulation to fluid) and a method of titrating the optimal dose of fluid to the individual's requirement.

Assessing the Response to a Fluid Challenge

The response of CVP or stroke volume and PAWP, should be monitored during a fluid challenge. Fluid challenges should be repeated while the response suggests continuing hypovolemia.

CVP or PAWP response

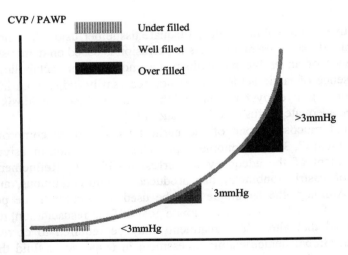

Figure 1. The response of CVP or PAWP to a 200 ml increment of blood volume. In the hypovolemic patient no significant rise in CVP or PAWP would be expected. In the optimally filled patient a rise in CVP or PAWP with no significant rise in stroke volume would be expected.

The change in CVP or PAWP after a 200 ml increment in circulating volume depends on the starting circulating volume (Figure 1). A 3 mm Hg rise in CVP or PAWP represents a significant increase and is probably indicative of an adequate circulating volume. It is important to assess the clinical response and the adequacy of tissue perfusion in addition; if inadequate it is appropriate to monitor stroke volume before further fluid challenges or considering further circulatory support.

Stroke volume response

In the inadequately filled left ventricle a fluid challenge will increase the stroke volume (Figure 2).

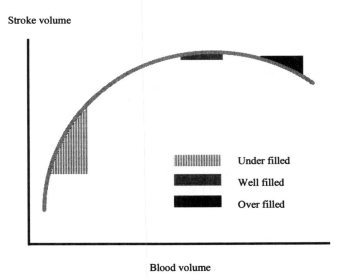

Figure 2. The response of stroke volume to small volume fluid challenges. In the hypovolaemic patient an increase in stroke volume would be expected. In the optimally filled patient no significant rise in stroke volume would be expected.

Failure to increase the stroke volume with a fluid challenge may represent an inadequate challenge, particularly if the PAWP or CVP fails to rise significantly (by at least 3 mm Hg). This indicates that cardiac filling was inadequate as the increment in circulating volume fills the depleted peripheral vascular space. In this case the fluid challenge should be repeated. It is important to monitor stroke volume rather than cardiac output during a fluid challenge. If the heart rate falls appropriately in response to a fluid challenge the cardiac output may not increase despite an increase in stroke volume.

CHOICE OF FLUID

An immediate transudation to the interstitial space of three quarters of the volume of saline [17, 42, 43] infused implies that edema is a necessary side effect of any increase in intravascular volume and therefore any correction of the shock state with crystalloid resuscitation. Although colloid will undoubtedly contribute to edema in states of capillary leak [43], the argument that the transfer of colloid to the interstitial space in capillary leak may contribute to further edema formation has been refuted consistently by experimental evidence [16, 44-46]. There is no difference in the process of edema formation whether the cause is an increase in capillary hydrostatic pressure or capillary leak. In the lung this process follows the sequence of interstitial fluid accumulation, followed by distension of the alveolar capillary barrier and finally alveolar flooding [47]. Thus, it is the intravascular Starling forces that are most relevant and any increase in capillary hydrostatic pressure through resuscitation will contribute to an increase in interstitial volume [48].

Recently, the crystalloid-colloid controversy has been fuelled by several meta-analyses demonstrating no benefit to mortality with colloid resuscitation [49-51]. It is of importance to note that the research on which these meta-analyses were based did not titrate fluid requirements by the dynamic fluid challenge method; in many cases titration was not a hemodynamic endpoint at all [52]. The aim of a fluid challenge is to produce a small but significant (200 ml) and rapid increase in circulating volume. Colloid fluids are ideal in that they give a reliable increase in plasma volume; crystalloids are rapidly lost from the circulation and larger volumes would be required to achieve an increase of 200 ml in circulating volume [17, 42]. Furthermore, fluid administration would have to be repeated more frequently to maintain microcirculatory blood flow [53].

A variety of colloid fluids are available for fluid resuscitation but none has been demonstrated to be superior to others in terms of outcome. In a study of retention of colloid across a standard leaking ultrafiltration membrane hydroxyethyl starch (HES) was superior to albumin, dextrans and gelatins [54]. If colloid fluids are to be used for resuscitation in sepsis it would seem appropriate to choose a fluid that is likely to be better retained in capillary leak. Studies with fractionated HES have demonstrated reduction of capillary leak for medium molecular weight pentastarches [55-57]. Although fractionated solutions are not available for clinical use there are studies suggesting reduced endothelial cell activation [58, 59] and preservation of microvascular cross-sectional area [60] with the currently available HES in sepsis.

CONCLUSION

Despite the plethora of physiological monitoring commonly available in the ICU there remain some challenges in the avoidance of hypovolemia in sepsis. Interpretation of physiological data assumes a reference point of normality or acceptability. Normality is a statistical concept from which 'acceptable' cannot be derived for the individual. Avoiding hypovolemia in sepsis requires a high degree of suspicion and a 'try it and see' approach with corrective treatment. The fluid challenge approach provides a safe method of confirming or refuting the diagnosis while titrating appropriate volume replacement.

REFERENCES

1. Parillo J, Parker M, Natanson C, et al. Septic shock in humans: advances in the understanding of pathogenesis, cardiovascular dysfunction and therapy. Ann Intern Med 1990; 113:227-242
2. Parker M, Shelhamer J, Bacharach S, et al. Profound but reversible myocardial depression in patients with septic shock. Ann Intern Med 1984; 100:483-490
3. Ognibene F, Parker M, Natanson C, et al. Depressed left ventricular performance: response to volume infusion in patients with sepsis and septic shock. Chest 1988; 93:903-910
4. Rackow E, Astiz M. Pathophysiology and treatment of septic shock. JAMA 1991; 266:548-554
5. Wilson M, Chou M, Spain D, et al. Fluid resuscitation attenuates early cytokine mRNA expression after peritonitis. J Trauma 1996; 41:622-627
6. von Ott aus St Petersburg. Über den Einfluß der kochsalzinfusion auf den verbluteten Organismus im Vergleich mit anderen zur Transfusion verwendeten Flüssigkeiten. Arch Path Anat 1883; 93:114-168
7. Bayliss W. Methods of raising a low arterial pressure. Proc Roy Soc London 1917; 89:380-393
8. Sugarman H, Diaco J, Pollak T, et al. Physiologic management of septicemic shock in man. Surg Forum 1971; 22:3-5
9. Cortez A, Zito J, Lucas C. Mechanism of inappropriate polyuria in septic patients. Arch Surg 1977; 172:471-476
10. Rackow E, Astiz M. Mechanisms and management of septic shock. Crit Care Clin 1993; 9:219-237
11. Weil M, Nishjima H. Cardiac output in bacterial shock. Am J Med 1978; 64:920-923

12. Dei CL, Metra M, Visioli O. Clinical pharmacology of inodilators. J Cardiovasc Pharmacol 1989; 14 (suppl 8):S60-S71
13. Takaoka H, Takeuchi M, Odake M, et al. Comparison of the effects on arterial-ventricular coupling between phosphodiesterase inhibitor and dobutamine in the diseases human heart. J Am Coll Cardiol 1993; 22:598-606
14. van Zwieten PA. Receptor-mediated inotropic drugs. Eur Heart J 1988; 9 (Suppl H):85-90
15. Webb A, Moss R, Tighe D, et al. The effects of dobutamine, dopexamine and fluid on hepatic histological responses to porcine faecal peritonitis. Intensive Care Med 1991; 17:487-493
16. Metildi LA, Shackford SR, Virgilio RW, et al. Crystalloid versus colloid in fluid resuscitation of patients with severe pulmonary insufficiency. Surg Gynecol Obstet 1984; 158:207-212
17. Falk J, Rackow E, Weil M. Colloid and crystalloid fluid resuscitation. Acute Care 1983; 10:59-94
18. Velanovich V. Crystalloid versus colloid fluid resuscitation: A meta-analysis of mortality. Surgery 1989; 105:65-71
19. Virgilio R, Rice C, Smith D, et al. Crystalloid vs. colloid resuscitation: is one better. Surgery 1979; 85:129-139
20. Gregersen ML, Rawson RA. Blood volume. Physiol Rev 1959; 39:307-342
21. Myhre L, Brown D, Hall F, et al. The use of carbon monoxide and T-1824 for determining blood volume. Clin Chem 1968; 14:1197-1205
22. Weil M, Shubin H, Rosoff L. Fluid repletion in circulatory shock - central venous pressure and other practical guides. JAMA 1965; 192:668-674
23. Barriot P, Riou B. Hemorrhagic shock with paradoxical bradycardia. Intensive Care Med 1987; 13:203-207
24. Hagan R, Diaz F, Horvath S. Plasma volume changes with movement to supine and standing positions. J Appl Physiol 1978; 45:414-418
25. Widgren B, Berglund G, Wikstrand J, et al. Reduced venous compliance in normotensive men with positive family histories of hypertension. J Hypertens 1992; 10:459-465
26. Amoroso P, Greenwood R. Posture and central venous pressure measurement in circulatory volume depletion. Lancet 1989; 2:258-260
27. Baek S, Makabali G, Byron-Brown C, et al. Plasma expansion in surgical patients with high central venous pressure; the relationship of blood volume to hematocrit, CVP, pulmonary wedge pressure, and cardiorespiratory changes. Surgery 1975; 78:304-315
28. Packman M, Rackow E. Optimum left heart filling pressure during fluid resuscitation of patients with hypovolemic and septic shock. Crit Care Med 1983; 11:165-169
29. Shasby D, Dauber I, Pfister S, et al. Swan-Ganz catheter location and left atrial pressure determine the accuracy of the wedge pressure when positive end-expiratory pressure is used. Chest 1981; 80:666-670
30. Elliot C, Zimmerman G, Clemmer T. Complications of pulmonary artery catheterisation in the care of critically ill patients. A prospective study. Chest 1979; 76:647-652
31. Connors A, Speroff T, Dawson N, et al. The effectiveness of right heart catheterization in the initial care of critically ill patients. JAMA 1996; 276:889-897
32. Kubicek W, Karnegis J, Patterson R, et al. Development and evaluation of an impedance cardiac output system. Aerosp Med 1966; 37:1208-1212
33. Singer M, Clarke J, Bennett E. Continuous hemodynamic monitoring by esophageal Doppler. Crit Care Med 1989; 17:447-452
34. Chiolero R, Gay L, Cotting J, et al. Assessment of changes in body water by bioimpedance in acutely ill surgical patients. Intensive Care Med 1992; 18:322-326

35. Singer M, Allen M, Webb A, et al. Effects of alterations in left ventricular filling, contractility, and systemic vascular resistance on the ascending aortic blood velocity waveform of normal subjects. Crit Care Med 1991; 19:1138-1145
36. Gutierrez G, Clark C, Brown SD, et al. Effect of dobutamine on oxygen consumption and gastric mucosal pH in septic patients. Am J Respir Crit Care Med 1994; 150:324-329
37. Dantzker D. The gastrointestinal tract: the canary of the body? JAMA 1993; 270:1247-1248.
38. Hamilton-Davies C, Mythen M, Salmon J, et al. Comparison of commonly used clinical indicators of hypovolaemia with gastrointestinal tonometry. Intensive Care Med 1997; 23:276-281
39. Grum C, Fiddian-Green R, Pittenger G, et al. Adequacy of tissue oxygenation in intact dog intestine. J Appl Physiol 1984; 56:1065-1069
40. Gutierrez G, Brown S. Gastric tonometry: a new monitoring modality in the intensive care unit. J Intensive Care Med 1995; 10:34-1044
41. Webb A. The fluid challenge. In Webb A, Shapiro M, Singer M, Suter P (Eds) Oxford textbook of Critical Care, Oxford University Press, Oxford, 1999, pp:32-34
42. Shoemaker W, Schluchter M, Hopkins JA, et al. Comparison of the relative effectiveness of colloids and crystalloids in emergency resuscitation. Am J Surg 1981; 142:73-84
43. Shoemaker W. Comparisons of the relative effectiveness of whole blood transfusions and various types of fluid therapy in resuscitation. Crit Care Med 1976; 4:71-78
44. Rackow E, Falk J, Fein I. Fluid resuscitation in shock: a comparison of cardiorespiratory effects of albumin, hetastarch and saline solutions in patients with hypovolemic shock. Crit Care Med 1983; 11:839-850
45. Nylander W, Hammon J, Roselli R, et al. Comparison of the effects of saline and homologous plasma infusion on lung fluid balance during endotoxemia in unanesthetized sheep. Surgery 1981; 90:221-228
46. Appel P, Shoemaker W. Evaluation of fluid therapy in adult respiratory failure. Crit Care Med 1981; 9:862-869
47. Staub N, Nagano H, Pearce M. Pulmonary edema in dogs, especially the sequence of fluid accumulation in the lung. J Appl Physiol 1967; 2:227-240
48. Rackow E, Astiz M, Janz T, et al. Absence of pulmonary edema during peritonitis and shock in rats. J Lab Clin Med 1989; 112:264-269
49. Schierhout G, Roberts I. Fluid resuscitation with colloids or crystalloids in critically ill patients: a systematic review of randomised trials. Br Med J 1998; 316:961-964
50. Cochrane Injuries Group Albumin Reviewers. Human albumin administration in critically ill patients: a systematic review of randomised controlled trials. Br Med J 1998; 317:235-239
51. Choi P, Yip G, Quinonez L, et al. Crystalloids versus colloids in fluid resuscitation: a systematic review. Crit Care Med 1999; 27:200-210
52. Webb A. Crystalloid or colloid resuscitation. Are we any the wiser? Crit Care 1999; 3:R25-R28
53. Funk W, Baldinger V. Microcirculatory perfusion during volume therapy. Anesthesiology 1995; 82:975-982
54. Webb A, Barclay S, Bennett E. In vitro colloid osmotic pressure of commonly used plasma expanders and substitutes: A study of the diffusibility of colloid molecules. Intensive Care Med 1989; 15:116-120
55. Zikria B, King T, Stanford J, et al. A biophysical approach to capillary permeability. Surgery 1989; 105:625-631
56. Webb A, Tighe D, Moss R, et al. Advantages of a narrow-range, medium molecular weight hydroxyethyl starch for volume maintenance in a porcine model of fecal peritonitis. Crit Care Med 1991; 19:409-416

57. Webb A, Moss R, Tighe D, et al. A narrow range, medium molecular weight pentastarch reduces structural organ damage in a hyperdynamic porcine model of sepsis. Intensive Care Med 1992; 18:348-355
58. Collis R, Collins P, Gutteridge C, et al. The effects of hydroxyethyl starch and other plasma volume substitutes on endothelial cell activation; an in vitro study. Intensive Care Med 1994; 20:37-41
59. Boldt J, Muller M, Heesen M, et al. Influence of different volume therapies and pentoxifylline infusion on circulatory soluble adhesion molecules in critically ill patients. Crit Care Med 1996; 24:358-391
60. Morisaki H, Bloos F, Keys J, et al. Compared with crystalloid, colloid therapy slows progression of extrapulmonary tissue injury in septic sheep. J Appl Physiol 1994; 77:1507-1518

23

BLOOD TRANSFUSION AND SEPSIS

David Neilipovitz
Paul C. Hébert

Septic shock is a common reason for admission to the intensive care unit (ICU). Despite recent medical advancements, mortality from sepsis remains around 40% [1] and can be as high as 85% in severe septic shock [2]. Since severe sepsis and septic shock result in significant oxygen delivery (DO_2) and extraction impairments, anemia may have serious clinical consequences in this population. The severe hemodynamic alterations require the administration of fluids, vasoactive drugs and frequently red blood cell (RBC) transfusions to maintain oxygen delivery. However, RBC transfusions may adversely affect immune function [3, 4], and potentially worsen the microvascular defects caused by infection. Recently, a large multicenter trial evaluating transfusion requirements in critical care (TRICC) concluded that a restrictive approach to RBC transfusion was at least as safe as a more liberal approach. Results from the trial were consistent with RBC transfusions either causing harm or being of limited benefit. In this chapter, we will review the potential benefits and risks of anemia and RBC transfusion in the critical care setting. We will also review the TRICC trial in the context of patients with severe sepsis and septic shock.

OXYGEN TRANSPORT, ANEMIA AND SEPSIS

The amount of oxygen delivered, either to the whole body or to specific organs, is the product of blood flow and arterial oxygen content. For the whole body, DO_2 is the product of cardiac output and arterial oxygen content [5-7]. Although anemia decreases arterial oxygen content, a number of adaptive mechanisms are initiated as a means of attempting to maintain DO_2.

These include increased cardiac output as a result of reduced blood viscosity and increased sympathetic output; redistribution of blood flow toward the cerebral and coronary circulation; and, an increase in 2,3-diphosphoglycerate (2,3-DPG) levels making it easier for hemoglobin to unload oxygen in peripheral tissue beds. Hébert and colleagues reviewed the evidence supporting the different adaptive mechanisms in response to anemia (Table 1) [5].

Inference	Quality of evidence
Oxyhemoglobin dissociation curve	
Anemia shifts the oxyhemoglobin curve to the right because of increased 2,3-DPG levels	Ci
Anemia causes clinically significant rightward shifts in the oxyhemoglobin curve because of the Bohr effect	Civ
The shift in the oxyhemoglobin curve has been clearly established in many forms of anemia (excluding hemoglobinopathies)	Cii
The shift in the oxyhemoglobin curve has been clearly established in a number of human diseases	Civ
Cardiac Output	
Cardiac output increases with increasing degrees of normovolemic anemia provided that blood volume is adequate	Ci
Increased cardiac output in normovolemic anemia is a result of increased stroke volume	Ci
The contribution of increased heart rate to the increase in cardiac output following normovolemic anemia is variable	Ci
Other hemodynamic alterations	
Changes in blood viscosity result in many of the hemodynamic changes in normovolemic anemia	Ci
Normovolemic anemia is accompanied by increased sympathetic activity	Ci
Normovolemic anemia causes increased myocardial contractility	Cii
Normovolemic anemia causes a decrease in systemic vascular resistance	Ci
Normovolemic anemia results in a redistribution of cardiac output toward the heart and brain and away from the splanchnic circulation	Ci
Maximum global O_2 delivery occurs at hemoglobin concentrations ([Hb]) of 100-110 g/l	Ciii
Global O_2 delivery declines above and below [Hb] of 100-160 g/l	Ci
Coronary and cerebral blood flow	
Coronary and cerebral blood flow is increased during anemia	Ci
Coronary artery disease in the presence of moderate degrees on anemia ([Hb] < 90 g/l) results in impaired left ventricle contractility or ischemia	Ci
Moderate anemia does not aggravate cerebral ischemia in patients with cerebrovascular disease	Ci

Note: 2,3-DPG=2,3-diphosphoglycerate.

Table 1. *Inferences drawn from the literature addressing physiologic mechanisms in anemia. Adapted from* [5]

However, it is unclear if and to what degree the complex effects of infection and inflammation may interfere with adaptive physiologic mechanisms initiated during anemia. During sepsis, the production of bacterial toxins and many of the cytokines released as a consequence of the host inflammatory responses result in increased cardiac output, impaired left ventricular contractility, decreased afterload from arterial vasodilatation and increased venous capacitance resulting in decreased preload [8-16]. Following adequate volume resuscitation, both anemia and sepsis result in decreased afterload and increased cardiac output but result in divergent effects on contractility and preload, decreased in sepsis and increased in anemia.

It is possible that the decreased contractility observed in sepsis may impair the increase in cardiac output required to maintain DO_2 in anemic patients. At this juncture, there are few laboratory studies examining the combined effects of anemia and sepsis on myocardial function. The interaction between sepsis and anemia may also modulate adaptive responses in the peripheral vasculature, particularly related to changes in the distribution of blood flow between organs [17]. Again, both pathologic processes result in the preferential redistribution of blood flow from the splanchnic circulation towards the brain and heart. However, the combined effects may not be similar to their independent effects.

Overwhelming infections and host immune responses not only modify the delivery of oxygen but have a number of clinically important effects on oxygen utilization. Indeed, sepsis results in increased basal metabolic rates and is also postulated to cause defects in microvascular flow and cellular respirations [18,19]. Studies using intra-vital microscopy suggest capillary occlusion occurs during sepsis [18]. The increase in inter-capillary area may result in increased diffusing distances and potentially cause cellular hypoxia [18,20,21]. A number of studies have also suggested that infection or inflammation as a consequence of infection impairs the ability to generate ATP through cellular respiration [22].

Normovolemic anemia or hemodilution may in fact improve the body's ability to deliver oxygen to the tissues through abnormal microvasculature beds in sepsis but will certainly have little or no effect on oxygen utilization if the predominant effect is an impairment of cellular respiration.

OXYGEN TRANSPORT, RBC TRANSFUSION AND SEPSIS

Over the past 30 years, the prevailing dogma in critical care has been to maintain DO_2 in the normal range and possibly to aim to maintain beyond normal values. Since hemoglobin is the principal oxygen carrier in blood,

RBC transfusion is potentially the most efficient method of augmenting DO_2; however, there are well established and theoretical risks to transfusion [23, 24]. There are a number of controversial issues surrounding oxygen kinetics which include the determination of optimal DO_2 and the ability to detect and optimally treat an oxygen debt in sepsis [25-27]. RBC transfusions have also been reported to result in clinically important immune suppression. There may be adverse clinical effects from the prolonged RBC storage time. These competing risks and benefits complicate any determination of optimal transfusion practice in critically ill patients with severe sepsis and septic shock.

In critical care, many opinion leaders have long advocated maintaining elevated hemoglobin concentrations as an adjunct in targeting oxygen transport to supranormal values [28-30]. The underlying rationale was based on a theory that disease processes, such as sepsis and acute respiratory distress syndrome (ARDS), induce tissue hypoxia by producing an abnormally elevated anaerobic threshold. Below this threshold or critical level of DO_2, O_2 consumption decreases as DO_2 decreases. This abnormal linear relationship is often referred to as 'pathologic supply dependence'. The resultant tissue hypoxia may eventually contribute to the evolution of irreversible multiple system organ failure (MOF) followed by death. Two prospective studies [25,31] have also documented a significant association between mortality and the finding of pathologic supply dependence.

Few studies, however, have examined the role of hemoglobin and red cell transfusions as a means of documenting and potentially alleviating supply dependency [32-37]. Ronco and colleagues [32,34] using red cell administration concluded that there was a pathologic dependence of oxygen consumption (VO_2) on DO_2 in ARDS. While systematically reviewing the literature, we identified 14 clinical studies evaluating the impact of RBC transfusions on oxygen kinetics. All studies measured DO_2 delivery and VO_2 before and after the transfusion of a pre-specified number of allogeneic RBC units. DO_2 uniformly increased but VO_2 was observed to change in only five of the studies (Table 2). Using blood transfusions, similar findings were noted in patients with sepsis [35]. There are no randomized clinical trials which examine the role of red cell transfusions in critically ill patients with potential 'pathologic supply dependence'.

In a study by Heyland et al. [38], the effect of interventions to achieve supraphysiologic values of cardiac index, DO_2 and VO_2 in critically ill patients were systematically reviewed. Mortality rates in this patient population were not significantly altered by these interventions; however, potential benefit was noted in patients in which therapy was initiated pre-operatively. The inferences drawn from this review may be limited by the methodologic limitations of the included studies. Six randomized open-labeled clinical trials [24,28,39-42] evaluated therapeutic interventions other than red cells to augment DO_2. These clinical trials involved the implementation of rigorous protocols using volume expansion with crystalloid and inotropic agents [24,28,40-42] or prostaglandin E_1 [39]. All but one [39] concluded that increasing DO_2 improves survival from sepsis [24], critical illness [42] and high risk surgery [28,40,41].

Concerns with all of these studies include small numbers, complex interventions, biased selection, over interpretation of subgroup analyses and a lack of blinded evaluations of outcomes. In the randomized trials that reported hemoglobin concentrations, transfusion triggers were set very high to maintain hemoglobin concentrations greater than 120 g/l [23].

The oxygen kinetics literature thus still has a number of unanswered questions. The identification of critical levels of DO_2 and, more importantly, optimal levels of DO_2 in various clinical conditions have not been well elucidated. From the overall results of the TRICC trial, transfused RBCs may be the best means of achieving optimal DO_2.

A prospective study which examined the effect of RBC transfusions in twenty-three septic patients had very different results [43] (Figure 1). The transfusion of 3 units of blood did not increase the oxygen uptake as measured by indirect calorimetry for up to 6 hours. A surprising result was a paradoxical decrease in splanchnic oxygen availability as measured by gastric tonometry after the transfusion. The decrease in gastric intramucosal pH (pHi) was inversely related to the age of the transfusion unit. The authors attributed the decrease to poorly deformable transfused red blood cells which caused microcirculatory ischemia. Presently unknown is whether or not a blood transfusion would improve DO_2 after 6 hours since the deformability of transfused RBCs can recover if given time [44,45].

RBC TRANSFUSION AS A CAUSE OF INFECTION

RBC transfusions may cause infections through direct transmission of viruses, bacteria or parasites or through indirect effects on the recipient's immune system. Although the cause of one of the most important epidemics of this century, the risk of transfusion-related viral infections has diminished greatly in developed nations as a consequence of improved collection procedures and testing of the donated blood [46]. The risk of bacterial contamination per unit transfused ranges from 1:100,000 and 1:150,000 for hepatitis B and C, respectively and 1:1,000,000 for human immunodeficiency virus (HIV) (Canadian Blood Services, personal communication, 2000). While the contamination of RBC transfusions by bacteria is quite rare, it is a much more frequent occurrence in platelet transfusions.

Study	Patients	No. of Patients	RBC Dose	HgB	Do$_2$	Vo$_2$	Lactate	Comments
Ronco et al [32] (1990)	PCP pneumonia	5	1.5 U	Yes	Yes	Yes	NA	All patients had lactate at baseline. Thermodilution used for DO$_2$ and Vo$_2$ measurements.
Fenwick, et al [34] (1990)	ARDS	24	1.5 U	Yes Yes	Yes Yes	No No	No Yes	Normal lactate group (n=1) was compared with high lactate group (n=13). Thermodilution catheter used for all measurements. Significant increases in Vo$_2$ in response to transfusion in high lactate group.
Ronco, et al [105] (1991)	ARDS	17	1.5 U	Yes	Yes	No	NA	Normal lactate group (n=7) was compared with high lactate group (n=10). No relationship between DO$_2$ and Vo$_2$ directly measured with expired gases.
Shah, et al [106] (1982)	Posttrauma	8	1 or 2 U	Yes	Yes	Yes	NA	Thermodilution used for DO$_2$ and Vo$_2$ measurements.
Steffes, et al [107] (1991)	Post-operative + Posttrauma	21	1-2 U	Yes	Yes	Yes	No	27 measurements sets in 21 patients. Thermodilution used for DO$_2$ and Vo$_2$ measurements. Increased lactate levels did not predict Vo$_2$ response.
Babineau, et al [108] (1992)	Post-operative	31	328±9 ml	Yes	Yes	No	NA	32 of 33 transfusions were single units. Thermodilution used for DO$_2$ and Vo$_2$ measurements. 58% of transfusions did not increase Vo$_2$.
Gilbert, et al [35] (1988)	Septic	17	20 g/L	Yes	Yes	No	No	33 measurement sets in 31 patients. 10 of 17 patients had increased lactate levels. Vo$_2$ increased significantly in high group only.

Dietrich, et al [37] (1990)	Medical shock (septic/cardiac)	32	577 ml	Yes	Yes	No	No	36 measurement sets in 32 patients. No change in Vo_2 after transfusion. Thermodilution used for DO_2 and Vo_2 measurements.
Conrad, et al [33] (1990)	Septic shock	19	30 g/L	Yes	Yes	No	No	Normal lactate group (n=8) compared with high lactate group (n=11). No increase in Vo_2 with transfusion in either group. Thermodilution used for DO_2 and Vo_2 measurements.
Marik, et al [43] (1993)	Septic	23	3 U	Yes	Yes	No	No	DO_2 measured independently of Vo_2. Using gastric tonometry, patients receiving old RBCs developed evidence of gastric ischemia.
Lorento, et al [109] (1993)	Septic	16	2 U	Yes	Yes	No	NA	Dobutamine significantly increased VO_2; RBCs did not. Thermodilution used for DO_2 and Vo_2 measurements.
Mink, et al [110] (1990)	Septic shock (2 mo - 6 yrs)	8	8-10 ml/kg x 1-2 h	Yes	Yes	No	NA	In pediatric patients, VO_2 did not increase with RBCs. Thermodilution used for DO_2 and Vo_2 measurements.
Lucking, et al [111] (1990)	Septic shock (4 mo - 15 yrs)	7	10-15 ml/kg x 1-3 h	Yes	Yes	Yes	NA	8 measurement sets in 7 patients. Thermodilution used for DO_2 and Vo_2 measurements.

Table 2. Studies examining oxygen delivery (DO_2), oxygen consumption (VO_2) and lactate before and after RBC transfusion

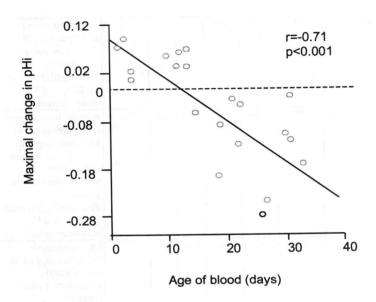

Figure 1: *Relationship of gastric intramucosal pH with increasing age of red blood cells (from [43])*

The immunosuppressive effects of allogeneic blood transfusions were first reported in the early 1970s. Opelz et al. [47] reported improved renal allograft survival in patients who had received multiple blood transfusions. Many laboratory studies have suggested that the immune suppression is primarily mediated by the white cells remaining in transfused RBCs. Altered host immune responses following allogeneic red cell transfusions may also predispose critically ill transfusion recipients to nosocomial infections [53,56-62] and increased rates of MOF [63,64] which may ultimately result in higher mortality rates. However, studies examining postoperative infections following transfusions have not been able to establish a causal association [65,66] due to weak study design and the lack of independence between allogeneic RBC transfusions and the potential complication.

Despite very compelling laboratory studies, observational and randomized controlled clinical trials have documented contradictory findings. We identified eight randomized controlled clinical trials evaluating the immune consequences of red cell transfusions, contrasting either rates of cancer recurrence (n=2) or postoperative infections (n=6). Investigators compared either leukocyte-depleted [62,67-70] or autologous [56,71] transfusions to allogeneic RBCs (Figure 2).

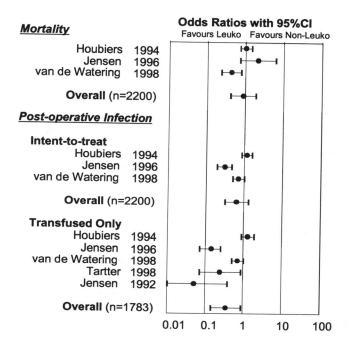

Figure 2: *Post-operative infection in the included studies*

Contradictory conclusions were drawn from the six RCTs examining postoperative infections. Two of the six studies [70,71] did not find any significant difference in the rates of infection among patients having undergone colorectal surgery. Houbiers et al. [70] found a higher rate of postoperative infections in patients receiving leukodepleted as opposed to allogeneic RBCs (42% versus 36%, p>0.05). The four remaining studies [56,62,68,69] documented clinically important decreases in postoperative infections in patients receiving leukodepleted allogeneic RBCs as compared to standard allogeneic RBC products. In a recent study, Jensen and colleagues [69] demonstrated that the rates of wound infections and intra-abdominal abscesses were significantly lower in patients receiving allogeneic RBCs compared to the untransfused groups (12% vs 1%, p<0.0001). The frequency of pneumonia was also lower in patients receiving leukodepleted RBCs (3%) or no transfusions (3%) compared to patients receiving buffy-coated leuko-depleted allogeneic transfusions (23%, p<0.001).

In summary, the six randomized controlled trials reached divergent conclusions concerning the risks of postoperative infections attributed to allogeneic red cell transfusions. A recent meta-analysis [72] combined the results from these trials and was unable to detect clinically important increases mortality and postoperative infections. Since the publication of the meta-analysis, van de Watering and colleagues have published another clinical trial in patients undergoing cardiovascular surgical interventions and observed a decrease in 30-day mortality from 7.8% in patients receiving buffy coat-depleted red cells compared to 3.6% and 3.3% (p=0.015) in patients receiving either fresh-filtered or stored-filtered RBCs, respectively [4]. Although the study was well conducted, the allogeneic RBC transfusion rates in the control group were on average 5.4 RBC units, well in excess of North American norms suggesting that the study results may have limited generalizability. In addition, the number of events were small, suggesting that the mortality estimates might be quite unstable.

To better understand the results of this study in the context of the rest of the literature, we have added the results of this new clinical trial to the meta-analysis by McAllister et al. [72]. In doing so, the relative risk for all-cause mortality was 1.05 (95% confidence interval ranging from 0.88 to 1.25) and 1.10 (95% confidence interval ranging from 0.85 to 1.43) for post-operative infections. In summary, despite convincing laboratory evidence, the clinical significance of the immunosuppressive effects of allogeneic RBC transfusions have not been clearly established [3].

RBC TRANSFUSIONS AS A CAUSE OF MICROCIRCULATORY DYSFUNCTION IN SEPSIS

A few recent reviews have summarized a large volume of literature characterizing well-defined biochemical and corpuscular changes to RBCs during storage, collectively referred to as the storage lesion [73-75]. From these reviews, it is evident that there are few data on the clinical consequences of transfusing old stored RBC product. Traditionally, the storage lesion has been restricted to changes occurring in the RBC rather than bioreactive substances as described by the media. Corpuscular changes include a depletion of ATP and 2,3-DPG, membrane vesiculation [76-78], lipid peroxidation of RBC membrane [79] and loss of deformability [80-82].

Depletion of 2,3-DPG is well described and has become an accepted occurrence during storage but its clinical relevance is debated. It has been repeatedly demonstrated in man and non-human primates that following transfusion of DPG-depleted RBCs, systemic DPG levels, as well as the p50 values (a measure of oxyhemoglobin affinity indicated by the oxygen tension at 50% hemoglobin saturation), fall significantly and then regenerate at a variable rate taking up to 24 hours to several days [83,84]. The potential consequences of transfusing older stored RBCs on DO_2 has not been adequately studied yet has led some clinicians to advocate the use of fresh blood in certain patients, such as those massively transfused. Under these circumstances, it has been speculated that transfusion of large amounts of stored blood low in 2,3-DPG may have an adverse clinical consequence on DO_2 in patients whose balance is precarious [85-88].

During RBC storage, there is a progressive fall in pH, an increase in plasma potassium and release of free hemoglobin from lysed RBCs [89]. The immediate clinical consequences of transfusing these storage by-products are probably limited (except in neonates) given the recipients capacity to buffer, dilute or remove these substances. However, their long-term effects are not known. In addition, there is generation of cytokines and other bioreactive substances [90], including histamine [91], complement [92,93], lipid [94], and cytokines [95], which have been found in the storage media and which may have deleterious effects when transfused.

There are no randomized clinical trials evaluating the clinical consequences of transfusing these bioreactive substances. The only prospective study in this area was designed to test the difference in gastric ischemic episodes between septic and nonseptic patients. Marik and colleagues [43] demonstrated an association between a fall in gastric pHi and transfusion of RBCs stored for greater than 15 days. Three retrospective clinical studies tested the association between the age of transfused blood and length of stay in the ICU [96] or mortality [97]. Martin et al. [96] observed a statistically significant association between the transfusion of aged blood (>14 days old) and increased length of ICU stay (p=0.003) in 698 critically ill patients. In patients receiving a transfusion, aged RBCs was the only predictor of length of stay (p<0.0001). In survivors, from this analysis, only median age of blood was predictive of length of stay (p<0.0001). Purdy et al. [97] demonstrated a negative correlation (r=-0.73) between the proportion of RBC units of a given age transfused to survivors and increasing age of RBCs in patients admitted to the ICU with a diagnosis of severe sepsis (n=31). Purdy et al. also noted that these latter units were more likely to be older. A recently published study evaluating the effect of length of RBC storage on postoperative pneumonia in 416 consecutive patients undergoing coronary artery bypass grafting noted an adjusted increase of 1% in the risk of postoperative pneumonia per day of average increase in the length of storage of RBCs (p<0.005) in transfused patients [98]. Each of these three studies also noted that patients receiving a large number of RBC units had a higher mortality.

SEPSIS, SEPTIC SHOCK AND THE TRICC TRIAL RESULTS

We recently completed and published the results of TRICC, a large multicenter clinical trial. The study was designed to determine whether a restrictive and a liberal transfusion strategy were equivalent in usual clinical ICU practice. We reasoned that if both transfusion strategies were found to be equivalent, then a lower threshold should be recommended in critically ill patients. Eight hundred and thirty-eight patients who: 1) were expected to stay more than 24 hours; 2) had a hemoglobin concentration less than or equal to 9.0 g/dl within 72 hours of ICU admission; and 3) were considered volume resuscitated or normovolemic by the attending staff were included in the study. Once randomized, a study patient's hemoglobin level was maintained using allogeneic red cell transfusions as required. Patients allocated to the restrictive strategy had their hemoglobin levels maintained between 7.0 and 9.0 g/dl, with a transfusion trigger at 7.0 g/dl. Patients allocated to the liberal transfusion strategy had their hemoglobin levels maintained between 10.0 and 12.0 g/dl, with a transfusion trigger at 10.0 g/dl. Blinding of treatment allocation was not feasible.

Average hemoglobin concentrations (8.5 ± 0.72 vs 10.7 ± 0.73 g/dl, $p<0.01$) and RBC units transfused (2.6 ± 4.1 vs. 5.6 ± 5.3 RBC units, $p<0.01$) were significantly lower in the restrictive as compared to the liberal group. Overall, 30-day mortality tended to be lower in the restrictive transfusion group (18.7 vs 23.3, $p = 0.11$). However, 30-day mortality rates were significantly decreased (8.7 vs 16.1%, $p=0.03$) in patients who were less acutely ill (APACHE II score < 20) and less than 55 years of age (5.7 and 13.0%, respectively, $p = 0.02$) but not in patients with significant cardiac disease (22.9 vs 20.5%, $p = 0.69$). Hospital mortality was significantly lower in the restrictive group (22.3 vs 28.1%, $p=0.05$). Other mortality rates, including ICU mortality (13.9 vs 16.2%, $p =0.29$) and 60-day mortality (22.8 vs 26.5%, $p =0.23$), were not significantly different but were always lower in absolute terms in the restrictive group. The multiple organ dysfunction score, modified to include mortality, was significantly less in the restrictive group overall (10.7 ± 7.5 vs 11.8 ± 7.7, $p = 0.03$). Therefore, in the TRICC trial, a trend towards decreased 30 day mortality was observed in patients treated according to a restrictive RBC transfusion strategy as compared to a more liberal approach to RBC transfusion. The significant differences noted in hospital mortality and in several subgroups, the increased rates of cardiac complications, and increased rates of combined organ dysfunction and mortality all favored the restrictive strategy. Thus, the use of an allogeneic red cell transfusion threshold as low as 7.0 g/dl combined with maintenance of hemoglobin concentrations in a low range was not only equivalent, but possibly superior, to a more liberal transfusion strategy in volume resuscitated critically ill patients.

Can the TRICC trial results be applied to patients sepsis and septic shock? In general, we suggest that the answer is yes because more than a third of all patients were admitted with an infection. In addition, all primary and secondary analyses conducted demonstrated that a restrictive policy was either equivalent or superior to a more liberal policy.

ALTERNATIVES TO RBC TRANSFUSION

Corwin et al. have reported that at least 30% of the transfusion requirement for patients in an ICU is due to blood sampling and testing [99]. A restricted blood testing policy with the elimination of routine laboratory tests will reduce the amount of blood transfused in critically ill patients. The routine use of pediatric sampling tubes can reduce the blood loss due to testing [100]. The use of pulse oximetry can reduce the need for blood gases. Furthermore, the practice of discarding the drawback blood from arterial sampling lines should be altered which can help reduce the amount of iatrogenic blood loss in critically ill patients. The use of new blood conservation systems along with in-line monitoring systems may further reduce the blood loss due to testing thus further reducing transfusion requirements. Erythropoietin (EPO), a hormone that stimulates the formation of RBCs in the bone marrow, may be used clinically to decrease transfusion needs by increasing endogenous erythrocyte production. A recently completed trial in 160 critically ill patients demonstrated that [101] EPO in high doses decreased transfusion requirements by 45% (p<0.002) with higher discharge hematocrits (35.1 vs 31.6, p<0.01). A larger trial is underway to assess whether a lower dose is effective and confirm that EPO is safe and possibly improves patient outcomes. All of these strategies may complement a restrictive transfusion strategy. Cell salvage, a non pharmacological intervention, may be useful in a small number of postoperative ICU patients while others, such as pre-operative autologous donation, have no place in this setting [102]. Finally, other pharmacological agents such as antifibrinolytics have limited usefulness in critically ill patients [103].

CONCLUSION AND RECOMMENDATIONS

The TRICC trial [104] demonstrated that a transfusion trigger of 7.0 g/dl and maintenance of hemoglobin concentrations between 7.0 and 9.0 g/dl was at worst equivalent and very likely superior to the more liberal use of red cells.

A restrictive strategy is truly a superior therapy because clinical outcomes are superior, transfusions are decreased by 54% and costs are minimized. Given conflicting evidence, the optimal transfusion policy for septic patients is not known. The increased demands imposed by sepsis along with its impairment of the normal adaptive process to anemia would suggest that severely infected patients should have a more liberal transfusion practice as compared to nonseptic patients. The potential problems with allogeneic blood products however limits one's enthusiasm for an aggressive transfusion practice. Thus, the best approach would be to limit the need to transfuse but to transfuse the best product available if a transfusion is required. We anxiously await the results of further trials with EPO, different RBC products, and other studies to confirm the results observed in the TRICC trial.

REFERENCES

1. Rangel-Frausto MS, Pittet D, Costigan M, Hwang T, Davis CS, Wenzel RP. The natural history of the systemic inflammatory response syndrome (SIRS). A prospective study. JAMA 1995; 273:117-123
2. Friedman G, Silva E, Vincent JL. Has the mortality of septic shock changed with time. Crit Care Med 1998; 26:2078-2086
3. Bordin JO, Heddle NM, Blajchman MA. Biologic effects of leukocytes present in transfused cellular blood products. Blood 1994; 84:1703-1721
4. van de Watering LMG, Hermans J, et al. Beneficial effects of leukocyte depletion of transfused blood on postoperative complications in patients undergoing cardiac surgery. Circulation 1998; 97:562-568
5. Hebert PC, Hu LQ, Biro GP. Review of physiologic mechanisms in response to anemia. Can Med Assoc J 1997; 156:S27-S40.
6. Barcroft J: The respiratory function of the blood. Part I: lessons from high altitudes. Cambridge University Press, 1925
7. Tuman KJ: Tissue oxygen delivery. The physiology of anemia. Anesth Clin N Am 1990; 8:451-469
8. Hall JB, Schmidt GA, Wood LDH. Principles of Critical Care, edn 1. Jeffers JD, McCurdy P (eds) McGraw-Hill, Inc., 1992
9. Turner A, Tsamitros M, Bellomo R. Myocardial cell injury in septic shock. Crit Care Med 1999; 27:1775-1780
10. Bernstein D, Sibbald WJ. Circulatory disturbances in multiple systems organ failure. Crit.Care Clin. 1989, 5:223-254
11. Hebert PC, Thompson CR, Gillis RP, Walley KR, Schellenberg RR. Histamine H2 stimulation decreases left ventricular contractility in humans. Circulation 2001 (In Press)
12. Walley KR, Hebert PC, Wakai Y, Wilcox PG, Road JD, Cooper DJ. Decrease in left ventricular contractility after tumor necrosis factor-alpha infusion in dogs. J Appl Physiol 1994; 76:1060-1067
13. Natanson C. Studies using a canine model to investigate the cardiovascular abnormality of, and potential therapies, for septic shock. Clin Res 1990; 38:206-214
14. Natanson C, Eichenholz PW, Danner RL. Endotoxin and tumor necrosis factor challenges in dogs simulate the cardiovascular profile of human septic shock. J Exp Med 1989; 169:823-832

15. Natanson C, Fink MP, Ballantyne HK, MacVittie TJ, Conklin JJ, Parrillo JE. Gram-negative bacteremia produces both severe systolic and diastolic cardiac dysfunction in a canine model that simulates human septic shock. J Clin Invest 1986; 78:259-270
16. Suffredini AF, Fromm RE, Parker MM, et al. The cardiovascular response of normal humans to the administration of endotoxin. N Engl J Med 1989; 321:280-287
17. Bersten AD, Sibbald WJ, Hersch M, Cheung H, Rutledge FS. Interaction of sepsis and sepsis plus sympathomimetics on myocardial oxygen availability. Am J Physiol 1992; 262:H1164-H1173
18. Lam C, Tyml K, Martin C, Sibbald W. Microvascular perfusion is impaired in a rat model of normotensive sepsis. J Clin Invest 1994; 94:2077-2083
19. Eklöf B, Neglén P, Thomson D. Temporary incomplete ischemia of the legs induced by aortic clamping in man: effects on central hemodynamics and skeletal muscle metabolism by adrenergic block. Ann Surg 1981; 193:89-98
20. Bersten AD, Sibbald WJ, Hersch M, Cheung H, Rutledge FS. Interaction of sepsis and sepsis plus sympathomimetics on myocardial oxygen availability. Am J Physiol 1992; 262:H1164-H1173
21. Sibbald WJ, Fox G, Martin CM. Abnormalities of vascular reactivity in sepsis syndrome. Chest 1991; 100 (Suppl):S155S-S159S
22. Rackow EC, Astiz ME, Weil MH. Cellular oxygen metabolism during sepsis and shock. The relationship of oxygen consumption to oxygen delivery. JAMA 1988; 259:1989-1993
23. Czer LSC, Shoemaker WC. Optimal hematocrit value in critically ill postoperative patients. Surg Gynecol Obstet 1978; 147:363-368
24. Tuchschmidt J, Fried J, Astiz ME, Rackow E. Elevation of cardiac output and oxygen delivery improves outcome in septic shock. Chest 1992; 102:216-220
25. Bihari D, Smithies M, Gimson A, Tinker J. The effects of vasodilation with prostacyclin on oxygen delivery and uptake in critically ill patients. N Engl J Med 1987; 317:397-403
26. Ronco JJ, Fenwick JC, Wiggs BR, Phang PT, Russell JA, Tweeddale MG. Oxygen consumption is independent of increases in oxygen delivery by dobutamine in septic patients who have normal or increased plasma lactate. Am Rev Respir Dis 1993; 147:25-31
27. Ronco JJ, Fenwick JC, Tweeddale MG, et al. Identification of the critical oxygen delivery for anaerobic metabolism in critically ill septic and nonseptic humans. JAMA 1993; 270:1724-1730
28. Boyd O, Ground M, Bennett D. A randomized clinical trial of the effect of deliberate perioperative increase of oxygen delivery on mortality in high-risk surgical patients. JAMA 1993; 270:2699-2707
29. Hayes MA, Timmins AC, Yau EHS, Palazzo M, Hinds CJ, Watson D. Elevation of systemic oxygen delivery in the treatment of critically ill patients. N Engl J Med 1994; 330:1717-1722
30. Gattinoni L, Brazzi L, Pelosi P, et al. A trial of goal-oriented hemodynamic therapy in critically ill patients. N Engl J Med 1995; 333:1025-1032
31. Gutierrez G, Pohil RJ. Oxygen consumption is linearly related to O2 supply in critically ill patients. J Crit Care 1986; 1:45-53
32. Ronco JJ, Montaner JSG, Fenwick JC, Ruedy J, Russell JA. Pathologic dependence of oxygen consumption on oxygen delivery in acute respiratory failure secondary to AIDS-related Pneumocystis carinii pneumonia. Chest 1990; 98:1463-1466
33. Conrad SA, Dietrich KA, Hebert CA, Romero MD. Effect of red cell transfusion on oxygen consumption following fluid resuscitation in septic shock. Circ Shock 1990; 31:419-429
34. Fenwick JC, Dodek PM, Ronco JJ, Phang PT, Wiggs B, Russell JA. Increased concentrations of plasma lactate predict pathologic dependence of oxygen consumption

on oxygen delivery in patients with adult respiratory distress syndrome. J Crit Care 1990; 5:81-86

35. Gilbert EM, Haupt MT, Mandanas RY, Huaringa AJ, Carlson RW. The effect of fluid loading, blood transfusion, and catecholamine infusion on oxygen delivery and consumption in patients with sepsis . Am Rev Respir Dis 1986; 134:873-878.

36. Kariman K, Burns SR. Regulation of tissue oxygen extraction is disturbed in adult respiratory distress syndrome. Am Rev Respir Dis 1985; 132:109-114

37. Dietrich KA, Conrad SA, Hebert CA, Levy GL, Romero MD. Cardiovascular and metabolic response to red blood cell transfusion in critically ill volume-resuscitated nonsurgical patients. Crit Care Med 1990; 18:940-944

38. Heyland DK, Cook DJ, King D, Kernerman P, Brun-Buisson C. Maximizing oxygen delivery in critically ill patients: a methodologic appraisal of the evidence. Crit Care Med 1996; 24:517-524

39. Silverman HJ, Slotman G, Bone RC, et al. Effects of prostaglandin E1 on oxygen delivery and consumption in patients with the adult respiratory distress syndrome. Chest 1990; 98:405-410

40. Shoemaker WC, Appel PL, Kram HB, Waxman K, Lee T-S. Prospective trial of supranormal values of survivors as therapeutic goals in high-risk surgical patients. Chest 1988; 94:1176-1186

41. Shoemaker WC, Appel PL, Kram HB. Role of oxygen debt in the development of organ failure sepsis, and death in high-risk surgical patients. Chest 1992; 102:208-215

42. Gutierrez G, Palizas F, Doglio G, et al. Gastric intramucosal pH as a therapeutic index of tissue oxygenation in critically ill patients. Lancet 1992; 339:195-199

43. Marik PE, Sibbald WJ. Effect of stored-blood transfusion on oxygen delivery in patients with sepsis. JAMA 1993; 269:3024-3029

44. Stuart J, Nash GB. Red cell deformability and haematological disorders. Blood Rev 1990; 4:141-147

45. Apstein CS, Dennis RC, Briggs L, Vogel WM, Frazer J, Valeri CR. Effect of erythrocyte storage and oxyhemoglobin affinity changes on cardiac function. Am J Physiol 1985; 248:H508-H515

46. Regan FAM, Hewitt P, Barbara JAJ, Contreras M, on behalf of the current TTI Study. Prospective investigation of transfusion transmitted infection in recipients of over 20000 units of blood. Br Med J 2000; 320:403-406

47. Opelz G, Sengar DPS, Mickey MR, Terasaki PI. Effect of blood transfusions on subsequent kidney transplants. Transplant Proc 1973; 5:253-259

48. Keown PA, Descamps B. Improved renal allograft survival after blood transfusion: a nonspecific, erythrocyte-mediated immunoregulatory process? Lancet 1979; 1:20-22

49. Kaplan J, Sarnaik S, Gitlin J, Lusher J. Diminished helper/suppressor lymphocyte ratios and natural killer activity in recipients of repeated blood transfusions. Blood 1984; 64:308-310

50. Kessler CM, Schulof RS, Goldstein AL, et al. Abnormal T-lymphocyte subpopulations associated with transfusions of blood-derived products. Lancet 1983; 1:991-992

51. Tartter PI, Quintero S, Barron DM. Perioperative transfusions associated with colorectal cancer surgery: clinical judgement versus the hematocrit. World J Surg 1986; 10.516-521

52. Fielding LP. Red for danger. blood transfusion and colorectal cancer. Br Med J 1985; 291:841-842

53. Nichols RL, Smith JW, Klein DB, et al. Risk of infection after penetrating abdominal trauma. N Engl J Med 1984; 311:1065-1070

54. Fischer E, Lenhard V, Seifert P, Kluge A, Johannsen R. Blood transfusion-induced suppression of cellular immunity in man. Hum Immunol 1980; 3:187-194

55. Lenhard V, Maassen G, Grosse-Wilde H, Wermet P, Opelz G. Effect of blood transfusions on immunoregulatory cells in prospective transplant recipients. Transplant

Proc 1983; 5:1011-1015

56. Heiss MM, Memple W, Jauch K-W, et al. Beneficial effects of autologous blood transfusion on infectious complications after colorectal cancer surgery. Lancet 1993; 342:1328-1333

57. Tartter PI. Blood transfusion and postoperative infections. Transfusion 1989; 29:456-459

58. Mezrow CK, Bergstein I, Tartter PI. Postoperative infections following autologous and homologous blood transfusions. Transfusion 1992; 32:27-30

59. Murphy P, Heal JM, Blumberg N. Infection or suspected infection after hip replacement surgery with autologous or homologous blood transfusions. Transfusion 1991; 31:212-217

60. Murphy PJ, Connery C, Hicks GLJr, Blumberg N. Homologous blood transfusion as a risk factor for postoperative infection after coronary artery bypass graft operations. J Thorac Cardiovasc Surg 1992; 104:1092-1099

61. Pinto V, Baldonedo R, Nicolas C, Barez A, Perez A, Aza J. Relationship of transfusion and infectious complications after gastric carcinoma operations. Transfusion 1991; 31:114-118

62. Jensen LS, Andersen AJ, Christiansen PM, et al. Postoperative infection and natural killer cell function following blood transfusion in patients undergoing elective colorectal surgery. Br J Surg 1992; 79:513-516

63. Marshall JC, Sweeney D. Microbial infection and the septic response in critical surgical illness. Sepsis, not infection, determines outcome. Arch Surg 1990; 125:17-23

64. Marshall JC. A scoring system for multiple organ dysfunction syndrome. In Sepsis. Current perspectives in pathophysiology and therapy. Edited by Reinhart K, Eyrich K, Sprung C. Berlin: Springer-Verlag, 1994:38-49

65. Crosby ET. Perioperative haemotherapy: I. Indications for blood component transfusion. Can J Anesth 1992; 39:695-707

66. Vamvakas E, Moore SB. Perioperative blood transfusion and colorectal cancer recurrence: a qualitative statistical overview and meta-analysis. Transfusion 1993; 33:754-765

67. Houbiers JGA, Brand A, van de Watering LMG, et al. Randomised controlled trial comparing transfusion of leucocyte-depleted or buffy-coat-depleted blood in surgery for colorectal cancer. Lancet 1996; 344:573-578

68. van de Watering LMG, Houbiers JGA, et al. Leukocyte depletion reduces postoperative mortality in patients undergoing cardiac surgery. Br J Haematol 1996; 93:312 (Abst)

69. Jensen LS, Kissmeyer-Nielsen P, Wolff B, Qvist N. Randomised comparison of leucocyte-depleted versus buffy-coat-poor blood transfusion and complications after colorectal surgery. Lancet 1996; 348:841-845

70. Houbiers JG, van de Velde CJ, van de Watering LM, et al. Transfusion of red cells is associated with increased incidence of bacterial infection after colorectal surgery: a prospective study. Transfusion 1997; 37:126-134

71. Busch ORC, Hop WCJ, Hoynck van Papendrecht MAW, Marquet RL, Jeekel J. Blood transfusions and prognosis in colorectal cancer. N Engl J Med 1993; 328:1372-1376

72. McAlister FA, Clark HD, Wells PS, Laupacis A. Perioperative allogeneic blood transfusion does not cause adverse sequelae in patients with cancer: a meta-analysis of unconfounded studies. Br J Surg 1998; 85:171-178

73. Chin-Yee I, Arya N, D'Almeida M. The red cell storage lesion and its implication for transfusion. Transfus Sci 1997; 18:447-458

74. Card RT. Red cell membrane changes during storage. Trans Med Rev 1988; 2:40-47

75. Wolfe LC. The membrane and the lesions of storage in preserved red cells. Transfusion 1985; 25:185-203

76. Greenwalt TJ, Bryan DJ, Dumaswala UJ. Erythrocyte membrane vesiculation and changes in membrane components during storage in citrate-phosphate-dextrose-adenine-

1. Vox Sang 1984; 47:261-270

77. Snyder LM, Fairbanks G, Trainor J, Fortier NL, Jacobs JB, Leb L. Properties and characterization of vesicules released by young and old human red cells. Br J Haematol 1985; 59:513-522

78. Wagner GM, Chiu DTY, Yee MC, Lubin BH. Red cell vesiculation-a common membrane physiologic event. J Lab Clin Med 1986; 108:315-324

79. Knight JA, Voorhees RP, Martin L, Anstall H. Lipid peroxidation in stored red cells. Transfusion 1992; 32:354-357

80. Card RT, Mohandas N, Perkins HA, Shohet SB. Deformability of stored red blood cells. Relationship to degree of packing. Transfusion 1982; 22:96-101

81. Card RT, Mohandas N, Mollison PL. Relationship of post-transfusion viability to deformability of stored red cells . Br J Haematol 1983; 53:237-240

82. Card RT, Fergusson DJ. Relationship of stored red cell deformability to survivability following transfusion: In vitro prediction of in vivo viability. Blood 1987; 70:327a (Abst)

83. Valeri CR, Rorth M, Zaroulis CG, Jakubowski MS, Vescera SV. Physiologic effects of transfusing red blood cells with high or low affinity for oxygen to passively hyperventilated, anemic baboons: systemic and cerebral oxygen extraction. Ann Surg 1975; 181:106-113

84. Valeri CR, Hirsh NM. Restoration in vivo of erythrocyte adenosine triphosphate, 2.3-diphosphoglycerate, potassium ion, and sodium ion concentrations following the transfusion of acid-citrate-dextrose-stored human red blood cells. J Lab Clin Med 1969; 73:722-733

85. Chaplin HJr, Beutler E, Collins JA, Giblett ER, Polesky HF. Current status of red-cell preservation and availability in relation to the development National Blood Policy. N Engl J Med 1974; 291:68-74

86. Bunn HF, May MH, Kocholaty WF, Shields CE. Hemoglobin function in stored blood. J Clin Invest 1969; 48:311-321

87. Sugerman HJ, Davidson DT, Vibul S, Delivoria-Papadopoulos M, Miller LD, Oski FA. The basis of defective oxygen delivery from stored blood. Surg Gynecol Obstet 1970; 137:733-741

88. Valeri CR, Collins FB. The physiologic effect of transfusing preserved red cells with low 2,3-diphosphoglycerate and high affinity for oxygen. Vox Sang 1971; 20:397-403

89. Latham JTJr, Bove JR, Weirich FL. Chemical and hematologic changes in stored CPDA-1 blood. Transfusion 1982; 22:158-159

90. Heddle NM. Febrile nonhemolytic transfusion reactions to platelets. Curr Opin Hematol 1995; 3:478-483

91. Smith KJ, Sierra ER, Nelson EJ. Histamine, IL-1b, and IL-8 increase in packed RBCs stored for 42 days but not in RBCs leukodepleted pre-storage. Transfusion 1993; 33:53S (Abst)

92. Miletic VD, Popovic O. Complement activation in stored platelet concentrates. Transfusion 1993; 33:150-154

93. Schleuning M, Bock M, Mempel W. Complement activation during storage of single-donor platelet concentrates. Vox Sang 1994; 67:144-148

94. Silliman CC, Clay KL, Thurman GW, Johnson CA, Ambruso DR. Partial characterization of lipids that develop during the routine storage of blood and prime the neutrophil NADPH oxidase. J Lab Clin Med 1994; 124:684-694

95. Muylle L, Peetermans ME. Effect of prestorage leukocyte removal on the cytokine levels in stored platelet concentrates. Vox Sang 1994; 66:14-17

96. Martin CM, Sibbald WJ, Lu X, Hebert P, Schweitzer I. Age of transfused red blood cells is associated with ICU length of stay. Clin Invest Med 1994; 17:124 (Abst)

97. Purdy FR, Tweeddale MG, Merrick PM. Association of mortality with age of blood transfused in septic ICU patients. Can J Anaesth 1997; 44:1256-1261

98. Vamvakas EC, Carven JH. Transfusion and postoperative pneumonia in coronary artery bypass graft surgery: effect of the length of storage of transfused red cells. Transfusion 1999; 39:701-710

99. Corwin HL, Parsonnet KC, Gettinger A. RBC transfusion in the ICU. Is there a reason? Chest 1995; 108:767-771

100. Smoller BR, Kruskall MS, Horowitz GL. Reducing adult phlebotomy blood loss with the use of pediatric sized blood collection tubes. Am J Clin Pathol 1989; 91:701-703

101. Corwin HL, Gettinger A, Rodriguez RM, et al. Efficacy of recombinant human erythropoietin in the critically ill patient. a randomized double blind placebo controlled trial. Crit Care Med 1999; 27:2346-2350

102. Huet C, Salmi LR, Fergusson D, Koopman-van Gemert AWMM, Rubens F, Laupacis A. A meta-analysis of the effectiveness of cell salvage to minimize perioperative allogeneic blood transfusion in cardiac and orthopedic surgery. Anesth Analg 1999; 89:861-869

103. Laupacis A, Fergusson D. Drugs to minimize perioperative blood loss in cardiac surgery: meta-analyses using perioperative blood transfusion as the outcome. Anesth Analg 1997; 85:1258-1267

104. Hebert PC, Wells G, Blajchman MA, et al. A multicenter, randomized, controlled clinical trial of transfusion requirements in critical care. N Engl J Med 1999; 340:409-417

105. Ronco JJ, Phang PT, Walley KR, Wiggs B, Fenwick JC, Russell JA. Oxygen consumption is independent of changes in oxygen delivery in severe adult respiratory distress syndrome. Am Rev Respir Dis 1991 ; 143:1267-1273

106. Shah DM, Gottlieb ME, Rahm RL, et al. Failure of red blood cell transfusion to increase oxygen transport or mixed venous PO2 in injured patients. J Trauma 1982; 22:741-746

107. Steffes CP, Bender JS, Levison MA. Blood transfusion and oxygen consumption in surgical sepsis. Crit Care Med 1991; 19:512-517

108. Babineau TJ, Dzik WH, Borlase BC, Baxter JK, Bistrian BR, Benotti PN. Reevaluation of current transfusion practices in patients in surgical intensive care units. Am J Surg 1992; 164:22-25

109. Lorente JA, Landin L, De Pablo R, Renes E, Rodriguez-Diaz R, Liste D. Effects of blood transfusion on oxygen transport variables in severe sepsis. Crit Care Med 1993; 21:1312-1318

110. Mink RB, Pollack MM. Effect of blood transfusion on oxygen consumption in pediatric septic shock. Crit Care Med 1990; 18:1087-1091

111. Lucking SE, Williams TM, Chaten FC, Metz RI, Mickell JJ. Dependence of oxygen consumption on oxygen delivery in children with hyperdynamic septic shock and low oxygen extraction. Crit Care Med. 1990; 18:1316-1319

24

CATECHOLAMINE THERAPY

Claude Martin
Joseph F. Dasta
Gregory M. Susla

Shock is caused by an inadequate supply, or inappropriate use of metabolic substrate (mainly oxygen) resulting in tissue damage and cellular death. When tissue perfusion is altered, treatment is targeted to the pathophysiologic changes: inadequate filling pressures, cardiac performance, or vascular resistance. Thus, therapeutic modalities for the hemodynamic support of sepsis can be broken down into three main categories: volume infusion, vasopressor therapy, and inotropic therapy.

Fluid resuscitation is the mainstay of initial hemodynamic management. Because septic shock is accompanied by fever, venodilation, and diffuse capillary leakage, virtually all septic patients present with inadequate preload and require infusion of large amounts of fluid. Thus, fluid resuscitation represents the best initial therapy for treatment of hypotension in sepsis. Patients with significant anemia may require blood transfusion to increase oxygen delivery (DO_2). The optimal left-heart filling pressure is still a matter of controversy, but values between 12 and 15 mmHg are considered adequate in most patients.

If fluid therapy alone fails to restore adequate arterial pressure and organ perfusion, therapy with vasopressor agents should be initiated. Potential vasopressor agents include dopamine, norepinephrine, epinephrine, or phenylephrine. These agents can be started before fluid resuscitation is considered optimal, if very low values of mean arterial blood pressure (MAP) compromise survival.

When adequately fluid resuscitated, most septic patients are hyperdynamic, but myocardial contractility, as assessed by ejection fraction, is impaired [1]. Some patients, especially those with pre-existing cardiac dysfunction, may have decreased cardiac output and may require inotropic agents such as dobutamine, dopamine, and epinephrine.

INDIVIDUAL VASOPRESSOR AGENTS

Dopamine

Dopamine possesses several dose-dependent pharmacologic effects (Table 1). At doses less than 5 µg/kg/min, the predominant effect of dopamine is to stimulate dopaminergic DA_1 and DA_2 receptors in the renal, mesenteric, and coronary beds, resulting in vasodilation. Infusion of low doses of dopamine causes an increase in glomerular filtration rate (GFR), renal blood flow, and sodium excretion [2]. At doses of 5 to 10 µg/kg/min, β_1-adrenergic effects predominate, producing an increase in cardiac contractility and heart rate. Dopamine causes the release of norepinephrine from nerve terminals, which contributes to its effects on the heart. At doses above 10 µg/kg/min, α_1-adrenergic effects predominate, leading to arterial vasoconstriction and an increase in blood pressure. However, it should be recognized that there is much overlap in these effects, particularly in critically ill patients.

	Isoprot	Dob	Epi	Dop	Norepi	Phenyl
Contractility (β_1, α_1)	++++	+++	+++	+ to ++	+ to ++	0 to +
Heart rate (β_1)	++++	+ to ++	+++	+ to ++	+ to ++	0 to ↓
Vasoconstriction (α_1)	0	0 to +	+ to +++	0 to +++	+ to +++	++
Vasodilation (β_2)	++++	+ to ++	+ to 0	0	0	0
Renal perfusion	↓ or ↑	↑ or ↓	↑ or ↓	↑ or ↓	↑ or ↓	↓ or ↑
Cardiac output	↑↑	↑↑	↑↑	↑	0 or ↑	0 or ↓
Resistance	↓↓	↓	↓ or ↑	↑	↑↑↑	↑↑
Blood pressure	↓ or ↑	0 or ↓ or ↑	↑↑	0 to ↑	↑ to ↑↑↑	↑
VO_2-VCO_2 REE	↑	↑	↑	↑	↑	↑

Table 1. Cardiovascular and metabolic effects of pressor and inotropic catecholamines. *Isoprot: isoproterenol; Dob: dobutamine; Epi: epinephrine; Dop: dopamine; Norepi: norepinephrine; Phenyl: phenylephrine*

Hemodynamic Effects

The hemodynamic effects of dopamine in patients with septic shock have been reported in a number of open labeled trials. Dopamine has been shown to produce a median increase in MAP of 24 % in patients who remained hypotensive after optimal fluid resuscitation [3-14]. Dopamine increased MAP primarily by increasing cardiac index with minimal effects on systemic vascular resistance. The increase in cardiac index was primarily due to an increase in stroke volume, and to a lesser extent, to increased heart rate [3-14]. The median dose of dopamine required to restore blood pressure was 15 μg/kg/min. In most studies central venous, pulmonary artery, pulmonary wedge pressures (PCWP), systemic vascular resistance index, and pulmonary artery resistance index were unchanged. In patients with elevated PCWP, dopamine may further increase wedge pressure by increasing venous return. Patients receiving dopamine infusion rates above 20 μg/kg/min did show increases in right heart pressures as well as heart rate. Dopamine has been shown to improve right ventricular contractility in patients with underlying right ventricular failure.

In a randomized, double-blind study, Martin et al. compared the ability of norepinephrine and dopamine to reverse hemodynamic abnormalities in 32 patients with hyperdynamic septic shock [9]. Targeted MAP and cardiac index were achieved with dopamine at doses between 10 and 25 μg/kg/min in 31% of patients; mean pulmonary pressure, PCWP, and urine flow were increased as well. In contrast, 93 % of patients treated initially with norepinephrine at a dose of 1.5 μg/kg/min reached the targeted endpoints, and 10 of 11 patients who did not respond to dopamine at 25 μg/kg/min were successfully treated with norepinephrine at a dose of 1.7 μg/kg/min. The authors concluded that norepinephrine was more efficient and reliable than dopamine to reverse the hemodynamic abnormalities seen in hyperdynamic septic shock.

Gas Exchange

In studying the effect of dopamine on pulmonary gas exchange, dopamine has been shown to consistently increase pulmonary shunt fraction (Qs/Qt), decrease arterial-venous oxygen difference, and increase mixed venous oxygen saturation (SvO$_2$) with the PaO$_2$ decreasing or remaining unchanged [7,8,10].

Oxygen Delivery

Dopamine has been shown to increase DO_2 above pretreatment levels or levels obtained with concurrently administered catecholamines [3-5]. Its effects on calculated or measured oxygen consumption, however, have been mixed. The oxygen extraction ratio typically decreases, suggesting no improvement in tissue oxygenation [3, 5]. This may be due to a failure to improve microcirculatory flow in vital organs or lack of a meaningful tissue oxygen debt in some patients [5].

Splanchnic Perfusion

The effect if dopamine on splanchnic perfusion as assessed by gastric tonometric parameters has also been mixed. Roukonen et al. [6] and Meier-Hellmann et al. [3] documented that dopamine can increase splanchnic blood flow. Roukonen et al. reported that splanchnic oxygen delivery increased as a result of the increase in splanchnic blood flow, with no significant increase in splanchnic oxygen consumption [6]. Meier-Hellmann et al. reported that dopamine increased fractional blood flow if the baseline was less than 0.30, but had no effect if the baseline fractional blood flow was greater than 0.30. They also reported an increase in splanchnic oxygen delivery without an effect on splanchnic oxygen consumption and a consequent reduction in splanchnic oxygen extraction [3]. There was no effect on pHi or systemic or splanchnic lactate values. Maynard et al. were unable to show any effect on splanchnic blood flow, intramucosal pH, lidocaine metabolism, or indocyanine clearance with low dose dopamine therapy [15].

Marik et al., on the other hand, reported a reduction in pHi associated with an increase in systemic DO_2 and oxygen consumption with dopamine [4]. They suggested that dopamine caused an increase in splanchnic oxygen utilization which was not compensated for by an increase in DO_2, resulting in an increase in splanchnic oxygen debt. They speculated that dopamine might have redistributed blood flow within the gut, reducing mucosal blood flow and increasing mucosal oxygen debt.

Neviere et al. reported that dopamine was associated with a reduction in gastric mucosal blood flow [16]. There were changes in gastric PCO_2, gastric-arterial PCO_2 difference, and calculated intramucosal pH (pHi). Because there were no changes in the acid-base parameters of the patients, the authors could not determine if the reduction in gastric mucosal blood flow was critical.

In summary, dopamine appears to be very effective in increasing MAP in patients who remain hypotensive after optimal volume expansion. Since MAP increases primarily as a result of increasing cardiac index, it should be most useful in patients who are hypotensive with reduced cardiac function. It may be used as an alternative agent in patients with hyperdynamic septic shock who require a vasopressor agent but would not benefit from a further increase in cardiac inotropic function. The major undesirable effects of dopamine are tachycardia, increased pulmonary artery occlusion pressure (PAOP), increased pulmonary shunt, decreased PaO_2, and the potential to decrease pHi.

Epinephrine (table 1)

In patients unresponsive to volume expansion or other catecholamine infusions, epinephrine can increase mean arterial pressure, primarily by increasing cardiac index and stroke volume with more modest increases in systemic vascular resistance and heart rate [17-19]. Epinephrine can increase DO_2, but oxygen consumption may be increased as well [17-21].

Epinephrine decreases splanchnic blood flow, with transient increases in arterial, splanchnic, and hepatic venous lactate concentrations, decreases in pHi, and increases in PCO_2 gap [3,22]. However, Levy et al. documented that the arterial lactate and pHi returned to normal values within 24 hours. [22]. These increases were thought to be due either to increases in splanchnic oxygen utilization and CO_2 production secondary to the thermogenic effect of epinephrine or to epinephrine-induced reduction in gut mucosal blood flow. The reduction in splanchnic blood flow has been associated with a decrease in DO_2 and a reduction in oxygen consumption. These effects may be due to a reduction in splanchnic DO_2 to a level that impairs nutrient blood flow and results in a reduction in global tissue oxygenation [3,22], and may potentially be reversed by the concomitant administration of dobutamine. [23]. The addition of dobutamine to epinephrine-treated patients has been shown to improve gastric mucosal perfusion, as assessed by improvements in pHi, arterial lactate concentration, and PCO_2 gap.

Epinephrine administration has been associated with increases in systemic and regional lactate concentrations [17,21,22]. The monitoring periods were short, and so it is unclear if these increases are transient. Other adverse effects of epinephrine include increases in heart rate, but electrocardiographic changes indicating ischemia [17] or arrhythmias [18] have not been reported in septic patients. Epinephrine has had minimal effects on pulmonary artery pressures and pulmonary vascular resistance in sepsis [17,18].

Norepinephrine (table 1)

Norepinephrine is a potent α-adrenergic agonist with less pronounced β-adrenergic agonist effects. In open labeled trials, norepinephrine has been shown to increase MAP in patients who remained hypotensive after fluid resuscitation and dopamine. Due to concerns about potential adverse vasoconstrictive effects on regional vascular beds such as the liver and the kidney, norepinephrine traditionally has either not been used or has been reserved as a last resort in a moribund patient, with predictably poor results.

The recent experience with norepinephrine in septic shock strongly suggests that this drug can successfully increase blood pressure without causing deterioration in organ function. In most studies, septic patients were given fluid to correct hypovolemia before dopamine, with or without dobutamine, was titrated to achieve the target blood pressure. When dopamine failed, norepinephrine was added to the dopamine regimen [9,24-26].

In most studies of septic patients, norepinephrine was used at a mean dose of 0.2 to 1.3 µg/kg/min. The initial dose can be as low as 0.01 µg/kg/min [25], and the highest reported norepinephrine dosage was 3.3 µg/kg/min [24]. Thus, large doses of the drug may be required in some patients with septic shock, possibly due to alpha-receptor down-regulation in sepsis [27].

Cardiovascular effects

Norepinephrine therapy usually causes a clinically significant increase in mean arterial pressure attributable to its vasoconstrictive effects, with little change in heart rate or cardiac output, leading to increased systemic vascular resistance (SVR). Several studies have demonstrated increases in cardiac output ranging from 10 to 20 % and increases of stroke volume index (SVI) of 10 to 15 % [9,24,25,28-30].Clinical studies have reported either no change [25,28-30] or modest increases [9,24,26], in PCWP. Mean pulmonary arterial pressure is either unchanged [9,28,30,24,26] or increases slightly [9,25,26].

Renal effects

In patients with hypotension and hypovolemia, e.g., during hemorrhagic or hypovolemic shock, the vasoconstrictive effects of norepinephrine can have severe detrimental effects on renal hemodynamics, with increased renal vascular resistance and renal ischemia [31-33]. Indeed, norepinephrine has been demonstrated to cause ischemia-induced acute renal failure in rats [34]. The situation is different in hyperdynamic septic shock, in which it is believed that urine flow decreases mainly as a results of lowered renal perfusion pressure [24]. Since norepinephrine has a greater effect on efferent arteriolar resistance and increases the filtration fraction, normalization of renal vascular resistance could effectively reestablish urine flow.

In the high output–low resistance state of septic shock patients, norepinephrine can markedly improve MAP and glomerular filtration. In the studies of Redl-Wenzl et al. [26], Desjars et al. [29], and Martin et al. [24] of septic shock patients treated with dopamine (and some also treated with dobutamine), addition of norepinephrine (0.5 to 1.5 µg/kg/min) significantly increased urine output, creatinine clearance, and osmolar clearance. In a study by Fukuoka et al. [35] addition of norepinephrine to dopamine and dobutamine increased SVR and urine flow only in patients with normal serum lactate concentrations, although this study was small and is at variance with other studies in which vascular resistance and urine flow were increased in patients with elevated lactate concentrations [9,40,36-38]. These studies support the hypothesis that renal ischemia observed during hyperdynamic septic shock is not worsened by norepinephrine infusion and even suggests that this drug may optimize effectively renal blood flow and renal vascular resistance [24,26,29].

Effects on lactate concentrations

The effects of norepinephrine on serum lactate concentrations have been assessed in few studies [4,6,9,30,36]. The results of these studies suggest that the use of norepinephrine does not worsen and can even improve tissue oxygenation of septic shock patients.

Effects on splanchnic circulation

The effects of norepinephrine on splanchnic blood flow have been evaluated in two studies. In a study by Ruokonen et al. [6] in septic shock patients receiving either norepinephrine (0.07 to 0.23 µg/kg/min) or dopamine (7.6 to 33.8 µg/kg/min) to correct hypotension, the effect of norepinephrine on splanchnic blood flow was considered unpredictable (increased in three patients, decreased in two), with no change in mean splanchnic blood flow, oxygen consumption, or oxygen extraction, while dopamine caused a consistent and statistically significant increase in splanchnic blood flow. Meier-Hellman et al. [3] showed that septic patients switched from dobutamine to norepinephrine or from dobutamine and norepinephrine to norepinephrine alone had a decrease in cardiac output and a decrease in splanchnic blood flow that paralleled the decrease in cardiac output. Splanchnic oxygen consumption remained unchanged due to a regional increase in oxygen extraction. The authors concluded that provided cardiac output is maintained, treatment with norepinephrine alone is without negative effects on splanchnic tissue oxygenation. This was confirmed by the study of Marik et al. [4] in which gastric mucosal pHi was significantly increased during a 3 hour treatment with norepinephrine while it was significantly decreased during treatment with dopamine. Reinelt et al. [38] showed that addition of dobutamine to norepinephrine to obtain a 20 % increase in cardiac index in septic shock patients could increase splanchnic blood flow and oxygen consumption and improve hepatic metabolic activity (as assessed by hepatic glucose production). Splanchnic blood flow and cardiac index increased in parallel, but there was no effect on splanchnic oxygen consumption and hepatic glucose production decreased.

Levy et al. [23] compared the effects of epinephrine to the combination of norepinephrine and dobutamine on gastric tonometric variables in 30 septic shock patients and found that while systemic hemodynamics were similar, pHi and gastric PCO_2 gap were normalized within 6 hours with norepinephrine and dobutamine while pHi decreased and gastric PCO_2 gaps increased in epinephrine-treated patients. Changes in the epinephrine group were transient and were corrected within 24 hours, but might have induced splanchnic ischemia and injury. The authors concluded that the splanchnic effects of the combination of norepinephrine-dobutamine were more predictable than epinephrine.

Phenylephrine

Phenylephrine, a selective α_1-adrenergic agonist, has been used by rapid intravenous administration to treat supraventricular tachycardia by causing a reflex vagal stimulation to the heart resulting from a rapid increase in blood pressure. It is also used intravenously in anesthesia to increase blood pressure. Its rapid onset, short duration, and primary vascular effects make it an attractive agent in the management of hypotension associated with sepsis. However, there are concerns about its potential to reduce cardiac output and lower heart rate in these patients (Table 1).

Unfortunately, there are only a few studies evaluating the clinical use of phenylephrine in hyperdynamic sepsis. As such, guidelines on its clinical use are limited. One study evaluated short-term phenylephrine therapy in hyperdynamic septic patients who were not hypotensive at the time of drug administration [39]. Phenylephrine, at a dosage of 70 µg/min, increased MAP, cardiac index, and stroke index. Heart rate was statistically significantly lower but the decrease averaged only 3 beats per minute. There was no change in SVR. In comparison, the response of normotensive patients with cardiac disease to the same phenylephrine dosing was an increase in MAP and SVR, a decrease in cardiac index and no change in heart rate. In a dose-response study, phenylephrine was administered to hyperdynamic septic patients who were normotensive at the time of drug therapy [40]. In incremental doses of 0.5 µg/kg/min to 8 µg/kg/min, phenylephrine increased MAP, SVR, and stroke index, while no change was seen in cardiac index. Heart rate was slightly but significantly lower, with a decrease ranging from 3 to 9 beats per minute. This study evaluated oxygen transport parameters and found no statistical changes in either DO_2 or oxygen consumption (VO_2). However, a clinically significant (>15 %) increase in VO_2 was seen in eight out of ten patients in at least one dosage.

There is only study evaluating the clinical effects of phenylephrine in treating hypotension associated with sepsis [41]. This was a small study of 13 patients with septic shock receiving either low-dose dopamine or dobutamine, who remained hypotensive despite fluid administration. Their baseline cardiac index was 3.3 l/min/m² and MAP was 57 mm Hg. Phenylephrine was begun at 0.5 µg/kg/min and was titrated to maintain a MAP of more than 70 mm Hg. Patients required phenylephrine for an average of 65 hours, and the maximum dosage in each patient averaged 3.7 µg/kg/min (range 0.4 to 9.1 µg/kg/min). Phenylephrine resulted in an increase in MAP, SVR, cardiac index, and stroke index. There was no change in heart rate. Clinically, a significant increase in urine output, and no change in serum creatinine were seen during phenylephrine therapy. Increases in DO_2 and consumption were reported.

The limited information available with phenylephrine suggests that this drug can increase blood pressure in fluid resuscitated septic shock patients. In addition, phenylephrine therapy does not impair cardiac or renal function. Phenylephrine may be a good choice when tachyarrhythmias limit therapy with other vasopressors. An increase in oxygen consumption and delivery may occur during therapy.

USE OF VASOPRESSOR THERAPY

Goal of Vasopressor Therapy

When fluid administration fails to restore an adequate arterial pressure and organ perfusion, therapy with vasopressor agents should be initiated [42]. Potential agents that can be selected include dopamine, norepinephrine, epinephrine and phenylephrine. Vasopressor therapy may be required transiently even while cardiac filling pressures are not yet adequate, in order to maintain perfusion in the face of life-threatening hypotension. Although the use of these drugs has the potential to reduce organ blood flow through arterial vasoconstriction, their final effects will depend upon the sum of the direct effects and any increase in organ perfusion pressure. In settings where organ autoregulation is lost, organ flow becomes linearly dependent on pressure [43,44] and organ perfusion pressure should be preserved if flow is to be optimized [35,45,46].

Whether or not a potent vasopressor also has positive inotropic effects is of clinical importance in patients with low cardiac output [47,48]. From a practical point of view, when a vasopressor infusion is started, doses should be carefully titrated to restore MAP, without impairing stroke volume. Should this occur, the dose of vasopressor should be lowered, or the use of dobutamine considered [48]. If right ventricular dysfunction occurs during vasopressor infusion one should keep pulmonary vascular resistance at the lowest values compatible with the restoration of normal systemic hemodynamics [49,51].

Attention should be paid to the renal and splanchnic circulation during vasopressor infusion. Although no prospective, randomized studies have demonstrated a significant improvement in renal function with increase in renal perfusion pressure, a number of open-label clinical series support this notion [9,24-26,28-30,52-54). Urine output and creatinine clearance are increased following the restoration of MAP. Thus, vasopressor agents can be effective tools for the augmentation of renal perfusion pressure. In some patients, the renal autoregulation curve may be shifted to the right, demanding a greater perfusion pressure for a given renal blood flow. The precise MAP level targeted depends upon the premorbid blood pressure but can be as high as 75 mm Hg [9,24-26,28-30,52-54). However, individual responses should be kept at the minimum level required to reestablish urine flow and in some patients this can be achieved with a MAP of 60 or 65 mm Hg.

The use of blood lactate concentrations to guide therapy in patients with septic shock has not been demonstrated conclusively but a trend toward decreased concentrations is a good prognostic indicator. In most forms of shock, elevated blood lactate concentrations reflect anaerobic metabolism due to hypoperfusion, but the interpretation of blood lactate concentrations in septic patients is not always straightforward. A number of studies have indicated that increasing either global [55] or regional [56] DO_2 fails to alter elevated lactate concentrations in patients with sepsis. Measurements of tissue PO_2 in septic patients have failed to demonstrate tissue hypoxia in the presence of lactic acidosis [57], and a number of studies have suggested that elevated lactate may result from cellular metabolic alterations rather than from global hypoperfusion in sepsis [58,59]. Nonetheless, although lactate concentrations should not be considered to represent tissue hypoxia in the strict sense, the prognostic value of elevations of blood lactate has been well established in septic shock patients [60-62]. The trend of lactate concentrations is a better indicator than a single value [60,62]. It is also of interest to note that blood lactate concentrations are a better prognostic indicator than oxygen-derived variables [63].

Mixed venous oxyhemoglobin levels have been suggested as an indicator of the balance between DO_2 and VO_2. SvO_2 can be measured by withdrawing a blood sample from the pulmonary artery in patients with a right heart catheter in place; continuous measurement of SvO_2 can be achieved using an oximetric right heart catheter. SvO_2 is dependent on cardiac output, VO_2, hemoglobin concentration, and arterial oxygen saturation. In patients with a stable oxygen demand, in the absence of hypoxemia and anemia, mixed venous desaturation can reflect decreased cardiac output. Normal SvO_2 is 70 % in critically ill patients, but in septic patients, SvO_2 can be elevated due to maldistribution of blood flow. The utility of using SvO_2 as an index of global perfusion to guide therapy in patients with septic shock has not been demonstrated conclusively, although saturations less than 65 % usually indicate decreased perfusion.

Interest has thus focused on methods of measuring regional perfusion more directly. The splanchnic circulation has been the focus of these investigations for several reasons: the countercurrent flow in the gut microcirculation increases the risk of mucosal hypoxia, the gut may have a higher critical DO_2 threshold than other organs [64], and gut ischemia increases intestinal permeability.

Gastric tonometry has been proposed as a simple method to assess regional perfusion in the gut by employing a balloon in the stomach to measure intramucosal PCO_2. From this PCO_2 measurement and the arterial bicarbonate concentration, one can then calculate gastric pHi using the Henderson-Hasselbalch equation, assuming that the bicarbonate concentration in the gastric mucosal tissue is in equilibrium with the systemic arterial bicarbonate [65]. Because this may not be the case in shock [66], and because remote systemic metabolic acidosis and alkalosis change systemic bicarbonate, gastric mucosal PCO_2, which is not confounded by arterial bicarbonate, may be more accurate than pHi. Gastric mucosal PCO_2 is influenced directly by systemic arterial PCO_2, however, and so the gastric-arterial PCO_2 difference has been proposed as the primary tonometric variable of interest, although even this measure is not a simple measure of gastric mucosal hypoxia [66].

Gastric tonometry is a good predictor for the ultimate outcome of critically-ill patients [67-70]. Its utility to guide therapy in patients with sepsis and septic shock, however, has not been proven. One study has shown decreased mortality with pHi-directed care in critically ill patients admitted to an ICU with initially normal pHi [69]. Interpretation of this study is complicated by the fact that mortality in the control group was high, and that therapy based on pHi was heterogeneous because they were made at the discretion of the clinicians and not by protocol. In addition, the degree to which the results of this trial are applicable to patients with septic shock is unclear. Gastric tonometry may prove to be a useful measure of regional perfusion in the splanchnic circulation, but further randomized controlled trials, with clear, reproducible treatment algorithms will be necessary to establish its utility in the management of patients with septic shock.

Complications of Vasopressor Therapy

All of the catecholamine vasopressor agents can cause significant tachycardia, especially in patients who are inadequately volume resuscitated. In patients with coexisting coronary disease, vasopressor-induced increases in myocardial VO_2 may precipitate myocardial ischemia and infarction. In the presence of myocardial dysfunction, excessive vasoconstriction can decrease stroke volume, cardiac output, and DO_2. When a vasopressor infusion is started, doses should be carefully titrated to restore MAP, without impairing stroke volume. Should this occur, the dose of vasopressor should be lowered, or the use of dobutamine considered [24]. In the presence of right ventricular dysfunction in septic shock, increased right ventricular afterload could worsen right ventricular function. During vasopressor infusion, one should keep pulmonary vascular resistance at the lowest values compatible with the restoration of normal systemic hemodynamics [9,36].

Potent vasopressors such as norepinephrine decrease renal blood flow in human and canine studies [31]. While on vasopressor therapy, cardiac index should be maintained at normal levels to optimize renal blood flow [24].

Administration of vasopressors may impair blood flow to the splanchnic system, and this can be manifested by stress ulceration, bowel ileus and malabsorption. Gut mucosal integrity occupies a key position in the pathogenesis of multiple organ failure (MOF), and countercurrent flow in splanchnic micro-circulation gives the gut a higher critical threshold for oxygen delivery than other organs. If possible, episodes of intramucosal acidosis, which might be detected either by a fall in gastric pHi or an increase in gastric mucosal PCO_2, should be avoided, although no prospective randomized controlled trial has demonstrated a decrease in mortality with pHi or gastric PCO_2-directed care in the management of patients with septic shock.

1) Criteria for prescribing a vasopressor agent (all 5 criteria simultaneously present)

- Adequate cardiac filling (CVP, PCWP : 12 to 15 mmHg).
  - Cardiac index > 3-4 l/min/m^2 or $SvO_2 \geq$ 65-70 %*
  - Mean arterial pressure $\leq$ 70 mmHg
  - Oliguria

2) Criteria of effectiveness

- Mean arterial pressure > 60-70 mmHg
  - No decrease in CI or SvO_2
  - Reestablishement of urine flow
  - Decrease in blood lactate level
  - Adequate skin perfusion
  - Adequate level of consciousness

3) Criteria for modulating the dose

- Decrease (15-20 %) in CI or SvO_2 (< 65 %)*
  (consider using dobutamine)
  - Mean blood pressure $\geq$ 80-90 mmHg

* no significant impairment in hemoglobin level and in SaO_2.

Table 2. Practical considerations for the use of vasopressor agents in patients with septic shock.

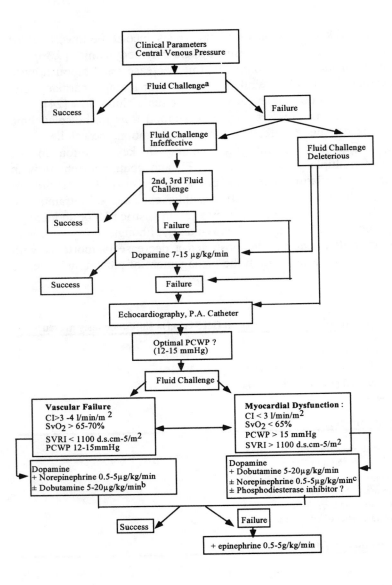

Figure 1. *Algorithm for the treatment of septic shock*
a : fluid challenge is 5-7 ml/kg of colloid or crystalloid in 15-20 min
b : when cardiac index and/or SvO$_2$ decrease by 15 % or more.
c : to maintain mean blood pressure > 75 mmHg.

Practical Considerations for the use of Vasopressors

Vasopressors should be considered as much more sophisticated pharmacologic tools than just agents used to constrict the vessels. Adequately used they can improve organ flow if the patient is correctly fluid resuscitated. Used in combination with a potent inotropic agent such as dobutamine, vasopressors are a key part of the hemodynamic management of the patients in septic shock. Tables 2 and 3 provide general consideration for the use of vasopressors during sepsis. Figure 1 summarizes the hemodynamic management of septic shock : fluid resuscitation, use of vasopressors, use of inotropes.

---

1) Goals for the treatment of patients with septic shock

---

    o Mean blood pressure $\geq$ 60-70 mmHg
    o Cardiac index $\geq$ 3.5.-4/min/m^2 or SvO_2 $\geq$ 65-70 %*
    o Urine flow $\geq$ 0.7 ml/kg
    o Decrease in blood lactate level
    o Improvement in skin perfusion and level of conciousness.

---

2) Selection of drugs

---

    o Cardiac index $\geq$ 3.5-4 l/min/m^2 or SvO_2 $\geq$ 65-70 %*:dopamine or norepinephrine titrated against mean blood pressure
    o Cardiac index < 3.5 l/min/m^2 or SvO_2 < 65 %* :dobutamine titrated against cardiac index (+ norepinephrine or dopamine if mean arterial pressure is < 70 mm Hg)
    o In case of failure, consider adding epinephrine, phenylephrine....

* No significant impairment in hemoglobin level and in SaO_2.

Table 3 . *Selection of adrenergic agents*

INDIVIDUAL INOTROPIC AGENTS

Isoproterenol

Isoproterenol is a β_1 and β_2 adrenergic agonist. Few studies have evaluated isoproterenol in sepsis and septic shock. In septic shock patients with a low cardiac index (mean < 2.0 l/min/m^2), isoproterenol (2-8 µg/min) will significantly increase cardiac index without decreasing blood pressure but at the expense of increasing heart rate [66] (Table 4).

In patients with a normal cardiac index, however, isoproterenol can decrease blood pressure through its β_2 adrenergic effects. In addition, the chronotropic effects of β_1 adrenergic stimulation can precipitate myocardial ischemia (Tables 1 and 4).

Drug	Dose range (µg/kg/m)	Heart rate	Cardiac index	Stroke volume index	Systemic Vascular Resistance Index	Left Ventricular Stroke Work Index
Isoproterenol	2–8	11–20	47–119	22–89	-24--44	74–157
Dopamine	2–55	1–23	4–44	7–32	-6–18	5–91
Epinephrine	0.06–0.47	-6–27	24–54	12	-7–34	32–95
Norepinephrine	0.03–3.3	-6–8	-3–21	5–15	13–111	42–142
Dobutamine	2–28	9–23	12–61	15	-6--21	23–28
Dopexamine	2–6	6–17	17–20	14	-15--27	6

Table 4. Cardiac effects (% change from baseline) of inotropes used in septic shock.

Dopamine

Dopamine is an adrenergic agonist with predominant dopaminergic properties at doses less than 5 µg/kg/m and increased β and α activity at doses in excess of 5 µg/kg/min. Even at low doses, significant α and β agonism may occur.

In patients with severe sepsis and/or septic shock, most studies [6, 7, 9, 11, 12, 91] have shown that dopamine will increase cardiac index in the range of 20-30 %, left ventricular stroke work index by 20-60 %, and right ventricular stroke work index by a modest 5-10 %. These improvements in cardiac performance come at the expense of an increase in the heart rate by approximately 15 % (Tables 1 and 4). The greatest increase in these variables occurs at doses ranging from 3-12 µg/kg/min. At higher doses, the rate of improvement in cardiac function decreases.

Dobutamine

Dobutamine is a racemic mixture of two isomers, a D isomer with β_1 and β_2 adrenergic effects, and an L isomer with β_1 and α_1 adrenergic effects; its predominant effect is inotropic via stimulation of β_1 receptors, with a variable effect on blood pressure. (tables 1 and 4)

A number of studies [48,71-76] have investigated the effect of dobutamine on cardiac function during sepsis or septic shock at doses ranging from 2 to 28 µg/kg/min. In the majority of these studies, increases in cardiac index ranged from 20 to 66 %. However, heart rate often increased significantly (10 to 25 %). Two studies [71,72] reported that left ventricular stroke work index increased by 23 to 37 % at mean dobutamine doses of 5 to 12 µg/kg/min. Similar increases in right ventricular stroke work were also observed in these studies.

Epinephrine

Epinephrine stimulates both α and β receptors. At low doses, the β adrenergic effects predominate. A few recent studies [17,18,21] have examined the hemodynamic effects of epinephrine in septic shock at doses ranging from 0.1-0.5 µg/kg/min. The increase in cardiac index varied from 23-54 %, and the heart rate response was variable. Only one study [18] reported LVSWI and noted a 95 % increase. Another study [21] suggested that lactic acidosis is increased and perfusion to the gut is altered with the use of epinephrine.

Norepinephrine

Like epinephrine, norepinephrine stimulates both α and β receptors; however, the α-adrenergic response is predominant (Tables 1 and 4).

The effect of norepinephrine on cardiac index is modest, with the majority of studies showing no change or increases of 10-12 % while heart rate is unaffected or even decreases by up to 10 % [7,9,25,36,51). However, several studies have shown a marked increase in left and right ventricular stroke work index due to increased blood pressure [4,25,36,51].

Dopexamine

Dopexamine is a dopamine analog that stimulates β_2 and DA_1 and DA_2 receptors (Table 4). Two studies [77,78] have evaluated short term infusions of dopexamine in sepsis or septic shock and demonstrated significant improvements in cardiac index and left ventricular stroke work index. In addition, mesenteric perfusion, as assessed by gastric tonometry, appeared to improve compared to baseline values.

Combination and Comparative Studies

A significant number of studies have investigated catecholamine combinations [22,26,28,38,79,82]. The majority of these studies did not study the catecholamine combination in a standardized fashion, thus limiting the conclusions that can be drawn about the effects of these catecholamine combinations on cardiac function. Patients who do not respond to dopamine with an increase in cardiac index may reach the desired endpoint with a dopamine/norepinephrine combination. Dobutamine and norepinephrine appear to be an effective combination to improve cardiac index and blood pressure [9,49].

A few investigations have been performed comparing different inotropic regimens [21,22,30,36,53-55]. Epinephrine appears to be as good, if not better, at improving cardiac performance than dopamine or a dobutamine/norepinephrine combination [21,22]. However, epinephrine is associated with increases in arterial lactate and decreases in pHi, suggesting that perfusion to regional vascular beds may be impaired [21,22] In several studies [4,36], dopamine increased cardiac index and stroke volume index to a greater extent than norepinephrine but increases in left and right ventricular stroke volume index were about the same with the two agents. There was less prominent tachycardia with norepinephrine, and one study suggested that mesenteric perfusion is impaired with dopamine compared to norepinephrine. [4,36].

USE OF INOTROPIC AGENTS

Goals of Inotropic Therapy

Although it is clear that myocardial performance is altered during sepsis and septic shock [83], endpoints for cardiac resuscitation are uncertain. Data from the 1980s and early 1990s suggested that a linear relationship between DO_2 and VO_2 ('pathologic supply dependency') was common in septic patients [84], i.e., DO_2 was insufficient to meet the metabolic needs of the patient. These observations led to the hypothesis that resuscitation to predetermined elevated end-points of cardiac index and DO_2 and VO_2 ('hyperresuscitation') might improve patient outcome. More recent investigations, however, have challenged the concept of pathologic supply-dependency and hyperresuscitation [83,85,86] Although cardiac index and DO_2 are correlated with outcome [87], it is unclear if increases in these variables are the cause of increased survival or represent underlying physiologic reserve of the patient.

Uncertainty exists in regard to other endpoints for inotropic therapy. Deficits in DO_2 can clearly cause a lactic acidosis, but the converse is not true; elevated lactate concentrations in patients with sepsis or septic shock do not necessarily reflect deficits in DO_2. In septic patients, SvO_2 is usually high, and this value correlates poorly with cardiac output, and several studies have questioned the value of SvO_2 as the endpoint for inotropic therapy in critically ill patients [88,89]. Low SvO_2 may indicate decreased global DO_2 [88]. However, global DO_2 may be adequate in many septic patients but regional perfusion may be suboptimal. Gastric tonometry monitors pHi as a proxy for determining the adequacy of gut perfusion. Although gastric tonometry is a good predictor for the ultimate outcome of critically-ill patients and may be useful in the resuscitation of such patients [67,70], its utility to guide therapy in patients with sepsis and septic shock has not been proven.

With the above considerations in mind, precise recommendations regarding specific endpoints for cardiac index, DO_2, VO_2 and SvO_2 are difficult to formulate based on currently available data. An inotropic agent should be considered to maintain an adequate cardiac index, MAP, SvO_2 and urine output (tables 2 and 3 and figure 1).

Complications of Inotropic Therapy

In the septic patient who has been inadequately volume resuscitated, all of the inotropic agents can cause significant tachycardia. In patients with coexisting coronary disease, the change in myocardial oxygen consumption may precipitate myocardial ischemia and infarction [86]. Excessive doses of catecholamines can also result in myocardial band necrosis independent of the presence of coronary disease. Sole use of inotropic agents that also have vasodilatory activity (e.g., isoproterenol) is likely to reduce blood pressure. In most patients a combination with a vasopressor is advocated (Figure 1). These alterations can be long-lasting with agents that have a long half-life. Administration of inotropic agents that have pressor activity may impair blood flow to other organ beds, such as the splanchnic circulation. Efforts to ensure adequate volume resuscitation and to assess end-organ function must be made.

CONCLUSION

In patients with septic shock not initially responsive to aggressive fluid challenge, dopamine and norepinephirne are both effective at increasing blood pressure. Norepinephrine may be a more effective vasopressor in some patients. Dobutamine is the first choice agent when cardiac index is low. Dobutamine and norepinephrine can be titrated separately to maintain both arterial pressure and cardiac output. Epinephrine can be considered for refractory hypotension or to increase cardiac output, although adverse effects are common. Clinical experience with phenylephrine is limited.

REFERENCES

1.   Parker M, Suffredini A, Natanson C, et al. Responses of left ventricular function in survivors and nonsurvivors of septic shock. J Crit Care 1989; 4:19-25
2.   Hoogenberg K, Smit AJ; Girbes ARJ. Effects of low-dose dopamine on renal and systemic hemodynamics during incremental norepinephrine infusion in healthy volunteers. Crit. Care Med. 1998; 26:260-265
3.   Meier-Hellmann A, Bredle DL, Specht M, et al. The effects of low-dose dopamine on splanchnic blood flow and oxygen utilization in patients with septic shock. Intensive Care Med 1997: 23:31-37
4.   Marik PE, Mohedin M. The contrasting effects of dopamine and norepinephrine on systemic and splanchnic oxygen utilization in hyperdynamic sepsis. JAMA 1994; 272:1354-1357
5.   Hannemann L, Reinhart K, Grenzer O, et al. Comparison of dopamine to dobutamine and norepinephrine for oxygen delivery and uptake in septic shock. Crit Care Med 1995; 23:1962-70
6.   Ruokonen E, Takala J, Kari A, et al. Regional blood flow and oxygen transport in septic shock. Crit Care Med 1993; 21:1296-1303
7.   Jardin F, Gurdjian F, Desfonds P, et al. Effect of dopamine on intrapulmonary shunt fraction and oxygen transmort in severe sepsis with circulatory and respiratory failure. Crit Care Med 1979; 7:273-277
8.   Jardin F, Eveleigh MC, Gurdjian F, et al. Venous admixture in human septic shock. Comparative effects of blood volume expansion, dopamine infusion and isoproterenol infusion in mismatching of ventilation and pulmonary blood flow in peritonitis. Circulation 1979; 60:155-159
9.   Martin C, Papazian L, Perrin G, et al. Norepinephrine or dopamine for the treatment of hyperdynamic septic shock. Chest 1993; 103:1826-1831
10. Regnier B, Safran D, Carlet J, et al. Comparative haemodynamic effects of dopamine and dobutamine in septic shock. Intensive Care Med. 1979; 5:115-120
11. Samii KL, Le Gall JR, Regnier B, et al. Hemodynamic effects of dopamine in septic shock with and without acute renal failure. Arch Surg 1978; 113:1414-1416

12. Drueck C, Welch GW, Pruitt BA, Jr. Hemodynamic analysis of septic shock in thermal injury : treatment with dopamine. Am Surg 1978; 44:424-427

13. Regnier B, Rapin M, Gory G, et al. Haemodynamic effects of dopamine in septic shock. Intensive Care Med 1977; 3:47-553

14. Wilson RF, Sibbald WJ, Jaanimagi JL. Hemodynamic effects of dopamine in critically ill septic patients. J Surg Res 1976; 20:163-172

15. Maynard ND, Bihari DJ, Dalton RN, al. Increasing splanchnic blood flow in the critically ill. Chest 1995; 108:1648-1654

16. Nevière R, Mathieu D, Chagnon JL, et al. The contrasting effects of dobutamine and dopamine on musocal perfusion in septic patients. Am J Respir Crit Care Med 1996; 154:1684-1688

17. Wilson W, Lipman J, Scribante J, et al. Septic shock : does adrenaline have a role as a first-line inotropic agents ? Anaesth Intensive Care 1992; 20:470-474

18. Moran JL, MS OF, Peisach AR, Chapman MH, Leppard P. Epinephrine as an inotropic agents in septic shock : a dose-profile analysis. Crit Care Med 1993; 21:70-77

19. Mackenzie SJ, Kapadia F, Nimmo GR, et al. Adrenaline in treatment of septic shock : effects on haemodynamics and oxygen transport. Intensive Care Med 1991; 17:36-39

20. Le Tulzo Y, Seguin P, Gacouin A, et al. effects of epinephrine on right ventricular function in patients with severe septic shock and right ventricular failure : a preliminary study. Intensive Care Med 1997; 23:664-670

21. Day NP, Phu NH, Bethell DP, et al. The effects of dopamine and adrenaline infusions on acid-base balance and systemic haemodynamics in severe infection. Lancet 1996; 348:219-223

22. Levy B, Bollaert PE, Charpentier C, et al. Compariosn of norepinephrine and dobutamine to epinerphrine for hemodynamics, lactate metabolism, and gastric tonomictric variables in septic shock : a prospective, randomized study. Intensive Care Med 1997; 23:282-287

23. Levy B, Bollaert PE, Lucchelli JP, et al. Dobutamine improves the adequacy of gastric mucosal perfusion in epinephrine-treated septic shock. Crit Care Med 1997; 25:1649-1654

24. Martin C, Eon B, Saux P, et al. Renal effects of norepinephrine used to treat septic shock patients. Crit Care Med 1990; 18:282-285

25. Meadows D, Edwards JD, Wilkins RG, et al. Reversal of intractable septic shock with norepinephrine therapy. Crit Care Med 1988; 16:663-667

26. Redl-Wenzl EM, Armbruster C, Edlmann G et al. The effects of norepinephrine on hemodynamics and renal function in severe septic shock states. Intensive Care Med 1993; 19:151-154

27. Chernow B, Roth BL. Pharmacologic manipulation of the peripheral vasculature in shock : clinical and experimental approaches; Circ Shock 1986; 18:141-155

28. Desjars P, Pinaud M, Tasseau F, et al. A reappraisal of norepinephrine therapy in human septic shock. Crit Care Med 1987; 15:134-137

29. Desjars P, Pinaud M, Brugnon D, et al. Norepinephrine therapy has no deleterious renal effects in human septic shock. Crit Care Med 1989; 17:426-429

30. Hesselvik JF, Brodin B. Low-dose norepinephrine in patients with septic shock and oliguria : effects on afterload, urine flow, and oxygen transport. Crit Care Med 1989; 17:179-180

31. Eckstein J, Abboud F. Circulation effect of sympathomimetic amines. Am Heart J 1962; 63:119-121

32. Mills L, Moyer J, Handley C. Effects of various sympathomimetic drugs on renal hemodynamics in normotensive and hypotensive dogs. Am J Physiol 1960; 198:1279-1284

33. Murakawa K, Kobayashi A. Effects of vasopressors on renal tissue gas tensions during hemorrhagic shock in dogs. Crit Care Med 1988; 16:789-92

34. Conger JD, Robinette JB, Guggenheim SJ. Effect of acetylcholine on the early phase of reversible norepinephrine-induced acute renal failure. Kidney Int 1981; 19:399-409

35. Bush HL, Huse JB, Johnson WC, et al. Prevention of renal insufficiency after abdominal aortic aneurysm resection by optimal volume loading. Arch Surg 1981; 116: 1517-1524

36. Schreuder WO, Scheiner AJ, Groeneveld ABJ, et al. Effect of dopamine vs norepinephrine on hemodynamics in septic shock. Chest 1989; 95:1282-1288

37. Winslow EJ, Loeb JS, Rahimtoola SH, et al. Hemodynamic studies and results of therapy in 50 patients with bacteremic shock. Am J Med 1973; 54:421-432

38. Reinelt H, Radermacher P, Fisher G, et al. Effects of a dobutamine-induced increase in splanchnic blood flow on hepatic metabolic activity in patients with septic shock. Anesthesiology 1997; 86:818-824

39. Yamazaki T, Shimada Y, Taenaka N, et al. Circulatory responses to afterloading with phenylephrine in hyperdynamic sepsis. Crit Care Med 1982; 10:432-435

40. Flancbaum L, Dick M, Dasta J, al. E. A dose-response study of phenylephrine in critically ill, septic surgical patients. Eur J Clin Pharmacol 1997; 51:461-465

41. Gregory J, Bonfiglio M, Dasta J, et al. Experience with phenylephrine as a component of the pharmacologic support of septic shock. Crit Care Med 1991; 19:1395-1400

42. Rudis MI, Basha MA, Zarowitz BJ. Is it time to reposition vasopressors and inotropes in sepsis ? Crit Care Med 1996; 24:525- 537

43. Bersten AD, Holt AW, et al. Vasoactive drug and the importance of renal perfusion pressure. New Horizons 1995; 3:650-661

44. Kircheim HR, Ehmke H, Hackenthal E. Autoregulation of renal blood flow, glomerular filtration rate and renin release in conscious dogs. Pflugers Arch 1987; 410: 441-449

45. Barry KG, Mazze RI, Schwarz FD. Prevention of surgical oliguria and renal hemodynamic suppression by sustained hydratation. N Engl J Med 1964; 270:1371-1377

46. Kelleher SP, Robinette JB, Bell PD, et al. Sympathetic nervous system in the loss of autoregulation in acute renal failure. Am J Physiol 1984; 246:F379-F386

47. Parker MM, Shelhamer JH, Bacharach SL, et al. Profound but reversible myocardial depression in patients with septic shock. Ann Intern Med 1984; 100:483-490

48. Martin C. Saux P, Eon B, et al. Septic Shock: a goal directed therapy using volume loading, dobutamine and/or norepinephrine. Acta Anaesthesiol Scand 1990; 34:413-417

49. Hoffman MJ, Greenflield LJ, Sugerman HJ, et al. Unsuspected right ventricular dysfunction in shock and sepsis. Arch Surg 1983; 198:307-319

50. Martin C, Perrin G, Saux P, et al. Effects of norepinephrine on right ventricular function in septic shock patients. Intensive Care Med 1994; 20:444-447

51. Vincent JL, Reuse C, Frank N, et al. Right ventricular dysfunction in septic shock : assessment by measurements of right ventricular ejection fraction using the thermodilation technique. Acta Anaesthesiol Scand 1989; 33:34-38

52. Bollaert PE, Baueur P, Audibert G, et al. Effects of epinephrine on hemodynamics and oxygen metabolism in dopamine-resistant septic shock. Chest 1990; 98:949-953

53. Fukuoka T, Nishimura M, Imanaka H et al. Effects of norepinephrine on renal function in septic patients with normal and elevated serum lactate levels. Crit Care Med 1989; 17:1104-1107

54. Lipman J, Roux A, Kraus P. Vasoconstrictor effects of adrenaline in human septic shock. Anaesth Intensive Care 1991; 19:61-65

55. Hayes MA, Timmins AC, Yau EH, et al. Oxygen transport patterns in patients with sepsis syndrome or septic shock : influence of treatment and relationship to outcome. Crit Care Med 1997; 25:46-52

56. Steffes CP, Dahn MS, Lange MP. Oxygen transport-dependent splanchnic metabolism in sepsis syndrome. Arch Surg 1994; 129:46-52

57. Boekstegers P, Weidenhofer S, Pilz G, et al. Peripheral oxygen availability within skeletal muscle in sepsis ans septic shock : comparison to limited infection and cardiogenic shock. Infection 1991; 5:317-323

58. Bredle D, Samsel R, Schumacker P. Critical O2 delivery to skeletal muscle at high and low PO2 in endotoxemic dogs . J Appl Physiol 1989; 66:2553-2558

59. Rackow E, Astiz ME, Weil MH. Increases in oxygen extraction during rapidly fatal septic shock in rats. J Lab Clin Med 1987; 109: 660-664

60. Friedman G, Berlot G, Kahn RJ, et al. Combined measurements of blood lactate levels and gastric intramucosal pH in patients with severe sepsis. Crit Care Med 1995; 23:1184-1193

61. Vincent JL, Dufaye P, Berre J et al. Serial lactate determinations during circulatory shock. Crit Care Med 1983; 11:449-451

62. Weil MH, Afifi AA. Experimental and clinical studies on lactate and pyruvate as indicators of the severity of acute circulatory failure. Circulation 1970; 41:989-1001

63. Bakker J, Coffernils M, Leon M et al. Blood lactate levels are superior to oxygen-derived variables in predicting outcome in human septic shock. Chest 1991; 99:956-962

64. Nelson D, Beyer C, Samsel R, et al. Pathologic supply dependence of systemic and intestinal O2 uptake during bacteremia in the dog. J Appl Physiol 1987; 63:1487-1489

65. Creteur J, Debacker D, Vincent JL. Monitoring gastric muscosal carbon dioxide presseur using gas tonometry : in vitro and in vivo validation studies. Anesthesiology 1997; 87:504-510

66. Russell JA. Gastric tonometry : Does it work ? Intensive Care Med 1997; 23:3-6

67. Marik PE. Gastric intramucosal pH. A better predictor of multiorgan dysfunction syndrome and death than oxygen-derived variables in patients with sepsis. Chest 1993; 104:225-229

68. Maynard N. Bihari D, Beale R, et al. Assessment of splanchnic oxygenation by gastric tonometry in patients with acute circulatory failure. JAMA 1993; 270:1203-1210

69. Gutierrez G, Palizas F, Doglio G, et al. Gastric intramucosal pH as a therapeutic index of tissue oxygenation in critically ill patients. Lancet 1992; 339:195-199

70. Doglio GR, Pusajo JF, Egurrola MA, et al. Gastric musocal pH as a prognostic index of mortality in critically ill patients. Crit Care Med 1991; 19:1037-1040

71. Jardin F, Sportiche M, Bazin M, et al. Dobutamine: a hemodynamic evaluation in human septic shock. Crit Care Med 1981; 9:329-332

72. De Backer D, Berre J, Zhang H, et al. Relationship between oxygen uptake and oxygen delivery in septic patients: effects of prostacyclin versus dobutamine. Crit Care Med 1993; 21:1658-1664

73. Vallet B, Chopin C, Curtis SE, et al. Prognostic value of the dobutamine test in patients with sepsis syndrome and normal lactate values: a prospective, multicenter study. Crit Care Med 1993; 21:1868-1875

74. Gutierrez G, Clark C, Brown SD, et al. Effects of dobutamine on oxygen consumption and gastric mucosal pH in septic patients. Am J Respir Crit Care Med 1994; 150:324-329

75. De Backer D, Moraine JJ, Berre J, et al. Effects of dobutamine on oxygen consumption in septic patients. Direct versus indirect determinations. Am J Respir Crit Care Med 1994; 150:95-100

76. Ronco JJ, Fenwick JC, Wiggs BR, et al. Oxygen consumption is independent of increases in oxygen delivery by dobutamine in septic patients who have normal or increased plasma lactate. Am Rev Respir Dis 1993; 147:25-31

77. Hannemann L, Reinhart K, Meier-Hellmann A, et al. Dopexamine hydrochloride in septic shock. Chest 1996; 109:756-760

78. Smithies M, Yee TH, Kackson L, et al. Protecting the gut and the liver in the critically ill: effects of dopexamine. Crit Care Med 1994; 22:789-795

79. Vincent JL, Roman A, Kahn RJ. Dobutamine administration in septic shock: addition to a standard protocol. Crit Care Med 1990; 18:689-693

80. Mira JP, Fabre JE, Baigorri F, et al. Lack of oxygen supply dependency in patients with severe sepsis. A study of oxygen delivery increased by military antishock trouser and dobutamine. Chest 1994; 106:1524-1531

81. Redl-Wenzl EM, Armbruster C, Edelmann G, et al. Noradrenaline in the "high output-low resistance" state of patients with abdominal sepsis. Anaesthesist 1990; 39:525-529

82. Tell B, Majerus TC, Flancbaum L. Dobutamine in elderly septic shock patients refractory to dopamine. Intensive Care Med 1977; 13:14-18

83. Gattinoni L, Brazzi L, Pelosi P, et al. A trial of goal-oriented hemodynamic therapy in critically patients. N Engl J Med 1995; 333:1025-1032

84. Haupt MT, Gilbert EM, Carlson RW. Fluid loading increases oxygen consumption in septic patients with lactic acidosis. Am Rev Respir Dis 1985; 131:912-916

85. Yu M, Levy MM, Smith P, et al. Effect of maximizing oxygen delivery on morbidity and mortality rates in critically ill patients: a prospective, randomized, controlled study. Crit Care Med 1993; 21:830-838

86. Hayes MA, Timmins AC, Yau EHS, et al. Elevation of systemic oxygen delivery in the treatment of critically ill patients. N Engl J Med 1994; 330:1717-1722

87. Tuchschmidt J, Fried J, Astiz M, et al. Elevation of cardiac output and oxygen delivery improves outcome in septic shock. Chest 1992; 102:216-220

88. Jain A, Shroff SG, Janicki JS, et al. Relation between mixed venous oxygen saturation and cardiac index. Nonlinearity and normalization for oxygen uptake and hemoglobin. Chest 1991; 99:1403-1409

89. Vaughn S, Puri VK. Cardiac output changes and continuous mixed venous oxygen saturation measurement in the critically ill. Crit Care Med 1988; 16:495-498

25

REGIONAL EFFECTS OF CATECHOLAMINES

Andreas Meier-Hellmann

The most important step in the supportive treatment of patients with sepsis is to restore and maintain oxygen transport and tissue oxygenation. Therefore, supportive treatment should be focused on adequate volume resuscitation and appropriate use of vasoactive drugs.

Tissue hypoxia, especially in the splanchnic area, is still considered to be an important cofactor in the pathogenesis of multiple organ failure (MOF) [1]. Therefore, the specific effects of the various therapeutic interventions on splanchnic perfusion and oxygenation are of particular interest.

Since the effects of the various vasoactive drugs on global and regional hemodynamics have been well studied, one would assume that the appropriate use of vasoactive drugs in the treatment of sepsis should be easily established. Unfortunately, the effects of vasoactive drugs on global and regional perfusion in patients with sepsis or septic shock may well differ from the effects in patients without sepsis [2], and studies measuring the effects of various fluids and catecholamines on splanchnic perfusion and oxygenation under the specific conditions of sepsis are, therefore, most relevant.

THE VARIOUS CATECHOLAMINES

Dobutamine

Under conditions of adequate volume replacement, dobutamine increases cardiac output and oxygen delivery (DO_2) to a greater extent than dopamine

[3]. Hannemann et al. [4] demonstrated in septic patients that a combination of dobutamine with norepinephrine when compared with dopamine alone, titrated to achieve a similar mean arterial pressure (MAP), was associated with a lower heart rate, lower filling pressures, and lower intrapulmonary shunt. A higher DO_2 with dopamine alone was not associated with a higher oxygen consumption (VO_2). Therefore, the authors concluded that dopamine did not improve tissue oxygenation but induced a greater myocardial stress and impaired pulmonary gas exchange. Also, Hayes et al. [5] demonstrated that an inappropriate use of dobutamine in very high dosages to elevate the DO_2 could be ineffective or even dangerous.

That dobutamine improves splanchnic perfusion and oxygenation has been supported by studies demonstrating an increased gastric mucosal pH (pHi) under dobutamine infusion [6,7]. Nevertheless, these effects paralleled an increase in whole body blood flow, as selective effects of dobutamine on splanchnic circulation, beyond the global hemodynamic effects, seem unlikely [8].

In conclusion, when dobutamine is used to increase DO_2, there is some evidence of improvement in tissue oxygenation. Nevertheless, there is no clear recommendation to what extent DO_2 should be increased, and it is doubtful that there is an optimal DO_2 appropriate for all septic patients. However, increasing the global DO_2 by the use of dobutamine often is associated with improved regional perfusion and oxygenation. There are as yet no data that demonstrate selective effects of dobutamine on regional perfusion. Therefore, the increase in DO_2 by dobutamine should be carefully monitored by using methods which indicate changes in tissue oxygenation such as lactate levels, regional CO_2 production or intramucosal pH (pHi), or changes in VO_2.

Norepinephrine

In experimental models, norepinephrine increased splanchnic vascular resistance and decreased splanchnic blood flow [9]. As a consequence, norepinephrine is most commonly used as a last resort when hemodynamic stabilization cannot be achieved with other catecholamines [10].

It has been demonstrated that treatment with norepinephrine in septic shock restores renal function [11,12]. However, it should be emphasized that these patients had markedly decreased blood pressures prior to the administration. Therefore, the potential unfavorable effects of vasopressors must be weighed against the known danger of inadequate perfusion pressure.

In fact, findings on the effects of norepinephrine on splanchnic perfusion in sepsis are inconsistent. Bersten et al. [2] compared the effects of several catecholamines on regional blood flow in septic and non-septic sheep. They found a redistribution of blood flow to the heart and away from the brain, kidneys, liver and pancreas with norepinephrine, dobutamine, dopamine, dopexamine or salbutamol treatment in the non-septic animals. In contrast, such a redistribution of regional blood flow was not observed in the septic animals.

A beneficial effect of norepinephrine on splanchnic oxygenation in septic patients was suggested in a pilot study by Marik and Mohedin [13] who compared norepinephrine and dopamine as vasopressors. Patients who were treated with norepinephrine had an increase in pHi whereas those treated with dopamine had a decrease in pHi.

We measured splanchnic blood flow in 10 patients with septic shock using the indocyaninegreen-dye dilution technique [14]. After changing the catecholamine treatment from a combination of dobutamine with norepinephrine to norepinephrine alone, we observed a parallel decrease in splanchnic perfusion and cardiac output, while splanchnic VO_2 remained unchanged.

In conclusion, as long as an adequate DO_2 is maintained, treatment with norepinephrine alone seems to be without negative effects on tissue oxygenation.

Epinephrine

The rationale for using epinephrine in the treatment of septic shock is its β-receptor mediated increase in cardiac output and α-receptor mediated increase in systemic perfusion pressure [15-17].

We [18] measured splanchnic perfusion, DO_2 and VO_2 in eight patients with septic shock who were treated with a combination of dobutamine and norepinephrine. After a change to epinephrine alone, titrated to achieve the same MAP as before, DO_2 and VO_2 remained unchanged. However, splanchnic perfusion decreased despite unchanged cardiac output. The decrease in splanchnic DO_2 was associated with a decrease in splanchnic VO_2. Furthermore, the deterioration in tissue oxygenation following the administration of epinephrine was evident by an increase in lactate levels and a decrease in pHi. Similar findings were reported by Levy et al. [19] who also found an increase in lactate and a decrease in pHi with epinephrine when compared to a combination of dobutamine and norepinephrine. These findings point to a very limited role for epinephrine in septic patients, and underline the recommendation that norepinephrine should be the vasopressor of first choice.

Dopamine

Low dose dopamine has been used for many years with the intention of increasing renal perfusion. In recently published recommendations concerning the treatment of sepsis [20], dopamine in higher dosages has been suggested as the primary drug of choice in the management of decreased mean arterial pressure (MAP) in patients in septic shock. Nevertheless, data on the regional effects of dopamine suggest careful use in either low or high dosages.

First, there are no data to demonstrate that low dose dopamine will improve renal function in septic patients. Only one study [21] demonstrated that low dose dopamine increased urine output and creatinine clearance in patients with severe sepsis, but no effects in patients with septic shock were found. Also, the beneficial effects in patients with severe sepsis were only seen for 48 hours.

Second, there is some evidence that low dose dopamine can have deleterious effects on gastrointestinal perfusion. Giraud and MacCannell [22] administered dopamine in dogs and measured an increase in superior mesenteric artery blood flow and in the muscle layer of the gut. However, they found a decreased blood flow to the gut mucosa accompanied by a decrease in splanchnic VO_2. In the already mentioned study by Marik and Mohedin [13], patients who were stabilized from septic shock using dopamine, had a lower pHi than patients who received norepinephrine. Moreover, dopamine at a dose of 5 µg/kg/min was equally effective when compared with dobutamine but led to a decrease in intestinal mucosa perfusion [23].

In 11 patients with septic shock treated with norepinephrine, we added dopamine in a dosage of 2.8 to 3.0 µg/kg/min. In those patients with a fractional splanchnic flow in the normal range, low dose dopamine increased splanchnic perfusion, whereas in patients with an elevated fractional splanchnic flow before treatment, no further increase or even a decrease in splanchnic flow was observed [24]. This suggests that the effects of dopamine depend on the individual baseline splanchnic flow, which in septic patients could vary from normal to markedly increased.

In addition, prolonged dopamine infusion can have important effects on the concentrations of various circulating pituitary-dependent hormones which may influence metabolic and immunological homeostasis in critically ill patients [25]. It remains questionable whether the management of septic shock with higher doses of dopamine alone is superior to the combination of dobutamine and norepinephrine.

Dopexamine

Dopexamine is a relatively new catecholamine with predominantly β_2 and dopaminergic receptor activity. Cain and Curtis [26] observed no difference in mesenteric venous blood flow in septic dogs treated with dopexamine when compared with a control group without catecholamine treatment. Since the gut of the dopexamine treated animals released less lactate, the authors concluded that dopexamine preferentially increased perfusion of the gut mucosa.

In another animal model of sepsis, the dopexamine infusion was associated with less damage in hepatic cells than an infusion of dobutamine [27]. Furthermore, dopexamine increased tissue PO_2 in various splanchnic organs in animals after the induction of sepsis [28]. Also, in a dosage of 2.5 μg/kg/min dopexamine prevented hypoperfusion of the intestinal villus after endotoxin infusion in rats [29].

In some clinical studies, dopexamine increased a pathological low pHi [30,31] as well as oxygen saturation in the mucosa of the upper gastrointestinal tract measured by reflectance spectrophotometry [32]. However, it remains unclear whether dopexamine had a selective effect on splanchnic perfusion or if this finding was simply the result of overall hemodynamic stabilization. Such an effect - an improved cardiac output but no selective effect on splanchnic perfusion - has been demonstrated in a recent study from Kiefer et al. [33].

Some studies have suggested that dopexamine may even have deleterious effects on splanchnic perfusion. Uusaro et al. [34] reported an increase in whole body DO_2 and splanchnic DO_2 to a similar extent after dopexamine infusion in cardiac surgery patients. They did not find a specific effect of dopexamine infusion on splanchnic blood flow, as indicated by an unchanged fractional splanchnic blood flow. In fact, they reported a decrease in pHi, which could reflects splanchnic hypoxia induced by the cardiac surgery. However, this effect could also be an indication of a redistribution of splanchnic blood flow and a hypoperfusion of gut mucosa similar to the possible effect from low dose dopamine. In our studies [35], dopexamine increased splanchnic perfusion to the same extent as whole body blood flow but was also associated with a decrease in pHi.

Although some investigators recommend dopexamine to improve splanchnic oxygenation and renal function, further studies are required to more clearly demonstrate the usefulness of dopexamine in the treatment of septic shock. At present, there are no convincing clinical data available to clearly justify the use of dopexamine in septic patients.

LIMITATIONS

Catecholamines may exhibit marked inter-individual variation in septic patients. Various factors, such as the fractional flow of the cardiac output to the splanchnic perfusion bed or therapy with other vasoactive substances, may influence the effects of catecholamines.

Unfortunately, studies concerning the effects of various catecholamines on outcome are lacking. Furthermore, available clinical techniques for the assessment of regional perfusion are rarely used and often only poorly evaluated. For example, it is still unclear whether the gastric mucosal pH (pHi) or the mucosal PCO_2 ($PgCO_2$) really reflects the whole splanchnic area [34,36]. It is well known that sepsis markedly changes the relationship between blood flow from the portal system and the hepatic artery [37], but the measurement of the hepatic blood flow by a hepatic venous catheter technique cannot separate these two.

These limitations underline that every concept for general use of catecholamines in sepsis only can be a rough suggestion. Until the above limitations can be overcome, it is impossible to give universally valid recommendations for the use of catecholamines.

CONCLUSION

Adequate fluid resuscitation is considered essential treatment in sepsis, before or with catecholamines. Any attempt to correct low cardiac output or hypotension due to hypovolemia by using catecholamines has to be strictly rejected.

When a normal value for DO_2 has already been achieved by fluid resuscitation, any further attempt to increase global DO_2 is questionable unless signs of inadequate tissue perfusion are still present. The clinical decision to further increase catecholamine dosages to elevate DO_2 should be guided by parameters that reflect organ function or tissue oxygenation, e.g., lactate, $PgCO_2$, and urine output. Due to the potentially harmful effects of dopamine and epinephrine, dobutamine seems to be the current catecholamine of choice to improve compromised cardiac function. The use of dobutamine in moderate dosages may further increase global DO_2, and thus also lead to an increase in DO_2 to the splanchnic area and to an improved gastric mucosal perfusion.

Based on the potential negative effects of dopamine and epinephrine, norepinephrine may be regarded as the first choice catecholamine to increase peripheral vascular resistance. The well documented negative effects of norepinephrine on kidney function in non-septic patients do not seem to be present in sepsis patients with adequate volume resuscitation. An inadequate perfusion pressure should not be tolerated just because of concerns over the use of norepinephrine.

There is no good evidence for routine treatment with dopamine in the so called 'renal dosage'. In septic patients with low fractional splanchnic blood flow, dopamine increased selective and absolute splanchnic blood flow. However, it remains unclear whether tissue oxygenation actually improves, since animal studies suggest a decrease in intestinal mucosal perfusion during dopamine infusion. In view of the lack of evidence of the benefits, and due to the potential adverse side-effects (selective impairment of mucosal perfusion, no or even negative effects on splanchnic blood flow in patients with primarily already increased blood flow, and its endocrinological effects) dopamine should only be used with extreme caution. For dopexamine, a selective effect on splanchnic blood flow has yet to be documented. Clinical studies that showed a positive effect for dopexamine on pHi could not be confirmed by others, who in fact reported a decrease in pHi with dopexamine. Accordingly, dopexamine cannot currently be recommended in the routine treatment of patients with sepsis.

To be sure, these recommendations remain quite limited due to the lack of outcome studies and methods of measurement of regional perfusion and oxidation. Until these limitations are addressed, other alternative treatments should not necessarily be dismissed as inappropriate.

Evidence-based Assessment

It is now well-documented that routine sepsis treatment to supranormal levels of DO_2 by using high doses of catecholamines is not beneficial (one multicenter, randomized, controlled study, n= 762 [38]; one randomized, controlled study, n= 109 [5]; one meta-analysis, 7 studies with in total n= 1016 [39]). The major role of adequate fluid resuscitation and an adequate arterial blood pressure has been proven in a large number of smaller trials and can be considered to have a high degree of evidence [20]. It has also been confirmed that epinephrine is not considered as a first choice catecholamine, and that there is no indication for the use of low-dose-dopamine [20,40]. However, due to the lack of evidence there is controversy concerning the use of high-dose dopamine. For dopexamine, only animal experiments and smaller clinical trials have been published; thus recommendations by an expert commission on the use of dopexamine are not yet available.

REFERENCES

1. Deitch EA, Berg R, Specian R. Endotoxin promotes the translocation of bacteria from the gut. Arch.Surg. 1987; 122:185-190
2. Bersten AD, Hersch M, Cheung H, et al. The effect of various sympathomimetics on the regional circulations in hyperdynamic sepsis. Surgery 1992; 112:549-561
3. Vincent JL, Van der Linden P, Domb M, et al. Dopamine compared with dobutamine in experimental septic shock: relevance to fluid administration. Anesth Analg 1987; 66:565-571
4. Hannemann L, Reinhart K, Grenzer O, et al. Comparison of dopamine to dobutamine and norepinephrine for oxygen delivery and uptake in septic shock. Crit Care Med 1995; 23:1962-1970
5. Hayes MA, Timmins AC, Yau EH, et al. Elevation of systemic oxygen delivery in the treatment of critically ill patients. N Engl J Med 1994; 330:1717-1722
6. Silverman HJ, Tuma P. Gastric tonometry in patients with sepsis. Effects of dobutamine infusions and packed red blood cell transfusions. Chest 1992; 102:184-188
7. Gutierrez G, Clark C, Brown SD, et al. Effect of dobutamine on oxygen consumption and gastric mucosal pH in septic patients. Am J Respir Crit Care Med 1994; 150:324-329
8. Reinelt H, Radermacher P, Fischer G, et al. Effects of a dobutamine-induced increase in splanchnic blood flow on hepatic metabolic activity in patients with septic shock. Anesthesiology 1997; 86:818-824
9. Granger DN, Richardson PD, Kvietys PR, et al. Intestinal blood flow. Gastroenterology 1980; 78:837-863
10. Shoemaker WC, Appel PL, Kram HB. Oxygen transport measurements to evaluate tissue perfusion and titrate therapy: dobutamine and dopamine effects. Crit Care Med 1991; 19:672-688
11. Hesselvik JF, Brodin B. Low dose norepinephrine in patients with septic shock and oliguria: effects on afterload, urine flow, and oxygen transport. Crit Care Med 1989; 17:179-180
12. Martin C, Eon B, Saux P, et al. Renal effects of norepinephrine used to treat septic shock patients. Crit Care Med 1990; 18:282-285
13. Marik PE, Mohedin M. The contrasting effects of dopamine and norepinephrine on systemic and splanchnic oxygen utilization in hyperdynamic sepsis. JAMA 1994; 272:1354-1357
14. Meier-Hellmann A, Reinhart K. Cardiovascular support by hemodynamic subset: Sepsis. In: Pinsky MR (ed) Applied Cardiovascular Physiology. Springer-Verlag, Berlin, 1997, pp: 230-245
15. Bollaert PE, Bauer P, Audibert G, et al. Effects of epinephrine on hemodynamics and oxygen metabolism in dopamine-resistant septic shock. Chest 1990; 98:949-953

16. Lipman J, Roux A, Kraus P. Vasoconstrictor effects of adrenaline in human septic shock. Anaesth.Intensive.Care 1991; 19:61-65
17. Mackenzie SJ, Kapadia F, Nimmo GR, et al. Adrenaline in treatment of septic shock: effects on haemodynamics and oxygen transport. Intensive Care Med 1991; 17:36-39
18. Meier-Hellmann A, Reinhart K, Bredle DL, et al. Epinephrine impairs splanchnic perfusion in septic shock. Crit Care Med 1997; 25:399-404
19. Levy B, Bollaert PE, Charpentier C, et al. Comparison of norepinephrine and dobutamine to epinephrine for hemodynamics, lactate metabolism, and gastric tonometric variables in septic shock: A prospective, randomized study. Intensive Care Med 1997; 23:282-287
20. Hollenberg SM, Ahrens TS, Astiz ME, et al. Practice parameters for hemodynamic support of sepsis in adult patients in sepsis. Crit Care Med 1999; 27:639-660
21. Lherm T, Troche G, Rossignol M, et al. Renal effects of low-dose dopamine in patients with sepsis syndrome or septic shock treated with catecholamines. Intensive Care Med 1996; 22:213-219
22. Giraud GD, MacCannell KL. Decreased nutrient blood flow during dopamine- and epinephrine- induced intestinal vasodilation. J Pharmacol Exp Ther 1984; 230:214-220
23. Neviere R, Mathieu D, Chagnon JL, et al. The contrasting effects of dobutamine and dopamine on gastric mucosal perfusion in septic patients. Am J Respir Crit Care Med 1996; 154:1684-1688
24. Meier-Hellmann A, Bredle DL, Specht M, et al. The effects of low dose dopamine on splanchnic blood flow and oxygen uptake in patients with septic shock. Intensive Care Med 1997; 23:31-37
25. Van den Berghe G, de Zegher F. Anterior pituitary function during critical illness and dopamine treatment. Crit Care Med 1996; 24:1580-1590
26. Cain SM, Curtis SE. Experimental models of pathologic oxygen supply dependency. Crit Care Med 1991; 19:603-612
27. Tighe D, Moss R, Heywood G, et al. Goal-directed therapy with dopexamine, dobutamine, and volume expansion: effects of systemic oxygen transport on hepatic ultrastructure in porcine sepsis. Crit Care Med 1995; 23:1997-2007
28. Lund N, de Asla RJ, Cladis F, et al. Dopexamine hydrochloride in septic shock: effects on oxygen delivery and oxygenation of gut, liver, and muscle. J Trauma 1995; 38:767-775
29. Schmidt H, Secchi A, Wellmann R, et al. Dopexamine maintains intestinal villus blood flow during endotoxemia in rats. Crit Care Med 1996; 24:1233-1237
30. Smithies M, Yee TH, Jackson L, et al. Protecting the gut and the liver in the critically ill: effects of dopexamine. Crit Care Med 1994; 22:789-795
31. Maynard ND, Bihari DJ, Dalton RN, et al. Increasing splanchnic blood flow in the critically III. Chest 1995; 108:1648-1654
32. Temmesfeld-Wollbrück B, Szalay A, Mayer K, et al. Abnormalities of gastric mucosal oxygenation in septic shock: Partial responsiveness to dopexamine. Am J Respir Crit Care Med 1998; 157:1586-1592
33. Kiefer P, Tugtekin I, Wiedeck H, et al. Effect of a dopexamine-induced increase in cardiac index on splanchnic hemodynamics in septic shock. Am J Respir Crit Care Med 2000; 161:775-779
34. Uusaro A, Ruokonen E, Takala J. Gastric mucosal pH does not reflect changes in splanchnic blood flow after cardiac surgery. Br J Anaesth 1995; 74:149-154
35. Meier-Hellmann A, Bredle DL, Specht M, et al. Dopexamine increases splanchnic blood flow but decreases gastric mucosal pH in severe septic patients treated with dobutamine. Crit.Care Med 1999; 27:2166-2171
36. Lang CH, Bagby GJ, Ferguson JL, et al. Cardiac output and redistribution of organ blood flow in hypermetabolic sepsis. Am J Physiol 1984; 246:R331-7

37. Imamura M, Clowes GH, Jr. Hepatic blood flow and oxygen consumption in starvation, sepsis and septic shock. Surg Gynecol Obstet 1975; 141:27-34
38. Gattinoni L, Brazzi L, Pelosi P, et al. A trial of goal-oriented hemodynamic therapy in critically ill patients. SvO2 Collaborative Group. N Engl J Med 1995; 333:1025-1032
39. Heyland DK, Cook DJ, King D, et al. Maximizing oxygen delivery in critically ill patients: a methodologic appraisal of the evidence. Crit Care Med 1996; 24:517-524
40. Sibbald WJ, Vincent JL. Round table conference on clinical trials for the treatment of sepsis. Crit Care Med 1995; 23:394-399

26

MANAGEMENT OF RESPIRATORY DYSFUNCTION IN PATIENTS WITH SEVERE SEPSIS

Greg S. Martin
Gordon R. Bernard

The development of respiratory dysfunction in patients with sepsis presents a myriad of complex interactions, which are yet to be completely understood. Similar to sepsis itself, the respiratory dysfunction that accompanies sepsis lies on a continuum from subclinical disease to overwhelming organ dysfunction. The most dreaded respiratory complication of sepsis is the acute respiratory distress syndrome (ARDS) - a severe form of acute lung injury (ALI) - at the end of the spectrum of respiratory dysfunction.

This article will address the respiratory system complications encountered in patients with sepsis, with a focus on clinically relevant diagnostic methods and management options for the practicing critical care physician.

BACKGROUND

Sepsis encompasses a range of inflammatory responses involving all organs of the body. As the criteria defining the sepsis syndrome have become more established, the determination of specific epidemiologic associations has become more feasible. The sepsis syndrome remains one of the most commonly recognized predisposing conditions for ALI, accounting for approximately 40% of cases [1,2]. In patients with sepsis preceding the diagnosis of ALI/ARDS, intra-abdominal infections are the most commonly associated sites, while patients suffering sepsis after ALI/ARDS are more likely to encounter a pulmonary source of infection [3]. The development of

ALI or ARDS in patients with sepsis is reported to occur in 25 to 42% of patients, increasing with persistent arterial hypotension [4].

Since its description in 1967, the defining criteria of ARDS have varied. Most physicians include the presence of bilateral pulmonary infiltrates on frontal chest radiograph, impaired gas exchange, and the absence of cardiac dysfunction. Many investigators believe reduced respiratory system compliance, increased extravascular lung water, or other biochemical markers of inflammation should be included [5]. The American-European Consensus Conference on ARDS created a uniform definition for ALI and ARDS in 1994, outlined in Table 1. These criteria have allowed for more precise epidemiologic estimates to be made, though the incidence has been reported to vary from 5 to 71 per 100,000 people in the United States [6, 7]. Imprecision in these statistics makes quantification of the financial burden of this disorder difficult, though rational yearly estimates approach $5 billion in the United States alone. Broad, cooperative studies to obtain more precise estimates are underway.

	ALI	ARDS
Timing	Acute	Acute
Oxygenation defect	$PaO_2/FiO_2 \leq 300$	$PaO_2/FiO_2 \leq 200$
Radiographic appearance	Bilateral infiltrates	Bilateral infiltrates
Hydrostatic pressure	$PAOP \leq 18$	$PAOP \leq 18$

PaO_2/FiO_2 = ratio of arterial to inspired oxygen, in mm Hg.
PAOP = pulmonary artery occlusion pressure, in mm Hg.

Table 1. Current definition for acute lung injury (ALI) and the acute respiratory distress syndrome (ARDS), adapted from the American-European consensus conference workshop.

The morbidity and mortality associated with ALI and ARDS is declining slowly, particularly in young patients with lung injury related to sepsis, though it remains near 40% [8]. Mortality is most often due to unresolved sepsis or multi-system organ failure (MOF) as opposed to progressive respiratory failure [3]. Several factors have been consistently found to affect mortality in patients with ALI/ARDS, including age, severity of illness, etiology of lung injury, presence of MOF, and pre-existing comorbid conditions [9]. Recently, investigators have shown chronic alcohol abuse to be associated with an increased incidence of ARDS in critically ill patients and to correlate with a higher mortality rate [10].

The degree of initial hypoxemia is not a reliable prognostic indicator, though changes in oxygenation over the first 48 hours appear to discriminate eventual outcomes. In 1988, the publication of the lung injury score [11] (LIS, Table 2) provided a method of grading the severity of lung injury – a system that has been validated prospectively for prognostic purposes. An initial LIS of > 3.5 correlates with a survival rate of 18%, while a score of 2.5-3.5 corresponds to a survival rate of 30%, a score of 1.1-2.4 with a 59% survival, and a score < 1.1 with a 66% rate of survival [12].

Points → Component ↓	0	1	2	3	4
Chest radiograph (No. of quadrants)	0	1	2	3	4
PaO_2/FiO_2 ratio (mm Hg)	> 300	225-299	172-224	100-174	< 100
PEEP (cm H_2O)	≤ 5	6 – 8	9 – 11	12 – 14	≥ 15
Static compliance (C_{STAT}=ml/cm H_2O)	≥ 80	60 – 79	40 – 59	20 – 39	≤ 19

Total Points	
Lung Injury Score	

Table 2. Calculation of the Lung Injury Score (LIS) is accomplished by dividing the total number of accumulated points by the number of components used.

PATHOPHYSIOLOGY

Biochemical and Cellular Mediators

The hallmark of ALI/ARDS is alveolar epithelial inflammation, airspace flooding with plasma proteins and cellular debris, surfactant depletion and inactivation, and a loss of normal endothelial reactivity [13]. This article is not intended to serve as a reference for the biochemical and cellular mediators of sepsis-induced respiratory dysfunction, though their interplay is indisputably critical to the pathophysiology common to the syndrome. The pathogenesis of ALI/ARDS is complex, with a consistently observed broad activation of the host inflammatory response. A well described pathophysiologic model of ALI/ARDS is one of acute lung inflammation mediated by neutrophils, cytokines, and oxidant stress [14]. Bronchoalveolar lavage (BAL) fluid from patients with ALI contains increased quantities of neutrophils and their enzymes, both of which correlate with the severity of lung injury [15]. While it is clear that neutrophils exert a critical role in the evolution of the host inflammatory response, neutropenic patients can develop ALI, thus supporting a pivotal role for other effector cells such as alveolar macrophages [16]. Both of these cell types produce inflammatory mediators, catalyze the generation of reactive oxygen species, and encourage lipid peroxidation through arachidonic acid metabolism pathways. Evidence of lipid peroxidation and oxidant stress is uniformly present in patients with sepsis, with reported elevations of hypoxanthine and arachidonic acid metabolites (e.g., isoprostanes) [17-19]. Plasma thiol levels have been found to directly correlate with survival in patients with ARDS, while lipid peroxidation products correlate with severity of disease and survival. Persistent elevations of the pro-inflammatory cytokines such as tumor necrosis factor (TNF)-α, interleukin (IL)-1, IL-6, and IL-8 correlate with reduced survival, while anti-inflammatory cytokines such as IL-10 correlate directly with survival [20-22].

Gas Exchange

The principal cause of hypoxemia associated with sepsis is extensive right-to-left intrapulmonary shunting of blood flow, thus accounting for the relative refractory nature of hypoxemia in ALI/ARDS. Intrapulmonary shunting is normally limited to less than five percent of the total cardiac output, whereas in ARDS it may consume more than 25% of the total cardiac output. In ARDS, shunting is due to persistent perfusion of atelectatic and fluid-filled alveoli. Ordinarily, compensation occurs through hypoxic pulmonary vasoconstriction to limit the amount of shunt by reducing perfusion to poorly ventilated lung units. In states of lung injury, however, hypoxic pulmonary vasoconstriction may be ineffective or absent, thereby increasing the magnitude of the intrapulmonary shunt. After the initial insult to the lung, gradients appear along a gravitational axis, in which the dependent lung is extensively consolidated and the main source of venous admixture [23].

Lung Mechanics

Decrements in lung compliance (the change in lung volume for a given change in transpulmonary pressure) related to small airway and alveolar collapse are nearly universal in patients with ALI/ARDS. When delivered by mechanical ventilation with no end-expiratory pressure, the static inflation pressure for typical tidal volumes of 8 ml/kg may exceed 25 cm H_2O. This implies lung compliance approaching 20 ml/cm H_2O, or less than ¼ of normal. To reflect the actual intrinsic elastic properties of lung tissue, compliance should be calculated with the quantity of lung participating in gas exchange. In early ARDS, the volume of aeratable lung is reduced by alveolar edema and surfactant dysfunction. These changes account for the need for higher inflation pressures, exclusive of any change in the intrinsic elastic properties of lung. As such, the inflation pressure may function as an estimation of the amount of edema and atelectasis early in the course of ARDS. This is reflected in the concept of a 'small' lung early in ARDS versus a 'stiff' lung later in the course. Only if fibrosis develops later do increases in inflation pressures reflect true changes in lung compliance. In a person with normal lungs, a transpulmonary pressure of 30 cm H_2O is sufficient to achieve total lung capacity – thus the recommended pressure limit adopted by a recent mechanical ventilation consensus conference [24]. Interestingly, this level of airway pressure has also been shown to induce lung injury in some animal models [25].

Whereas the static inflation pressure is the best index of transalveolar pressure during mechanical ventilation, the mean airway pressure is the best predictor of an overall effect on oxygenation or hemodynamics. As the mean airway pressure increases, progressively greater amounts of potentially recruitable lung are recruited. Unfortunately, at the same time, venous return can be impeded and cardiac output depressed. Because volume-related alveolar overdistension is now recognized to play a major role in airway pressure-associated injury in ARDS, the term 'volutrauma' (instead of barotrauma) has been coined.

At times, peak airway pressures during mechanical ventilatory support of patients with ARDS are increased out of proportion to the increase in static inflation pressures. This finding, when present, suggests an increase in airway resistance. Airway secretions, edema, mediators that provoke bronchospasm, narrow endotracheal tubes, etc., can all increase airway resistance. Airway resistance, like compliance, should be normalized for the amount of aeratable lung volume available and, though abnormal in part due to bronchoconstriction, the extent to which airway resistance is increased in ARDS is not completely known [26].

Work of Breathing

Because these changes in mechanical properties increase the airway pressure necessary to achieve a given tidal volume, the work of breathing (measured as the pressure-volume product during spontaneous breaths) is also increased in ARDS – an effect that is multiplied by coincident tachypnea. One cause of increased dead-space ventilation is hyperventilation of still normal or relatively normal alveolar units, a process exaggerated by differences in the distribution of ventilation with mechanical ventilatory support and by overinflation of normal lung units when mean airway pressure is increased by PEEP or other maneuvers. Normally, the dead space-to-tidal volume ratio (VD/VT) is 0.3, but in severe ARDS as much as 90% (VD/VT=0.9) of each tidal volume may fail to participate in effective gas exchange. As a consequence, minute ventilation greater than five times normal may be necessary to maintain normal arterial CO_2 concentrations.

Extravascular Lung Water

The equation described by Starling in 1896 characterizes fluid flux across a semi-permeable membrane and has been applied both experimentally and clinically to predict pulmonary edema formation in humans. The primary factors in this equation are the hydrostatic and oncotic gradients between the vasculature and interstitium coupled with the degree of capillary permeability. Simplistically, when fluid deposition exceeds the capacity of the lung to remove such fluid (i.e., lymphatic flow), extravascular water accumulates. Patients with sepsis demonstrate variable degrees of capillary permeability to solutes, thus increasing the relative effect of the hydrostatic pressure gradient to the oncotic pressure gradient as molecules responsible for maintaining oncotic pressure may be allowed to freely cross such leaky barriers. Accumulation of extravascular lung water and exudation of blood products with plasma proteins into the alveolar space creates the interstitial edema recognized as a complication of sepsis (i.e., ALI/ARDS).

Pulmonary Hemodynamics

Increased pulmonary artery pressure is common in patients with ARDS, but pulmonary vascular resistance is usually only mildly to moderately elevated as a consequence of increased cardiac output. The prognosis of patients with significant elevations in pulmonary vascular resistance is worse, whether related to depressed cardiac function or worsening pulmonary hypertension. The etiology of pulmonary hypertension in ARDS is multifactorial [27]. Vasoconstriction caused by alveolar hypoxia or other vasoactive mediators like thromboxane and endothelin and intravascular obstruction from platelet thrombi or perivascular edema probably dominate initially. Later, sustained or worsening pulmonary hypertension probably reflects the degree to which fibrosis is responsible for obliteration of the vascular bed. Thus the poor prognosis associated with late pulmonary hypertension in ARDS may simply reflect the severity of fibrosis.

Pathology and Lung Repair

The pathologic hallmark of ALI/ARDS, diffuse alveolar damage (DAD), changes dynamically as ARDS evolves [28-29]. This occurs gradually over days to weeks, depending on the severity and resolution of the insult, and may not resolve for months or may result in chronic fibrotic changes along the alveolar interstitium. The changes that develop are conveniently divided into three phases: the early exudative phase (days 1 to 5), the fibroproliferative phase (days 6 to 10), and the fibrotic phase (after 10 days). These times are approximate, and the characteristic features in each phase often overlap. The initial pathologic abnormalities are interstitial swelling, proteinaceous alveolar edema, hemorrhage, and fibrin deposition. Basement membrane disruption and denudation, especially of alveolar epithelial cells, can be seen with electron microscopy. After 1 to 2 days, hyaline membranes (sloughed alveolar cellular debris mixed with fibrin) are commonly observed by light microscopy. Cellular infiltrates may be minimal or may be dominated by neutrophils. Fibrin thrombi can be seen in some of the alveolar capillaries and small pulmonary arteries.

Although type I alveolar epithelial cells cover 95% of the alveolar surface, they are terminally differentiated cells that cannot regenerate. Instead, several days after the onset of ARDS, type II cells (the cell responsible for surfactant production) proliferate and then differentiate into new type I cells to reline the alveolar walls.

After approximately one week, most of the alveolar edema has resolved, hyaline membranes are much less prominent, mononuclear cells have replaced the neutrophilic infiltrate, and fibroblasts are proliferating within the interstitium and depositing new collagen. Pulmonary fibrosis in ARDS is often referred to as 'interstitial' because structures between airspaces appear to be markedly widened by fibrotic material. Detailed inspection has revealed, however, that this fibrosis is often the result of either alveolar collapse or intra-alveolar fibrosis in which the proteinaceous edema and cellular debris of the exudative stage have been incorporated into the alveolar wall. Actual deposition of new collagen within the interstitial space appears to be relatively uncommon [30]. Eventually, this healing of injured tissue may result in lung fibrosis, but the extent to which scarring develops is enormously variable. When parenchymal fibrosis does develop, intimal fibrosis and medial hypertrophy of pulmonary arterioles, along with complete obliteration of portions of the vascular bed, are also common.

CLINICAL PRESENTATION

Initial Signs and Symptoms

When clinical manifestations of sepsis first appear, between 28% and 33% of patients will meet the criteria for ARDS [31]. Few data exist regarding respiratory abnormalities prior to this time, though progression through a clinical spectrum of dysfunction is likely the case. Patients may experience severe dyspnea, tachypnea, and unremitting hypoxemia prior to meeting all the criteria for ALI/ARDS. Hypoxemia results from myriad causes, including cardiocirculatory dysfunction affecting global oxygen delivery (DO_2) and shifts in the oxy-hemoglobin dissociation curve. Respiratory dysfunction contributes to hypoxemia as well, with increased work of breathing. The multi-faceted increase in work of breathing is easier to recognize than to quantify. Changes occur through increased dead space ventilation, related to ventilation-perfusion mismatching, respiratory muscle dysfunction, decreased thoracic compliance and increased airway resistance (bronchoconstriction). Both increased physiologic dead-space ventilation and intrapulmonary shunting are responsible for the tachypnea and elevated minute ventilation required to achieve effective CO_2 excretion in patients with ARDS. Patients may also experience altered mental status or extrapulmonary organ failure confounding their respiratory dysfunction.

The early physiologic changes in pulmonary and cardiocirculatory function are most often radiographically unapparent. In practice, the radiographic findings associated with sepsis vary widely [32]. During the course of sepsis, pulmonary edema may develop as a combination of increased pulmonary vascular permeability as described earlier, increased hydrostatic pressures related to resuscitation efforts, and/or lowered oncotic pressure gradients from any cause. Bilateral infiltrates may appear on the chest x-ray without overt radiographic evidence of fluid overload. When coupled with appropriate thresholds of hypoxemia, the diagnosis of ALI or ARDS is secured. The supine portable chest radiographs commonly available in the ICU are incompletely described, but appear to be poor predictors of the severity of oxygenation defect or clinical outcome. Computed tomography (CT) scans will demonstrate the gravitational nature of permeability pulmonary edema and may provide information regarding unrecognized complications [33, 34]. Though the classic pulmonary parenchymal changes associated with ALI are diffuse, bilateral, peripheral, and interstitial in nature, they may be asymmetric or even patchy and focal, making diagnostic consensus difficult [35].

Clinical Course

The natural history of ALI/ARDS tends to be dominated by the inciting event rather than the lung injury itself. In patients who resolve ARDS relatively rapidly (over a period of 10 to 14 days), minute ventilation and dead-space ventilation both decrease in tandem with improvements in oxygenation. Given the substantial delay in peak incidence of pneumothoraces, the lung appears to withstand exposure to higher pressures in the earliest phases of ARDS without radiographically evident barotrauma [36,37]. Further improvements in oxygenation depend on restoration of normal lung architecture via the fibroproliferative response. In patients with more severe ARDS, i.e., those in whom significant lung fibrosis eventually develops, increased ventilatory requirements persist as oxygenation improves. As fibrosis develops, progressive amounts of the vascular bed are obliterated, which contributes to the increase in dead-space ventilation even as alveolar edema and the intrapulmonary shunt resolve.

Prognostication

As discussed previously, respiratory dysfunction related to sepsis exists on a continuum from subclinical aberrations to overt respiratory failure. Quantifying the severity of respiratory system involvement has been of keen interest for more than a decade. To streamline the ability to conduct research in this area, a clinical definition of lung injury was proposed and adopted in 1994 (Table 1). The consensus conference definition of ARDS emphasizes the spectrum of abnormalities present from ALI to ARDS, using readily available clinical criteria to make the necessary distinction. Though the exact role of respiratory failure in multiple organ failure (MOF) is not clear, it has been demonstrated that injurious modes of mechanical ventilation can produce cytokine release with associated end-organ damage [38,39].

A number of detailed models have been created in an attempt to accurately predict the clinical outcomes in respiratory failure and/or sepsis (APACHE, MODS, SOFA, ISS). Unfortunately, the prospective ability to recognize those patients who will survive is much closer to being an art than a science. For the first two decades since ARDS was first reported, mortality remained relatively constant at 60 to 70%. More recent reports, however, suggest that mortality may have declined to near 40% [8]. The explanation for this apparent improvement in patient outcomes is not clear but could be due to differences in patient populations, changes in ventilator support strategies, greater attention to fluid management, improved hemodynamic and nutritional support, improved antibiotics for nosocomial infection, corticosteroid use later in ARDS, or the potential benefits of protocol-driven patient management systems now implemented in many intensive care units.

General scoring systems provide an estimate of the probability of mortality on admission to the ICU [40]. The lung injury score (see above) functions as a specific scoring system for ARDS, however, its predictive accuracy is debated. The number of acquired organ system failures is often the most important prognostic indicator for patients requiring intensive care, including patients with ARDS. Liver failure in association with ARDS carries a particularly poor prognosis [3]. Not surprisingly, patients in whom pulmonary fibrosis develops have a poorer outcome than do other patients.

More specific predictors of outcome for patients with ARDS have been sought from measurements of various serum and lung lavage factors. The integrity of the epithelial barrier in relation to resolution of alveolar edema also appears to be a determinant of outcome in patients with ARDS [41]. Individuals capable of concentrating the protein in their edema fluid during the first 12 hours of illness (indicating an intact epithelial barrier with the ability to actively transport fluid out of the alveoli) are more likely to recover. Concentrations of pro-inflammatory cytokines and other factors appear to correlate with outcome, including von Willebrand factor antigen, neutrophil activating factor type 1, and procollagen peptide. Increases in unsaturated serum acyl chain ratios appear to discriminate severity of illness, and may serve as a marker of those most at risk of developing ALI/ARDS [42]. Similarly, the change in the PaO_2/FiO_2 ratio following initial treatment of ARDS can discriminate between survivors and nonsurvivors [43]. At the present time, none of these markers has been validated as an accurate method for predicting outcome in individual patients with ARDS.

The long-term functional outlook for survivors of ARDS is generally good [44]. Long-term abnormalities in pulmonary function are more common if lung function is impaired for more than a few days after the onset of ARDS. Most of the improvement in pulmonary function and perceived health will occur in the first 3 months following an episode of ARDS. Recently, more complete data concerning long-term outcomes in patients suffering severe respiratory complications suggest a reduction in the quality of life relative to their premorbid level of function, often attributed to objective or subjective declines in pulmonary function [45].

MANAGEMENT OPTIONS

No therapeutic intervention has proven effective in reducing the incidence or mortality of respiratory failure in sepsis. Prevention of complications is of utmost importance while general supportive measures (e.g., antimicrobial therapy, nutrition, etc.) are undertaken. Control of the upper airway and consideration of the need for ventilatory assistance is an important first step in the management of patients with respiratory dysfunction related to sepsis. If patients cannot adequately protect their airway, placement of an endotracheal tube is indicated. It is important to recognize that placement of an endotracheal tube is not a therapeutic maneuver. This step carries the attendant risks of anesthesia for the procedure and subsequent morbid events such as ventilator-associated pneumonia (VAP), and thus by itself does not improve outcome in this clinical circumstance. In addition, mechanical ventilation (independent of airway protection, etc.) has not been shown to improve outcome in patients with sepsis and respiratory failure, though this has not been studied in depth. In comparison with historical controls (i.e., the polio epidemic), mechanical ventilation does indeed provide significant tangible clinical benefits [46].

Based on increased rates of sinusitis, orotracheal intubation is preferred to the nasotracheal route [47,48]. Mounting evidence implicates nosocomial sinusitis in the development of VAP [49], an entity with a significant independent contribution to mortality [50,51]. Commonly accepted indications for institution of mechanical ventilation from other causes of respiratory failure apply equally to this patient population, including refractory hypoxemia (PaO_2 < 60 mm Hg despite high flow supplemental oxygen), respiratory rate > 35 breaths/minute, vital capacity < 15 ml/kg, and altered mental status, among others. Limited and conflicting data exist such that non-invasive positive-pressure ventilation (NIPPV) has not been proven effective in this clinical circumstance [52,55]. In addition, it is critically important to not impede the timing of other appropriate respiratory interventions, such as institution of mechanical ventilation, regardless of the availability and/or seeming adequacy of NIPPV.

No specific mode of ventilation is superior to others in terms of outcomes in patients with sepsis-related respiratory failure, though complete ventilatory support is appropriate immediately after institution of mechanical ventilation. For this reason, volume-cycled ventilation using the 'assist-control' mode (controlled mandatory ventilation) is an appropriate mode to choose at the outset. Similar degrees of respiratory support can probably be achieved with intermittent mandatory ventilation (IMV) or pressure-regulated volume-controlled ventilation (PRVC).

Tidal volume should be chosen based on *ideal* body weight, and should be targeted to prevent end-inspiratory plateau pressures from exceeding 30 cm H_2O whenever possible. Trials designed to alter inspiratory pressure through variations in tidal volume have been conducted with varying results [56-59]. It is not completely understood why these results conflict, though the intergroup differential in airway pressure is a likely contributor. In a recent trial in the United States, absolute all-cause mortality was reduced by 10% in ALI patients receiving mechanical ventilation with tidal volumes of 6 ml/kg of ideal body weight [60]. Permissive hypercapnia, the method of allowing PCO_2 to rise while reducing tidal volume and minute ventilation to prevent alveolar overdistension or propagation of lung injury, has been shown to be safe and effective at reducing mortality without adverse consequences in small non-randomized series [61-63]. Gradual increases in PCO_2 are generally well-tolerated, particularly if significant acidosis does not occur, though the reduction in mean airway pressure may adversely affect indices of oxygenation [63]. In cases of severe acidosis, intravenous bicarbonate or extracorporeal CO_2 removal ($ECCO_2R$) may be employed.

Supplemental oxygen should be employed to maintain an oximetric saturation of 90% (PaO_2 approximating 60 mm Hg) with non-toxic concentrations of oxygen ($FiO_2 < 0.60$) [64]. To ameliorate the changes in closing volume and lung derecruitment, application of positive end-expiratory pressure (PEEP) is appropriate and may provide dramatic improvements in PaO_2. Though it may be beneficial to apply PEEP at levels above the lower inflection point of the respiratory system pressure-volume curves, this is impractical in current clinical practice because of the inability to make these measures at the bedside [65]. Until additional data and sophisticated measuring devices become available, PEEP should be applied progressively between 5 and 20 cm H_2O, increasing with higher oxygen requirements.

Prone positioning has been shown to safely improve oxygenation in approximately 65% of patients with ALI/ARDS in a number of small randomized controlled trials [66, 67]. Unfortunately, no data exist to predict which patients will respond in this manner. Those who do respond (defined as an improvement in $PaO_2 > 10\%$ from baseline) often maintain higher oxygenation levels for up to 18 hours after resuming supine positioning, and are more likely to respond to subsequent attempts at prone positioning. [68]

No trials have been conducted to specifically define the most effective method of liberating septic patients from mechanical ventilation, though clinical trials have included this patient population in adequate numbers to make their findings applicable [69-71]. In patients with significant hemodynamic instability or altered mental status, attempts at discontinuing mechanical ventilation are not recommended. Thus, a two-step method of identifying patients ready to discontinue mechanical ventilation is required. A daily screening test (consisting of a brief evaluation of the resolution of the primary indication for mechanical ventilation and adequacy of oxygenation and ventilation) is the most efficient way to identify those patients potentially capable of breathing spontaneously [72]. The following criteria may be employed to identify patients ready to accept a trial of spontaneous breathing:

FiO$_2$ < 0.50, PEEP ≤ 5 cm H$_2$O, intact airway reflexes (i.e., cough and gag), hemodynamic stability and adequate mental status. Patients with adequate respiratory recovery according to the screening information should progress to a spontaneous breathing trial (through a T-piece connection or with minimal ventilatory support such as flow-by with PEEP of 5 cm H$_2$O) to assess their true ability to be liberated from mechanical ventilation [73-75]. In trials lasting 30 minutes, 50% of patients will fail extubation, while trials lasting 60-120 minutes will accurately identify 85% of patients capable of breathing spontaneously [75]. In some circumstances, pressure support may help 'bridge' patients in the weaning process, by slow reductions in the applied level of support to determine the ability of the patient to effectively breath spontaneously before a trial with minimal support as described above.

EXPERIMENTAL OPTIONS

It is well-known that numerous agents have challenged the unyielding morbidity and mortality of ALI/ARDS associated with sepsis in clinical trials, only to be added to the growing list of failed therapies. Use of systemic corticosteroids has been thoroughly tested for both prevention of lung injury as well as treatment of early phase ALI/ARDS and found not to be efficacious in either setting with possible increased mortality in patients with established ALI/ARDS [76-78]. Uncontrolled or small randomized trials have suggested benefit with intravenous corticosteroid therapy in patients with prolonged (fibroproliferative phase) ALI/ARDS [79], with a large scale trial underway to definitively answer this important question [80]. Ketoconazole, having demonstrated potential benefit in the prevention of sepsis-induced lung injury [81], was intensely evaluated in a multi-center trial supported by the National Institute of Health (NIH)-sponsored ARDS network in the United States and found to lack efficacy in treating established ARDS [82]. Intravenous prostaglandin E$_1$ [83-84] and aerosolized prostaglandin I$_2$ (prostacyclin) [85,86] have been shown to improve pulmonary physiology without improving outcome. Also completely tested has been intravenous lisofylline and strategies to achieve supranormal DO$_2$ [87, 88]. Immunomodulation continues to be a difficult but promising area of intervention, with incompletely tested strategies including N-acetylcysteine (NAC) [89], blocking of TNF-α, IL-10 therapy [90] and platelet activating factor (PAF) antagonists [91,92]. A number of experimental therapies exist on the horizon for patients with sepsis-induced lung injury, including gene therapy [93,94].

Strong data exist to confirm the physiologic benefits of inhaled nitric oxide (NO, either alone, or in combination with the selective pulmonary vasoconstrictor almitrine), which has been shown to improve oxygenation without any reduction in duration of mechanical ventilation or mortality [95-98]. Inhaled NO improves oxygenation and may reduce edema formation in patients with ALI/ARDS through effects on hydrostatic pressure. Unfortunately, it has not been found to significantly affect mortality.

Extracorporeal membrane oxygenation (ECMO) [99] or $ECCO_2R$ [100-102] have been shown to result in significant physiologic improvements in severely ill patients with ARDS, without clear beneficial effects on the development of organ failure or survival. Liquid ventilation has been shown to reduce inflammation and improve physiology, with phase III trials underway to evaluate its efficacy in humans with ALI/ARDS [103-105]. Similarly, phase III trials are underway to evaluate the promising results of surfactant replacement therapy [106].

OTHER RELEVANT RESPIRATORY ISSUES

Despite the enormous potential of future therapies, we should not ignore simple and readily available *potentially* beneficial therapies. This includes the use of inhaled beta-agonists, which have been shown to reduce inspiratory pressure and increase lung compliance by reducing airway resistance without significant benefits on dead-space ventilation, oxygenation, or overall outcome [107]. The recognition that mechanical ventilation may initiate or propagate lung injury has been recently reviewed by an international expert consensus conference [108], recognizing that injurious ventilation may contribute to mortality by inducing MOF.

The greatest morbidity associated with endotracheal tube placement relates to the risk of VAP, which is increased in patients with burns, trauma, central nervous system disease, respiratory disease, cardiac disease, and witnessed aspiration [109]. Potentially, VAP may be decreased by use of orotracheal intubation, subglottic secretion removal, kinetic hospital beds, and increased by heated respiratory circuit humidifiers and histamine-2 receptor antagonists [110,111]. Simple measures such as elevating the head of the bed at least 30 degrees at all times has been shown to reduce the incidence of gastric material migrating to the trachea [112].

Given our knowledge of fluid flux in states of altered capillary permeability (i.e., complete equalization of oncotic forces with attendant magnification of effective hydrostatic forces predicted by Starling's equation), it seems prudent to advocate judicious fluid resuscitation and/or fluid restriction when possible in this condition [113]. Recently, investigators have noted heightened mortality in ICU patients with poor fluid handling capabilities (i.e., fluid overload or reduced oncotic pressure) [114,115].

Furthermore, improvements in physiology and outcome occur in patients who lose weight or whose microvascular pressures fall as a result of diuresis or fluid restriction [116]. These improvements can be produced by strategies employing fluid restriction without any higher incidence of complications such as renal failure or hemodynamic compromise [117]. The intravenous solution of choice (i.e., crystalloid versus colloid) is still unclear despite years of detailed investigation. In hypo-oncotic patients with established lung injury, treatment with the combination of albumin and furosemide appears to improve physiology and may reduce the duration of mechanical ventilation, though evidence of improved outcomes requires further investigation [118].

Hospital beds capable of patient rotation and/or diffuse distribution of pressure points may prevent decubitus ulceration in patients requiring prolonged intensive care [119]. Finally, specific enteral nutritional formulae with antioxidants and amino acid compositions designed to reduce inflammatory mediators have recently been suggested to improve gas exchange and reduce the duration of mechanical ventilation and intensive care stay in patients with ARDS, though these benefits require confirmation [120].

POST-EXTUBATION PERIOD

After removal of the endotracheal tube, patients should be monitored closely for signs of respiratory compromise for a period of 6-24 hours depending on the etiology and severity of respiratory failure. Endotracheal intubation may cause upper airway injuries that result in immediate or delayed airway compromise. Insertion of an endotracheal tube with an internal stylet may tear the pyriform recesses beside the larynx and result in bleeding and hematoma formation [121]. Use of a tube that is too large can result in vocal cord injury, edema, and hematoma and overinflation or malpositioning of the endotracheal tube cuff can cause peri-glottic injury and stenosis. Prolonged intubation, coughing, or repeated endotracheal tube placements can cause the formation of obstructive arytenoid granulation tissue [122]. Stridor, related to upper airway injury or inflammation, may occur in 25-75% of pediatric extubations, but is rare in adults, comprising a small fraction of endotracheally intubated patients [123]. Although in some circumstances this may be managed expectantly, a low level of tolerance should exist before replacement of an adequate airway to prevent respiratory compromise. Flexible fiber-optic examination of the larynx before extubation is often prudent in such patients.

Typically, within a few hours, patients will tolerate reintroduction of oral nutrition, though this should progress through stages demonstrating adequate swallowing and airway protective reflexes. For patients with significant respiratory secretions, assistance with 'pulmonary toilet' may be required either through airway suctioning (naso-tracheal or oro-tracheal) or chest percussion with postural drainage. A subset of patients requiring prolonged mechanical ventilation will demonstrate significant respiratory muscle weakness, in which case assisted coughing and/or hyperinflation therapy (e.g., intermittent positive pressure breathing [IPPB]) may be of benefit.

CONCLUSION

Respiratory dysfunction related to sepsis is not uncommon and is associated with significant independent mortality, making heightened awareness and vigilance for such respiratory complications more critical. Until a direct and effective therapy appears on the horizon, the focus of care remains on supportive measures and prevention of complications.

Despite significant advances in both the knowledge of sepsis-related respiratory failure and the care of critically ill patients, ALI/ARDS continues to be a complex problem with high mortality. The recommendations above represent the current state of knowledge for this condition, but equally serve to highlight the vast deficiencies of knowledge that remain. To provide our patients with the best possible outcome, a continued focus on physiologic, therapeutic, and outcomes research is necessary.

REFERENCES

1. Fowler AA, Hamman RF, Good JT, et al. Adult respiratory distress syndrome: risk with common predispositions. Ann Intern Med 1983; 98:593-597
2. Pepe PE, Potkin RT, Reus DH, Hudson LD, Carrico CJ. Clinical predictors of the adult respiratory distress syndrome. Am J Surg 1982; 144:124-130
3. Montgomery AB, Stager MA, Carrico CJ, Hudson LD. Causes of mortality in patients with the adult respiratory distress syndrome. Am Rev Respir Dis 1985; 132:485-489
4. Bernard GR, Artigas A, Brigham KL, et al. The American-European consensus conference on ARDS. Definitions, mechanisms, relevant outcomes, and clinical trial coordination. Am J Respir Crit Care Med 1994; 149:818-824
5. Kollef MH, Schuster DP. The acute respiratory distress syndrome. N Engl J Med 1995; 332:27-37
6. National Heart and Lung Institute, National Institutes of Health. Respiratory Distress Syndromes: Task force on Problems, Research Approaches, Needs. US Government Printing Office, Washington, DC. 1972; DHEW Publication No. (NIH) 73-432, pp 165-180
7. Thomsen GE, Morris AH. Incidence of the adult respiratory distress syndrome in the State of Utah. Am J Respir Crit Care Med 1995; 152:965-971

8. Milberg JA, Davis DR, Steinberg KP, Hudson LD. Improved survival of patients with acute respiratory distress syndrome (ARDS): 1983-1993. JAMA 1995; 273:306-309

9. Doyle RL, Szaflarski N, Modin GW, Wiener-Kronish JP, Matthay MA. Identification of patients with acute lung injury. Predictors of mortality. Am J Respir Crit Care Med 1995; 152:1818-1824

10. Moss M, Bucher B, Morre FA, Moore EE, Parsons PE. The role of chronic alcohol abuse in the development of acute respiratory distress syndrome in adults. JAMA 1996; 275:50-54

11. Murray JF, Matthay MA, Luce JM, et al. An expanded definition of the adult respiratory distress syndrome. Am Rev Respir Dis 1988; 138:720-723

12. Vasilyev S, Schaap RN, Mortensen JD. Hospital survival rates of patients with acute respiratory failure in modern respiratory intensive care units: an international, multi-center, prospective survey. Chest 1995; 107:1083-1088

13. Artigas A, Bernard GR, Carlet J, et al. The American-European Consensus Conference on ARDS, part 2: Ventilatory, pharmacologic, supportive therapy, study design strategies, and issues related to recovery and remodeling. Am J Respir Crit Care Med 1998; 157:1332-1347

14. Demling RH. The modern version of the adult respiratory distress syndrome. Annu Rev Med 1995; 46: 193-202

15. Steinberg KP, Milberg JA, Martin TR, et al. Evolution of bronchoalveolar cell populations in the adult respiratory distress syndrome. Am Rev Respir Dis 1988; 138:720-723

16. Rinaldo JE, Christman JW. Mechanisms and mediators of the adult respiratory distress syndrome. Clin Chest Med 1990; 11:621-632

17. Quinlan GJ, Lamb NJ, Tilley R, Evans TW, Gutteridge JM. Plasma hypoxanthine levels in ARDS: implications for oxidative stress, morbidity, and mortality. Am J Respir Crit Care Med 1997; 155:479-484

18. Carpenter CT, Price PV, Christman BW. Exhaled breath condensate isoprostanes are elevated in patients with acute lung injury or ARDS. Chest 1998; 114:1653-1659

19. Christman BW, Bernard GR. Antilipid mediator and antioxidant therapy in adult respiratory distress syndrome. New Horiz 1993; 1:623-630

20. Marks JD, Marks CB, Luce JM, et al. Plasma tumor necrosis factor in patients with septic shock: Mortality rate and incidence of adult respiratory distress syndrome. Am Rev Respir Dis 1990; 141:94-97

21. Calandra T, Baumgartner JD, Grau GE, et al. Prognostic values of tumor necrosis factor/cachectin, interleukin-1, interferon alpha, and interferon gamma in the serum of patients with septic shock. J Infect Dis 1990; 161:982-987

22. Roumen RMH, Hendriks T, van der Ven-Jongekrijg J, et al. Cytokine patterns in patients after major vascular surgery, hemorrhagic shock, and severe blunt trauma: relation with subsequent adult respiratory distress syndrome and multiple organ failure. Ann Surg 1993; 218:769-776

23. Gattinoni L, Pesenti A, Bombino M, et al. Relationships between lung computed tomographic density, gas exchange, and PEEP in acute respiratory failure. Anesthesiology 1988; 69:824-832

24. Slutsky AS. Mechanical ventilation: American College of Chest Physicians' Consensus Conference. Chest 1993; 104:1833-1859

25. Tsuno K, Prato P, Kolobow T. Acute lung injury from mechanical ventilation at moderately high airway pressures. J Appl Physiol 1990; 69:956-61.

26. Wright PE, Bernard GR. The role of airflow resistance in patients with the adult respiratory distress syndrome. Am Rev Respir Dis 1989; 139:1169-74.

27. Jones R, Reid LM, Zapol WM, et al. Pulmonary vascular pathology: Human and experimental studies. In Falke KJ (ed) Lung Biology in Health and Disease. WB Saunders, Philadelphia, 1992.

28. Meyrick B. Pathology of the adult respiratory distress syndrome. Crit Care Clin 1986; 2:405-28

29. Tomashefski JF Jr. Pulmonary pathology of the adult respiratory distress syndrome. Clin Chest Med 1990; 11:593-620

30. McDonald JA. Idiopathic pulmonary fibrosis: A paradigm for lung injury and repair. Chest 1991; 99 Suppl:87-93

31. Bernard GR, Wheeler AP, Russell JA, et al. The effects of ibuprofen on the physiology and survival of patients with sepsis. The Ibuprofen in Sepsis Study Group. N Engl J Med 1997; 336:912-918

32. Wheeler AP, Carroll FE, Bernard GR. Radiographic issues in the adult respiratory distress syndrome. New Horiz 1993; 1:471-477

33. Maunder RJ, Shuman WP, McHugh JW, Marglin SI, Butler J. Preservation of normal lung regions in the adult respiratory distress syndrome. JAMA 1986; 255:2463-2465

34. Mirvis SE, Tobin KD, Kostrubiak I, Belzberg H. Thoracic CT in detecting occult disease in critically ill patients. Am J Roentgenol 1987; 148:685-9

35. Rubenfeld GD, Caldwell E, Granton J, Hudson LD, Matthay MA. Interobserver variability in applying a radiographic definition for ARDS. Chest 1999; 116:1347-53

36. Gammon RB, Shin MS, Buchalter SE. Pulmonary barotrauma in mechanical ventilation: patterns and risk factors. Chest 1992; 102:568-72

37. Gammon RB, Shin MS, Groves RH, Hardin M, Hsu C, Buchalter SE. Clinical risk factors for pulmonary barotrauma: a multivariate analysis. Am J Respir Crit Care Med 1995; 152:1235-40

38. Ranieri VM, Suter PM, Tortorella C, et al. Effect of mechanical ventilation on inflammatory mediators in patients with acute respiratory distress syndrome: a randomized controlled trial. JAMA 1999; 282:54-61

39. Ranieri VM, Giunta F, Suter PM, Slutsky AS. Mechanical ventilation as a mediator of multisystem organ failure in acute respiratory distress syndrome. JAMA 2000; 284:43-4

40. Schuster DP. Predicting outcome after ICU admission. The art and science of assessing risk. Chest 1992; 102:1861-1870

41. Matthay MA, Wiener-Kronish JP. Intact epithelial barrier function is critical for the resolution of alveolar edema in humans. Am Rev Respir Dis 1990; 142:1250-7

42. Bursten SL, Federighi DA, Parsons P, et al. An increase in serum C18 unsaturated free fatty acids as a predictor of the development of acute respiratory distress syndrome. Crit Care Med 1996; 24:1129-36

43. Sloane PJ, Gee MH, Gottlieb JE, et al. A multicenter registry of patients with acute respiratory distress syndrome: physiology and outcome. Am Rev Respir Dis 1992; 146:419-26

44. McHugh LG, Milberg JA, Whitcomb ME, et al. Recovery of function in survivors of the acute respiratory distress syndrome. Am J Respir Crit Care Med 1994; 150:90-4

45. Davidson TA, Caldwell ES, Curtis JR, Hudson LD, Steinberg KP. Reduced quality of life in survivors of acute respiratory distress syndrome compared with critically ill control patients. JAMA 1999; 281:354-60

46. Petty TL. A historical perspective of mechanical ventilation. In: Tobin MJ (ed) Critical Care Clinics: Mechanical Ventilation. W.B. Saunders Company, Philadelphia, 1990, 489-504

47. Salord F, Gaussorgues P, Marti-Flich J, et al. Nosocomial maxillary sinusitis during mechanical ventilation: a prospective comparison of orotracheal versus the nasotracheal route for intubation. Intensive Care Med 1990; 16:390-3

48. Holzapfel L, Chevret S, Madinier G, et al. Influence of long-term oro- or nasotracheal intubation on nosocomial maxillary sinusitis and pneumonia: results of a prospective, randomized, clinical trial. Crit Care Med 1993; 21:1132-8

49. Holzapfel L, Chastang C, Demingeon G, Bohe J, Piralla B, Coupry A. A randomized study assessing the systematic search for maxillary sinusitis in nasotracheally mechanically ventilated patients. Influence of nosocomial maxillary sinusitis on the occurrence of ventilator-associated pneumonia. Am J Respir Crit Care Med 1999; 159:695-701

50. Cook D, De Jonghe B, Brochard L, Brun-Buisson C. Influence of airway management on ventilator-associated pneumonia: evidence from randomized trials. JAMA 1998; 279:781-7

51. Heyland DK, Cook DJ, Griffith L, Keenan SP, Brun-Buisson C. The attributable morbidity and mortality of ventilator-associated pneumonia in the critically ill patient. The Canadian Critical Trials Group. Am J Respir Crit Care Med 1999; 159:1249-56

52. Alsous F, Amoateng-Adjepong Y, Manthous CA. Noninvasive ventilation: experience at a community teaching hospital. Intensive Care Med 1999; 25:458-63

53. Antonelli M, Conti G, Rocco M, et al. A comparison of noninvasive positive-pressure ventilation and conventional mechanical ventilation in patients with acute respiratory failure. N Engl J Med 1998; 339:429-35

54. Meduri GU, Turner RE, Abou-Shala N, Wunderink R, Tolley E. Noninvasive Positive Pressure Ventilation Via Face Mask: First-Line Intervention in Patients With Acute Hypercapnic and Hypoxemic Respiratory Failure. Chest 1996; 109:179-93

55. Patrick W, Webster K, Ludwig L, Roberts D, Wiebe P, Younes M. Noninvasive positive-pressure ventilation in acute respiratory distress without prior chronic respiratory failure. Am J Respir Crit Care Med 1996; 153:1005-11

56. Amato MBP, Barbas CS, Medeiros DM, et al. Effect of a protective-ventilation strategy on mortality in the acute respiratory distress syndrome. N Engl J Med 1998; 338:347-54

57. Stewart TE, Meade MO, Cook DJ, et al. Evaluation of a ventilation strategy to prevent barotrauma in patients at high risk for acute respiratory distress syndrome. Pressure- and Volume-Limited Ventilation Strategy Group. N Engl J Med 1998; 338:355-61

58. Brochard L, Roudot-Thoraval F, Roupie E, et al. Tidal volume reduction for prevention of ventilator-induced lung injury in acute respiratory distress syndrome. The Multicenter Trail Group on Tidal Volume reduction in ARDS. Am J Respir Crit Care Med 1998; 158:1831-8

59. Brower RG, Shanholtz CB, Fessler HE, et al. Prospective, randomized, controlled clinical trial comparing traditional versus reduced tidal volume ventilation in acute respiratory distress syndrome patients. Crit Care Med 1999; 27 8:1661-3

60. The ARDS Network Investigators. Ventilation with lower tidal volumes as compared with traditional tidal volumes for acute lung injury and the acute respiratory distress syndrome. The Acute Respiratory Distress Syndrome Network. N Engl J Med 2000; 342:1301-8

61. Hickling KG, Walsh J, Henderson S, Jackson R. Low mortality rate in adult respiratory distress syndrome using low-volume, pressure-limited ventilation with permissive hypercapnia: a prospective study. Crit Care Med 1994; 22:1568-78

62. Bidani A, Tzouanakis AE, Cardenas VJ, Zwischenberger JB. Permissive hypercapnia in acute respiratory failure. JAMA 1994; 272:957-62

63. Thorens JB, Jolliet P, Ritz M, Chevrolet JC. Effects of rapid permissive hypercapnia on hemodynamics, gas exchange, and oxygen transport and consumption during mechanical ventilation for the acute respiratory distress syndrome. Intensive Care Med 1996; 22:182-91

64. Jenkinson SG. Oxygen toxicity. New Horiz 1993; 1:504-511

65. Amato MB, Barbas CS, Medeiros DM, et al. Beneficial effects of the "open lung approach" with low distending pressures in acute respiratory distress syndrome. A prospective randomized study on mechanical ventilation. Am J Respir Crit Care Med 1995; 152:1835-46

66. Stocker R, Neff T, Stein S, Ecknauer E, Trentz O, Russi E. Prone positioning and low-volume pressure-limited ventilation improve survival in patients with severe ARDS. Chest 1997; 111:1008-17

67. Lamm WJ, Graham MM, Albert RK. Mechanism by which prone position improves oxygenation in acute lung injury. Am J Respir Crit Care Med 1994; 150:184-93

68. Jolliet P, Bulpa P, Chevrolet JC. Effects of the prone position on gas exchange and hemodynamics in severe acute respiratory distress syndrome. Crit Care Med 1998; 26:1977-85

69. Esteban A, Frutos F, Tobin MJ, et al. A comparison of four methods of weaning patients from mechanical ventilation. N Engl J Med 1995; 332:345-50

70. Brochard L, Rauss A, Benito S, et al. Comparison of three methods of gradual withdrawal from ventilatory support during weaning from mechanical ventilation. Am J Respir Crit Care Med 1994; 150:896-903

71. Yang KL, Tobin MJ. A prospective study of indexes predicting the outcome of trials of weaning from mechanical ventilation. N Engl J Med 1991; 324:1445-50

72. Ely EW, Baker AM, Dunagan DP, et al. Effect on the duration of mechanical ventilation of identifying patients capable of breathing spontaneously. N Engl J Med 1996; 335:1864-9

73. Kollef MH, Shapiro SD, Silver P, et al. A randomized, controlled trial of protocol-directed versus physician-directed weaning from mechanical ventilation. Crit Care Med 1997; 25:567-74

74. Esteban A, Alia I, Gordo F, et al. Extubation outcome after spontaneous breathing trials with T-tube or pressure support ventilation. The Spanish Lung Failure Collaborative Group. Am J Respir Crit Care Med 1997; 156:459-65

75. Esteban A, Alia I, Tobin MJ, et al. Effect of spontaneous breathing trial duration on outcome of attempts to discontinue mechanical ventilation. Spanish Lung Failure Collaborative Group. Am J Respir Crit Care Med 1999; 159:512-8

76. Bone RC, Fisher CJ Jr, Clemmer TP, Slotman GJ, Metz CA, Balk RA. A controlled clinical trial of high-dose methylprednisolone in the treatment of severe sepsis and septic shock. N Engl J Med 1987; 317:653-8

77. Bone RC, Fisher CJ Jr, Clemmer TP, Slotman GJ, Metz CA. Early methylprednisolone treatment for septic syndrome and the adult respiratory distress syndrome. Chest 1987 92:1032-6

78. Luce JM, Montgomery AB, Marks JD, Turner J, Metz CA, Murray JF. Ineffectiveness of high-dose methylprednisolone in preventing parenchymal lung injury and improving mortality in patients with septic shock. Am Rev Respir Dis 1988; 138:62-8

79. Meduri GU, Headley AS, Golden E, et al. Effect of prolonged methylprednisolone therapy in unresolving acute respiratory distress syndrome: a randomized controlled trial. JAMA 1998; 280:159-65

80. LateSteroids Rescue Study (LaSRS). *http://hedwig.mgh.harvard.edu/ardsnet/ards02.html.*

81. Yu M, Tomasa G. A double-blind, prospective, randomized trial of ketoconazole, a thromboxane synthetase inhibitor, in the prophylaxis of the adult respiratory distress syndrome. Crit Care Med 1993; 21:1635-42

82. The ARDS Network. Ketoconazole for early treatment of acute lung injury and acute respiratory distress syndrome: a randomized controlled trial. JAMA 2000; 283:1995-2002

83. Abraham E, Park YC, Covington P, et al. Liposomal prostaglandin E1 in acute respiratory distress syndrome: a placebo-controlled, randomized, double-blind, multicenter clinical trial. Crit Care Med 1996; 24:10-5

84. Meyer J, Theilmeier G, Van Aken H, et al. Inhaled prostaglandin E1 for treatment of acute lung injury in severe multiple organ failure. Anesth Analg 1998; 86,4:753-8.

85. Walmrath D, Schneider T, Pilch J, et al. Aerosolized prostacyclin in adult respiratory distress syndrome. Lancet 1993; 342:961-2

86. Zwissler B, Kemming G, Habler O, et al. Inhaled prostacyclin (PGI2) versus inhaled nitric oxide in adult respiratory distress syndrome. Am J Respir Crit Care Med 1996; 154:1671-7

87. Hayes MA, Timmins AC, Yau EHS, et al. Elevation of systemic oxygen delivery in the treatment of critically ill patients. N Engl J Med 1994; 330:1717-22

88. Gattinoni L, Brazzi L, Pelosi P, et al. A trial of goal-oriented hemodynamic therapy in critically ill patients. N Engl J Med 1995; 333:1025-32

89. Bernard GR, Wheeler AP, Arons MM, et al. A trial of antioxidants N-acetylcysteine and procysteine in ARDS. The Antioxidants in ARDS Study Group. Chest 1997; 112:164-72

90. Bernard GR, Wheeler AP, Naum CC, et al. A placebo controlled randomized trial of IL-10 in acute lung injury. Chest 1999; 116:260S (Abst)

91. Vincent JL, Spapen H, Bakker J, Webster NR, Curtis L. Phase II multicenter clinical study of the platelet-activating factor receptor antagonist BB-882 in the treatment of sepsis. Crit Care Med. 2000; 28:638-42

92. Dhainaut JF, Tenaillon A, Hemmer M, et al. Confirmatory platelet-activating factor receptor antagonist trial in patients with severe gram-negative bacterial sepsis: a phase III, randomized, double-blind, placebo-controlled, multicenter trial. BN 52021 Sepsis Investigator Group. Crit Care Med. 2000; 26:1963-71

93. Brigham KL, Stecenko AA. Gene therapy in acute critical illness. New Horiz 1995; 3:321-9

94. Bhattacharya J. Gene Therapy for Pulmonary Edema. Am J Respir Cell Mol Biol 2000; 22:640-1

95. Rossaint R, Gerlach H, Schmidt-Ruhnke H, et al. Efficacy of inhaled nitric oxide in patients with severe ARDS. Chest 1995; 107:1107-15

96. Troncy E, Collet J-P, Shapiro S, et al. Should we treat acute respiratory distress syndrome with inhaled nitric oxide? Lancet 1997; 350:111-2

97. Dellinger RP, Zimmerman JL, Taylor RW, et al. Effects of inhaled nitric oxide in patients with acute respiratory distress syndrome: results of a randomized phase II trial. Inhaled Nitric Oxide in ARDS Study Group. Crit Care Med 1998; 26:15-23

98. Gallart L, Lu Q, Puybasset L, Umamaheswara Rao GS, Coriat P, Rouby JJ. Intravenous almitrine combined with inhaled nitric oxide for acute respiratory distress syndrome. The NO Almitrine Study Group. Am J Respir Crit Care Med 1998 158:1770-7

99. Zapol WM, Snider MT, Hill JD, et al. Extracorporeal membrane oxygenation in severe acute respiratory failure. JAMA 1979; 242:2193-6

100. Morris AH, Wallace J, Menlove RL, et al. Randomized clinical trial of pressure controlled inverse ratio ventilation and extracorporeal CO_2 removal for adult respiratory distress syndrome. Am J Respir Crit Care Med 1994; 149:295-305

101. Brunet F, Belghith M, Mira JP, et al. Extracorporeal carbon dioxide removal and low-frequency positive-pressure ventilation. Improvement in arterial oxygenation with reduction of risk of pulmonary barotrauma in patients with adult respiratory distress syndrome. Chest 1993; 104:889-98

102. Gattinoni L, Pesenti A, Mascheroni D, et al. Low frequency positive pressure ventilation with extracorporeal CO_2 removal In severe acute respiratory failure. JAMA 1986; 256:881-6

103. Hirschl RB, Tooley R, Parent A, Johnson K, Bartlett RH. Evaluation of gas exchange, pulmonary compliance, and lung injury during total and partial liquid ventilation in the acute respiratory distress syndrome. Crit Care Med 1996; 24:1001-8

104. Hirschl RB, Pranikoff T, Wise C, et al. Initial experience with partial liquid ventilation in adult patients with the acute respiratory distress syndrome. JAMA 1996; 275:383-9

105. Bartlett RH, Croce M, Hirschl RH, et al. A phase II randomized, controlled trial of partial liquid ventilation (PLV) in adult patients with acute hypoxemic respiratory failure. Crit Care Med 1997; (Suppl) 25:A35

106. Anzueto A, Baughman RP, Guntupalli KK, et al. Aerosolized surfactant in adults with sepsis-induced acute respiratory distress syndrome. Exosurf Acute Respiratory Distress Syndrome Sepsis Study Group. N Engl J Med 1996; 334:1417-21

107. Wright PE, Carmichael LC, Bernard GR. Effect of bronchodilators on lung mechanics in the acute respiratory distress syndrome (ARDS). Chest 1994; 106:1517-23

108. Anonymous. International Consensus Conferences in Intensive Care Medicine: Ventilator-associated Lung Injury in ARDS. Am J Respir Crit Care Med 1999; 160:2118-24

109. Cook DJ, Walter SD, Cook RJ, et al. Incidence of and risk factors for ventilator-associated pneumonia in critically ill patients. Ann Intern Med 1998; 129:433-40

110. Cook DJ, De Jonghe B, Brochard L, Brun-Buisson C. Influence of airway management on ventilator-associated pneumonia: evidence from randomized trials. JAMA 1998; 279:781-7

111. Kollef MH. The prevention of ventilator-associated pneumonia. N Engl J Med 1999; 340:627-34

112. Torres A, Serra-Batlles J, Ros E, et al. Pulmonary aspiration of gastric contents in patients receiving mechanical ventilation: the effect of body position. Ann Intern Med 1992; 116:540-3

113. Schuster DP. The case for and against fluid restriction and occlusion pressure reduction in adult respiratory distress syndrome. New Horiz 1993; 1:478-88

114. Mangialardi RJ, Martin GS, Bernard GR, et al. Hypoproteinemia predicts acute respiratory distress syndrome development, weight gain, and death in patients with sepsis. Crit Care Med 2000; 28:3137-45

115. Simmons RS, Berdine GG, Seidenfeld JJ, et al. Fluid balance and the adult respiratory distress syndrome. Am Rev Respir Dis 1987; 135:924-9

116. Humphrey H, Hall J, Sznajder I, Silverstein M, Wood L. Improved survival in ARDS patients associated with a reduction in pulmonary capillary wedge pressure. Chest 1990; 97:1176-80

117. Mitchell JP, Schuller D, Calandrino FS, Schuster DP. Improved outcome based on fluid management in critically ill patients requiring pulmonary artery catheterization. Am Rev Respir Dis 1992; 145:990-8
118. Martin GS, Mangialardi RJ, Wheeler AP, Bernard GR. Albumin and diuretics in ARDS [abstract]. Am J Respir Crit Care Med 1999; 159:A376 (Abst)
119. Ferrell BA, Osterweil D, Christenson P. A randomized trial of low-air-loss beds for treatment of pressure ulcers. JAMA 1993; 269:494-7
120. Gadek JE, DeMichele SJ, Karlstad MD, et al. Effect of enteral feeding with eicosapentaenoic acid, gamma-linolenic acid, and antioxidants in patients with acute respiratory distress syndrome. Enteral Nutrition in ARDS Study Group. Crit Care Med 1999; 27:1409-1420
121. Laporta D, Kleiman S, Begin L, et al. Traumatic perforation of the cervical esophagus: A complication of endotracheal intubation. Intensive Care Med 1993; 19:59-60
122. Keiser GJ, Bozentka NE, Gold BD. Laryngeal granuloma: A complication of prolonged endotracheal intubation. Anesth Prog 1991; 38:232-234
123. Demling RH, Read T, Lind TJ, et al. Incidence and morbidity of extubation failure in surgical intensive care patients. Crit Care Med 1988; 16:573-77

27

THE ROLE OF NUTRITIONAL SUPPORT IN SEPSIS

Daren K. Heyland
James K. Lukan
Stephen A. McClave

The proinflammatory metabolic response to sepsis is characterized by dramatic increases in energy expenditure, accelerated catabolism, and hyperdynamic circulatory changes. If persistent, this response can lead to severe wasting of the lean body mass, impairment of visceral organ function, and decreases in the body's reparative and immune functions [1,2]. Such processes, especially if exaggerated, can lead to protein-calorie malnutrition, increased infectious morbidity, prolonged ventilatory dependence, greater length of hospital stay, and increased mortality [3-5].

Following a proinflammatory phase of sepsis (induced by release of tumor necrosis factor-alpha [TNF-α], interleukin [IL]-1β, IL-6, IL-8 and other cytokines), patients with sepsis may evolve into an anti-inflammatory phase of their illness, which is characterized by suppression of the immune system [6]. During this phase, anti-inflammatory mediators may cause anergy to skin test antigens, impaired antibody production and diminished phagocytosis rendering patients at increased risk for additional infectious morbidity and mortality [7]. Certain nutrients with immune-enhancing properties may be helpful at this phase in reducing infectious complications.

Finally, the gastrointestinal tract is recognized for its key role in the initiation or perpetuation of the inflammatory response associated with sepsis. Abnormalities in the immunologic role and barrier function of the gastrointestinal tract are associated with alterations in the inflammatory response to illness, resulting in greater infectious morbidity [8,9].

These findings have led to a shift in the paradigm of nutritional therapy from simply supporting the hypermetabolic state and meeting nutrient requirements, to an important opportunity to manipulate local and systemic immune and inflammatory responses. The implications of nutritional therapy are not just dietary support, but rather a pharmacological means by which to improve gut structure and function, enhance the immune system, and modify the inflammatory response to sepsis. In this chapter, we will review the general principles surrounding the provision of nutritional support and examine the relationship between nutritional support and infectious morbidity and mortality in the septic, critically ill patient.

PATHOPHYSIOLOGY OF SEPSIS DICTATES THE PRINCIPLES OF NUTRITIONAL SUPPORT

The pathophysiologic effects of sepsis on metabolism and fuel utilization may be difficult to distinguish from the overall changes seen in the stress response to any injury (from processes such as trauma, burns, major surgery or pancreatitis). The injury disrupts the orderly physiologic changes of starvation (which are otherwise characterized by conservation of protein, increased fat utilization, reduced energy expenditure, and increased production and use of ketone bodies for fuel of the central nervous system, white blood cells, and renal medulla). Disruption of this process by injury leads initially to a brief 'ebb' phase of injury, which is associated with the release of counter-regulatory hormones (ACTH, cortisol, catecholamines, glucagon), and is characterized by normometabolism and hemodynamic stability [10,11]. Within twelve to twenty-four hours, this process evolves into the 'flow' phase characterized by a hypermetabolic, dynamic, catabolic response [12,13]. There is rapid acceleration of gluconeogenesis, acute phase protein synthesis, fatty acid mobilization, depletion of glycogen, accelerated protein breakdown, and ureagenesis. These changes are accompanied by a moderate hyperglycemia, increased insulin resistance in the liver and periphery, increased glucose turnover, and accelerated hepatic uptake of amino acids for gluconeogenesis [14].

In sepsis, an exaggerated stress response may be due to the fact that infection by itself may contribute to further release of counter-regulatory hormones and endogenous mediators (TNF, prostaglandins, leukotrienes, cytokines), or the fact that the effects of endotoxin released by the microorganisms themselves are similar to TNF [14].

Late phase, uncontrolled sepsis leading to organ failure, circulatory compromise, and septic shock results in metabolic failure, which resembles in some respect the features of liver failure [14]. Progression of this pre-terminal pattern results in decreased hepatic glucose production, reduced uptake of amino acids, and diminished ketogenesis. Decreases in fat utilization and protein metabolic failure lead to "septic auto-cannibalism" [14]. Energy expenditure progressively decreases from simple infection to septic shock, as the delivery and uptake of oxygen by tissues diminish [15,16].

Design of the nutritional support regimen must account for these physiologic changes. For the clinician, the exaggerated response in the patient with sepsis means worsening hyperglycemia and insulin resistance and possibly even higher protein and caloric requirements, compared to the stressed patient without sepsis [14]. In general, the increased need for protein (to stimulate maximal hepatic protein synthesis) out of proportion to the increased need for provision of calories (due to poor substrate utilization), necessitates a design for the nutritional support regimen that provides a non-protein calorie:nitrogen ratio of 60-80:1.

In the critically ill septic patient, many of the tenants of traditional nutritional assessment are virtually meaningless. The reprioritization of hepatic protein synthesis, increased vascular permeability, and propensity to edema from third-spacing of fluids seen in the basic stress response to injury, may all be exacerbated by the development of sepsis [17,18]. As a result, standard clinical markers for nutritional assessment such as visceral proteins, weight as a percentage of usual or ideal body weight, and anthropometric studies are not useful in evaluating baseline nutritional status, adequacy of the nutrition support regimen, determining which patients are candidates for nutritional supplementation, or in predicting risk of further deterioration [17,18].

Careful estimates of caloric requirements by predictive equations or specific measurement by indirect calorimetry are important to avoid the consequences of inappropriate feeding [19]. Clearly, for the septic critically ill patient, overfeeding may have greater adverse effects than underfeeding, due to associated worsening of hyperglycemia, lipogenesis leading to excessive carbon dioxide production and respiratory load, steatosis and hepatic dysfunction, and greater energy expenditure causing increased physiologic stress [19-22]. Permissive underfeeding has been advocated by some investigators in this patient group specifically and has been shown to lead to improved outcomes in animal models [23]. Underfeeding is not without concern however, due to risk of further deterioration of nutritional status and immune compromise, failure to maximize hepatic protein synthesis, and the possibility of further loss of gut integrity [24]. In animal studies, only 25% of goal calories were required to maintain gut integrity and inhibit bacterial translocation in the unstressed mouse [25], whereas twice that amount was required to do the same in the stressed animal [26]. The estimate of 25 kcal/kg /day and 1.5-2.0 gms of protein/kg/day provides a reasonable prediction for most patients. Use of corrective factors with the Harris-Benedict equation routinely results in overestimation of requirements and overfeeding [27]. The value for the measured resting energy expenditure (REE) obtained from a 5 minute steady state period by indirect calorimetry is the most accurate means of defining goal and should not be adjusted for activity, degree of illness, anabolism, diet induced thermogenesis, degree of metabolism, or wound requirements (unpublished data). A mixed fuel regimen (carbohydrate:fat ratio of 50:50 to 60:40) should be used [2]. Even if overall caloric provision is appropriate, an excessive percentage of carbohydrate may worsen hyperglycemia, hepatic dysfunction, and respiratory impairment [19-21]. Excessive percentage of fat may clog the reliculoendothelial system, cause macrophage dysfunction, or lead to jaundice [19-21].

Selection of an enteral access device and level of the GI tract into which nutrients are infused is based upon the clinician's assessment of segmental contractility. By vigilantly maintaining normal electrolytes and avoiding drugs (such as opiode narcotics) that inhibit gastric emptying, approximately 85% of patients may be fed successfully by the intragastric route [28]. A pattern of ileus with diminished bowel sounds should not deter the initiation of enteral feeds. Rapid advancement is important as early attainment of goal feeding promotes delivery of a sufficient amount of nutrients to meet requirements, and may actually decrease the incidence and duration of ileus (through the release of promotility agents such as gastrin, motilin and bombesin). Patients with severely impaired gastric emptying, and patients with pancreatitis, generally require jejunal access prior to initiation of the nutritional therapy. Enteral nutrition should be withheld in patients who are at risk for intestinal ischemia due to inadequate resuscitation or hemodynamic instability requiring pressor support, and in patients with mechanical obstruction below the access site.

ENTERAL FEEDING: DOES IT MODIFY THE COURSE OF SEPSIS AND RESULT IN IMPROVED CLINICAL OUTCOMES?

Over the past few decades, the gastrointestinal tract has emerged to play a central role in the pathogenesis of acquired infection in the critically ill patient. Alterations in the normal gut flora, function and structure, due to illness or intervention, have been implicated in the pathogenesis or perpetuation of sepsis, multiple organ failure (MOF), and other complications of critical illness [29]. The gut 'motor' hypothesis suggests that loss of the protective function of the gut barrier leads to translocation of bacteria and/or endotoxin across the intestinal epithelium, which triggers or perpetuates the inflammatory response seen in sepsis and multiple organ dysfunction.

There are numerous studies in animal models of critical illness that suggest that enteral nutrition may have beneficial effects on gut structure and function. Compared to parenteral nutrition, animal studies demonstrate that enteral nutrition results in higher levels of secretory IgA in biliary tract secretions [30], greater preservation of gut-associated lymphoid tissue (GALT) [31], greater gastrointestinal mucosal weight and thickness, decreased secretion of catabolic hormones following a burn injury [32], less bacterial leak through the intestinal barrier (translocation) [33], greater preservation of upper respiratory tract immunity [34], greater wound strength after abdominal surgery [35], reductions in hypermetabolism and catabolism following injury [36], and reduced mortality following a septic [37] or hypotensive [38] insult.

While studies suggest that gut integrity in humans is much more resilient with less atrophy and deterioration in response to injury of the host compared to animal models, the issues are still relevant as suggested by improved outcomes with use of enteral nutrition compared to parenteral nutrition. Compared to parenteral nutrition, critically ill patients receiving enteral nutrition have demonstrated better wound healing [39], a decrease in gastrointestinal tract mucosal permeability [40], increased levels of visceral protein synthesis, less hepatic dysfunction, better substrate utilization and better nutritional status [41]. While the data in head-injured patients are less conclusive [42,43], trauma patients without head injury have shown consistent reductions in infectious morbidity with use of enteral nutrition compared to parenteral nutrition [44-45]. In patients with pancreatitis, enteral nutrition results in rapid recovery from the systemic inflammatory response, reduced requirements for intensive care, lower incidence of organ failure, and fewer septic complications [46,47].

The optimal timing and dose of enteral nutrition is not clear. While one study in trauma patients showed that early (within 6 hours) institution of enteral nutrition resulted in less gut permeability, less organ dysfunction and improved tolerance to enteral nutrition compared to delayed enteral nutrition (>24 hours) [48], another study of trauma patients of similar design failed to demonstrate a difference between the two groups in the metabolic response to trauma (as measured by plasma lactate, catecholamines, cortisol and urinary nitrogen) [49]. Neither of these two studies demonstrated a reduction in complications, length of stay or mortality associated with the early institution of enteral feeding. While these findings prevent making strong inferences as to the timing of enteral nutrition, current guidelines recommend that enteral nutrition should be initiated as soon as hemodynamic stability is restored.

PARENTERAL NUTRITION: DOES IT HAVE A ROLE IN THE MANAGEMENT OF CRITICALLY ILL PATIENTS WITH SEPSIS?

Despite the evidence that route of nutritional support does impact patient outcome (favoring use of enteral nutrition over parenteral nutrition), a large percentage of physicians still take advantage of the convenience of parenteral nutrition. A common misconception is that parenteral nutrition is better 'tolerated'. Delivery is independent of altered bowel function and intestinal pathology (with regard to ischemia and risk of aspiration). Access may be gained easily, independent of the operating room, and is often already in place in the septic patient prior to consideration for nutritional supplementation. Parenteral nutrition is perceived to be free of tolerance issues such as diarrhea and high residual volumes that often limit the amount of nutrients actually delivered when feeding enterally.

There are limited data to evaluate the effect of parenteral nutrition on clinically important outcomes in critically ill patients specifically with sepsis. The majority of studies evaluating parenteral nutrition are in elective surgical patients; the results of which are not necessarily generalizable to critically ill patients [50]. In a recent meta-analysis of parenteral nutrition in the critically ill patient, the effect of parenteral nutrition in the elective surgical patient was systematically different to the effect in critically ill patients. The overall estimate effect derived from those few studies of critically ill patients (6, none in patients with sepsis) was associated with an increased mortality and a trend toward increased complications [50].

Is it plausible that parenteral nutrition may do more harm than good in the critically ill patient? While supporting the metabolic demands of critically ill septic patients seems to follow logical rationale, there is little support for the notion that parenteral nutrition translates into an improvement in clinical outcomes. There are several reports that demonstrate that lipids may adversely affect immune status and clinical outcomes [51-53]. This is consistent with the findings of a recent randomized trial of parenteral nutrition with lipids compared to parenteral nutrition without lipids in critically ill trauma patients [54]. Patients who received lipids had depressed T-cell function and a higher rate of infectious complications. This resulted in a longer duration of mechanical ventilation and longer intensive care unit (ICU) and hospital stay.

Alternative explanations as to why parenteral nutrition is associated with worse outcomes in critically ill patients may relate to the lack of enteral stimulation rather than anything intrinsic in the parenteral nutrition. Work done by Kudsk and colleagues demonstrates that parenteral nutrition has adverse effects on GALT. GALT plays an important role in natural defense mechanisms influencing cytokine and IgA production and endothelial cell activation and recruitment [55]. Intravenous nutrition reduces GALT cell mass and function, which seems to reduce respiratory tract immunity and ability to overcome an infectious challenge [56]. This is supported by the clinical trials in trauma patients that demonstrate that enteral nutrition, compared to parenteral nutrition, results in fewer intraabdominal abscesses and less pneumonia in trauma patients [44,45].

Perhaps the adverse effects of parenteral nutrition in sepsis relate to resultant hyperglycemia. Abnormalities in glucose metabolism in sepsis have been well-described [57] and hyperglycemia occurs commonly during parenteral nutrition administration [58]. Hyperglycemia results in some degree of cellular immune dysfunction and increased infection in seriously ill patients [59]. Finally, increased levels of TNF-α [60] seen with the use of parenteral nutrition may have deleterious effects in patients with sepsis.

It would seem prudent, given the lack of data demonstrating benefit, that parenteral nutrition be given a very limited role in the management of critically ill patients with sepsis; it should be reserved for patients with gastrointestinal failure in whom enteral feeds are contraindicated or not tolerated.

IS THERE A ROLE FOR IMMUNE-ENHANCING DIETS?

In recent years, there has been an enormous amount of interest in the immunomodulating properties of various nutrients (branch-chained amino acid, nucleotides, arginine, glutamine, taurine, glycine, and omega-3 fatty acids). While each of these nutrients may have effects on the cellular immune function, cytokine production and gastrointestinal structure and function, there are very few randomized, controlled trials evaluating the effect of each individual supplement on clinically important infectious outcomes in critically ill humans.

However, several trials using a combination of various nutrients have been reported. These trials have recently been aggregated in three separate meta-analyses [61-63], reporting on various combinations of 22 randomized trials involving 2,419 patients, where use of immune-enhanced enteral formulas was compared to standard formulas [61-63]. Based on these three meta-analyses, use of immune-enhanced formulas (compared to standard enteral formulas) in properly selected patients might be expected to reduce the incidence of nosocomial infection by 34-53% [61-63], duration of mechanical ventilation by 2.6 days [61] and length of hospitalization by 0.6-2.9 days [61-63].

There is some evidence that some subgroups of critically ill patients may be harmed by immunonutrtion. The meta-analysis by Heys et al. [62] suggested an effect on mortality that was consistent with more harm than good (OR 1.77, 95% confidence intervals 1.00, 3.12), as did the largest meta-analysis by Heyland et al. (high quality studies in critically ill patients RR 1.46; 95% CI 1.01-2.11) [63]. In one large multi-centered, double-blinded, randomized trial included in these meta-analyses, Bower et al. compared Impact to Osmolite HN in 326 critically ill patients [64]. When only those patients who received feeds were evaluated, more patients receiving the experimental formula died (24/153, 15.7%) than in the control group given standard formula (12/143, 8.4%) (chi-square, p=0.055). In patients stratified as septic at baseline, hospital stay was reduced by 10 days. However, the mortality rate in the septic group who received the experimental feed was three times that of septic patients who received control feeds (25% vs 8.9%, p=0.051).

In an unpublished study of immunonutrition, there is another signal that immunonutrition may be associated with increased mortality in patients with pre-existing infection [65]. One hundred and seventy critically ill patients were randomized to receive either an experimental diet consisting of arginine, omega-3 fatty acids and vitamins A,E and beta carotene or an isonitrogenous control feed. There were significantly more deaths in the group that received the experimental immune-enhanced formula (20/87, 23.0%) compared to the control group (8/83, 9.6%, p= 0.03). However, most of the excess deaths occurred in patients with pneumonia at baseline. Despite similar baseline demographics, more elderly patients with pneumonia at baseline were included in the group that received the experimental immune formula than the control group that received standard formula. There were no deaths in the group of patients with pneumonia at baseline that received the control formula (0/9) compared to 10/26 (38.5%) of patients with pneumonia who received the experimental formula.

The above results contrast with the recently completed multicenter study by Galban and colleagues [66]. In this study, 181 ICU patients, with APACHE II score $\geq$ 10 with laboratory or clinical signs of infection, were randomized either to receive Impact or a standard enteral diet. Five patients were excluded from the analysis. In this unblinded study, there was no report on cointerventions (the extent to which antibiotics, ventilation, oxygen and transfusions were being equally applied across groups). The results suggested that use of Impact was associated with a significant decrease in ICU mortality (28/87, 32.2%) compared to the control group (17/89, 19.1 %, p= 0.05). There was no follow up after discharge to assess the effect of the experimental formula following ICU discharge. The methodological weaknesses of this study limit the inferences we can make from these results. Furthermore, in the subgroup analysis, it was apparent that all the treatment benefit was in the least sick patients (baseline APACHE II score <15) whereas there was no effect in sicker patients (baseline APACHE II > 15). The effect of immunonutrition on sick, critically ill septic patients remains unanswered.

Currently, over 40 novel therapeutic interventions in the treatment of sepsis have been studied. Almost universally, these agents either block or inhibit some aspect of the inflammatory cascade. Immune-enhancing formulas that increase cytokine production and stimulate cellular immune function may not achieve desirable outcomes in a patient who already is septic. Arginine, a precursor to nitric oxide (NO), is associated with increased mortality in animal models of sepsis [67] and worsening hemodynamics in a study of patients with sepsis syndrome [68]. Given the potential to do more harm than good in critically ill patients with pre-existing infection, immune-enhancing diets have limited, if any, role in the current management of sepsis.

CONCLUSION

The critically ill patient with sepsis experiences a unique pathophysiologic state that promotes deterioration of organ function and systemic immunity. Beyond its effect on nutritional status, providing nutritional support by the enteral route may modify the course of sepsis through maintenance of gut structure and function, thereby reducing the inflammatory response to sepsis, and improving clinical outcomes. Parenteral nutrition seems to have little role and may even worsen outcomes in sepsis. While use of immune-enhancing nutrients may be helpful in a variety of patient groups who are non-septic, evidence for possible deleterious effects may prevent their use in patients who have pre-existing infection. Careful selection and close monitoring should maximize efficacy and benefit from the nutritional support regimen in this complex patient population.

REFERENCES

1.   Barton RG. Nutrition support in critical illness. Nutr Clin Pract 1994; 9:127-139
2.   Wojnar, MM, William WG, Lang CH. Nutritional support of the septic patient. Crit Care Clin 1995; 3:717-733
3.   Reinhardt GF, Myscofski JW, Wilkens DB, et al. Incidence and mortality of hypoalbuminemic patients in hospitalized veterans. J Parenter Enteral Nutr 1980; 4:357-359
4.   Windsor JA, Hill GL. Risk factors for postoperative pneumonia. The importance of protein depletion. Ann Surg 1988; 208:209-214
5.   Herrmann FR, Safran C, Levkoff SE, et al. Serum albumin level on admission as a predictor of death, length of stay, and readmission. Arch Intern Med 1992; 152:125-130
6.   Bone RC. Sir Isaac Newton, sepsis, SIRS and CARS. Crit Care Med 1996; 24:1125-1128
7.   Zedler S, Bone RC, Baue AE, et al. T cell reactivity and its protective role in immunosuppression after burns. Crit Care Med 1999; 27: 66-72
8.   Border JR, Hassett J, LaDuca J, et al. The gut origin septic states in blunt multiple trauma (ISS=40) in the ICU. Ann Surg 1987; 206:427-448
9.   Deitch EA, Winterton J, Li M, et al. The gut as a portal of entry for bacteremia: Role of protein malnutrition. Ann Surg 1987; 205:681-690
10. Bursztein S, Elwyn DH, Askanazi J, et al. Energy metabolism, indirect calorimetry, and nutrition. Williams & Wilkins, Baltimore, 1989:; pp 15-65 and 219-220
11. Cerra FB. Hypermetabolism, organ failure, and metabolic support. Surgery 1987; 101:1
12. Cunningham JJ. Factors contributing to increased energy expenditure in thermal injury: A review of studies employing indirect calorimetry. J Parenter Enteral Nutr 1990; 14:649-656
13. Wilmore DW, Long JM, Mason RD. Catecholamines: Mediators of the hypermetabolic response to thermal injury. Ann Surg 1974; 180:653-669
14. Baue AE. Nutrition and metabolism in sepsis and multisystem organ failure. Surg Clin North Am 1991; 71:549-563
15. Kreymann G, Grosser S, Buggisch P, et al. Oxygen consumption and resting metabolic rate in sepsis, sepsis syndrome, and septic shock. Crit Care Med 1993; 21:1012-1019
16. McClave SA, Snider HL. Understanding the metabolic response to critical illness: Factors which cause patients to deviate from the expected pattern of hypermetabolism. New Horiz 1994; 2:139-146
17. Grant JP. Nutritional assessment in clinical practice. Nutr Clin Pract 1986; 1:3-11
18. Fleck A. Acute phase response: implications for nutrition and recovery. Nutrition 1988; 4: 109-117
19. McClave SA. The consequences of overfeeding and underfeeding. J Respir Care Pract 1997; April/May: 57-64
20. Jenkinson S. Nutritonal problems during mechanical ventilation in acute respiratory failure. Respir Care 1983; 28:641-644
21. Lowry S, Brennan M. Abnormal liver function during parenteral nutrition; relation to infusion excess. J Surg Res 1979; 26:300-307
22. Liposkey JM, Nelson LD. Ventilatory response to high caloric loads in critically ill patients. Crit Care Med. 1994; 22:796-802
23. Alexander JW, Gonce SJ, Miskell PW, et al. A new model for studying nutrition in peritonitis; the adverse effects of over feeding. Ann Surg 1989; 209: 334-340
24. Reilly JJ, Hull SF, AlbertN et al. Economic impact of malnutrition: A model system for hospitalised patients. J Parenter Enteral Nutr 1988; 12: 371-376

25. Sax HC, Illig KA, Ryan CK, et al. Low-dose enteral feeding is beneficial during total parenteral nutrition. Am J Surg 1996; 171:587-590

26. Nelson JL, Foley-Nelson TL, Gianotti L, et al. Caloric intake and bacterial translocation following burn trauma in guinea pigs. Nutrition. In press.

27. McClave SA, Snider HL. Use of indirect calorimetry in clinical nutrition. Nutr Clin Pract 1992; 7:207-221

28. Heyland DK, Cook D, King D et al. Do critically ill patients tolerate early intragastric nutrition. Clin Intensive Care 1996; 768-773

29. Carrico CJ, Meakins JL, Marshall JC, et al. Multiple organ failure syndrome. The gastrointestinal tract: the motor of MOF. Arch Surg 1986; 121:196-208

30. Alverdy J, Chi HS, Sheldon G. The effect of parenteral nutrition on gastrointestinal immunity: the importance of enteral immunity. Ann Surg 1985; 202:681-684

31. Li L, Kudsk KA, Gocinski B, et al. Effects of parenteral and enteral nutrition on gut-associated lymphoid tissue. J Trauma 1995; 39: 44-51

32. Saito H, Trocki O, Alexander JW, et al. The effect of route of administration on the nutritional state, catabolic hormone secretion and gut mucosal integrity after burn injury. J Parenter Enteral Nutr 1987; 11:1-7

33. Alverdy JC, Aoys E, Moss GS. TPN promotes bacterial translocation from the gut. Surgery 1988; 104:185-190

34. Kudsk KA, Li J, Renegar KB. Loss of upper respiratory immunity with parenteral feeding. Ann Surg 1996; 223: 629-635

35. Zaloga GP, Bortenschlager L, Black KW, et al. Immediate postoperative enteral feeding decreases weight loss and improves healing after abdominal surgery in rats. Crit Care Med 1992; 20:115-119

36. Mochizuki H, Trocki O, Dominioni L, et al. Mechanism of prevention of postburn hypermetabolism and catabolism by early enteral feeding. Ann Surg 1984; 200:297-308

37. Kudsk KA, Stone JM, Carpenter G, et al. Enteral and parenteral feeding influences mortality after hemoglobin-E. coli peritonitis in normal rats. J Trauma 1983; 23:605-609

38. Zaloga GP, Knowles R, Black KW, et al. Total parenteral nutrition increases mortality after haemorrhage. Crit Care Med 1990; 19:54-59

39. Schroeder D, Gillanders L, Mahr K, et al. Effects of immediate postoperative enteral nutrition on body composition, muscle function, and would healing. J Parenter Enteral Nutr 1991; 15:376-383

40. Hadfield RJ, Sinclair DG, Houldsworth PE, et al. Effects of enteral and parenteral nutrition on gut mucosal permeability in the critically ill. Am J Respir Crit Care Med 1995; 152:1545-1548

41. Suchner U, Senftleben U, Eckart T, et al. Enteral versus parenteral nutrition: Effects on gastrointestinal function and metabolism. Nutrition 1996; 12:13-22

42. Rapp RP, Young B, Twyman D, et al. The favourable effect of early parenteral feeding on survival in head-injured patients. J Neurosurg 1983; 58:906-912

43. Young B, Ott L, Twyman D, et al. The effect of nutritional support on outcome from severe head injury. J Neurosurg 1987; 67:668-676

44. Moore FA, Moore EE, Jones TN, et al. TEN versus TPN following major abdominal trauma – reduced septic morbidity. J Trauma 1989; 29: 219-223

45. Kudsk KA, Croce MA, Fabian TC, et al. Enteral versus parenteral feeding. Ann Surg 1992; 215:503-513

46. Windsor ACJ, Kanwar S, Li AGK, et al. Compared with parenteral nutrition, enteral feeding attentuates the acute phase response and improves disease severity in acute pancreatitis. Gut 1998; 42:431-435

47. Kalfarentzos F, Kehagias J, Mead N, et al. Enteral nutrition is superior to parenteral nutrition in severe acute pancreatitis: Results of a randomized prospective trial. Br J Surg 1997; 84:1665-1669

48.   Kompan L, Kremzar B, Gadzijev E, et al. Effects of early enteral nutrition on intestinal permeability and the development of multiple organ failure after multiple injury. Intensive Care Med 1999; 25:157-161

49.   Eyer SD, Micon LT, Konstantinides FN, et al. Early enteral feeding does not attenuate metabolic response after blunt trauma. J Trauma 1993; 34:639-643

50.   Heyland DK, MacDonald S, Keefe L, et al. Total parenteral nutrition in the critically ill patient. A meta-analysis. JAMA 1998; 280: 2013-2019

51.   Nordenstrom J, Jarstarand C, Wirniek A. Decreased chemotactic and random migration of leukocytes during intralipid infusion. Am J Clin Nutr 1979; 32: 2416-2420

52.   Seidener DL, Mascioli EA, Istfan NW, et al. Effects of long-chain triglyceride emulsions on reticuloendothelial system function in humans. J Parenter Enteral Nutr 1989; 13:614-619

53.   Freeman J, Goldmann DA, Smith NE, et al. Association of intravenous lipid emulsion and coagulase-negative staphylococcal bacteremia in neonatal intensive care units. N Engl J Med 1990; 323:301-308

54.   Basttistella FD, Widergren JT, Anderson JT, et al. A prospective, randomized trial of intravenous fat emulsion administration in trauma victims requiring total parenteral nutrition. J Trauma 1997; 43:52-58

55.   Kudsk KA. Influence of nutrition on mucosal immunity. In: Vincent JL (ed) Yearbook of Intensive Care and Emergency Medicine. Springer, Berlin; pp: 64-72

56.   King BK, Kudsk KA, Li J, et al. Route and type of nutrition influence mucosal immunity to bacterial pneumonia. Ann Surg 1999; 229:272-278

57.   Saeed M, Carlson GL, Little RA, et al. Selective impairment of glucose storage in human sepsis. Br J Surg 1999; 86:813-821

58.   Trujillo EB, Young LS, Chertow GM, et al. Metabolic and monetary costs of avoidable parenteral nutrition use. J Parenter Enteral Nutr 1999; 23:109-113

59.   Pomposelli JJ, Baxter JK, Babineau TJ, et al. Early postoperative glucose control predicts nosocomial infection rate in diabetic patients. J Parenter Enteral Nutr 1998; 22:77-81

60.   Fong Y, Marano MA, Barber A, et al. Total parenteral nutrition and bowel rest modify the metabolic response to endotoxin in humans. Ann Surg 1989; 210:449

61.   Beale RJ, Bryg DJ, Bihari DJ. Immunonutrition in the critically ill: a systematic review of clinical outcome. Crit Care Med 1999; 27:2799-2805

62.   Heys SD, Walker LG, Smith I, et al. Enteral nutritional supplementation with key nutrients in patients with critical illness and cancer: a meta-analysis of randomized controlled clinical trials. Ann Surg 1999; 229:467-477

63.   Heyland DK, Novak F, Drover J, et al. Enteral immunonutrition in the critically ill patient: A meta-analysis. Clin Invest Med 2000. In press.

64.   Bower RH, Cerra FB, Bershadsky B, et.al. Early enteral administration of a formula (Impact) supplemented with arginine, nucelotides, and fish oil in intensive care unit patients: Results of a multicenter, prospective, randomized, clinical trial. Crit Care Med 1995; 23:436-449

65.   Ross Products Division of Abbott Laboratories: Comparison of Option One and a Polymeric Enteral Feeding: Effect on Length of Stay and Clinical and Immune Parameters, 1996. Study Protocol.

66.   Galbán C, Montejo JC, Mesejo A, et al. An immune-enhancing enteral diet reduces mortality rate and episodes of bacteremia in septic intensive care unit patients. Crit Care Med 2000; 28:643-648

67.   Gonce SJ, Peck MD, Alexander JW, et al. Arginine supplementation and its effect on established peritonitis in guinea pigs. J Parenter Enteral Nutr 1990; 14:237-244

68.   Lorente JA, Landin L, De Pablo R, et al. L-arginine pathway in the sepsis syndrome. Crit Care Med 1993; 21:1287-1295

28

THE SOURCES OF SEPSIS

Corinne Alberti
Christian Brun-Buisson

The term 'sepsis' has long been used interchangeably with bacteremia, severe sepsis or even septic shock, undoubtedly a source of some confusion and difficulty in comparing results from published studies [1]. By producing a consensus statement on definitions for the septic syndromes in 1992, the ACCP/SCCM panel of experts helped to characterize the various stages of the associated inflammatory response and to differentiate infectious from non infectious processes [2]. Since then, a number of studies using these definitions have been published, whether clinical trials (Table 1) or epidemiological studies (Table 2). These studies have helped in our understanding of the clinical features and interplay of the syndromes thus defined. In this chapter, we shall review these studies, focusing on the distribution of the source of sepsis according to the type of study and selection of patients, and discuss the relationships between the source of sepsis and patient outcome.

DOCUMENTATION OF INFECTION DURING SEPSIS

Examining the (infectious) sources of sepsis requires that infection be documented, either from clinically gross evidence of infection (e.g., peritonitis confirmed at surgery), or more often, via microbiological documentation. A major problem with the definitions of the septic syndromes must be emphasized at the outset, which is that the definition includes documentation of infection [2].

	Angus 2000 [25]*	Dhainaut 1998 [24]*	Abraham 1998 [23]†	Opal 1997 [22]	Abraham 1997 [21]	Bernard 1997 [20]	Cohen 1996 [19]†	Abraham 1995 [18]	Bone 1995 [17]*	Mean
No. Pts	1090	608	1879	696	444	455	420	994	530	
% documented	84	73	74	85	61	76	77	73	100	78
% shock	84	73	-	-	44	64	79	48	-	-
% respiratory	19	26	30	37	-	47	24	28	42	32
% primary bacteremia,	23	-	27	-	34	-	23	22	-	26
% genito-urinary	22	11	12	11	-	10	9	18	33	16
% abdomen/peritoneum	31	37	12	31	-	15	23	15	22	23
% unknown source	1.6	22	-	14	-	-	-	1.6	-	-
% bacteremia	-	35	41	37	-	35	38	39	40	38

* Clinical trials focusing on clinical evidence of Gram-negative infections
† Clinical trials focusing on septic shock

Table 1 - Clinical trials including patients with 'evidence of severe sepsis or septic shock', 1995-2000

However, it is apparent that all clinically septic patients fulfilling criteria for one or the other of the septic syndromes may not have documented infection. Strictly speaking, these patients cannot be qualified as having sepsis or one of its more advanced forms of severe sepsis or septic shock, even though they may have clinical evidence of infection (e.g., community-acquired pneumonia).

Conversely, it has also become clear that a fraction of patients with clearly documented infection (e.g., bacteremia) do not fulfil criteria for one of the septic syndromes. From the point of view of clinical trials of new adjunctive therapies for sepsis aimed at modulating the systemic response to infection, this may not actually be a major problem, as such patients have little or no systemic response to infection and would not be candidates for such therapies. It does however, obscure the analysis of the relationships between infection and the septic syndromes.

DISTRIBUTION OF SOURCES OF INFECTION DURING SEPSIS

Since the underlying hypothesis of the new ACCP/SCCM classification was that infection, whatever its characteristics, would lead to a "final common pathway" of various cellular and humoral derangements of graded severity, clinically reflected in organ system dysfunction, an obvious consequence of the classification is that categorization of intensive care unit (ICU) patients into the various stages of sepsis categories results in heterogeneous populations in terms of infection, reflecting the fact that sepsis depicts a clinical syndrome and not a disease.

INCIDENCE OF INFECTION AND RELATED SEPTIC SYNDROMES IN ICUS

Clinical symptoms characterizing the systemic inflammatory response are present at some point in time in a large proportion of ICU patients. For example, Rangel-Frausto et al. [3], in a prospective surveillance study, found that 68% of patients met at least two criteria for the systemic inflammatory response syndrome (SIRS). Likewise, Sands et al. [4] found that criteria for SIRS were met during 44% of 15,515 surveillance episodes in 12,759 patients.

Author, yr [Ref]	Inclusion criteria	Units	Country
Gatell 1988 [26]	Nosocomial bacteremia	Wards / ICUs (1 H)	Spain
Kieft 1993 [11]	Sepsis / sepsis syndrome	Wards / 5 ICUs (1 H)	Netherlands
Rello 1994 [27]	Nosocomial bacteremia	1 ICU (1 H)	Spain
Pittet 1994 [28]	Nosocomial bacteremia	4 surgical ICUs (1 H)	Switzerland
Pittet 1995 [10]	SIRS / sepsis syndrome	1 ICU (1 H)	Switzerland
Brun-Buisson 1995 [13]	Severe sepsis / septic shock	170 ICUs	France
Vincent 1995 [6]*	Nosocomial infections	1417 ICUs	14 European countries
Rangel-Frausto 1995 [3]	SIRS / sepsis syndrome	3 wards / 3 ICUs (1 H)	USA
Brun-Buisson 1996 [8]	Bacteremia and sepsis/severe sepsis	Wards / 29 ICUs (24 H)	France
Pittet 1996 [12]	Bacteremia and sepsis syndrome	1 surgical ICU	Switzerland
Sands 1997 [4]	Sepsis syndrome	Wards / ICUs (8 H)	USA
Valles 1997 [9]	Nosocomial bacteremia and sepsis syndrome	30 ICUs	Spain
Reyes 1999 [15]	Septic shock	1 ICU	Belgium
Richards 1999 [14]	Nosocomial infections	122 ICUs (97 H)	USA
Ponce 2000 [5]*	Infections and sepsis syndrome	254 ICUs	Mexico
Alberti 2000 [7]	Infections and sepsis syndrome	28 ICUs	8 European countries

H : hospital
* prevalence study

Table 2 - Epidemiological studies of sepsis

In such patients, documentation of infection was recorded in less than 50% of cases (Table 3). However, documentation of infection is more often obtained in the more severe presentations of the septic syndromes, i.e., severe sepsis and septic shock.

Two recent studies have examined the problem from the viewpoint of infection in ICUs. In a one-day prevalence study, Ponce de Leon et al. [5] studied 895 patients from 254 ICUs in Mexico; they found a 58% prevalence of infection (521 patients and 752 episodes), of which 294 (56.5%) were associated with sepsis, severe sepsis or septic shock.

Study [Ref]	No. admissions (No. patients/ episodes)	% documented	% bacteremia	% primary bacteremia	% respiratory	% UTI	% digestive tract/ abdominal	% unknown
Pittet, 1995 [8]								
Sepsis syndrome	170 (83/83)	-	-	16	19	9	-	-
Kieft, 1993 [9]	6,762							
Sepsis	(290/448)	-	12	5	24	12	-/7	38
Severe sepsis	(92/119)	-	28	3	53	8	-/17	7
Brun-Buisson, 1995 [11]	11,470							
Severe sepsis	(1052/1064)	70	37	3	40	8	32	5
Rangel-Frausto, 1995	3708							
Sepsis (61%)	(-/2729)	45	16.5	-	9	26	-	-
Severe sepsis (39%)		42	25	-	25	38	-	-
Septic shock (7%)		47	69	-	26	25	-	-
		57						
Sands, 1997 [5]	12,759							
Sepsis	(1063/1342)	64.5	32.5	12	42	11	10	8
Reyes, 1999 [14]	-							
Septic shock	227/227	67	36	3	38	6	33	13
Ponce, 2000 [13]	895							
All Infections	(521/752)	49	-	2	39	16	7	4
Alberti, 2000 [4]	8,353 (3564/4277)							
no SIRS (18%)		64	9	8	68	12	8	-
Sepsis (28%)		66	16	10	63	10	13	-
Severe Sepsis (24%)		77	30	18	85	15	12	-
Septic shock (30%)		78	27	16	54	11	21	-

Table 3. Sources of infection and sepsis

The prevalence rate is consistent with that recorded in the large European Prevalence of Infection in Intensive Care (EPIC) study [6] performed in 1992 across 1417 ICUs and including 10,038 patients, of whom 4081 patients (45%) had infection; unfortunately, the distribution of septic syndromes among infected patients was not reported in that study. In a more recent and detailed incidence study [7], including 28 ICUs from 8 countries, and 14,364 ICU patients, the overall incidence of infection was 21 %, of which 12% was community-acquired, and 9 % hospital-acquired (including ICU-acquired infections). The rates of sepsis, severe sepsis, and septic shock among infected patients were, respectively, 28 %, 24 %, and 30 % (thus leaving 18 % infectious episodes not associated with one of the septic syndromes). Of note, microbiological documentation of infection was obtained in that study in only 55 % of community-acquired infections and in 71 % of hospital-acquired infections; respiratory, digestive tract, urinary tract infection and primary bloodstream infections represented 80 % of all infectious episodes. Several conclusions regarding the relationships between infection and sepsis can be derived from this study. First, only about 80 % of clinically documented infections were classified in sepsis categories from which about one-half have manifestations of either severe sepsis or septic shock. Second, one-fifth of infections do not fulfil criteria for any sepsis category (Table 3). Therefore, besides sepsis categorization, it appears important to focus epidemiological studies on infection itself for a better understanding of the associated conditions, risks and outcomes of septic patients. Indeed, many community-acquired infections cannot be microbiologically documented because of antimicrobial therapy prior to ICU admission and sampling, whereas appropriate microbiologic samples are more likely to be obtained during the ICU course. Conversely, a clinical diagnosis of infection may be easier to ascertain in the former than in the latter case, in the absence of interference of previous events occurring during the ICU stay. Therefore, the sepsis definitions result in eliminating nearly one-half of ICU patients having community-acquired infection, which is a major problem for the evaluation of new therapeutic approaches.

BACTEREMIA AND SEPSIS

To assess the influence of the sepsis categorization on the source of sepsis, it is useful to contrast the epidemiology of bacteremia, the most indisputable evidence for infection, to those of the septic syndromes. Table 4 shows the sources of infections recorded in studies that have examined the relationships between bacteremia and sepsis in hospital and/or ICU populations.

Author, yr [Ref]	No. admissions	No. patients	No. episodes	Incidence	% IV lines	% UTI	% respiratory	% abdominal	% unknown/primary
Brun-Buisson,1996 [6]	85,750								
Bacteremia		842	842	1%	11	21	16	18	14
Sepsis (74%)		621	621		12	25	14	15	16
Severe sepsis 26%)		221	221		9	12	20	25	9
Pittet, 1996 [10]	5457								
Bacteremia		246	246	3.2%	-	-	-	-	-
Sepsis (71%)		176	176						21
Valles, 1997 [7]	1626								
Bacteremia		481	590	3.6%	37	6	17	6	28
Sepsis (63%)					40	6	14	3	31
Severe Sepsis (18%)					38	5	25	8	19
Septic shock (19%)					25	6	21	14	27

UTI: urinary tract infection

Table 4. Sources of bacteremic infections and associated sepsis syndrome

In bacteremic patients, a clinical syndrome of sepsis occurs in about 2/3 to 3/4 of patients, as shown by Sands et al. [4] and by the larger studies performed in ICUs or general wards in France and in Spain by our group [8] and by Valles et al. [9], the latter focusing on nosocomial bacteremia in ICUs. A similar figure was recorded by Pittet in Geneva, with 71 % of bacteremic patients having sepsis [8]. Severe sepsis occurs in about a quarter of bacteremic patients. When looking at the distribution of sources recorded, a slightly different distribution is noted between all patients with bacteremia and those with sepsis, especially severe sepsis. In the latter group, the prevalence of primary bacteremia and urinary tract infection is lower, while those of other sources, especially respiratory and abdominal sources, is higher. This is reflected in the analysis of risk factors for severe sepsis during bacteremia, where we found that a respiratory or abdominal source of bacteremia were respectively 2.2 and 3.1 times more likely to be associated with severe sepsis or septic shock than an intravascular or urinary tract source of infection [6]. When infection occurred as a consequence of multiple source of infection, this was also associated with a 3.6 fold increased risk of severe sepsis.

SEPSIS AND INFECTION

Epidemiological Studies

A number of epidemiological studies have been performed in the past 10 years looking at the problem from the side of sepsis itself (Table 2). In these studies, patients hospitalized in ICUs and sometimes hospital wards have been included. The studies by Kieft et al. [9], Brun-Buisson et al. [6], and Sands et al. [5], included patients from both ICUs and wards in the same hospital or in multicenter hospital wide studies, whereas those conducted by Pittet et al. [10], Brun-Buisson et al. [11], Valles et al. [7], Richards et al. [12], Ponce et al. [13] and Alberti et al. [4] were restricted to ICUs. Sands et al. [5] evaluated the incidence of sepsis syndromes in 12,759 patients from 8 hospitals in the USA, and found an incidence of SIRS, sepsis, and severe sepsis of, respectively, 18 %, 4.5 %, and 1 to 3.3 %; the latter estimate is consistent with that found by Kieft et al. [9], who studied 6,762 admissions in one hospital in the Netherlands, and found sepsis in 290 patients (incidence 5.6 %), of whom only 92 had severe sepsis (incidence 1.4 % admissions); this incidence of severe sepsis in these studies is somewhat higher than that found in the French multicenter study (0.6 %). In ICUs, however, figures also vary widely across studies, with incidences of severe sepsis ranging from 2.4 % to 13.6 %, and that of septic shock from 6.1 % to 20.3 % of patients admitted.

Despite these variations in incidence, the distribution of sources of sepsis is fairly consistent across these studies. The major sources of infection associated with sepsis are the respiratory and urinary tract. However, the proportion of infections of the urinary tract declines as the severity of the systemic response increases, whereas that originating from the respiratory tract increases. Likewise, intra-abdominal infection accounts for about 20% (10% to 30%) episodes of severe sepsis or septic shock, and a smaller proportion of cases with sepsis only (Table 3). The proportion of associated bacteremia also increases with the severity of the systemic response to infection, with only about 10% of patients with sepsis having positive blood cultures, and 20 to 30% or more patients with severe sepsis or septic shock having bacteremia. Finally, it should be noted that patients with unidentified source of septic shock have a worse prognosis than their counterparts with identified source [14].

Etiologic organisms involved in bacteremia and sepsis have been described in several studies. In bacteremia, major shifts in the distribution of organisms have occurred in the recent years, with an increasing prevalence of gram-positive organisms, largely caused by the increased use of intravascular catheters and other invasive devices. A similar less pronounced trend can be recorded in the septic syndromes. There is *in vitro* and experimental evidence that Gram-negative and Gram-positive bacteria differ in terms of pathophysiology of the host response [15]. Whether these differences are clinically important in terms of outcome of patients remains debated, but they may imply different therapeutic approaches.

Clinical Trials of New Adjunctive Therapies

It is interesting to contrast these data with those recorded during clinical trials of adjunctive therapies in sepsis performed recently. Most such trials have focused on severe sepsis, although slightly different criteria for inclusion have been used in the various studies. Some of these have focused on patients having Gram-negative infection, and some only on patients with septic shock (Table1). In these studies, strict inclusion and exclusion criteria have been used, which result in a more homogeneous pattern of infection than in epidemiological studies where virtually all patients fulfilling criteria fro septic syndromes have been included. Therefore, the epidemiology of sepsis appears much more consistent across the clinical trials than in the epidemiological studies reviewed above.

Table 1 shows the mean distribution of infection reported in phase III clinical trials published between 1995 and 2000, in which patients were usually included on the basis of "clinical evidence of infection with clinical features of severe sepsis or septic shock". Similar to the epidemiological studies, the proportion of cases with documented infection represents about three-fourths of the patients included. In clinical trials, the rate of bacteremia varied in a narrow range, from 35 to 41 % of patients. Although the respiratory tract still leads the sources identified, accounting for about one third of cases (range 24-37), other sources account for a somewhat higher proportion than in the epidemiological studies, with intra-abdominal infection accounting for 23 %, and genito-urinary tract infection for 16 %; a high mean proportion of primary bacteremia is also noted (26 %). It is likely that the bias toward selection of patients not having severe underlying disease in clinical trials, as well as of infections with less overall acute severity (i.e., excluding patients with refractory shock), explains in large part the relatively lower mortality recorded in phase III clinical trials as compared with the epidemiological studies.

CONCLUSION

The usefulness of the sepsis classification has been challenged, because it requires microbiologic documentation of infection, which is often available only in retrospect, and because some patients with definite infection do not fulfil criteria for any of the sepsis categories. Whereas this is not a major problem for the least severe forms of the syndrome (i.e., SIRS), where the prognosis does not differ markedly from that of non-infected patients, it may be more important for patients with non-documented clinical infection and organ dysfunction. Such patients may be qualified as having severe SIRS - which is not very helpful clinically - and this classification has the major theoretical drawback of precluding inclusion into clinical trials where 'sepsis' (with documented infection) is one of the inclusion criteria. This is, however, somewhat theoretical, because patients have been included in such trials on the basis of clinical evidence for infection and systemic response to suspected infection, whether microbiogical documentation was or was not available. Indeed, only about 70% of patients included in most phase III clinical trials were found to have microbiologically documented infection.

The heterogeneity of populations defined according to sepsis criteria has led some investigators to suggest that focusing on some of the specific infections and sources would reduce the heterogeneity of clinical trials and probably facilitate the interpretation of outcome of therapy. It is apparent that overall, different sites of infection are associated with different risk in terms of evolution towards sepsis and its severe forms. This is likely due in large part to the ease of diagnosis (earlier recognition) and accessibility to therapy of the involved focus. It is apparent that IV line infection can be most often easily controlled via pulling out the catheter, and urinary tract infection are usually more amenable to diagnosis and treatment, although sometimes via surgical drainage. Peritonitis or pneumonia are more difficult-to-treat infections. From a pathophysiological viewpoint, infection caused by various organisms, from various sources, can indeed elicit a similar systemic response to infection in terms of cellular and humoral reactions. There is however some (mostly experimental) evidence that different responses to adjunctive therapies may be elicited according to the site of infection, or according to pathogens involved. Whether these differences are clinically important remains at present equivocal. Another potentially important factor of variability of response between patients is the cellular responsiveness at time of infection, part of which is likely dependent on host and genetic factors. These factors are likely more important than the source itself or the organisms involved.

REFERENCES

1. Sibbald WJ, McCormack D, Marshall JC. Sepsis: clarity of existing terminology...or more confusion? Crit Care Med 1991; 19:996-998
2. Bone RC, Balk RA, Cerra FB, et al. Definitions for sepsis and organ failure and guidelines for the use of innovative therapies in sepsis. Chest 1992; 101:1656-1662
3. Vincent JL, Bihari DJ, Suter PM, et al. The prevalence of nosocomial infection in intensive care units in Europe. Results of the European Prevalence of Infection in Intensive Care (EPIC) Study. JAMA 1995; 274: 639-644
4. Alberti C, Soufir L, Brun-Buisson C, et al. Assessing the incidence of ICU-acquired events: overestimation by the Kaplan-Meier estimation. Intensive Care Med 2000; 26:S272 (Abst)
5. Sands KE, Bates DW, Lanken PN, et al. Epidemiology of sepsis syndrome in 8 academic medical centers. JAMA 1997; 1997:234-240
6. Brun-Buisson C, Doyon F, Carlet J. Bacteremia and severe sepsis in adults: A multicenter prospective survey in ICUs and wards of 24 hospitals. Am J Respir Crit Care Med 1996; 154:617-624
7. Vallés J, Leon C, Alvarez-Lerma F, The Spanish Collaborative Group for Infections in Intensive Care Units of SEMIUC. Nosocomial bacteremia in critically ill patients: A

multicenter study evaluating epidemiology and prognosis. Clin Infect Dis 1997; 24:387-395

8. Pittet D, Rangel-Frausto MS, Tarara D, et al. Systemic inflammatory response syndrome, sepsis, severe sepsis and septic shock: incidence, morbidities and outcomes in surgical ICU patients. Intensive Care Med 1995; 21:302-309

9. Kieft H, Hoepelman AIM, Zhou W, et al. The sepsis syndrome in a Dutch University Hospital. Clinical observations. Arch Intern Med 1993; 153:2241-2247

10. Pittet D, Thiévent B, Wenzel RP, et al. Bedside prediction of mortality from bacteremic sepsis. A dynamic analysis of ICU patients. Am J Respir Crit Care Med 1996; 153:684-693

11. Brun-Buisson C, Doyon F, Carlet J, et al. Incidence, risk factors, and outcome of severe sepsis and septic shock in adults. A multicenter prospective study in intensive care units. JAMA 1995; 274:968-674

12. Richards MJ, Edwards JR, Culver DH, et al. Nosocomial infections in medical intensive care units in the United States. National Nosocomial Infections Surveillance System. Crit Care Med 1999; 27:887-892

13. Ponce de Leon-Rosales SP, Molinar-Ramos F, Dominguez-Cherit G, et al. Prevalence of infections in intensive care units in Mexico: a multicenter study. Crit Care Med 2000; 28:1316-1321

14. Reyes WJ, Brimioulle S, Vincent JL. Septic shock without documented infection: an uncommon entity with a high mortality. Intensive Care Med 1999; 25:1267-1270

15. Opal SM, Cohen J. Clinical gram-positive sepsis: does it fundamentally differ from gram-negative bacterial sepsis? Crit Care Med 1999; 27:1608-1616

16. Bone RC, Balk RA, Fein AM, et al. A second large controlled clinical study of E5, a monoclonal antibody to endotoxin: results of a prospective, multicenter, randomized, controlled trial. The E5 Sepsis Study Group. Crit Care Med 1995; 23:994-1006

17. Abraham E, Wunderink R, Silverman H, et al. Efficacy and safety of monoclonal antibody to human tumor necrosis factor α in patients with sepsis syndrome. A randomized, controlled, double-blind; multicenter clinical trial. J A M A 1995; 273: 934-941

18. Cohen J, Carlet J, the INTERSEPT Study Group. INTERSEPT: an international, multicenter, placebo-controlled trial of monoclonal antibody to human tumor necrosis factor-α in patients with sepsis. Crit Care Med 1996; 24:1431-1440

19. Bernard GR, Wheeler AP, Russell JA, et al. The effects of ibuprofen on the physiology and survival of patients with sepsis. The Ibuprofen in Sepsis Study Group. N Engl J Med 1997; 336:912-918

20. Abraham E, Glauser MP, Butler T, et al. p55 tumor necrosis factor receptor fusion protein in the treatment of patients with severe sepsis and septic shock. J A M A 1997; 277:1531-1538

21. Opal SM, Fisher CJ, Jr., Dhainaut JF, Vincent JL, et al. Confirmatory interleukin-1 receptor antagonist trial in severe sepsis: a phase III, randomized, double-blind, placebo-controlled, multicenter trial. The Interleukin-1 Receptor Antagonist Sepsis Investigator Group. Crit Care Med 1997; 25:1115-1124

22. Abraham E, Anzueto A, Gutierrez G, et al. Double-blind randomised controlled trial of monoclonal antibody to human tumour necrosis factor in treatment of septic shock. Lancet 1998; 351:929-933

23. Dhainaut J-F, Tenaillon A, Hemmer M, et al. Confirmatory platelet-activating factor receptor antagonist trial in patients with severe Gram-negative bacterial sepsis: a phase III, randomized, double-blind, placebo-controlled, multicenter trial. Crit Care Med 1998; 26:1963-1971

24. Angus DC, Birmingham MC, Balk RA, et al. E5 murine monoclonal antiendotoxin antibody in gram-negative sepsis: a randomized controlled trial. E5 Study Investigators. JAMA 2000; 283:1723-1730
25. Gatell JM, Trilla A, Latorre X, et al. Nosocomial bacteremia in a large spanish teachning hospital: analysis of factors influencing prognosis. Rev Infect Dis 1988; 10:203-210
26. Rello J, Ricart M, Mirelis B, et al. Nosocomial bacteremia in a medical-surgical intensive care unit: Epidemiologic characteristics and factors influencing mortality in 111 episodes. Intensive Care Med 1994; 20:94-98
27. Pittet D, Tarara D, Wenzel RP. Nosocomial bloodstream infection in critically ill patients: excess length of stay, extra costs, and attributable mortality. JAMA 1994; 271:1598-601
28. Rangel-Frausto MS, Pittet D, Costigan MD, et al. The natural history of the systemic inflammatory response syndrome. JAMA 1995; 273:117-123

29

CATHETER-RELATED SEPSIS

Jean-François Timsit

Central venous catheters (CVCs) inserted for short term use are common and indispensable tools in caring for critically ill patients. The infectious risk of exposure to these devices is 48 % per intensive care unit (ICU) day. However, short-term CVCs are also associated with serious complications, the most common of which is infection. Catheter-related infection is the third most frequent cause of nosocomial infections in the ICU [1]. Attention to simple, practical details can reduce the infectious risk.

EPIDEMIOLOGY

Definition

Catheter colonization is defined by a growth of greater than 15 colony forming units (cfu) using the semi-quantitative roll-plate culture [2] or the presence of more than 1000 cfu/ml per catheter tip segment culture using catheter sonication [3] or vortexing [4] in sterile solution.

Catheter-related infections can be subdivided into two subsets: local infection and bacteremic infection. Local infection is defined as the presence of pus at the catheter exit site [1]. Catheter-related bloodstream infection is defined as a positive blood culture and evidence implying catheter involvement: i.e., 1) presence of pus at the insertion site or the catheter tunnel, growing the same microorganism as blood cultures; 2) positive culture of both the catheter tip and bloodstream with the same microorganism; or 3) clinical evidence of sepsis that does not respond to antibiotic therapy but resolves once the catheter is removed [1]. Some authors have proposed additional methods, including paired blood cultures drawn from the CVC and a peripheral vein [5], or a technique in which time to culture positivity for blood drawn from the CVC is compared to that for blood drawn from percutaneous venipuncture [6]. Probable catheter-related sepsis should also be defined as: 1) a positive quantitative tip culture associated with clinical symptoms of sepsis that resolves after catheter removal; or 2) a common skin organism, e.g., *Staph. aureus* or *Candida,* isolated from one or more blood cultures from a patient with clinical manifestations of sepsis and no apparent source of sepsis apart from the catheter.

Incidence

CVCs are a leading source of bacteremia in ICUs [7]. The so-called primary bacteremias, most of which are actually secondary to catheter infection, are responsible for about 10-20 % of nosocomial infections in ICUs in the USA. Catheter-related infections occur in about 5-10 % of nosocomial infections. The reported ICU incidence of catheter-related bacteremia is variable, ranging from 0.28 to 1.28 per 100 catheter-days for all ICU types and average rates of 0.45 per 100 catheter-days for medical-surgical ICUs [8]. Catheter-related blood-stream infections are less frequent in respiratory ICUs. On the contrary, the incidence may reach 3 per 100 days of catheterization in burn centers. The rate of Swan-Ganz catheter-related blood-stream infections is higher than for central lines. The rate of Swan-Ganz catheter colonization and blood-stream infection ranged between 5.9 and 29.1 per 100 catheter days (median: 21.9), and from 0 to 4.6 per 100 catheter days (median 1), respectively, in 14 prospective studies [9].

The most common organisms causing catheter-related blood-stream infections are Staphylococci, *Candida* spp and Gram-negative rods. However, coagulase negative staphylococci are frequently recovered from systematic culture of no longer needed catheters in asymptomatic patients [10]. On the contrary, positive quantitative catheter cultures with *Staph. aureus, P. aeruginosa,* and *A. baumannii* are more frequently associated with bacteremia, severe sepsis and complications [11-13].

Mechanisms of Infection

Colonization of the catheter may occur by two main pathways: the extra-luminal route or the intra-luminal route. Colonization of the catheter from its cutaneous entry site is the predominant route of colonization for short-term CVCs (<15-20 days) whereas colonization via the endoluminal route resulting from hub contamination predominates for prolonged catheterization [14]. In both cases, the source of microorganism is the patient's own skin commensal bacteria. Accordingly, the occurrence of bacteremia caused by common skin organisms is a major criterion for the diagnosis of catheter-related blood-stream infection. Most infections are caused by Gram-positive cocci.

The other sources of microorganisms, which are considered to be relatively minor contributors to sepsis, are either via hematogeneous spread from other body sites or from a contaminated infusate [15].

Attributable Morbidity, Mortality

The mortality attributable to catheter-related blood-stream infections is generally considered the lowest among nosocomial bacteremias [16,17]. Catheter-related blood-stream infection is also less frequently associated with severe sepsis than bacteremia from urinary, pulmonary or abdominal origin [18]. The estimated attributable mortality of nosocomial bloodstream infections usually ranges between 20 and 45 % in case-control studies matched on severity scores at admission. In the subgroup of catheter-related bloodstream infections, the attributable mortality is lower, between 10 and 30 % [19-21]. However, these estimations should be interpreted with caution: First, the size of studies looking at attributable mortality is far too low to use severity scores to demonstrate that prognosis of cases and controls were similar at admission; second, severity scores are not correlated very strongly with the length of stay in the ICU, and thus to the time for exposure to invasive devices, which are known to be important risk factors for catheter related blood-stream infections. Thus, adjusting for severity at admission may not be appropriate. The case-control studies performed until now thus have some weaknesses and cannot really give a definitive answer on the 'real' attributable mortality of nosocomial blood-stream infections.

Soufir et al. [13] showed, in an exposed-unexposed study, that adjusting for severity at 3 or 7 days before the onset of a catheter-related bloodstream infection decreased dramatically the attributable mortality of this event when compared to adjusting only for admission severity (relative risk from 2.1 [1.08-3.73] to 1.3 [0.69-2.46]). Similar results were obtained by Digiovine et al. [17] who matched patients according to severity on admission and severity the day before primary nosocomial bloodstream infection. They found that the crude mortality of the blood-stream infection group was

35.3 % as compared to 30.9 % for the control group (OR 1.33; 95% CI: 0.56-3.16). Although the results of the last study could be biased by an overmatching phenomenon, They are consistent with an 1.3 increased risk of death which would need a very large sample size to be statistically different.

Intravascular catheter sepsis may lead to infectious complications that are life-threatening and difficult to treat. In the study by Arnow et al. [11], septic shock occurred in 12 % of cases, suppurative thrombophlebitis in 7 %, metastatic infection in 5 %, with two episodes of right sided endocarditis. Major complications were highest in episodes of catheter sepsis caused by *Staph. aureus, Candida spp* and *P. aeruginosa.* Although catheter-related blood-stream infections may have more benign consequences than other bacteremic infections, this category of nosocomial infection is typical of device-associated iatrogenic infection and therefore mostly accessible to prevention, if rigorous policies are adopted.

Economic Evaluation of CVC-related Infection

Catheter-related infection is associated, in case-control studies, with a 7-21 day excess hospital stay [17,19]. Catheter-related blood-stream infections undoubtedly increase healthcare costs for affected patients, but the exact extent is imprecisely known. According to previously published data, the most recent cost-effectiveness study estimated a total additional cost of about $10,000 per catheter-related blood-stream infection [22]. The estimated extra cost is more than two-fold higher in ICUs [19]. Similarly, the cost of symptomatic local catheter-related infection has been estimated at $400 [22].

DIAGNOSIS OF CATHETER-RELATED INFECTIONS

Establishing the diagnosis of catheter-related infection is often difficult. Diagnosis is typically based on clinical and/or laboratory criteria, each having significant diagnostic limitations.

Value of Clinical Criteria

Fever or erythema at the catheter entry site are non specific and usually of little help in diagnosing catheter-related blood-stream infection. Usually, when catheter-related blood-stream infection is suspected, it is common practice to remove the CVC and replace it at a new site. However, only about

15 to 25 % of CVCs so removed actually prove to be infected on quantitative tip culture. Moreover, in our experience, erythema was not associated with an increased risk of the catheter origin of a new sepsis [23].

Catheter-related infections can be subdivided into local and bacteremic infections. Superficial infections are defined by inflammation or the presence of pus at the CVC exit site or along the catheter tunnel. These signs of deep venous inflammation may have high diagnostic value and mandate removal of the CVC. Most often, local signs are minor and the suspicion of catheter-related blood-stream infection is based on the occurrence of an unexplained sepsis and/or positive blood culture in a patient with a CVC.

Diagnostic Tests for Catheter-related Bloodstream Infections

Diagnostic Tests after Removal of the Catheter

Qualitative broth culture has a high sensitivity but a very low specificity and is unable to distinguish contamination from infection. Therefore, Maki et al. have proposed a semi-quantitative culture technique, whereby the external surface of the catheter segment is rolled on a blood agar plate. A threshold of 15 cfu/ml was found to be associated with local signs of inflammation, and corresponded to catheter colonization [2]. This method can only explore the external surface of the catheter and endoluminal infection may be undetected. The technique has been widely used since the 1980s, and has very good sensitivity but lacks specificity (20 to 50 %); for this reason a higher threshold of 100 cfu/ml has been proposed by others [24].

Quantitative culture techniques have been also tested. Using serial dilution of a catheter rinse, Cleri et al. [25] found a good correlation between catheter-related infections and catheter culture yelding $\geq 10^3$ cfu/ml. This technique explores only the internal surface of the catheter. The technique has been modified by Brun-Buisson et al. [4] and tested for short-term catheter-related sepsis, in a French ICU. The distal 5 cm catheter segment is vortexed vigorously in a tube containing 1ml sterile water. Then, 0.1 ml of this solution is cultured. Using a 10^3 cfu/ml threshold, this technique exhibited a 88 % sensitivity and a 97 % specificity in predicting catheter-related sepsis with or without bacteremia. A quantitative technique using sonication gave similar results [3]. Using a 10^3 CFU/ml threshold, this latter technique predicted the catheter origin of *C. albicans* or *Staph. aureus* bacteremia in more than 70% cases. The prediction was lower for *Staph. epidermidis* (44.4 %) and *P. aeruginosa* (43.5 %).

Overall, quantitative culture techniques appear to be more accurate than semi-quantitative ones [10].

Diagnosis of Infection with the Catheter in Place

In cases of severe sepsis, the treatment of catheter-related bloodstream infection necessitates catheter removal in most cases. In these cases, the diagnosis of catheter-related blood-stream infection should be performed as previously described.

However, most of the situations in which catheter-related infections are suspected are not life-threatening. Assuming that the catheter is still needed, diagnostic techniques enabling accurate diagnosis while keeping the catheter still in place would be attractive, especially when the insertion of a new catheter would be hazardous.

Quantitative Culture of the Catheter Exit Site

Quantitative culture of the catheter exit site reflects the extra-luminal contamination pathway, which predominates for short term catheters. Using a threshold of 15-50 cfu/ml, culture of the skin insertion site appears to be very sensitive in detecting colonization, but since all colonized patients will not develop catheter-related infection, it may not be systematically indicated in the absence of local signs of thrombophlebitis [26-28]. Nevertheless, the absence of micro-organisms at the insertion site may have a good negative diagnostic value. In case of suspicion of catheter-related infection, this technique allows the diagnosis of catheter-related infection to be excluded and avoids unnecessary catheter replacement.

However, routine surveillance culture is useless as a positive cutaneous culture is closely related to cutaneous signs at the insertion site [29]. The specificity of the technique is good but the negative predictive value of a systematic cutaneous culture remained as low as 25 % in this setting because of the low prevalence of the disease [30].

Quantitative Blood Culture

Quantitative culture of the blood drawn from the catheter is 99 % specific but not sensitive using a 1000 cfu/ml threshold [31]. Simultaneous samples, drawn through the catheter and a peripheral vein without removal or exchange of the catheter, are more accurate in predicting catheter-related blood-stream infection. A differential colony count of 10:1 is indicative of catheter-related blood-stream infection [5,29,32,33]. The major limitation of the technique is that organisms are retrieved from the internal surface of the catheter. Consequently, it is probably more accurate for diagnosis of long-term catheter-related blood-stream infection. However, Quilici et al. [34] found a very good diagnostic accuracy of this technique using a 8:1 threshold in ICU patients. Overall, this technique is very specific but is limited by its complexity and cost.

An attractive alternative of this technique is to measure the differential time to positivity between hub-blood and peripheral blood cultures [6]. Using a cut off of 120 minutes, sensitivity and specificity was greater than 90 %. However, this result needs to be confirmed, since the correlation between quantitative count and time to detection of culture positivity is variable according to pathogen. This method needs to be tested in critically ill patients with short-term catheters.

Another technique of rapid diagnosis of catheter-related blood-stream infection using an acridine orange leukocyte cytocentrifugation (AOLC) has been tested recently in surgical patients and provided sensitivity and specificity greater than 90 % [35]. The Gram stain and AOLC is rapid (30 min), inexpensive, and requires only 100 µl catheter blood (treated with edetic acid) and the use of light and ultraviolet microscopy. The accuracy of this technique has been improved by the use of an endoluminal brushing of the catheter before blood sample. However, the theoretical risk of embolization or subsequent bacteremia limits its further use before confirmatory studies are available [36].

Guidewire Exchange of the Catheter

Catheters may be changed using guidewire exchange in cases of catheter malfunction, a positive blood culture obtained since the catheter was last changed, a septic clinical pattern when there is no other likely source of sepsis in the absence of skin site infection (purulent drainage at the skin puncture site, cellulitis (erythema, tenderness and oedema) at the skin puncture site or the association of erythema at the skin puncture site and a positive qualitative skin culture at 24 hours). If guidewire exchange occurs in the setting of an infection, the newly placed catheter should be removed. Guidewire exchange is associated with fewer mechanical complications (RR 0.48, 95%CI: 0.12-1.91) than catheter replacement at a new site. However, as compared to new-site replacement, guidewire esxchange is associated with a trend toward a higher rate of catheter colonization (RR 1.26, 95% CI:0.87-1.84). Guidewire exchange is also associated with a trend toward a higher rate of catheter exit site infection (RR 1.52, 95%CI [0.34-6.73]) and catheter-related bacteremia RR= 1.72, 95%CI: [0.89-3.33]) [37].

MANAGEMENT OF CATHETER-RELATED SEPSIS (Figure 1)

Catheter Removal or a More Conservative Attitude?

In case of suspicion of catheter infection, the diagnostic strategy must be either to change the catheter or to adopt a more conservative strategy. The physician's attitude must be guided by the ease of new catheter insertion, the immune status, the severity of the underlying illness of the patient and the severity of the clinical sepsis. In this field, relevant data are very rare as there is few randomized studies and because of uncontrolled biases in most of the cohort studies. Decisions about catheter removal and the type and duration of antibiotic therapy should be made after careful evaluation of each case, in the light of these variables.

In cases of septic shock or severe sepsis of undetermined origin, or when frank local signs of infection are found, the catheter should be removed. In the absence of severe sepsis or local signs, two conservative strategies might be proposed, especially when a new catheter insertion is hazardous:
1) To change the catheter over a guidewire
2) To perform catheter exit site culture (high negative predictive value) with or without paired blood cultures (high positive predictive value).
When a conservative strategy has been initially decided on, the decision for catheter removal mainly depends on microorganisms and on the evolution of the patient's status during the first 48 hours.

For *Staph. aureus* and *P. aeruginosa* infections the catheter should be removed, given the high risk of septic thrombophlebitis and deep-seated infection with these bacteria [1,38]. The attitude should be similar for catheter-related blood-stream infection with *Pseudomonas* spp, *A. baumannii*, and multiresistant Gram-negative bacilli [39]. One comparative study in patients undergoing hemodialysis concluded that during *Staph. aureus* catheter-related blood-stream infection, together with an appropriate antibiotic treatment the change of the catheter over a guidewire was as effective as catheter exchange at a new site [40]. For *Candida spp* catheter-related blood-stream infection, Rex et al [41], in a subgroup analysis, have shown that failure to remove the catheter resulted in a prolonged duration of candidemia. Similarly, a prospective cohort study suggested that catheter removal is associated independently with a lower rate of complications and a better survival [42].

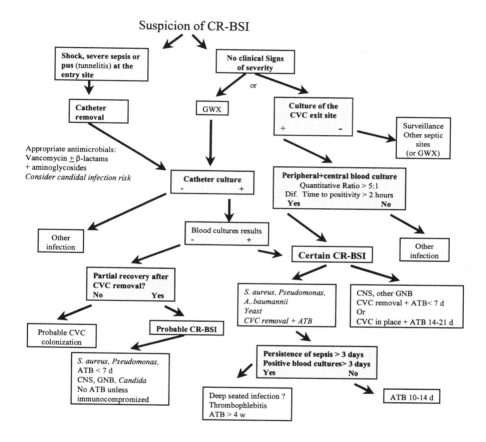

Figure 1. *Suggestions for diagnosis and therapeutic strategies for suspected catheter-related blood stream infection (CR- BSI). GWX: Guidewire exchange, ATB: antimicrobial therapy, CNS: Coagulase negative staphylococci, GNB: Gram-negative bacilli, CVC: central venous catheter (adapted from [74])*

Overall, conservative strategies are always risky. For example, in 62 episodes of catheter-related blood-stream infection in hemodialyzed patients, the relative risk of persistent bacteremia was 4-fold higher when the catheters were left in place [43]. When the decision is made to leave the catheter in

place, patients must be carefully monitored. The catheter must be removed
when a complicated course is suggested by persistent fever or bacteremia > 3
days [1]. Results from studies, mainly performed in cancer patients, suggest
that coagulase-negative staphylococci might be treated successfully without
catheter removal. However, if the CVC is not removed, there is a 20 %
chance of bacteremia recurrence (as compared to 3 % if the CVC is
removed) [44].

Antimicrobial Therapy

When catheter-related blood-stream infection is associated with severe sepsis
or shock, antimicrobials must be administered immediately, together with
catheter replacement. Appropriate treatment should include vancomycin, a
broad spectrum beta-lactamase and an aminoglycoside. In case of previous
Candida colonization or in high risk patients [45], antifungal therapy should
be started.

Treatment must be adapted according to the results of catheter tip culture
and blood culture. The duration of treatment should be at least ten days for
uncomplicated blood-stream infection (regression of septic signs and
bacteremia < 3 days, no persistent infectious site) due to *Staph. aureus,
Pseudomonas* spp, *A. baumanni*, and *Candida* spp. Therapy must be
prolonged for at least four weeks in case of complicated course [1]. For other
micro-organisms, antimicrobial therapy should not exceed one week if the
catheter has been removed.

Relapse, continuous fever, or bacteremia, despite removal of the catheter
is consistent with a persistent focus of infection. This implies prolonged or
modified antimicrobial treatment and an active search for a catheter-related
infection of another vascular line, metastatic abscess, septic thrombophlebitis
or endocarditis [11].

PREVENTION OF CATHETER-RELATED SEPSIS

Risk factors of CVC-blood-stream infection can be divided into host related
and catheter related factors. The underlying condition of the patient
influences the risk of catheter-related infection. Malignancy,
immunodeficiency, severe burns, and malnutrition, all problems that
compromise host defense, lead to a higher rate of infection. Similarly, severe
sepsis, or severe and sustained multiple organ dysfunction, are associated
with a higher risk of CVC infections [10].

However, a large number of risk factors are device-related, suggesting that CVC related infection is accessible to prevention, if rigorous policies are adopted.

Strategies of prevention have been extensively reviewed in two recent publications (Tables 1 and 2) [46,47]. Some key points will be developed in this chapter.

Recommended preventive strategies	Grade[1]	Mermel [47]	HICPAC [46]
Full barrier precautions for CVC insertion	IIa	Yes	Yes
Contamination shield for PAC	IIa	Yes	No reco.
Preparation of cutaneous site with chlorhexidine	IIa	Yes	No reco.
Subclavian rather than jugular access	III	Yes	Yes
Femoral access	III	No	No reco.
Subcutaneous tunneling for internal jugular or femoral short-term CVCs	IIa	Yes	No reco.
I.V. antibiotic prophylaxis	IIa	No	No

CVC: central venous catheter, PAC: pulmonary artery catheter, No reco.: no recommendation
(1) Grade of evidence: I: well designed meta-analysis from randomized controlled trials, IIa: at least one randomized control trial, IIb: at least one randomized trial allowing catheter guidewire exchange, III: at least one well design trial without randomization, IV: evidence from experience of authority on subject.

Table 1. *Main recommendations (grade of evidence) for prevention of intravascular infections during insertion (adapted from [46] and [47])*

Cutaneous Antisepsis

Rigorous cleansing and disinfection of the insertion site is a key point. Povidone iodine 10% and alcohol 70% are less effective than chlorhexidine 2% [46-47]. An alcohol-based preparation of chlorhexidine gluconate (0.5%) is also superior to povidone iodine [49].

Site of Insertion of the Catheter

Subclavian catheters carry a lower risk of infection than internal jugular or femoral vein catheters [12,50]. This result is only based on cohort studies and is partly explained by the higher risk of skin colonization and a better occlusion of dressings. However subclavian catheters are associated with a 1-3 % incidence of pneumothorax, and accidental puncture of the artery might have severe consequences in the critically ill patient with acute respiratory distress syndrome (ARDS), severe emphysema or disorders of hemostasis [51].

It is commonly believed that femoral vein catheters carry a greater risk of catheter related infection and septicemia. Some studies performed recently argue that a properly placed femoral catheter, in which the site is appropriately managed, is at no higher risk for infection than one placed in the subclavian or internal jugular route. However, the risk of deep vein thrombosis (DVT) is higher with femoral vein insertion [52]. For example in a recent observational study , the risk of ilio-femoral vein DVT was 6 fold higher (confidence interval, 1.5 to 23.5) in the cannulated leg than in the uncannulated one [53]. In other studies using phlebography, femoral DVT occurred in 8.5 % of patients and was never associated with clinical symptoms [54].

Catheter Tunneling

Subcutaneous tunneling of short-term catheters inserted into the jugular [23] or the femoral vein [55] decreased more than 3-fold the risk of catheter-related blood-stream infection, probably by reducing the extra-luminal migration of micro-organisms into the bloodstream and by allowing a better occlusion of dressings. This technique should be recommended if subclavian access is undesirable.

Prophylactic Treatments

Antithrombotic Prophylaxis

Both experimental [56] and cohort studies [57,58] suggest a close relationship between catheter-thrombosis and infection. Several thrombus proteins are able to increase adherence of *Staphylococci* and *Candida* spp to catheters. Thrombus formation on indwelling intravascular catheters is associated with catheter-related blood-stream infection.

Recommended preventive strategies	Grade[1]	Mermel [47]	HICPAC [46]
Routine replacement of CVCs	I	No	No
Remove catheters as soon as possible after intended use	IV	Yes	Yes
Continuing quality improvement programs	IV	Yes	Yes
Adequate nurse to patient ratio	III	Yes	No reco.
Specialized nursing teams for CVC care (TPN only)	IV	Yes	Yes
Transparent gauze dressings for CVCs	IIb	Yes	Yes
Gauze when blood is oozing from the insertion site	IIb	Yes	No reco.
Triple antibiotic ointments applied to insertion sites	IIa	No	No
Disinfect catheter hub and sampling ports before assessing	IV	Yes	Yes
Hub with antiseptic chamber for CVCs >2 weeks	IIa	Yes	No reco.
Antiseptic in plastic casing fitted around the hub of CVCs (>2 weeks)	IIa	Yes	No reco.
Low-dose heparin for short-term CVCs	I	Yes	Yes
Low dose warfarin for long-term CVCs	IIa	Yes	No reco.
PAC heparin-bonded with benzalkonium chloride	IV	Yes	No reco
Chlorhexidine-sulfadiazine impregnated short-term CVCs	I	Yes	Yes
Rifampin-minocycline impregnated short term CVCs	IIa	Yes	Yes
Silver-impregnated subcutaneous collagen-cuff	IIa	No	Yes

CVC: central venous catheter, PAC: pulmonary artery catheter, No reco.: no recommendation
(1) Grade of evidence: I: well designed meta-analysis from randomized controlled trials, IIa: at least one randomized control trial, IIb: at least one randomized trial allowing catheter guidewire exchange, III: at least one well design trial without randomization, IV: evidence from experience of authorities.

Table 2. *Main recommendations (grade of evidence) for prevention of intravascular infections during maintenance (adapted from 46 and 47)*

Very low-dose warfarin reduces by 4-fold ($p<0.05$) venographically documented thrombosis with long-term use of central venous catheters [59]. In a meta-analysis, prophylactic heparin reduces catheter-related thrombosis

(RR=0.4 [95%CI: 0.2-0.8], catheter colonization (RR=0.6 [95%CI: 0.06-0.6]) and, although non-significantly, catheter-related blood-stream infection (RR=0.26 [95% CI: 0.07-1.03]) [60]. It also strongly reduced pulmonary artery catheter thrombosis (RR=0.08 [95%CI: 0.02-0.37]). Subcutaneous low-molecular-weight heparins appear to be as effective as non-fractioned heparins.

Catheter Care

Catheter Replacement

Although not accessible to preventive measures, one should be aware that repeated catheterization increases the risk of catheter infection. This finding, together with a randomized study, against routine replacement of CVCs [61]. The physician and nurses should assess a patient's need for intravascular catheter on a daily basis. It is recommended that pulmonary artery catheters be removed after no longer than 5 days [9,62] .

Catheter Dressings

Semi-permeable transparent dressings are widely used and allow continuous observation of the skin insertion site and reduce the risk of extrinsic colonization. However, the old generation transparent dressings promoted moisture and bacterial proliferation and have been associated with higher rates of infection when compared with traditional gauze dressings [63]. Maki et al. using highly semi-permeable transparent dressings did not find any differences with gauze dressings [64]. Gauze dressing is preferred if blood is oozing from the catheter insertion site [47]. Catheter dressings should be changed immediately if the dressing becomes damp, loosened or soiled. The frequency of routine CVC dressing changes should be at least 48-72 hours.

A 5-fold reduction in the rate of catheter-related blood-stream infection was reported in a cohort study with the use of a new antiseptic hub model in a surgical unit [65]. This finding calls for further prospective randomized study in this field.

Overall, any excessive manipulation of CVCs independently increases the risk for catheter-related blood-stream infection and must be avoided [46,47]. The effect of a 'hands-off' system of manipulation have been tested for pulmonary artery catheters. The use of this system decreased the rate of PAC-blood-stream infection dramatically [62].

Educational Programs

Specific prevention strategies and improved guidelines for the use of intravascular devices can decrease the rate of infection; however, the impact of a combination of these strategies on rates of vascular-access infection in ICUs is not known. In a cohort study involving more than 3500 ICU patients, an educational campaign for vascular-access insertion and on device use and care decreased the incidence density of exit-site catheter infection (9.2 episodes per 1000 patient-days before the intervention, and 3.3 episodes per 1000 patient-days afterwards (relative risk 0.36 [95 % CI: 0.20-0.63])) and of bloodstream infection (11.3 before and 3.8 episodes per 1000 patient-days after the intervention, (RR: 0.33 [95 % CI 0.20-0.56]) due to decreased rates of both microbiologically documented infections and clinical sepsis [66].

Similarly, improved knowledge of young physicians after a one day course on infectious control practices and procedures was associated with a 28 % decrease in the rate of catheter-related blood-stream infection in 6 ICUs, corresponding to an estimate cost-saving of at least $63000 [67]. Educational programs are probably more cost-effective that the implementation of a specialized IV team [68], however, the efficacy of educational programs is reduced when the nurse or physician workload is too high [69].

Antimicrobial-coated or -impregnated Catheters

The efficacy of catheters impregnated with chlorhexidine and silver sulfadiazine on the external surface has been tested in many randomized studies. A well-conducted meta-analysis concluded that this technique reduces the risk of catheter-related blood-stream infection (RR=0.4, 95 % CI: 0.2-0.8) for short-term (<2 weeks) central venous catheterization [70]. This technique is cost-saving in settings in which the incidence of catheter-related-blood-stream infection of short-term CVCs is more than 3.3 per 1000 catheter-days. Resistance to chlorhexidine-sulfadiazine has not been demonstrated in clinical studies. However, resistance to chlorhexidine has been induced in *in vitro* studies [71]. Rare reports of anaphylactic reactions to the chlorhexidine component of this catheter has been reported [47]. Consequently, the use of chlorhexidine-silver-sulfadiazine impregnated catheters should be used when the catheter is expected to last less than two weeks and when the rate of infection is high despite adherence to other strategies such as maximal barrier precautions and implementation of educational program [72].

Catheters impregnated intraluminally and extraluminally with minocycline rifampin reduced the risk of catheter-related blood-stream infection as compared to chlorhexidine-silver-sulfadiazine-impregnated catheters (0.3 vs 3.4 %, p<0.002) [73]. The superiority of the antimicrobial impregnated catheter was probably due to the absence of intraluminal impregnation with chlorhexidine sulfadiazine. Internal and external chlohexidine-silver-sulfadiazine CVCs are now available and require further studies. The impact of antimicrobial-impregnated CVCs on resistance among skin microbes is not sufficiently known to recommend its use.

CONCLUSION

Catheter-related bloodstream infection remains a leading cause of nosocomial infections, particularly in ICUs. It is the most frequent cause of hospital bacteremia. Although catheter-related blood-stream infection may have more benign consequences than other bacteremic infections, it is typical of device-associated iatrogenic infection and therefore mostly accessible to prevention, if rigorous policies are adopted. Prevention of catheter-related blood-stream infection should be one of the main targets of a quality improvement program.

REFERENCES

1. Raad II, Bodey GP. Infectious complications of indwelling vascular catheters. Clin Infect Dis 1992 ; 15:197-210
2. Maki DG, Weise CE, Sarafin HW. A semiquantitative culture method for identifying intravenous-catheter-related infection. N Engl J Med 1977; 296:1305-1309
3. Sherertz RJ, Raad II, Belani A et al. Three-year experience with sonicated vascular catheter cultures in a clinical microbiology laboratory. J Clin Microbiol 1990; 28:76-82
4. Brun-Buisson C, Abrouk F, Legrand P, et al. Diagnosis of central venous catheter-related sepsis. Critical level of quantitative tip cultures. Arch Intern Med 1987; 147:873-877
5. Flynn P, Sheneb J, Strokes D, Barrett F. "In situ" management of confirmed central venous catheter-related bacteremia. Pediatr Infect Dis 1987; 6:729-734
6. Blot F, Nitenberg G, Chachaty E, et al. Diagnosis of catheter-related bacteraemia : a prospective comparison of the time to positivity of central vs. peripheral blood cultures. Lancet 1999; 354:1071-1077
7. Edgeworth JD, Treacher DF, Eykin SJ, et al. A 25-year study of nosocomial bacteremia in an adult intensive care unit. Crit Care Med 1999; 27:1421-1428
8. National Nosocomial infection surveillance system report, data summary from October 1986-April 1998. Am J Infect Control 1998; 26:522-525

9. Mermel LA, Maki DG. Infectious complications of Swan Ganz pulmonary artery catheters: Pathogenesis, epidemiology, prevention and management. Am J Respir Crit Care Med 1994; 149:1020-1036

10. Raad I. Intravascular-catheter-related infections. Lancet 1998; 351:893-898

11. Arnow C, Quimosing EM, Beach M. Consequences of intravascular catheter sepsis. Clin Infect Dis 1993; 16:778-784

12. Richet H, Hubert B, Nitenberg G, et al. Prospective multicenter study of vascular-catheter-related complications and risk factors for positive central-catheter cultures in intensive care unit patients. J Clin Microbiol 1990; 28:2520-2525

13. Soufir L, Timsit JF, Mahe C, et al. Attributable morbidity and mortality of catheter-related septicemia in critically ill patients: a matched, risk-adjusted, cohort study. Infect Control Hosp Epidemiol 1999; 20:396-401

14. Stiges Sera A, Linares J, Perez JL, et al. A randomized trial on the effect of tubing changes on hub contamination and catheter sepsis during parenteral nutrition. J Parenter Enteral Nutr 1985; 9:322-325

15. Goldmann DA, Pier GB. Pathogenesis of infections related to intravascular catheterization. Clin Microbiol Rev 1993; 6:176-192

16. Valles J, Leon C, Alvarez-lerma F, et al. Nosocomial bacteremia in critically ill patients: a multicenter study evaluating epidemiology and prognosis. Clin Infect Dis 1997; 24:387-395

17. DiGiovine B, Chenoweth C, Watts C et al. The attributable mortality and costs of primary nosocomial bloodstream infections in the ICU. Am J Respir Crit Care Med 1999; 160:976-981

18. Brun-Buisson C, Doyon F, Carlet J. Bacteremia and severe sepsis in adults: a multicenter prospective survey in ICUs and wards of hospital. Am J Respir Crit Care Medicine 1996; 154:617-624

19. Pittet D, Wenzel RP. Nosocomial bloodstream infection in the critically ill. JAMA 1994; 272-1819-1820

20. Renaud B, Brun-Buisson C. Bactériémies nosocomiales acquises dans les services de réanimation : mortalité et durée de séjour. Reanim Urg 1997; 1:62S (Abst)

21. Smith RL, Meixler SM, Simberkoff MS. Excess mortality in critically ill patients with nosocomial bloodstream infections. Chest 1990; 100:164-167

22. Saint S, Veenstra DL, Lipsky BE. The clinical and economic consequences of nosocomial central venous catheter related infection: are antimicrobial catheters useful? Infect Control Hosp Epidemiol 2000; 21:375-380

23. Timsit JF, Sebille V, Farkas JC, et al. Effect of subcutaneous tunneling on internal jugular catheter-related sepsis in critically ill patients. A prospective randomized multicenter study. JAMA 1996; 276:1416-1420

24. Colignon PJ, Soni N, Pearson IY, et al. Is semi-quantitative culture of central vein catheter tips usefull in the diagnosis of catheter associated bacteremia. J Clin Microbiol 1986; 24:532-535

25. Cleri DJ, Corrado ML, Seligman SJ. Quantitative culture of intravenous catheters and other intravascular inserts. J Infect Dis 1980; 141:781-786

26. Fan ST, Teoh-Tchan CH, Lau KF, et al. Predictive value of surveillance skin and hub cultures in central venous catheter sepsis. J Hosp Infect 1988; 12:191-198

27. Guidet B, Nicola I, Barakett V, et al. Skin versus hub cultures to predict colonization and infection of central venous catheter in intensive care patients. Infection 1994; 22:43-52

28. Snydman DR, Gorbea HF, Pober BR, et al. Predictive value of surveillance skin cultures in total-parenteral-nutrition-related infection. Lancet 1982; ii:1385-1388

29. Armstrong CW, Mayhall CG, Miller KB, et al. Clinical predictors of infection of central venous catheters used for total parenteral nutrition. Infect Control Hosp Epidemiol 1990; 11:71-78

30. Raad II, Baba M, Bodey GP. Diagnosis of catheter-related infections: the role of surveillance and targeted quantitative skin cultures. Clin Infect Dis 1995; 20:593-597

31. Andremont A, Paulet R, Nitenberg G, et al. Value of semiquantitative cultures of blood drawn through catheter hubs for estimating the risk of catheter tip colonization in cancer patients. J Clin Microbiol 1988; 26:2297-2299

32. Mosca R, Curtas S, Forbes B, et al The benefits of Isolator cultures in the management of suspected catheter sepsis. Surgery 1987; 102:718-723

33. Capdevila JA, Planes AM, Palomar M, et al. Value of differential quantitative blood cultures in the diagnosis of catheter-related sepsis. Eur J Clin Microbiol Infect Dis 1992; 11:403-407

34. Quilici N, Audibert G, Conroy MC, et al. Differential quantitative blood cultures in the diagnosis of catheter-related sepsis in intensive care units. Clin Infect Dis 1997; 25:1066-1070

35. Kite P, Dobbins BM, Wilcox MH, et al. Rapid diagnosis of central-venous catheter-related bloodstream infection without catheter removal. Lancet 1999; 354:1504-1507

36. Tighe MJ, Kite P, Thomas D, et al. Rapid diagnosis of catheter-related sepsis using the acridine orange leukocyte cytospin test and an endoluminal brush. J Parenter Enteral Nutr 1996; 20:215-218

37. Cook D, Randolph A, Kernerman P, et al. Central venous catheter replacement strategies: a systematic review of the literature. Crit Care Med 1997; 25:1417-1424

38. Elting LS, Bodey GP. Septicemia due to *Xanthomonas species* and non-aeruginosa *Pseudomonas* species : increasing incidence of catheter-related infections. Medicine 1990; 69:296-306

39. Benezra D, Kiehn TE, Gold GWM, et al. Prospective study of infections in indwelling central venous catheters using quantitative blood cultures. Am J Med 1988; 85:495-498

40. Tanriover B, Carlton D, Saddekni S, et al. Bacteremia associated with tunneled dialysis catheters: comparison of two treatment strategies. Kidney Int 2000; 57:2151-2155

41. Rex JH, Bennett JE, Sugar AM, et al. Intravascular catheter exchange and duration of candidemia. Clin Infect Dis 1995; 21:994-996

42. Nguyen MH, Peacock JE Jr, Tanner DC, et al. Therapeutic approaches in patients with candidemia: evaluation in a multicenter, prospective, observational study. Arch Intern Med 1995; 155:2429-2435

43. Marr KA, Sexton DJ, Conlon PJ, et al. Catheter-related bacteremia and outome of attempted catheter salvage in patients undergoing hemodialysis. Ann Intern Med 1997; 127:275-280

44. Raad I, Davis S, Khan A, et al. Catheter removal affects recurrence of catheter-related coagulase-negative staphylococci bacteremia. Infect Control Hosp Epidemiol 1992; 13:215-221

45. Pittet D, Monod M, Suter, et al. *Candida* colonization and subsequent infections in critically ill surgical patients. Ann Surg 1994; 220:751-758

46. Pearson ML. Guidelines for prevention of intra-vascular device-related infections Hospital Infection Control Practices Advisory Committee. Infect Control Hosp Epidemiol 1996; 17:438-473

47. Mermel LA. Prevention of intravascular catheter-related infections. Ann Intern Med 2000; 132:391-402

48. Raad II, Hohn DC, Gilbreath J, et al. Prevention of central venous catheter-related infection by using maximal sterile barrier precautions during insertion. Infect Control Hosp Epidemiol 1994; 15:231-238

49. Mimoz O, Pieroni L, Lawrence C, et al. Prospective, randomized trial of two antiseptic solutions for prevention of central venous or arterial catheter colonization and infection in intensive care unit patients. Crit Care Med 1996; 24:1818-1823

50. Moro ML, Vigano EF, Cozzi Lepri A, et al. Risk factors for central venous catheter-related infections in surgical and intensive care units. Infect Contol Hosp Epidemiol 1994; 15:253-264

51. Mansfield PF, Hohn DC, Fornage BD, et al. Complications and failures of subclavian-vein catheterization. N Engl J Med 1994; 331:1735-1738

52. Trottier SJ, Veremakis C, O'Brien J, et al. Femoral deep vein thrombosis associated with central venous cathetrization: results from a prospective randomized trial. Crit Care Med 1995; 23:52-59

53. Joynt GM, Kew J, Gomersall CD, et al. Deep venous thrombosis caused by femoral venous catheters in critically ill adult patients. Chest 2000; 117:178-183

54. Durbec O, Viviand X, Potie F, et al. A prospective evaluation of the use of femoral venous catheters in critically ill adults. Crit Care Med 1997; 25:1986-1989

55. Timsit JF, Bruneel F, Cheval C, et al. Use of tunneled femoral catheters to prevent Catheter-related infection. A randomized controlled trial. Ann Intern Med 1999; 130:729-735

56. Hermann M, Lai QJ, Albrecht RM, et al. Adhesion of staphylococcus aureus to surface bound platelets: role of fibrinogen fibrin and platelets integrins. J Infect Dis 1993; 167:312-322

57. Raad II, Luna M, Khalil SA, et al. The relationship between the thrombotic and infectious complications of central venous catheters. JAMA 1994; 271:1014-1016

58. Timsit JF, Farkas JC, Boyer JM, et al. Central vein catheter related thrombosis in intensive care patients: Incidence, risk factors and relationship with catheter related sepsis- Chest 1998;114:207-213

59. Bern MM, Lockich JJ, Wallach SR, et al. Very low doses of warfarin can prevent thrombosis in central venous catheters. A randomized, prospective trial. Ann Intern Med 1990; 112:423-428

60. Randolph AG, Cook DJ, Gonzales CA, et al. Benefit of heparin in central venous and pulmonary artery catheters. A meta-analysis of randomized controlled trials. Chest 1998; 113:165-171

61. Timsit JF. Scheduled replacement of central venous catheter is not necessary - Infect Control Hospit Epidemiol 2000; 21:371-374

62. Cohen Y, Fosse JP, Karoubi P, et al. The "hands-off" catheter and the prevention of systemic infections associated with pulmonary artery catheter. A prospective study. Am J Respir Crit Care Med 1998; 157:284-287

63. Hoffmann KK, Weber DJ, Samsa GP, et al. Transparent polyurethane film as an intravenous catheter dressing. A meta-analysis of the infection risks. JAMA 1992; 267:2072-2076

64. Maki DG, Stolz S, Wheeler S, et al. A prospective, randomized trial of gauze and two polyurethane dressings for site care of pulmonary artery catheters : implications for catheter management. Crit Care Med 1994; 22:1729-1737

65. Segura M, Alvarez-Lerma F, Tellado JM, et al. A clinical trial on the prevention of catheter-related sepsis using a new hub model. Ann Surg 1996; 223: 363-369

66. Eggimann P, Harbarth S, Constantin MN, et al. Impact of a prevention strategy targeted at vascular-access care on incidence of infections acquired in intensive care. Lancet 2000; 355:1864-1868

67. Sherertz RJ, Ely EW, Westbrook DM, et al. Education of physicians-in-training can decrease the risk for vascular catheter infection. Ann Intern Med 2000; 132:641-648

68. Meier PA, Fredrickson M, Catney M, et al. Impact of a dedicated intravenous therapy team on nosocomial blood stream infection rates. Am J Infect Control 1998; 26:388-392
69. Fridklin SK, Pear SM, Williamson TH, et al. The role of understaffing in central venous catheter-associated bloodstream infections. Infect Control Hosp Epidemiol 1996; 17:150-158
70. Veenstra DL, Saint S, Saha S, Lumley T, Sullivan SD. Efficacy of antiseptic-impregnated central venous catheters in preventing catheter-related bloodstream infection: a meta-analysis. JAMA 1999; 281:261-267
71. Tattawasart U, Maillard JY, Furr JR. Development of resistance to chlorhexidine diacetate and cetylpyridium chloride in *Pseudomonas stutzeri* and changes in antibiotic susceptibility. Infect Control Hosp Epidemiol 1999; 42:219-229
72. Civetta JM, Hudson-Civetta J, Ball S. Decreasing catheter-related infection and hospital costs by continuous quality improvement. Crit Care Med 1996; 24:1660-1665
73. Darouiche RO, Raad II, Heard SO, et al. A comparison of two antimicrobial-impregnated central venous catheters. Catheter Study Group. N Engl J Med 1999; 340:1-8
74. Blot F, Brun-Buisson C. Current approaches to the diagnosis and prevention of catheter-related infections. Curr Opin Crit Care 1999; 5:341-349

30

CONTROL OF THE SOURCE OF SEPSIS

John C. Marshall

The management of life-threatening infection is grounded in three principles:
- Resuscitation and physiologic support
- Administration of appropriate systemic antimicrobial therapy
- Definitive control of foci of ongoing microbial contamination.

The term 'source control' encompasses the spectrum of physical interventions used to accomplish the third objective. But, while source control measures are critical to the successful outcome of therapeutic intervention in sepsis, the rational basis for such measures is poorly established, both theoretically, and empirically.

This chapter reviews the principles that guide the use of source control measures in the septic patient, recognizing that the decision-making processes involved are often complex, and that optimal management of the septic patient requires the co-ordinated interaction of the surgeon and the intensivist.

PRINCIPLES OF SOURCE CONTROL

Source control can be defined as all those physical measures undertaken to eradicate a focus of invasive infection, and to correct the anatomic derangement responsible for ongoing microbial contamination [1]. These can be further classified into three broad categories of intervention (Table 1).

Intervention	Examples
Drainage: Converts an abscess to a controlled sinus or fistula	❑ Opening of an infected wound ❑ Percutaneous cholecystostomy or nephrostomy ❑ Tube thoracostomy for drainage of empyema ❑ Surgical drainage of mediastinal abscess secondary to esophageal perforation ❑ Open abdomen management of diffuse peritonitis
Debridement and Device Removal: Removes dead tissue, permitting entry of host immune cells and antibiotics; eliminates established microbial colonies on infected foreign bodies	❑ Surgical debridement of necrotizing fasciitis ❑ Debridement of open wound for wound infection ❑ Surgical excision of infected peripancreatic necrosis ❑ Sequestrectomy for osteomyelitis ❑ Line removal for catheter-related bacteremia ❑ Urinary catheter removal for UTI ❑ Valve replacement for endocarditis
Definitive Management or Diversion: Eliminates source of ongoing contamination from anatomic breach of epithelial surface	❑ Patch repair or duodenal ulcer ❑ Pyloric exclusion for complex duodenal or pancreatic injuries ❑ Resection of perforated diverticulitis ❑ Proximal colostomy for colon perforation ❑ Cholecystectomy for gangrenous cholecystitis ❑ Decortication for empyema

Table 1. Principles of source control

Drainage

The expression of a local host inflammatory response results in the activation of a co-ordinated series of processes that serve to contain an infectious challenge, isolating it from the host through the formation of an *abscess*. The objective of drainage is to convert this localized and well-defined focus of invasive infection into a controlled *sinus* (a communication with an epithelial surface) or *fistula* (an abnormal communication between two epithelially lined surfaces). Once that objective has been satisfactorily accomplished, the residual cavity will contract and obliterate, and the focus of infection will resolve.

Drainage can be accomplished by several approaches; in general, the best approach is that which achieves its objective with the least degree of physiologic upset to the host. Drainage may occur spontaneously, a fact that led surgeons of an earlier era to manage appendiceal abscesses expectantly, awaiting spontaneous drainage into the adjacent rectum [2]. However, expectant management carries the risk that drainage will occur into the peritoneal cavity, and result in generalized peritonitis, rather than externally, or into the gastrointestinal tract. Operative drainage, therefore, has been the standard approach to the treatment of abscesses, and a number of strategies have evolved to drain abscesses in discrete anatomic sites while minimizing the contamination of adjacent uninfected tissues. Recent improvements in diagnostic imaging techniques have permitted percutaneous access to increasingly complex and deep-seated foci of infection, and the approach of the interventional radiologist has become the strategy of choice for the initial management of most abscesses [3].

Debridement and Device Removal

Necrotic tissue serves as an excellent culture medium for microorganisms, providing a source of nutrients, and isolating the organism from host immune cells or circulating antibiotics. Surgical removal of devitalized tissue, a process termed *debridement,* plays an important role in the management of discrete foci of infection. Rapid debridement is critical to the successful management of certain infections such as clostridial myonecrosis in which the infecting organism both proliferates in an anaerobic environment, and produces toxins that promote microvascular thrombosis and tissue destruction. Similarly, intestinal infarction is a devastating disease that is rapidly lethal unless the dead bowel is surgically excised [4]. In other situations, notably infected peripancreatic necrosis, the benefits of removing necrotic tissue must be weighed against the risks of intervention, principally the occurrence of significant bleeding at the interface of viable and non-viable tissues.

The presence of a foreign body contributes to the persistence of infection in two ways [5]. First, certain micro-organisms, for example coagulase-negative *staphylococci*, are able to form biofilms on prosthetic materials, and to establish stable colonies producing a focus of ongoing infection. Second, the presence of a foreign body has been shown to impair local host phagocytic defences, thus favoring microbial proliferation. Removal of a colonized foreign body is important to the achievement of successful source control. For the patient with an infected central venous catheter, removal of the colonized foreign body is curative. However the risks associated with surgical removal of an infected heart valve or intravascular prosthesis are considerable, and justify initial attempts at the non-operative management of endocarditis or prosthetic graft infection.

Definitive Management of Foci of Ongoing Contamination

When infection arises as a consequence of an anatomic breach of the gastrointestinal tract, drainage will create a controlled fistula, however ongoing contamination will occur until the defect is managed definitively. Usually, as in the patient with perforated diverticultis or acute cholecystitis, control necessitates surgical excision of the involved organ. When excision is not possible, further contamination can be minimized by surgical closure of the defect (for example, patch closure of a duodenal perforation) or exclusion of the defect through the creation of a proximal diverting stoma.

ESTABLISHING THE NEED FOR SOURCE CONTROL

Source control measures should be considered an integral component of the management of any localized infectious focus. They also play an unappreciated role in the management of many medical infectious diseases. For example, in the patient with pneumonia, suctioning of tracheal secretions represents a form of debridement, while nursing in the semirecumbent position and elimination of unneeded nasogastric or endotracheal tubes are established preventive measures. Moreover discrete foci of infection - a lung abscess or empyema - may complicate the course of the disease, and necessitate active intervention.

In the initial assessment of the septic patient, therefore, it is crucial to address the need for source control through consideration of a series of questions:
- Is there a discrete focus of infection (for example, a septic arthritis, duodenal perforation, or pneumonia) responsible for the systemic syndrome of sepsis?
- Does the patient have a foreign body (for example, an intravenous catheter, vascular graft, or intraventicular drain) in situ?

- Has there been an anatomic breach of an epithelial surface (for example, traumatic injury to an extremity, perforation of a colonic malignancy, or perforation of an ulcer)?
- Is there dead or ischemic tissue present (for example, intestinal infarction or necrotizing fasciitis)?

In general, the diagnosis of an infection requiring source control can be readily established on the basis of history, physical examination, and appropriate radiographic investigations. The development of ultrasonography and computerized tomography (CT) have revolutionized both the diagnosis and the management of the septic patient with a localized focus of infection, and missed or delayed diagnoses, a relatively common and catastrophic occurrence in the past [6,7], should be largely avoidable.

TIMING OF INTERVENTION

While expeditious intervention is critical to the successful management of life-threatening infection, source control measures rarely form part of the initial resuscitation of the patient. Control of exsanguinating hemorrhage in the patient with a mycotic vascular aneurysm may necessitate surgical intervention to stabilize the patient. More commonly, however, source control measures should be deferred until the patient has been resuscitated and stabilized, and an anatomic diagnosis has been made, events that, even in the most complex patient, can usually be accomplished rapidly. It must be appreciated that transfer to the radiology suite for investigation is potentially risky for the critically ill patient, and that such investigations should only be undertaken following stabilization, and that an intensivist or emergentologist should accompany the patient.

On the other hand, intervention should not be delayed once the patient has been resuscitated, and the anatomic problem defined. Timely intervention is particularly important in the patient with infected necrosis, for example, gangrenous bowel or necrotizing fasciitis [8,9]. Occasionally it will not be possible to stabilize the patient without surgical intervention to control the source of sepsis. Under these circumstances, intervention despite hemodynamic instability may be life-saving, and should not be withheld; if the patent is considered too unstable to transfer to the operating room, surgical intervention to provide temporary control can be undertaken in the intensive care unit (ICU).

The objective of source control in the management of sepsis is to prevent ongoing microbial contamination. Definitive management of the consequences of source control - for example, closure of fistulae, reversal of stomas, or closure of soft tissue defects - should be deferred until the patient has recovered from the acute episode of sepsis.

SOURCE CONTROL IN INFECTIONS COMMONLY CAUSING SEPSIS

Intra-abdominal Infection

Infections within the abdominal cavity arise as a consequence of perforation of the gastrointestinal tract, obstruction of a hollow viscus, ischemia and infarction, bacteremic spread from a distant site, or contamination from the exterior as a result of surgery or trauma.

Primary Peritonitis

In the adult, infection of pre-existing ascites in the patient with advanced liver disease is the most common cause of primary peritonitis [10]. Sterile peritonitis may also arise during the course of inflammatory conditions such as systemic lupus erythematosus. Because there is no distinct locus of bacterial contamination producing the infection, and no localized abscess to drain, source control measures are not indicated.

Gastrointestinal Perforations

Breach of the gastrointestinal tract, resulting, for example, from perforation of a duodenal ulcer or of a sigmoid diverticulum, results in leakage of intestinal contents into the peritoneal cavity. Treatment, therefore, entails drainage of the resulting intraperitoneal collection, and control of the perforation. In the patient with perforated diverticulitis, case series [11-13] and a single randomized trial [14] have shown that outcome is improved if the involved segment of colon is resected at the time of intervention. Usually the proximal end is exteriorized as a colostomy, an operation known as the Hartmann procedure, however several clinical series suggest that primary anastomosis, even in the face of peritoneal inflammation, results in less morbidity [15-17]. If the perforation has created a well-localized peridiverticular abscess, then radiologically-guided percutaneous drainage of the abscess, followed later by definitive resection of the colon is the approach of choice. On the other hand, if free perforation with diffuse peritoneal contamination has occurred, then operative intervention is indicated. Some authors advocate an open abdomen approach, or a policy of planned repeat abdominal exploration [18], however the merits of this more aggressive surgical approach remain unproven [19].

Perforation of a duodenal ulcer is usually managed by laparotomy and drainage, closing the perforation with an omental patch. When ongoing contamination cannot be controlled with an omental patch, diverticularization of the duodenum, by closure of the pylorus, tube drainage of the duodenum and common bile duct, and diversion with a gastrojejunostomy is an option [20]. For the patient with a walled off duodenal perforation, non-operative management awaiting spontaneous drainage into the duodenal lumen is a reasonable approach; surgical intervention is indicated for worsening of clinical status over the first 12 to 24 hours of conservative therapy [21].

Intestinal Ischemia or Infarction

Intestinal ischemia develops as a result of arterial occlusion by embolus or thrombus, venous occlusion by thrombus (typically in association with a hypercoagulable state), intestinal obstruction with vascular occlusion, or splanchnic hypoperfusion [22]. Acute mesenteric ischemia is rapidly lethal unless blood flow is restored, or ischemic and necrotic bowel excised. The history provides important diagnostic information, whereas physical examination is notoriously unreliable. Atrial fibrillation, recent myocardial infraction, or recent aortography suggest arterial embolism, while a history of peripheral vascular disease should suggest a diagnosis of arterial thrombosis, and of venous thrombosis, the possibility of mesenteric venous thrombosis. The classic laboratory manifestations - acidosis and marked leukocytosis - are late phenomena, and generally portend frank intestinal infarction. Transmural intestinal ischemia is an emergency; the diagnosis must be made rapidly, often by exploratory laparotomy, and the underlying problem corrected - by restoring blood flow to ischemic bowel, or excising bowel that is no longer viable. When intestinal viability is uncertain, planned re-exploration in 24 hours is recommended.

Post-operative Peritonitis

Peritonitis developing after an elective abdominal procedure commonly results from an anastomotic leak, a missed or unappreciated intestinal injury, or inadvertent incorporation of a loop of bowel into the abdominal closure. The clinical presentation is often subtle, the earliest manifestations often being unexplained respiratory insufficiency, new onset of a supraventricular arrhythmia, or other evidence of acute organ system dysfunction [23]. The mortality of postoperative peritonitis tends to be high, in part because the diagnosis is delayed [24]. CT scanning is the most effective means of establishing a diagnosis. Re-operation is commonly indicated, although a localized focus of infection, or a contained anastomotic leak can be managed by percutaneous drainage.

Tertiary Peritonitis

Tertiary peritonitis is defined as persistent or recurrent peritonitis developing after apparently adequate treatment of primary or secondary peritonitis. The morbidity and mortality of this condition is substantial, and it is unclear whether outcome can be improved by aggressive source control measures [25-27]. Nonetheless, radiographic diagnosis and subsequent management as suggested by the results is indicated. Blind exploration, in the absence of radiologic evidence of infection, is rarely, if ever, justified [28].

Appendicitis, Cholecystitis, and Cholangitis

Both acute cholecystitis and appendicitis develop as a result of inflammation and bacterial growth in an obstructed hollow viscus. The diagnosis is established by history and physical examination, and confirmed by ultrasound or CT scan. Although both disorders are common, they rarely lead to the severe systemic derangements of sepsis. When they do, emergent operative intervention with excision of the affected organ is usually indicated. In patients with appendicitis, a well-localized appendiceal abscess can be managed by percutaneous drainage, with subsequent interval appendectomy. Similarly, for the unstable or high-risk patient with gangrenous cholecystitis or empyema of the gall bladder, percutaneous cholecystostomy may be the safer initial management option [29]. As discussed earlier, the initial objective of therapy is to convert an infection evolving in an enclosed space (the lumen of the appendix or gall bladder) into a controlled fistula. Percutaneous drainage accomplishes this objective with minimal morbidity, at the cost, however, of leaving injured, ischemic, or necrotic tissue *in situ*.

Bacterial cholangitis results from bacterial proliferation in an obstructed common bile duct. The classical features of Charcot's triad (jaundice, right upper quadrant pain, and fever and chills) or, in more severe cases, Reynold's pentad (Charcot's triad plus hypotension and mental changes) are commonly present, and the diagnosis is established by ultrasound examination revealing dilatation of the common bile duct [30]. Because of the elevated pressures within the bile duct, blood cultures are frequently positive. Although antibiotics can provide early improvement, source control measures to decompress the obstructed bile duct should be undertaken emergently. Endoscopic retrograde cholangiopancreatography (ERCP) permits both extraction of the obstructing stone, and decompression of the bile duct, and is the therapy of choice, when it is available [31,32]. Percutaneous transhepatic cholangiography in the radiology suite is an alternative, however it necessitates leaving a percutaneous drain in place, and is less effective in removing the cause of the obstruction. Surgical intervention consists of common bile duct exploration with stone removal and tube drainage of the common bile duct; its role has diminished with the more widespread availability of ERCP or percutaneous cholangiography.

Infected Pancreatic Necrosis

Evolving approaches to the management of the patient with infected peripancreatic necrosis derive from the principles of source control enunciated earlier in this chapter. On the one hand, infection and tissue necrosis suggest the need for urgent surgical intervention; on the other, the risks of such intervention - bleeding from inflamed tissue with poorly demarcated margins - may be substantial. A randomized trial of the timing of surgery in patients with infected pancreatic necrosis showed that outcome is improved when surgery is delayed [33], and current practice is to defer intervention in the hemodynamically stable patient until adequate demarcation of viable and non-viable tissues has occurred, usually a minimum of three to four weeks following the onset of the episode of pancreatitis [34].

Urinary Tract Infections

Uncomplicated cystitis is an uncommon cause of sepsis, although the physiologic sequelae of lower urinary tract infection are often more severe in the patient with paraplegia or quadriplegia. Colonization of an indwelling urinary catheter commonly contributes to persistent infection, and removal of the catheter is an important aspect of source control for cystitis.

Pyelonephritis resulting from obstruction of the upper urinary tract typically responds to systemic antibiotic therapy, however definitive management requires relief of the urinary tract obstruction, initially by percutaneous nephrostomy [35], and definitively by relief of the obstruction.

Skin and Soft Tissue Infections

In the absence of tissue necrosis, infections of the skin and subcutaneous tissues are well controlled with antibiotics alone. However necrotizing soft tissue infections are life threatening, and prognosis is directly related to the rapidity with which necrotic tissue is debrided surgically. Establishing the presence of tissue necrosis can be difficult. Necrotizing fasciitis characteristically arises in a patient with compromised host defenses secondary to diabetes, malnutrition, obesity, cirrhosis, or renal failure, although group A streptococcal infections and clostridial myonecrosis show no such selectivity, and arise in otherwise healthy patients. Physical examination usually reveals some degree of erythema or discoloration of the overlying skin, and in the case of Fournier's gangrene of the scrotum, a small area of skin necrosis. However the process is often much more extensive in the deeper tissues, and the extent of tissue necrosis is best established by surgical exploration under general anesthesia.

Management consists of rapid operative debridement, excising necrotic tissues back until healthy bleeding tissue is encountered [8,36]. It is frequently difficult to assess the extent of tissue necrosis, and a policy of planned daily re-exploration is often advisable. Amputation of an extremity is occasionally indicated, particularly if the extent of debridement of necrotic muscle is such that function is lost. However, for most patients with necrotizing fasciitis, muscle involvement is minimal, and the limb can be spared.

Bacteremia and Endovascular Infection

Although bacteremia has classically been considered a hallmark of disseminated and uncontrolled infection, in the septic critically ill patient, it often reflects infection of an intravascular device, most commonly a central venous catheter. If that foreign body is a central venous or pulmonary artery catheter, removal is both simple and curative. Tunneled central venous lines pose a somewhat more difficult decision, as do catheter infections in the patient with limited venous access, since their removal risks loss of vascular access; a trial of systemic antibiotics alone is indicated. Similarly, in the patient with a vascular graft infection or endocarditis, removal of the infected foreign body necessitates a major operation and its attendant risks [37]. Initial management is usually conservative, with surgery indicated for persistent non-resolving infection, hemodynamic compromise, or, in the case of an infected vascular graft, the risk of uncontrolled hemorrhage [38].

Intrathoracic Infections

Empyema

Infection of the pleural cavity is diagnosed by CT, and confirmed by demonstration of white cells and organisms in the pleural fluid. If the empyema contents are liquid, and there has been minimal fibrotic reaction around the infectious focus, tube thoracostomy alone can result in resolution of the empyema [39]. Open drainage is indicated for infections that have become organised, while surgical decortication may be required when the fibrotic abscess cavity prevents re-expansion of the underlying lung [40,41].

Mediastinitis

Infection within the mediastinum can result from inferior tracking of infection in the head and neck, from perforation of the esophagus, or following mediastinal surgery. Source control management consists of drainage of defined collections, usually operatively, debridement of necrotic mediastinal tissues, and control of the source of the perforation by resection, repair, or proximal diversion [42,43].

Septic Arthritis

Source control measures for infections arising within a joint space include repeated transcutaneous aspiration, or, occasionally, operative drainage with joint debridement. When the infection involves a prosthetic joint, removal of the foreign body is indicated for definitive control [44].

Infections of the Central Nervous System

Source control measures are indicated for patients with meningitis secondary to infection of an intracranial pressure monitoring device or other foreign body. Epidural abscesses are an uncommon cause of sepsis, but when they occur, drainage must be instituted.

CONCLUSION

There are few rigorous studies of the role of source control, or of the relative advantages of differing approaches, for example, the merits of operative versus percutaneous drainage, or of open abdomen approaches in comparison to more conservative kinds of intervention. The reasons for this lack of strong data are numerous, and include the inherent difficulties in standardizing approaches in complex infections, and the relative rarity of the conditions involved. In general, the best approach is that which accomplishes the objectives of drainage, device removal, debridement, and definitive control with the least degree of physiologic risk to the patient. On the other hand, for the patient whose instability arises form uncontrolled infection, intervention as a heroic and life-saving measure should not be withheld.

Successful source control usually results in resolution of the clinical manifestations of sepsis; conversely, their persistence or recurrence, or the development of new organ dysfunction, should suggest the need for further intervention and prompt appropriate investigation and therapy.

REFERENCES

1. Marshall JC, Lowry SF. Evaluation of the adequacy of source control in clinical trials in sepsis. In: Clinical Trials for the Treatment of Sepsis. Sibbald WJ, Vincent JL (eds) Springer-Verlag, 1995; 327-344
2. Nitecki S, Assalia A, Schein M. Contemporary management of the appendiceal mass. Br J Surg 1993; 80:18-20
3. Montgomery RS, Wilson SE. Intraabdominal abscesses: image-guided diagnosis and therapy. Clin Infect Dis 1996; 23:28-36
4. Montgomery RA, Venbrux AC, Bulkley GB. Mesenteric vascular insufficiency. Curr.Prob.Surg. 1997; 34:941-1025
5. Dougherty SH. Pathobiology of infection in prosthetic devices. Rev Infect Dis 1988; 10:1102-1117
6. Volk HC, Shields CL. Remote organ failure: a valid sign of occult intraabdominal infection. Surgery 1977; 81:310-313
7. Fry DE, Pearlstein L, Fulton RL, Polk HC. Multiple system organ failure. The role of uncontrolled infection. Arch Surg 1980; 115:136-140

8. Bilton BD, Zibari GB, McMillan RW, Aultman DF, Dunn G, McDonald JC. Aggressive surgical management of necrotizing fasciitis serves to decrease mortality: A retrospective study. Am Surg 1998; 64:397-400
9. Moss RL, Musemeche CA, Kosloske AM. Necrotizing fasciitis in children: prompt recognition and aggressive therapy improve survival. J Pediatr Surg 1996; 31:1142-1146
10. Crossley IR, Williams R. Spontaneous bacterial peritonitis. Gut 1985; 26:325-331
11. Tucci G, Torquati A, Grande M, Stroppa I, Siaesi M, Farinon AM. Major acute inflammatory complications of diverticular disease of the colon: planning of surgical treatment. Hepatogastroenterology 1996; 43:839-845
12. Finlay IG, Carter DC. A comparison of emergency resection and staged management in perforated diverticular disease. Dis Col Rect 1987; 30:929-933
13. Nagorney DM, Adson MA, Pemberton JH. Sigmoid diverticulitis with perforation and generalized peritonitis. Dis Col Rect 1985; 28:71-75
14. Kronborg O. Treatment of perforated sigmoid diverticulitis: a prospective randomized trial. Br J Surg 1993; 80:505-507
15. Umbach TW, Dorazio RA. Primary resection and anastomosis for perforated left colon lesions. Am Surg 1999; 65:931-933
16. Saccomani GE, Santi F, Gramegna A. Primary resection with and without anastomosis for perforation of acute diverticulitis. Acta Chir Belg 1993; 93:169-172
17. Alanis A, Papanicolaou GK, Tadros RR, Fielding LP. Primary resection and anastomosis for treatment of acute diverticulitis. Dis Col Rect 1989; 21:933-939
18. Wittmann DH, Aprahamian C, Bergstein JM: Etappenlavage. Avanced diffuse peritonitis managed by planned multiple laparotomies utilizing zippers, slide fastener, and velcro analogue for temporary abdominal closure. World J Surg 1990; 14:218-226
19. Christou NV, Barie PS, Dellinger EP, Waymack JP, Stone HH. Surgical Infection Society intra-abdominal infection study. Prospective evaluation of management techniques and outcome. Arch Surg 1993; 128:193-198
20. Ivatury RR, Nassoura ZE, Simon RJ, Rodriguez A. Complex duodenal injuries. Surg Clin North Am 1996; 76:797-812
21. Crofts TJ, Park KG, Steele RJ, Chung SS, Li AK. A randomized trial of nonoperative treatment for perforated peptic ulcer. N Engl J Med 1989; 321:970-973
22. Kaleya RN, Boley SJ. Acute mesenteric ischemia. Crit Care Clin 1995; 11:479-512
23. Fry DE, Garrison RN, Heitsch RC, Calhoun K, Polk HC. Determinants of death in patients with intraabdominal abscess. Surgery 1980; 88:517-523
24. Bohnen J, Boulanger M, Meakins JL, Mclean APH. Prognosis in generalized peritonitis. Relation to cause and risk factors. Arch Surg 1983; 118:285-290
25. Rotstein OD, Pruett TL, Simmons RL. Microbiologic features and treatment of persistent peritonitis in patients in the intensive care unit. Can J Surg 1986; 29:247-250
26. Nathens AB, Rotstein OD, Marshall JC. Tertiary peritonitis: Clinical features of a complex nosocomial infection. World J Surg 1998; 22:158-163
27. Anderson ID, Fearon KC, Grant IS. Laparotomy for abdominal sepsis in the critically ill. Br J Surg 1996; 83:535-539
28. Bunt TJ. Non-directed relaparotomy for intraabdominal sepsis: a futile procedure. Am Surg 1986; 52:294-298
29. Lillemoe KD. Surgical treatment of biliary tract infections. Am Surg 2000; 66:138-144
30. Hanau LH, Steigbigel NH. Cholangitis: Pathogenesis, diagnosis, and treatment. Curr Clin Top Infect Dis 1995; 15:153-178
31. Boender J, Nix GA, de Ridder MA, et al. Endoscopic sphincterotomy and biliary drainage in patients with cholangitis due to common bile duct stones. Am J Gastroenterol 1995; 90:233-238

32. Lau JY, Chung SC, Leung JW, Ling TK, Yung MY, Li AK. Endoscopic drainage aborts endotoxemia in acute cholangitis. Br J Surg 1996; 83:181-184
33. Mier J, Leon EL, Castillo A, Robledo F, Blanco R. Early versus late necrosectomy in severe necrotizing pancreatitis. Am J Surg 1997; 173:71-75
34. Urbach DR, Marshall JC. Pancreatic abscess and infected pancreatic necrosis. Curr Opin Surg Infect 1996; 4:57-66
35. Watson RA, Esposito M, Richter F, Irwin RJJr, Lang EK. Percutaneous nephrostomy as adjunct management in advanced upper urinary tract infection. Urology 1999; 54:234-239
36. Freischlag JA, Ajalat G, Busuttil RW. Treatment of necrotizing soft tissue infections. A need for a new approach. Am J Surg 1985; 149:751-755
37. Blaustein AS, Lee JR. Indications for and timing of surgical intervention in infective endocarditis. Cardiol Clin 1996; 14:393-404
38. Calligaro KD, DeLaurentis DA, Veith FJ. An overview of the treatment of infected prosthetic vascular grafts. Adv Surg 1996; 29:3-16
39. Ulmer JL, Choplin RH, Reed JC. Image-guided catheter drainage of the infected pleural space. J Thorac Imag 1991; 6:65-73
40. Martella AT, Santos GH. Decortication for chronic postpneumonic empyema. J Am Coll Surg 1995; 180:573-576
41. Ferguson DK. Surgical management of intrapleural infections. Semin Respir Infect 1999; 14:73-81
42. Marty-Ane CH, Berthet JP, Alric P, Pegis JD, Rouviere P, Mary H. Management of descending necrotizing mediastinitis: an aggressive treatment for an aggressive disease. Ann Thorac Surg 1999; 68:212-217
43. Cherveniakov A, Cherveniakov P. Surgical gtreatment of acute purulent mediastinitis. Eur J CardioThorac Surg 1992; 6:407-410
44. Donatto KC. Orthopedic management of septic arthritis. Rheum Dis Clin North Am 1998; 24:275-286

31

EMPIRICAL ANTIBIOTIC THERAPY FOR PATIENTS WITH SEVERE SEPSIS AND SEPTIC SHOCK

Pierre-Yves Bochud
Michel P. Glauser
Jean Carlet
Thierry Calandra

Treatment of patients with sepsis necessitates a multifaceted approach combining the use of optimal diagnostic tools, prompt initiation of appropriate antimicrobial therapy, and adequate supportive care. Antimicrobial therapy is the basis of the treatment of the septic patient, but whenever indicated drainage of abscesses and removal of infected necrotic tissues or prosthetic material is also essential for recovery. Several recent articles and other chapters of this book have reviewed different aspects of the management of patients with severe sepsis and septic shock [1-3]. In the present chapter we will focus our attention on antimicrobial therapy.

Two striking observations were made when reviewing the literature on this topic. One was the lack of unifying definitions for the terms bacteremia, septicemia, severe sepsis or septic shock, that were often used interchangeably. Although not flawless, the definitions of the Consensus Conference of the American College of Chest Physicians and the Society of Critical Care Medicine published in 1992 have contributed to group patients into categories according to the severity of disease [4]. The other observation was the limited number of large studies on the efficacy and safety of various antimicrobial regimens in septic patients without neutropenia. While the original studies performed in the 1960s and 1970s included a majority of non-neutropenic patients [5,6], most recent studies on antibiotic therapy have been conducted in neutropenic cancer patients. Treatment recommendations for patients with severe sepsis and septic shock have been based primarily on the results of multicenter studies performed in neutropenic cancer patients treated with extended-spectrum penicillins, third- or fourth-generation cephalosporins, or carbapenem antibiotics [7,8]. However, critically ill septic patients differ considerably from neutropenic cancer patients. For example, capillary leak syndrome and multi-organ dysfunction are much more frequent in patients with severe sepsis or septic shock than in neutropenic cancer patients. These conditions are likely to have profound effects on the volume of distribution and turn-over of the antibiotics, altering the pharmacokinetic profile, which ultimately may affect both the efficacy and the toxicity of the agents used. Thus, treatment guidelines derived from observations made in the neutropenic host may not apply to patients with severe sepsis or septic shock. Therefore, the pharmacokinetic profile, efficacy and toxicity of new antibiotics should also be assessed in large, prospective, randomized trials performed in patients with severe sepsis and septic shock.

EPIDEMIOLOGY

The monitoring of bloodstream infections by surveillance networks provides a critical source of information on which to base epidemiological studies of patients with sepsis [9]. A recent report of the National Nosocomial Infection Surveillance (NNIS) in the United States has revealed a significant change in the proportion of bloodstream infections caused by Gram-negative and by Gram-positive bacteria. Whereas Gram-negative bacteria were predominant in the 1960s and early 1970s, the frequency of Gram-positive bacteremia has increased during the last two decades [10]. However, even though blood cultures are positive in only 30-40 % of patients with severe sepsis and septic shock, it is likely that the shift observed for bloodstream infections also reflects changes occurring at the primary site of infection. In a recent study, coagulase-negative staphylococci were the most frequent blood isolates (38 %), but were considered to be the causative agent of sepsis in only 12 % of the cases [11].

We have analyzed microbiological data from 27 clinical trials of different anti-inflammatory and immunomodulatory agents and three epidemiological studies [12]. Most of these articles used standard definitions of severe sepsis and septic shock and provided comparable clinical and microbiological data. A pathogen was identified in 72 % of 8097 episodes of sepsis and blood cultures were positive in 34 % of the cases. Consistent with the results obtained in the NNIS survey, Gram-negative organisms were responsible for a majority of severe infections in studies performed in the 1960s and 70s, while Gram-positive organisms have increased considerably in the last decade (Figure 1). In some studies, Gram-positive bacteria were even more frequent than Gram-negative bacteria.

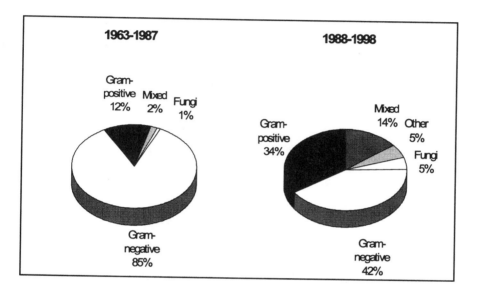

Figure 1. Etiology of infections in patients with severe sepsis and septic shock [12].

The number of fungal infections is also increasing. *Candida* was the fourth most common isolate in all recent US studies of nosocomial bloodstream infections [13], outnumbering all Gram-negative bacteria [14]. The pathogens isolated most frequently from the blood of patients with severe sepsis and septic shock are reported in Table 1.

There has also been a change in the relative frequency of the primary sites of infection in the last decade (Figure 2). For over two decades, the abdominal cavity and the urinary tract were the most frequent sites of infections. Recent studies have shown that lung infections are now predominant, followed by infections of the bloodstream, the abdominal cavity and the urinary tract.

Organism	Number/total
Escherichia coli	13%
Staphylococcus aureus	12%
Klebsiella species	8%
Pseudomonas aeruginosa	8%
Enterococcus species	8%
Coagulase-negative staphylococci	7%
Enterobacter species	5%
Fungi	5%
Streptococcus pneumoniae	4%
Anaerobes	2%

Table 1. *Pathogens most commonly isolated from patients with severe sepsis and septic shock (1988-1998) [12].*

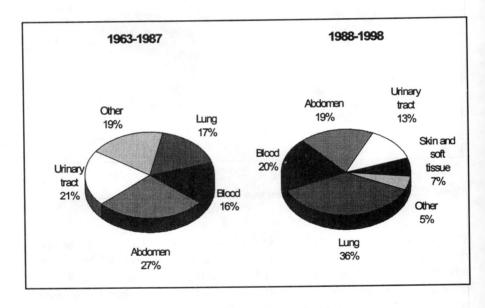

Figure 2. *Sites of infections in patients with severe sepsis and septic shock [12]*

ROLE OF ANTIBIOTICS IN SEVERE SEPSIS

Retrospective studies performed in the 1960s and in the 1970s showed that appropriate antimicrobial therapy reduced the mortality of patients with Gram-negative sepsis. In 173 patients with Gram-negative bacteremia, appropriate antibiotic therapy, defined as the use of at least one antibiotic active *in vitro* against the causative bacteria, was observed to reduce mortality from 48 to 22 % [15]. Three subsequent studies gave similar results [16-18]. In a recent prospective study of 2124 patients with Gram-negative bacteremia, mortality was 34 % in 670 patients given inappropriate antibiotics, whereas it was 18 % in 1454 patients who had received appropriate antibiotics (p<0.0001) [19]. Similar results were obtained in a prospective observational study of 129 adults with *Enterobacter* species bacteremia [20]. In a prospective study evaluating 189 episodes of *P. aeruginosa* bacteremia, the appropriateness of the antibiotics influenced the outcome, since 24 of 170 subjects receiving appropriate treatment died (14 %) as compared to 10 of 19 who received inappropriate treatment (54 %, p<0.001) [21]. A case-control study compared 31 patients with ceftazidime-resistant *K. pneumonia* or *E. coli* bacteremia to 31 control patients with ceftazidime-sensitive *K. pneumoniae* or *E. coli* [22]. Of the 19 patients who received appropriate therapy within three days of the onset of bacteremia, only one died of sepsis (5 %) compared to five of 12 patients who received inappropriate antibiotics (42 %, p=0.02).

Very few data have been published on the impact of appropriate antibiotic therapy in patients with Gram-positive sepsis. Recently, three studies evaluated the advantage of appropriate antimicrobial therapy in patients with Gram-negative and Gram-positive bacteremias [11,23,24]. In a prospective cohort study, 436 of 2158 (20 %) patients with bloodstream infections given appropriate antibiotics died, compared to 432 of 1255 (34 %) patients given inappropriate treatment (p<0.001) [23]. Even in the subset of patients with septic shock, the fatality rate was lower in subjects given appropriate antibiotics (148/199, 74 %) than in those given inappropriate treatment (127/154, 83 %, p=0.07). The highest benefit of antimicrobial therapy was observed for patients with infections due to *K. pneumoniae* and *Strep. pneumoniae*. Weinstein et al. reviewed 843 episodes of bloodstream infection in 707 patients. The most common organisms were *Staph. aureus*, *E. coli*, coagulase-negative staphylococci, *K. pneumoniae* and enterococci [11]. The mortality rate was 10.5 % (65/620) among patients who received appropriate antibiotics throughout the course of infection. In contrast, the mortality rate was 13.3 % (6/45, relative risk 1.27 when compared with patients treated with appropriate antibiotics) among patients who received inappropriate empirical antibiotics initially followed by appropriate antibiotics upon identification of the pathogen and susceptibility testing. A small group of patients who received inappropriate antibiotics throughout the follow-up had a mortality of 33 % (3/9, relative risk 3.18). A multivariate analysis showed that inappropriate antibiotic therapy was an independent risk factor for death.

In a prospective surveillance study, 492 patients with a bloodstream infection were identified among 4913 patients hospitalized in a medical and surgical intensive care unit [24]. The mortality rate for patients receiving adequate antimicrobial treatment was statistically lower than that of patients receiving inadequate antimicrobial therapy (12 vs. 30 %, p<0.001). Multivariate analysis of risk factors demonstrated that inadequate antimicrobial treatment was the most important risk factor for hospital mortality (p<0.001).

Similar results have been obtained for patients with fungal infections. The occurrence of candidemia is also associated with high morbidity and mortality. In a multicenter, prospective observational study of 427 patients with candidemia, antifungal therapy significantly reduced mortality [25]. The mortality rate was 27 % in 369 patients who received antifungal therapy compared to 74 % in 58 who did not. This beneficial effect of therapy remained even when patients were stratified according to severity of illness, underlying disease or *Candida* species.

ANTIMICROBIAL THERAPY

Historical Background

Having shown that early, appropriate antibiotic therapy improved the outcome of patients with Gram-negative sepsis, clinical investigators then examined whether therapy with two, instead of one, active antibiotics (usually a beta-lactam plus an aminoglycoside) would further improve patient survival. The rationale for the use of a combination of antimicrobial agents relies on three main considerations summarized in Table 2, which have been challenged with the advent of the newest broad-spectrum antibiotics.

Two clinical studies failed to demonstrate the advantage of combination therapy versus monotherapy for patients with Gram-negative bacteremias [5,6]. However, subgroup analyses revealed a benefit of combination therapy in patients with severe underlying conditions (i.e., rapidly or ultimately fatal diseases) [6], and when the synergistic effect of the two antimicrobial agents could be demonstrated *in vitro* [5].

Despite the absence of definite evidence supporting the use of combination therapy over monotherapy, for many years the association of a beta-lactam agent and an aminoglycoside was considered to be standard empirical treatment of severe sepsis and septic shock. Different antibiotic combinations with a beta-lactam agent (i.e., penicillin, carbenicillin, mezlocillin or ceftazidime) and an aminoglycoside (i.e., amikacin, sisomycin or isepamycin) were shown to be equally efficacious for the treatment of Gram-negative infections [35-37]. Some investigators even evaluated combinations of three rather than two antibiotics [38]. Yet, triple therapy did not improve outcome further and was associated with an increased frequency of adverse events.

Pro	Con
1. Combination therapy offers a broader antimicrobial spectrum: - pathogens are not yet identified when the treatment is initiated - polymicrobial infections may occur	1. Newer broad-spectrum antibiotics (i.e., carbapenems, extended-spectrum penicillins, or third-and fourth-generation cephalosporins) offer adequate empirical treatment for most pathogens
2. Additive or synergistic antibiotic effect - may be associated with improved clinical response [26] - may allow to reduce the dosage of the most toxic drug [27]	2. Newer broad spectrum antibiotics - have a high bactericidal activity - are less toxic than aminoglycoside-containing combination therapy [28-31]
3. Combination therapy may prevent the emergence of resistance and/or superinfections [32]	3. Emergence of resistance or superinfections does not occur more frequently in patients treated with monotherapy [28-30,33,34]

Table 2. Arguments in favor of, and against, the use of antibiotic combinations

Monotherapy versus Combination Therapy

Over the last 15 to 20 years, broad-spectrum and highly bactericidal antibiotics with an excellent safety profile, such as the extended-spectrum penicillins, third- or fourth-generation cephalosporins, and the carbapenems have become available, invalidating most of the arguments supporting the use of aminoglycoside-containing regimens (Table 2).

Carbapenems

Three prospective trials evaluated the efficacy of a carbapenem (i.e., imipenem or meropenem) to that of a combination of a third-generation cephalosporin and amikacin in patients with severe sepsis and septic shock [33,34,39]. Similar results were obtained in all these studies in terms of clinical efficacy and mortality (Table 3). Of note, in all but one study different beta-lactams were used in the two treatment arms, which makes it difficult to evaluate the true impact of the addition of an aminoglycoside. In the study that compared imipenem monotherapy to the combination of imipenem plus netilmicin, both regimens were shown to be equally efficacious, but the aminoglycoside-containing regimen was more nephrotoxic [28].

	Mouton et al. 1990 [33]	Cometta et al. 1994 [28]	Solberg et al. 1995 [34]	Mouton et al. 1995 [39]
Number of patients	140	280	153	237
Treatment	Imipenem vs. cefotaxime + amikacin	Imipenem vs. imipenem + netilmicin	Meropenem vs. ceftazidime +/- amikacin	Meropenem vs. Ceftazidime + amikacin
Clinical success	=	=	=	=
Overall mortality	n.a.	n.a.	n.a.	=
Mortality due to infection	=	=	n.a.	n.a.
Eradication of primary pathogen	=	n.a.	n.a.	=
Relapse of infection	n.a.	n.a.	=	=
Superinfections	=	=	=	n.a.
Nephrotoxicity	=	<	n.a.	n.a.

=: not statistically different; <: less frequent in monotherapy arm, n.a. : not available

***Table 3.** Studies comparing monotherapy with a carbapenem to a combination of a beta-lactam and an aminoglycoside.*

One of the arguments supporting the use of antibiotic combinations is that combination therapy may prevent the emergence of resistance and/or the occurrence of superinfections. Interestingly, the rate of superinfections was not increased in patients receiving monotherapy [28,33,34]. Moreover, the addition of netilmicin to imipenem did not prevent the emergence of imipenem-resistant *Pseudomonas aeruginosa* [28].

Third- or Fourth-generation Cephalosporins

Five prospective randomized studies have compared the efficacy and safety of treatment with third-generation cephalosporin or with combination therapy in patients with severe sepsis (Table 4) [29-31,40,41].

	Oblinger et al. 1982 [29]	Arich et al. 1987 [30]	White et al. 1989 [40]	Extermann et al. 1995 [41]	McCormick et al. 1997 [42]
Number of patients	97	47	161	128	128
Treatment	Moxalactam vs. conventional therapy	Cefotaxime vs. cefazolin + tobramycin	Ceftazidime vs. doxycycline + chloramph. + TMT/SMX	Ceftazidime vs. "best guess" combination	Ceftazidime vs. mezlocilin + netilmicin
Clinical success	=	=	n.a.	=	=
Overall mortality	=	=	<	=	=
Mortality due to infection	=	n.a.	n.a.	=	n.a.
Eradication of primary pathogen	n.a.	n.a.	n.a.	=	n.a.
Relapse of infection	n.a.	n.a.	=	n.a.	n.a.
Superinfections	=	=	n.a.	n.a.	n.a.
Nephrotoxicity	<	<	n.a.	n.a.	<

=: *Not statistically different;* <: *less frequent in monotherapy arm, n.a.: not available; chloramph.:chloramphenicol, TMT/SMX= trimethoprim/sulfamethoxazole.*

Table 4. *Studies comparing monotherapy with a third-generation cephalosporin to combination therapy.*

However, two of these studies included patients with specific clinical conditions: one study was performed in cirrhotic patients [31] and the other in patients with severe melioidosis [40]. In two studies, patients receiving monotherapy with a cephalosporin were compared to a group of patients treated with different combinations of antibiotics [29,41], which made it difficult to compare the results obtained in the various treatment groups. In all but one of these studies [40], clinical success and mortality rates were similar in both treatment arms. For the treatment of patients with severe melioidosis, ceftazidime monotherapy was associated with a 50% reduction in mortality when compared to combination therapy (74 versus 34%, p=0.009). The most striking observation in all these studies was the fact that monotherapy was associated with a significantly lower nephrotoxicity than aminoglycoside-containing antibiotic combinations [29-31].

Extended-spectrum Penicillins

Extended-spectrum penicillins combined with beta-lactamase inhibitors have a broad spectrum of activity encompassing most bacterial pathogens implicated in severe sepsis, including Gram-negative aerobic bacilli, Gram-positive cocci and anaerobes. Piperacillin/tazobactam monotherapy has been shown to be effective for the treatment of febrile, neutropenic cancer patients [42] and patients with suspected peritonitis [43-45] or with nosocomial pneumonia [46]. However, only two randomized, prospective studies were identified that compared extended-spectrum penicillin monotherapy with combination therapy in patients with severe sepsis. In the first study, 396 premature neonates at risk of early onset sepsis were treated with piperacillin or with ampicillin plus amikacin. Mortality rates were similar in both treatment groups (8.5% and 13.8%) [47], suggesting that piperacillin was as efficacious as combination therapy for the empirical therapy of sepsis in premature newborns. In the other study, piperacillin/tazobactam monotherapy was compared to piperacillin/tazobactam plus amikacin for the treatment of 227 patients with severe peritonitis [48]. More than half of the patients entered in this French multicenter trial had severe sepsis according to standard definitions [4]. Clinical success and mortality rates were equivalent in the two treatment arms, suggesting that piperacillin/tazobactam monotherapy is effective in the treatment of severe abdominal sepsis.

Monobactams

Aztreonam is a monobactam antibiotic that is active only against Gram-negative aerobes. In a small randomized study, aztreonam was shown to be as efficacious as monotherapy with aminoglycosides for the treatment of microbiologically proven or clinically suspected Gram-negative infections [49]. Superinfections with *Enterococcus faecalis* were more frequent in patients treated with aztreonam than in those treated with aminoglycosides. In a multicenter study, aztreonam monotherapy was associated with a higher clinical cure rate than amikacin given either alone or in combination with a broad-spectrum beta-lactam [50]. These studies thus suggested that aztreonam was an effective treatment of documented Gram-negative infection. However, aztreonam monotherapy should not be used as empirical therapy in patients with severe sepsis or septic shock, since it is devoid of activity against Gram-positive bacteria.

Single Antibiotic Therapy

Three studies have compared the efficacy and safety of different third- and fourth-generation cephalosporins in patients with severe sepsis [51-53]. Clinical success and mortality rates were similar among patients treated with ceftazidime, cefpirome or cefepime (Table 5).

	Hartenauer et al. 1990 [54]	Norrby et al. 1993 [51]	Schrank et al. 1995 [52]	Norrby et al. 1998 [53]
Number of patients	45	224	28	372
Treatment	Ceftazidime vs. imipenem	Cefpirome vs. ceftazidime	Cefepime vs. ceftazidime	Cefpirome vs. ceftazidime
Clinical success	=	=	=	=
Overall mortality	n.a.	=	=	=
Infection related mortality	n.a.	n.a.	n.a.	n.a.
Eradication of pathogen	=	=	n.a.	=
Relapse of infection	=	=	n.a.	=
Superinfection	n.a.	=	n.a.	n.a.

=: not statistically different; < : less frequent in monotherapy arm, n.a. : not available

Table 5. *Studies comparing monotherapy with a carbapenem or a third- or fourth- generation cephalosporin.*

In a small prospective trial, imipenem was shown to be as effective as ceftazidime for the empirical treatment of patients with severe pneumonias or bacteremias [54]. Third- and fourth-generation cephalosporins and carbapenem antibiotics appear to be equally effective as empirical therapy for severe sepsis. Piperacillin/tazobactam monotherapy was as effective as monotherapy with imipenem for the treatment of 371 patients with nosocomial pneumonia or peritonitis [46]. However, a significant proportion of the patients recruited in this study did not have severe sepsis or septic shock. Ciprofloxacin therapy has been shown to be as efficacious as several beta-lactam agents (administered either alone or in combination with aminoglycosides) for the treatment of severe infections [55]. However, there was a great diversity in antibiotics used (aztreonam, ceftazidime, ticarcillin-clavulanate or imipenem), which limits the impact of this study [55]. Whereas first-generation fluoroquinolones, such as ciprofloxacin and norfloxacin, exert limited activity against Gram-positive organisms, the newest fluoroquinolones have a broader spectrum of activity covering most Gram-positive organisms. Further studies are needed to evaluate the role of these new quinolones (i.e., levofloxacin, gatifloxacin and moxifloxacin) in non-neutropenic patients with severe sepsis.

GLYCOPEPTIDE ANTIBIOTICS FOR THE TREATMENT OF GRAM-POSITIVE INFECTIONS

As discussed previously, half of the infections associated with severe sepsis or septic shock are caused by Gram-positive bacteria. In some centers, a majority of staphylococcal infections are caused by methicillin-resistant *Staphylococcus aureus* (MRSA) or coagulase-negative staphylococci. Moreover, penicillin-resistant pneumococci are increasing in many regions of the world. To what extent does this epidemiological context justify a liberal use of glycopeptide antibiotics (i.e., vancomycin or teicoplanin)? The question of the role of glycopeptide antibiotics has been addressed in neutropenic cancer patients, in whom coagulase-negative staphylococci and viridans streptococci are leading bacterial pathogens. While some studies have suggested that the addition of vancomycin or teicoplanin at the initiation of empirical therapy is preferable, others have not supported this concept. Although there may still be some controversy as to the place of glycopeptides in the management of neutropenic cancer patients, it appears that there is no need for up-front use of glycopeptide antibiotics in the majority of febrile neutropenic cancer patients. In contrast to the cancer patient, no study has examined prospectively whether adding a glycopeptide antibiotic to the empirical antibiotic regimen would improve the outcome of patients with severe sepsis. What recommendations can be made in the absence of relevant studies? The indiscriminate use of glycopeptide antibiotics for presumed Gram-positive infections in patients with severe sepsis or septic should be strongly discouraged. Yet, treatment with glycopeptides is appropriate in critically ill patients who present with catheter-related infections and who are hospitalized in centers with a high prevalence of MRSA infections. One also should emphasize that glycopeptide monotherapy will hardly ever be appropriate in severely ill septic patients, as anti-Gram-negative coverage is indicated until results of microbiological cultures are available. These recommendations are in agreement with the guidelines of the CDC which suggest that vancomycin is appropriate for the treatment of severe documented infections caused by beta-lactam–resistant Gram-positive microorganisms [56]. The clinical gain associated with the empirical use of vancomycin or teicoplanin should be balanced against the risk of increased toxicity, especially nephrotoxicity when these agents are used in combination with aminoglycosides, or the emergence of glycopeptide-resistant microorganisms, particularly enterococci [57,58]. To help minimize these risks, empirical glycopeptides should be discontinued in patients in whom beta-lactam–resistant Gram-positive infections have been ruled out.

ANTIFUNGALS FOR THE TREATMENT OF CANDIDA INFECTIONS

Candida has emerged as an increasingly frequent cause of bloodstream infections, especially in ICU patients, and is associated with severe morbidity and a high mortality [59]. However, the proportion of bloodstream infections due to *Candida* varies in different areas of the world. *Candida* is the fourth most common cause of bloodstream infections in the US [13], but is much less common in Europe. Recent epidemiological studies have revealed that fungi accounted for only 2-6 % of all cases of severe sepsis and septic shock [60,61]. Therefore, *Candida* are responsible for only a small number of infections and antifungal agents should not be used on a routine basis in patients with severe sepsis and septic shock. Another argument in favor of the cautious use of antifungal agents of the azole class is the observation of an increased proportion of non-albicans *Candida* infections with reduced sensitivities to azoles in patients who have been exposed previously to fluconazole [62].

The efficacy and safety of fluconazole and amphotericin B for the treatment of candidemia was compared in three prospective [63-65] and two observational studies [25,66]. Overall mortality rates were similar in patients treated with fluconazole or with amphotericin B, but fewer cases of renal failure, hypokalemia, fever and chills occurred with fluconazole than with amphotericin B. According to the practice guidelines of the Infectious Diseases Society of America and a report of an International Conference for the Development of a Consensus on the Management and Prevention of Severe Candidal Infections, fluconazole is an appropriate treatment option for the initial management of clinically stable patients with candidemia, who have not been treated recently with azoles and who are likely to be infected with a sensitive *Candida* strain [67]. However, most experts would use amphotericin B for the treatment of clinically unstable patients infected with an isolate of unknown species. Treatment may then be adjusted based on the identification of the *Candida* species and the results of susceptibility tests. *C. albicans*, *C. tropicalis* and *C. parapsilosis* are usually sensitive to both fluconazole and amphothericin B. Amphotericin B is preferred for the treatment of infections caused by *C. krusei*, which is intrinsically resistant to fluconazole. Most experts would use amphotericin B for the initial treatment of infections due to *C. glabrata*, but high-dose fluconazole may be an alternative therapy. Fluconazole should be used to treat infections caused by *C. lusitaniae*, which is resistant to amphotericin B.

PHARMACOLOGICAL ISSUES

Antibiotic levels must be high enough to kill bacteria both in blood and infected tissues. Thus, it is very important to select appropriate doses of antibiotics at the onset of treatment. Apart from teicoplanin and a few other drugs, the effect of a high initial bolus, has been poorly studied. The importance of the ratio between the antibiotic level in either blood or infected tissue and the minimum inhibitory concentration (MIC) of the pathogen has been increasingly emphasized in the literature in recent years. It is well assessed by measuring the area under the curve (AUC) over time. A relationship between treatment failures and plasma levels of aminoglycosides was demonstrated many years ago in neutropenic patients with severe infections [68]. More recently, Forrest et al. [69] have shown an association between the number of clinical and bacteriological failures and the AUC of ciprofloxacin in patients with severe pneumonia. The ability of antibiotics to diffuse within the infected tissues is likely to be very important. This could be one of the reasons why good results have been obtained with fluroquinolones for the treatment of severe infections, including pneumonia [70,71]. The mode of administration of the antibiotics could also be of crucial importance. In fact, certain classes of antibiotics display primarily time-dependent effects (cephalosporins, glycopeptides), while others exhibit primarily concentration-dependent effects (aminoglycosides). The clinical relevance of this '*in vitro*' concept is unclear at the present time, since very few clinical studies have addressed this issue.

Another key component of the management of the critically ill septic patient is the need to measure blood levels of antibiotics. Indeed, one should not assume that the administration of standard doses of antibiotics will always result in appropriate levels in a given patient. Monitoring of antibiotic levels should not be restricted only to patients with either renal or hepatic failure, or to patients in whom drug interactions may occur, but should also be performed when patients fail to respond to an appropriate antimicrobial agent as assessed by *in vitro* susceptibility tests.

ECOLOGICAL ISSUES

The effect of various antibiotics on endogenous flora should be considered when selecting an empirical regimen or when reassessing the appropriateness of the initial therapy. The digestive tract is likely to be the main reservoir of resistant strains that may emerge under therapy. Very few data are available on this topic. It would be especially important to know if fourth-generation cephalosporins, like cefepime or cefpirome, that are known to penetrate quickly into the bacteria and to be weak inducers of cephalosporinases, might be as efficient as third-generation cephalosporins, yet exert lower selection pressure for resistance. Preliminary encouraging results have been published in abstract forms [72,73], suggesting that the concept should be tested further in a prospective, randomized study.

CONCLUSION

For many years combination therapy with a beta-lactam and an aminoglycoside was considered to be standard therapy for patients with severe sepsis or septic shock. Prospective trials performed in the last decade have shown that broad-spectrum antibiotics, such as the carbapenems, third-generation and fourth-generation cephalosporins or extended-spectrum penicillins are as efficacious as and less toxic than aminoglycoside-containing antibiotic combinations. Superinfections or the emergence of resistant bacteria were not more frequent in patients treated with single antibiotics. However, monotherapy is not a universal panacea. Beta-lactams used in combination with aminoglycosides or possible with a quinolone may still be preferred as empirical treatment of Gram-negative sepsis in centers with a high incidence of multi-resistant Gram-negative bacilli or of nosocomial Gram-negative pneumonia. Moreover, the results of these studies should be interpreted with some caution for several reasons. First, very few studies have used the same beta-lactam antibiotic in both treatment arms, which affects the interpretation of the intrinsic effect of the aminoglycoside component of the combined therapy. Second, fewer and much smaller studies have been conducted in critically ill patients with severe sepsis or septic shock than in febrile neutropenic cancer patients. Many of the clinical trials have included less than 200 patients which limits the statistical power of these studies. Third, treatment recommendations derived from studies in the neutropenic host may not necessarily be relevant for the management of severely ill septic patients. Multiple organ dysfunction, a common feature in septic ICU patients, is likely to affect the pharmacokinetics, pharmacodynamics, efficacy and safety profiles of the antibiotic. Thus, any antibiotics aimed at treating patients with severe sepsis or septic shock should be evaluated in the appropriate clinical context. Last, one should not assume that the administration of standard doses of antibiotics to critically ill patients will result in appropriate blood and tissue levels in every single patient. Monitoring of antibiotic levels is an integral part of the management of the severely ill septic patient, and should not be restricted only to patients with renal or hepatic failure or to patients in whom drug interactions are a concern, but be performed in any patient who fails to improve after administration of appropriate antimicrobials.

Whatever the choice of initial empirical antibiotics, it is of paramount importance to reassess the appropriateness of antibiotic therapy within 24-48 hours, at a time when bacteriological data become available and the initial clinical response can be evaluated. Whenever possible, one should try to use the least expensive antibiotic with the narrowest possible spectrum of activity in order to lessen the "ecological" impact and minimize the risk of selecting resistant organisms.

REFERENCES

1. Astiz ME, Rackow EC. Septic shock. Lancet 1998; 351:1501-1505
2. Wheeler AP, Bernard GR. Treating patients with severe sepsis. N Engl J Med 1999; 340:207-214
3. Shenep JL. Septic shock. Adv Pediatr Infect Dis 1996; 12:209-241
4. Bone RC, Sibbald WJ, Sprung CL. The ACCP-SCCM consensus conference on sepsis and organ failure. Chest 1992; 101:1481-1483
5. Anderson ET, Young LS, Hewitt WL. Antimicrobial synergism in the therapy of gram-negative rod bacteremia. Chemotherapy 1978; 24:45-54
6. Kreger BE, Craven DE, McCabe WR. Gram-negative bacteremia. IV. Re-evaluation of clinical features and treatment in 612 patients. Am J Med 1980; 68:344-355
7. Young LS. Sepsis syndrome. In: Mandell GL, Bennett JE, Dolin R (eds) Principles and Practice of Infectious Diseases. Churchill Livingstone, New York, 1995: pp 690-705
8. Calandra T, Cometta A. Antibiotic therapy for gram-negative bacteremia. Infect Dis Clin North Am 1991; 5:817-834
9. Rangel-Frausto MS. The epidemiology of bacterial sepsis. Infect Dis Clin North Am 1999; 13:299-312
10. National Nosocomial Infections Surveillance (NNIS) report, data summary from October 1986-April 1997, issued May 1997. A report from the NNIS System. Am J Infect Control 1997; 25:477-487
11. Weinstein MP, Towns ML, Quartey SM, et al. The clinical significance of positive blood cultures in the 1990s: a prospective comprehensive evaluation of the microbiology, epidemiology, and outcome of bacteremia and fungemia in adults. Clin Infect Dis 1997; 24:584-602

12. Bochud PY, Glauser MP, Calandra T. Antibiotics in sepsis. Intensive Care Med 2001; 27 (suppl 1):S33-S48

13. Edmond MB, Wallace SE, McClish DK, et al. Nosocomial bloodstream infections in United States hospitals: a three- year analysis. Clin Infect Dis 1999; 29:239-244

14. Pfaller MA, Jones RN, Messer SA, et al. National surveillance of nosocomial blood stream infection due to species of Candida other than Candida albicans: frequency of occurrence and antifungal susceptibility in the SCOPE Program. SCOPE Participant Group. Surveillance and Control of Pathogens of Epidemiologic. Diagn Microbiol Infect Dis 1998; 30:121-129

15. McCabe WR, Jackson GG. Gram negative bacteremia. Arch Intern Med 1962; 110:92-100

16. Bryant RE, Hood AF, Hood CE, et al. Factors affecting mortality of gram-negative rod bacteremia. Arch Intern Med 1971; 127:120-128

17. Young LS, Martin WJ, Meyer RD, et al. Gram-negative rod bacteremia: microbiologic, immunologic, and therapeutic considerations. Ann Intern Med 1977; 86:456-471

18. Freid MA, Vosti KL. The importance of underlying disease in patients with gram-negative bacteremia. Arch Intern Med 1968; 121:418-423

19. Leibovici L, Paul M, Poznanski O, et al. Monotherapy versus beta-lactam-aminoglycoside combination treatment for gram-negative bacteremia: a prospective, observational study. Antimicrob Agents Chemother 1997; 41:1127-1133

20. Chow JW, Fine MJ, Shlaes DM, et al. Enterobacter bacteremia: clinical features and emergence of antibiotic resistance during therapy. Ann Intern Med 1991; 115:585-590

21. Vidal F, Mensa J, Almela M, et al. Epidemiology and outcome of Pseudomonas aeruginosa bacteremia, with special emphasis on the influence of antibiotic treatment. Analysis of 189 episodes. Arch Intern Med 1996; 156 :2121-6.

22. Schiappa DA, Hayden MK, Matushek MG, et al. Ceftazidime-resistant Klebsiella pneumoniae and Escherichia coli bloodstream infection: a case-control and molecular epidemiologic investigation. J Infect Dis 1996; 174:529-536

23. Leibovici L, Shraga I, Drucker M, et al. The benefit of appropriate empirical antibiotic treatment in patients with bloodstream infection. J Intern Med 1998; 244:379-386

24. Ibrahim EH, Sherman G, Ward S, et al. The influence of inadequate antimicrobial treatment of bloodstream infections on patient outcomes in the ICU setting. Chest 2000; 118:146-155

25. Nguyen MH, Peacock JE, Jr., Tanner DC, et al. Therapeutic approaches in patients with candidemia. Evaluation in a multicenter, prospective, observational study. Arch Intern Med 1995; 155:2429-2435

26. Calandra T, Glauser MP. Immunocompromised animal models for the study of antibiotic combinations. Am J Med 1986; 80:45-52

27. Gribble MJ, Chow AW, Naiman SC, et al. Prospective randomized trial of piperacillin monotherapy versus carboxypenicillin-aminoglycoside combination regimens in the empirical treatment of serious bacterial infections. Antimicrob Agents Chemother 1983; 24:388-393

28. Cometta A, Baumgartner JD, Lew D, et al. Prospective randomized comparison of imipenem monotherapy with imipenem plus netilmicin for treatment of severe infections in nonneutropenic patients. Antimicrob Agents Chemother 1994; 38:1309-1313

29. Oblinger MJ, Bowers JT, Sande MA, et al. Moxalactam therapy vs. standard antimicrobial therapy for selected serious infections. Rev Infect Dis 1982; 4 (Suppl):S639-S649

30. Arich C, Gouby A, Bengler C, et al. Comparison of the efficacy of cefotaxime alone and the combination cefazolin-tobramycin in the treatment of enterobacterial septicemia. Pathol Biol 1987; 35:613-615

31. McCormick PA, Greenslade L, Kibbler CC, et al. A prospective randomized trial of ceftazidime versus netilmicin plus mezlocillin in the empirical therapy of presumed sepsis in cirrhotic patients. Hepatology 1997; 25:833-836

32. Ceftazidime combined with a short or long course of amikacin for empirical therapy of gram-negative bacteremia in cancer patients with granulocytopenia. The EORTC International Antimicrobial Therapy Cooperative Group. N Engl J Med 1987; 317:1692-1698

33. Mouton Y, Deboscker Y, Bazin C, et al. Prospective, randomized, controlled study of imipenem- cilastatin versus cefotaxime-amikacin in the treatment of lower respiratory tract infection and septicemia at intensive care units. Presse Medicale 1990; 19:607-612

34. Solberg CO, Sjursen H. Safety and efficacy of meropenem in patients with septicaemia: a randomised comparison with ceftazidime, alone or combined with amikacin. J Antimicrob Chemother 1995; 36 (Suppl A):157-166

35. Klastersky J, Meunier-Carpentier F, Prevost JM. Significance of antimicrobial synergism for the outcome of gram negative sepsis. Am J Med Sci 1977; 273:157-167

36. Hanson B, Coppens L, Klastersky J. Comparative studies of ticarcillin and mezlocillin plus sisomicin in Gram-negative bacillary bacteraemia and bronchopneumonia. J Antimicrob Chemother 1982; 10:335-341

37. Beaucaire G. Evaluation of the efficacy and safety of isepamicin compared with amikacin in the treatment of nosocomial pneumonia and septicaemia. J Chemother 1995; 7 Suppl 2:165-173

38. Klastersky J, Coppens L, Meunier-Carpentier F, et al. Carbenicillin plus cefazolin with or without mecillinam as an early treatment of bacteremia caused by gram-negative organisms: randomized double-blind study. Antimicrob Agents Chemother 1980; 18:437-442

39. Mouton YJ, Beuscart C. Empirical monotherapy with meropenem in serious bacterial infections. Meropenem Study Group. J Antimicrob Chemother 1995; 36 (Suppl A):145-156

40. White NJ, Dance DA, Chaowagul W, et al. Halving of mortality of severe melioidosis by ceftazidime. Lancet 1989; 2:697-701

41. Extermann M, Regamey C, Humair L, et al. Initial treatment of sepsis in non-neutropenic patients: ceftazidime alone versus 'best guess' combined antibiotic therapy. Chemotherapy 1995; 41:306-315

42. Hess U, Bohme C, Rey K, et al. Monotherapy with piperacillin/tazobactam versus combination therapy with ceftazidime plus amikacin as an empiric therapy for fever in neutropenic cancer patients. Support Care Cancer 1998; 6:402-409

43. Brismar B, Malmborg AS, Tunevall G, et al. Piperacillin-tazobactam versus imipenem-cilastatin for treatment of intra-abdominal infections. Antimicrob Agents Chemother 1992; 36:2766-2773

44. Eklund AE, Nord CE. A randomized multicenter trial of piperacillin/tazobactam versus imipenem/cilastatin in the treatment of severe intra-abdominal infections. Swedish Study Group. J Antimicrob Chemother 1993; 31 (Suppl A):79-85

45. Polk HC, Jr., Fink MP, Laverdiere M, et al. Prospective randomized study of piperacillin/tazobactam therapy of surgically treated intra-abdominal infection. The Piperacillin/Tazobactam Intra-Abdominal Infection Study Group. Am Surg 1993; 59:598-605

46. Jaccard C, Troillet N, Harbarth S, et al. Prospective randomized comparison of imipenem-cilastatin and piperacillin-tazobactam in nosocomial pneumonia or peritonitis. Antimicrob Agents Chemother 1998; 42:2966-2972

47. Hammerberg O, Kurnitzki C, Watts J, et al. Randomized trial using piperacillin versus ampicillin and amikacin for treatment of premature neonates with risk factors for sepsis. Eur J Clin Microbiol Infect Dis 1989; 8:241-244

48. Dupont H, Carbon C, Carlet J. Monotherapy with a broad-spectrum beta-lactam is as effective as its combination with an aminoglycoside in treatment of severe generalized peritonitis: a multicenter randomized controlled trial. Antimicrob Agents Chemother 2000; 44:2028-2333

49. Gudiol F, Pallares R, Ariza X, et al. Comparative clinical evaluation of aztreonam versus aminoglycosides in gram-negative septicaemia. J Antimicrob Chemother 1986; 17:661-671

50. Rabinad E, Bosch-Perez A. A multicenter comparative trial of aztreonam in the treatment of gram-negative infections in compromised intensive-care patients. Chemotherapy 1989; 35 (Suppl 1):1-7

51. Norrby SR, Geddes AM. Efficacy of cefpirome in the treatment of septicaemia. Scand J Infect Dis 1993; 91:51-59

52. Schrank JH, Jr., Kelly JW, McAllister CK. Randomized comparison of cefepime and ceftazidime for treatment of hospitalized patients with gram-negative bacteremia. Clin Infect Dis 1995; 20:56-58

53. Norrby SR, Geddes AM, Shah PM. Randomized comparative trial of cefpirome versus ceftazidime in the empirical treatment of suspected bacteraemia or sepsis. Multicentre Study Group. J Antimicrob Chemother 1998; 42:503-509

54. Hartenauer U, Weilemann LS, Bodmann KF, et al. Comparative clinical trial of ceftazidime and imipenem/cilastatin in patients with severe nosocomial pneumonias and septicaemias. J Hosp Infect 1990; 15 (Suppl A):61-64

55. Krumpe PE, Cohn S, Garreltes J, et al. Intravenous and oral mono- or combination-therapy in the treatment of severe infections: ciprofloxacin versus standard antibiotic therapy. Ciprofloxacin Study Group. J Antimicrob Chemother 1999; 43 (Suppl A):117-128

56. CDC. Recommendations for preventing the spread of vancomycin resistance: recommendations of the Hospital Infection Control Practices Advisory Committee (HICPAC). MMWR Morb Mortal Wkly Rep 1995; 44:1-13

57. Rubin LG, Tucci V, Cercenado E, et al. Vancomycin-resistant Enterococcus faecium in hospitalized children. Infect Control Hosp Epidemiol 1992; 13:700-705

58. Handwerger S, Raucher B, Altarac D, et al. Nosocomial outbreak due to Enterococcus faecium highly resistant to vancomycin, penicillin, and gentamicin. Clin Infect Dis 1993; 16:750-755

59. Wenzel RP. Nosocomial candidemia: risk factors and attributable mortality. Clin Infect Dis 1995; 20:1531-1534

60. Brun-Buisson C, Doyon F, Carlet J. Bacteremia and severe sepsis in adults: a multicenter prospective survey in ICUs and wards of 24 hospitals. French Bacteremia-Sepsis Study Group. Am J Respir Crit Care Med 1996; 154:617-624

61. Sands KE, Bates DW, Lanken PN, et al. Epidemiology of sepsis syndrome in 8 academic medical centers. Academic Medical Center Consortium Sepsis Project Working Group. JAMA 1997; 278:234-240

62. Nguyen MH, Peacock JE, Jr., Morris AJ, et al. The changing face of candidemia: emergence of non-Candida albicans species and antifungal resistance. Am J Med 1996; 100:617-623

63. Rex JH, Bennett JE, Sugar AM, et al. A randomized trial comparing fluconazole with amphotericin B for the treatment of candidemia in patients without neutropenia. Candidemia Study Group and the National Institute. N Engl J Med 1994; 331:1325-1330

64. Phillips P, Shafran S, Garber G, et al. Multicenter randomized trial of fluconazole versus amphotericin B for treatment of candidemia in non-neutropenic patients. Canadian Candidemia Study Group. Eur J Clin Microbiol Infect Dis 1997; 16:337-345

65. Abele-Horn M, Kopp A, Sternberg U, et al. A randomized study comparing fluconazole with amphotericin B/5- flucytosine for the treatment of systemic Candida infections in intensive care patients. Infection 1996; 24:426-432

66. Anaissie EJ, Vartivarian SE, Abi-Said D, et al. Fluconazole versus amphotericin B in the treatment of hematogenous candidiasis: a matched cohort study. Am J Med 1996; 101:170-176

67. Rex JH, Walsh TJ, Sobel JD, et al. Practice guidelines for the treatment of candidiasis. Clin Infect Dis 2000; 30:662-678

68. Moore RD, Smith CR, Lietman PS. Association of aminoglycoside plasma levels with therapeutic outcome in gram-negative pneumonia. Am J Med 1984; 77:657-662

69. Forrest A, Nix DE, Ballow CH, et al. Pharmacodynamics of intravenous ciprofloxacin in seriously ill patients. Antimicrob Agents Chemother 1993; 37:1073-1081

70. Fink MP, Snydman DR, Niederman MS, et al. Treatment of severe pneumonia in hospitalized patients: results of a multicenter, randomized, double-blind trial comparing intravenous ciprofloxacin with imipenem-cilastatin. The Severe Pneumonia Study Group. Antimicrob Agents Chemother 1994; 38:547-557

71. Caldwell JW, Singh S, Johnson RH. Clinical and economic evaluation of subsequent infection following intravenous ciprofloxacin or imipenem therapy in hospitalized patients with severe pneumonia. J Antimicrob Chemother 1999; 43 (Suppl A):129-34

72. Struelens MJ, Byl B, Govaerts D, et al. Modification of antibiotic policy associated with decrease in antibiotic-resistant Gram-negative bacilli in an intensive care unit. In: Abstracts of the 38th Interscience Conference on Antimicrobial Agents and Chemotherapy (San Diego). Washington, DC: American Society for Microbiology, 1998.

73. Hamza L, Benali A, Cheval C, et al. Effect of an antibiotic intervention upon resistance of Enterobacteriaceae producing inducible cephalosporinases in two intensive care units of a 430 bed hospital. In: Abstracts of the 40th Interscience Conference on Antimicrobial Agents and Chemotherapy (Toronto). Washington, DC: American Society for Microbiology, 2000.

32

CANDIDA INFECTIONS IN THE INTENSIVE CARE UNIT

Joseph S. Solomkin
Elias J. Anaissie
Bishara B Albair

The infectious diseases most commonly encountered in the intensive care unit (ICU) are acute events accompanied by the appearance of signs of inflammation such as fever, leukocytosis, and localized tenderness. In this situation, physical, laboratory and radiographic findings are sufficient to indicate an infection and the need for antimicrobial chemotherapy. However, patients with *Candida* infections routinely have had antecedent infections treated with antibacterial agents. Many have diseases, or have received therapy, suppressing immunologic responses. Previous operative intervention may have left surgical wounds or drainage tracts. These circumstances result in colonization by various opportunistic pathogens, with the risk of overgrowth or invasion by microorganisms such as *Candida* species.

This chapter provides a brief review of *Candida* infections in the ICU and provides recommendations for prophylaxis and therapy. We will review data from various patient groups, including neutropenic and leukemic patients. We believe these patients provide mechanistic information relevant to the non-neutropenic patients most commonly seen by intensivists.

MAGNITUDE OF THE PROBLEM

The incidence of fungal infections, particularly with *Candida* species, has increased substantially over the past two decades [1]. *Candida* species have become the fourth leading cause of nosocomial bloodstream infection, preceded only by coagulase-negative staphylococci, *Staphylococcus aureus,* and enterococci. Data from National Nosocomial Infections Surveillance (NNIS) hospitals show that between 1980 and 1989, the incidence of primary bloodstream infections attributable to *Candida* species increased by 487 % in large teaching hospitals and by 219 % in small (<200 bed) hospitals [1]. The greatest increase occurred in surgical patients, particularly in burn and trauma patients, but including both cardiac and general surgery patients.

Nosocomial bloodstream infections caused by *Candida* species carry a high mortality. In a case-controlled study, there was an excess 38% mortality directly attributable to *Candida* infection [2]. Survivors had 30 additional days of hospitalization compared to controls. In a more recent prospective study, *Candida* species were the only microorganisms that independently influenced the outcome of nosocomial primary bloodstream, and were associated with the highest mortality rates (35 % at 28 days and 69 % at discharge) [3].

The reasons for this excess mortality are not fully understood, but are real. Mortality from infectious disease occurs most commonly because of the physiologic derangement resulting from the host response to the organism. This can be due to circumstances of the infection (e.g., the density of organisms, the location of the infection) and may also be related to specific virulence mechanisms of the microorganism.

CLINICAL ASPECTS OF CANDIDA INFECTION

Only four species of *Candida* are commonly associated with infection: *C. albicans, C. tropicalis, C. parapsilosis,* and *C. glabrata.* Of these, *C. albicans* has long been the most common (>60 % of infections). The other three major species are seen at rates varying from 5–20 %. There has been a reduction in the incidence of *C. albicans* in favor of the *non-albicans* species, in particular *C. glabrata and C. krusei* [4]. This is presumed to be due to wide usage of fluconazole, and is important because several strains of *C. glabrata* have reduced susceptibility to fluconazole, an event termed dose-dependent susceptibility. *C. krusei* is highly resistant to the triazoles such as fluconazole and itraconazole.

Candidemia

Candidemia is defined as the isolation of any pathogenic species of *Candida* from at least one blood culture specimen. The recovery of *Candida* species from the bloodstream is a significant observation even in the absence of clinical signs and symptoms, especially if the patient is debilitated, uremic or is receiving immunosuppressive therapy.

Many if not most candidemias seen in the ICU are catheter-associated. This is defined as candidemia occurring in a patient with an intravascular catheter and no other obvious site of origin of infection after careful clinical and laboratory evaluation. Several procedures have been developed to aid in the diagnosis of catheter-associated candidemia. While these provide some insight into mechanisms of infection, they are not commonly used in routine clinical practice. If the catheter is removed, a quantitative culture of the tip should recover at least 15 colony-forming units (cfu) of the same *Candida* species as that found in blood culture by the roll-plate technique, or at least 100 cfu of the same *Candida* species as that found in blood culture by the sonication technique [5]. If the catheter is not removed, a quantitative blood culture collected through a central catheter should contain at least a 10-fold greater concentration of *Candida* species than a simultaneously collected quantitative peripheral blood culture. Routine catheter tip cultures are of no value [6].

Catheter Management in Candidemic Patients

Little controversy remains regarding the role of central venous catheters as a factor predicting outcome in candidemia. Nguyen et al. [7] reported that catheter-related candidemia had a more favorable prognosis compared with candidemia from other sources, but that prognosis was worse in patients whose catheters were retained. This was supported by a study of duration of candidemia as function of catheter removal in patients entered in a clinical trial of fluconazole vs amphotericin B [8].

The formation of a biofilm in these infections is likely an important determinant of the need to remove the catheter. Histologically, biofilms consist of a dense network of yeasts, germ tubes, pseudohyphae, and hyphae. The ability of an a species of *Candida* to form biofilm *in vitro* correlates with its pathogenicity *in vivo*. Antifungal therapy is not highly effective in removing biofilm from catheters [9].

In cases of candidemia, we recommend removal of all intravascular catheters placed three or more days prior to the positive culture. Retention of an infected catheter will result in persistent fever and persistent fungemia. This is particularly important in patients infected with *Candida parapsilosis* (which is more likely to be catheter-related than infection with other *Candida* species). If culture results are not available, there appears little harm in leaving catheters in place until this diagnosis is established. This decision must be individualized and depends in part upon the difficulty of inserting a catheter at a new site.

The use of thrombolytic therapy for infections of surgically implanted catheter has been reported with variable success, particularly in pediatric hematology patients. While the technique appears particularly useful in bacterial infection, failures are more common with *Candida* [10-11].

Disseminated Candidiasis

Persisting candidemia results in the formation of microabscesses in multiple organs, and avoidance of this unique disease state is a primary motivation for the treatment of all candidemias. *Candida* produces microabscesses and, frequently, noncaseating granulomas. The histologic picture suggests that blood-borne fungi are lodged in the microvasculature, resulting in vasculitis. This is consistent with the ability of hyphal forms to adhere to endothelial cells. This multifocal microscopic disease explains the absence of localizing findings despite the progressive cerebral, renal, and cardiac dysfunction seen in infected persons.

The evolution of *Candida* microabscesses after hematogenous distribution has been studied in animal models. After intravenous infusion in nonneutropenic animals, the liver, the kidneys, the heart, the eyes, the brain, and the skin show a pattern of intracapillary fungi (yeasts and pseudohyphae) with an accumulation of neutrophils. In time, focal areas of necrosis occur, resulting in organ dysfunction that ultimately leads to death. In nonneutropenic patients, a similar histologic picture and a similar pattern of organ involvement may be seen [12]. The organs most frequently involved are the brain, the heart, the kidneys, and the eyes

As in the animal models, ocular involvement is a common finding in patients with disseminated candidiasis and by itself is an indication for systemic therapy. It occurs in approximately 10 % of patients with candidemia. The eye pathology is a chorioretinitis with microabscess formation. Funduscopic examination, mandatory in patients suspected of having systemic *Candida* infection, reveals patchy, wool-like tufts.

It is apparent that greater awareness of the pathogenicity of *Candida*, perhaps improved diagnostics, better understanding of amphotericin B dosing, and the availability of less toxic agents has greatly reduced the incidence of these pathological syndromes, first defined in the 1970s.

SOURCES OF CANDIDA IN THE INTENSIVE CARE PATIENT

In humans, as well as in animals, the gastrointestinal tract is considered to be an important portal of entry for microorganisms, including yeasts, into the bloodstream. Although yeast cells have no intrinsic motility, they are able to translocate across the intestinal mucosa within a few hours of ingestion if present in high enough concentration. That *Candida* species can translocate from the gut into the bloodstream in humans was demonstrated in a study where signs and symptoms of sepsis developed in a healthy volunteer two hours after ingestion of a suspension containing 10^{12} *C. albicans* organisms, and blood cultures taken 3 and 6 hours after ingestion were positive for *Candida* [13].

Microbial translocation has been demonstrated in several animal models, using a range of stresses. These include, most notably, malnutrition, parenteral nutrition, endotoxemia, bacterial overgrowth, and burn injury. It is enhanced by fasting (which induces complex changes in host defenses), and protein deficiency (which results in intestinal microbial overgrowth, increased intestinal absorption of intact proteins, and decreased intracellular killing of bacteria and fungi) [14].

Colonization as a Major Risk Factor for Subsequent Candidemia

An important implication of this work on translocation from the intestinal tract is the potential utility of prophylaxis. Identification of an intestinal reservoir has led to a broader concept of progression from intestinal to various extra-intestinal sites as a prelude to infection.

This notion is supported by studies demonstrating that 95 % of neutropenic patients and 84 % of non-neutropenic patients with documented fungal infection were infected with the same strains that had previously colonized them [15-16]. Patients who were not colonized were significantly less likely to develop infection.

In a prospective study among patients admitted to surgical and neonatal intensive care units, Pittet et al. [17] demonstrated that the intensity of *Candida* colonization (as determined by an ad hoc *Candida* colonization index) was significantly higher in patients who subsequently became infected than in those who did not. Other case-control studies have demonstrated that colonization by *Candida* species at various body sites and exposure to several antibiotics are independent risk factors for candidemia [18].

The typical endogenous intestinal flora inhibits gastrointestinal colonization and overgrowth by potentially pathogenic bacteria and fungi, by forming what may be thought of as living wallpaper in the large intestine. Current wisdom is that suppression of endogenous microflora as a consequence of antimicrobial administration may permit overgrowth of pathogenic strains in the GI tract and selection of resistant strains, which may result in enterocolitis, systemic infection and/or the septic response.

Nonetheless, the consequences of antibiotic exposure are overstated. In a case-controlled study, antibiotic administration was shown to be only marginally associated with candidemia, and substantially less important than prior *Candida* colonization [18]. There are multiple other factors that result in changes in the gastrointestinal flora. These include ileus, antacid therapy, and contamination with a hospital flora. The particular concern is that appropriate anti-infective therapy for a bacterial infection should not be stopped because *Candida* is identified at one or more sites. In intra-abdominal infections, mixed flora infections involving *Candida* and bacteria are the norm, rather than the exception.

It is also important to recognize that contamination of vascular catheter hubs is an important source of organisms resulting in candidemia, and the relationship between gastrointestinal colonization and catheter contamination is not obvious.

LABORATORY ASSESSMENT OF CANDIDA INFECTION

Cultures

The workup of the intensive care patient suspected of having a *Candida* infection begins with a complete set of cultures of sputum, oropharynx, stool, urine, all drain sites, and blood. Obtaining more than three sets of blood cultures has little value, and there is no evidence to support doing arterial cultures.

An important concern is whether blood culture is a sufficient technique for identifying clinically significant candidal infection. The incidence of positive ante mortem blood cultures in patients found to have candidiasis at autopsy has been reported to be 30 to 50 % [12]. There are numerous possible explanations for this, including a low inoculum and/or intermittent candidemia. However, candidemia should not be used as a necessary element in the diagnosis of significant infection. As with their bacterial counterparts, these organisms cause clinical illness by extensive local infection.

Because *Candida* species grow poorly under anaerobic conditions, venting the blood culture bottles is thought to improve the yield. Improved sensitivity and time to recognition of positive fungal blood cultures has been achieved with the development of new media, including: biphasic media, automated radiometric and non-radiometric systems and the lysis-centrifugation technique (the latter allowing an estimation of the number of colony forming units of *Candida* per milliliter of blood). There is, however, little evidence that use of these newer methods provides a clinical advantage in the management of patients with candidemia. In a study by Berenguer et al. [19], the sensitivity of the lysis-centrifugation method increased with increasing numbers of involved organs, but was still only 58 % overall.

Antibody Detection

Previous studies have reported the detection anti-*Candida* antibodies in human sera using incompletely characterized antigenic extracts of *C. albicans*. Difficulties with consistent production of uniform materials have limited the usefulness of these tests. Recent work has attempted to detect antibodies directed towards defined purified antigen using a variety of detection technologies (ELISA, immunodiffusion, and latex agglutination). However, the sensitivity and specificity of these methods remain low [20-23].

Antigen Detection and Polymerase Chain Reaction (PCR)

A simple and commercially available test (CAND-TEC *Candida* Detection System, Ramco Laboratories, Texas, USA) relies on the detection of a heat-labile antigen However, the low sensitivity (as low as 19 %) and specificity of this test have limited its clinical use [24-26].

A more recently studied antigen is an immunodominant 48 kDa cytoplasmic protein, *Candida* enolase [23]. As cytoplasmic antigens are thought to be released during invasive infection, detection of this antigen may distinguish between colonization and invasive infection [23]. Unfortunately, this test is not commercially available.

A commercial kit (Bichro-latex albicans) for the rapid diagnosis of *Candida*isis uses monoclonal antibodies against cell wall extracts of *Candida albicans* mannoprotein and appears to have high sensitivity and specificity for *Candida* albicans.

Another antigen studied is (1->3)-beta-D-glucan, an important cell wall constituent of fungi not shared with bacteria [27-28]. This assay indicates the presence of fungi but does not identify the fungal genus causing infection. Studies with this antigen, have been promising. This antigen can be detected in the blood in patients with colonization only. However, its concentration remains lower than 20 pg/ml in such setting.

Amplification of DNA of *Candida* spp. appears to be a quick and specific diagnostic tool. Several limitations still need to be overcome before this methodology can be routinely used [29].

Metabolites

Systems detecting D-arabinitol have been extensively developed [30]. D-arabinitol is a pentose produce by the major *Candida* species except *C. krusei* and *C. glabrata*. D-arabinitol is excreted by the kidneys at the same rate as creatinine, and the ratio of D-arabinitol to creatinine is used to interpret any observed concentration of D-arabinitol. The sensitivity of the serum D-arabinitol-creatinine ratio for diagnosis of invasive candidiasis has been reported in the range of 40–83 %, and rises with repeated sampling. Sensitivity is highest in patients with fungemia (74–83 %) and lowest (40–44%) in patients with tissue invasive *Candida* infections. The magnitude of the D-arabinitol-creatinine ratio is strongly related to the degree of tissue invasion.

Histologic analyses

Fungal smears are relatively insensitive methods of diagnosing *Candida* infection in otherwise sterile sites (e.g., joint fluid, peritoneal fluid, vitreous humor, or cerebrospinal fluid). Centrifugation of these fluids and examination of the sediment may improve the diagnostic yield. Conventional fungal stains, such as hematoxylin-eosin, periodic acid–Schiff (PAS), and Gomori's methenamine-silver (GMS), are useful. The most sensitive stain is calcofluor white, but unfortunately, it requires fluorescent microscopy. Deep tissue biopsy provides a definitive diagnosis of invasive infection.

CLINICAL DIAGNOSIS OF CANDIDA INFECTION

Candidemia has no characteristic clinical picture. Three clinical findings that may lead to an early diagnosis of candidemia in the surgical patient are candidal endophthalmitis, suppurative phlebitis, and candiduria in the absence of bladder instrumentation. If the patient is colonized with *Candida*, the onset of systemic inflammatory response should prompt a careful eye examination to identify the presence of candidal infection. All patients with candidemia should undergo examination. A repeat examination should be performed after therapy for proven candidemia. Approximately 10 % of patients with candidemia will be found to have endophthalmitis. Candidal endophthalmitis may remain asymptomatic until late in the course of infection.

The presence of peripheral suppurative phlebitis that fails to yield bacteria or does not respond to antibacterial agents may be an early clue to the presence of hematogenous candidiasis. Gentle squeezing of the venous catheter exit site or needle aspiration of a palpable cord may demonstrate pus that yields *Candida* species on a smear or culture [31-32]. Surgical excision of the infected vein usually reveals *Candida* infection in its lumen.

A much rarer form of thrombophlebitis involves the central veins [33]. This is diagnosed by recognition of persisting candidemia and central vein thrombosis, and requires surgical treatment.

The presence of high-grade candiduria in surgical patients who have not had instrumentation of the renal pelvis or the bladder suggests hematogenous candidiasis and should prompt a work-up for this infection [34]. In this setting, candiduria may result from seeding of or filtering through the kidney. Fever may be the only sign of infection but may be absent in patients who are receiving corticosteroids. a patient with hematogenous candidiasis presents with he systemic inflammatory response syndrome (SIRS) or septic shock. The diagnosis should be seriously considered in high-risk patients who are persistently febrile. Because of the high mortality associated with this infection, empirical antifungal therapy for the early treatment of clinical occult fungal infection or for the prevention of new fungal infections is recommended.

SELECTION OF PATIENTS FOR EMPIRICAL ANTIFUNGAL THERAPY

The most common dilemma is suspicion of fungal infection in patients without positive blood cultures or histologic evidence of tissue invasion. At-risk patients typically manifest fever, leukocytosis, and other potential indicators of infection because of non-infectious inflammatory disease, and often are under treatment for bacterial infection without resolution of the signs of infection.

It is a clinical truism that ICU patients do not tolerate well the further physiologic stress imposed by untreated infection. Recent progress in the measurement of severity of illness and its close correlation with subsequent mortality has underscored the importance of physiologic disturbance accompanying infection in determining outcome. Physiologic deterioration is a much stronger determinant of outcome than is the provision of effective anti-infective therapy. This creates strong pressure to provide early treatment for possible infection.

As the magnitude of this problem has increased, there has been considerable effort expended to better understand the epidemiology of fungal infection in the intensive care unit, and to thereby define indications for treatment of early infection, prior to candidemia. There are now available guidelines for optimizing antifungal therapy, put together by various working groups [35].

The patients at risk of *Candida* infection are those with prolonged ICU stay. The average hospital length of stay for patients developing candidemia is 18 days [2].Various other risk factors have been identified, including prior antibiotic treatment, presence of intravascular catheters, and parenteral nutrition [18]. However, these factors generally serve only as markers for prolonged ICU stay and are not sufficiently discriminatory to serve as a guide to patients who might benefit from some form of prophylaxis or early therapy.

The indications for treatment have recently been expanded as more experience has accumulated. Candidemia, defined as one or more positive blood cultures for any *Candida* species, is now viewed as a clear indication for anti-fungal therapy. There is strong evidence that patients colonized with *Candida*, that is, who grow the same species from the same site (urine, sputum, surgical drain sites) on two or more occasions, are at an approximate 30-50% risk of progressing on to candidemia [17]. The risk of subsequent infection increases as more sites become positive. This is particularly true for patients found to have *Candida* in the peritoneal cavity of either recurrent intra-abdominal infection or following elective operation[36].

It is now well established that the minimum adult dosage of fluconazole is 400 mg qd. Because of an increase in the incidence of non-*albicans* species, with lessened susceptibility to fluconazole, dosages of 600 to 800 mg may be useful if the particular ICU has a high incidence of such organisms [37-39]. Various studies have demonstrated the excelllent absorption of fluconazole in enterally fed ICU patients, and this is therefore the preferred route.

Peritonitis and Intra-abdominal Abscess

A controversial aspect of *Candida* infectious syndromes in surgical patients is whether systemic therapy is required to eradicate *Candida* found within intra-abdominal abscesses, peritoneal fluid, or fistula drainage. *Candida* is frequently cultured from intra-abdominal infectious foci but should be considered a serious threat only in specific patient groupss. Four risk factors for intra-abdominal *Candida* infection have been identified including failed treatment for intra-abdominal infection, anastomotic leakage following elective or urgent operation, surgery for acute pancreatitis, and splenectomy [36,40,41].

Systemic antifungal therapy should be provided for these patients found to have *Candida* at the site of recurrent of intra-abdominal infection or previous operation, and we would include patients with extensive areas of communication between the abdominal cavity and the external environment via either fistulas or drain tracts. Anti-bacterial therapy should be provided if bacteria are identified either by Gram stain or culture. Most of these patients will have polymicrobial infection.

Occasionally, *Candida* species may cause acalculous cholecystitis or cholangitis. This problem is increasingly found in patients with percutaneously placed drainage catheters for malignancy [42]. Such patients must be given systemic therapy for clinical evidence of infection, including candidemia, and the drainage catheter must be changed.

There is an increasing appreciation of the role of *Candida* in infections following acute pancreatitis [43]. A large series of patients undergoing operation for infected pancreatic necrosis found *Candida* present in approximately 10% of the patients at their initial operation for infection. These patients had received prophylaxis with amoxicillin/clavulanate, a factor which might explain intestinal overgrowth and translocation of *Candida*. This is a particular issue because of the interest in the use of broad spectrum antibiotics, especially imipenem/cilastatin, as prophylaxis for patients with necrotizing pancreatitis. The results of contemporary randomized clinical trials restricted to patients with prognostically severe acute pancreatitis have demonstrated improvement in outcome associated with antibiotic treatment [44]. Given the apparently high incidence of *Candida* at the site of pancreatic necrosis in patients receiving anti-bacterial prophylaxis, the notion of additional anti-fungal prophylaxis has arisen. At this time we would recommend against this approach, unless the patient is known to be colonized with *Candida*.

Urinary Tract Infection

The recovery of *Candida* species from the urinary tract most commonly results from contamination from the perirectal or the genital area. Persistent candiduria in the surgical ICU may be an early marker of disseminated infection in critically ill high-risk patients.

If *Candida* colonization persists, antifungal therapy should be considered. Amphotericin B bladder irrigation only provides temporary clearance of funguria and systemic agents (single-dose IV amphotericin B or a-5-day course of oral fluconazole) are usually needed. Recently, a large multicenter prospective study has evaluated fluconazole vs amphotericin B bladder irrigations for this condition [45]. This study included very few ICU patients and thus was unable to specifically address the issue of progression to candidemia. Candiduria cleared by day 14 in 79 (50 %) of 159 patients receiving fluconazole and 46 (29 %) of 157 receiving placebo (p<.001).

ANTIFUNGAL THERAPY

During the 1960s and 1970s, the standard approach to managing candidemia was to classify patients according to the degree of risk of disseminated candidiasis and to withhold antifungal treatment from those in whom dissemination appeared to be unlikely. This approach was based on the rarity of candidemia in non-neutropenic and non-immunosuppressed surgical patients and an acute awareness of the toxicities of amphotericin B, the only systemic antifungal agent available at the time. Reports of an increase in candidal infection in surgical patients led to a re-examination of this approach. It is now recommended that all candidemic patients be treated [35].

Therapeutic Recommendations

The role of amphotericin B in the treatment of candidemia in surgical patients has been difficult to determine -- first, because most of the studies that evaluated amphotericin B were retrospective with small sample sizes, and second, because varying definitions of *Candida* infection were used. In one study, treatment with amphotericin B had no effect on overall outcome in a mixed population of patients; however, the timing of therapy and the dose administered were not clearly stated [46]. In general, mortality was found to be lower in patients who received amphotericin B than in those who did not

[36,47,48]. Significant amphotericin B-related nephrotoxicity was identified [49].

The discovery of the azole antifungal agents has changed the management of *Candida* infections. The first two azoles, clotrimazole and miconazole, were not suitable for systemic use. The lack of a parenteral formulation of ketoconazole and the erratic bioavailability of the drug in patients receiving H_2 receptor blockers or antacids have limited its use in the treatment of hematogenous candidiasis in surgical patients [50].

Fluconazole is a well-tolerated triazole, with good activity in candidemia. The data available from several clinical trials demonstrate that the drug is as effective as and better tolerated than amphotericin B. Overall, four comparative studies have been completed in various patient populations: randomized, prospective observational, and matched cohort [7,51,52] Fluconazole dosages were generally 400mg/day (range 200 to 800) orally or intravenously while intravenous amphotericin B was given at doses of 0.3 to 1.2 mg/kg.

The primary evidence for the efficacy of fluconazole has come from two prospective, randomized multicenter studies. In one, 164 patients with documented or presumed invasive candidiasis received either amphotericin B, 0.7 mg/kg/day, or fluconazole, 400 mg/day [52]. The response rate for fluconazole (62 %) was virtually identical to that for amphotericin B (63 %), and fluconazole was better tolerated. In another prospective, randomized multicenter study, 206 non-immunocompromised candidemic patients received either amphotericin B or fluconazole [51]. Once again, the two drugs were comparable in their efficacy, and fluconazole had a better safety profile.

Newer therapeutic options have now become available with the advent of the lipid-associated formulations of amphotericin B, which are less nephrotoxic than the parent compound [53,54]. So far, three lipid products of amphotericin B have been marketed in Europe or the USA: Abelcet (Amphotericin B Lipid Complex), Amphocil (Amphotericin B Colloidal Dispersion) and Amphotericin Bisome (Liposomal Amphotericin B). A prospective randomized trial showed that Abelcet was as efficacious as conventional amphotericin B in hematogenous candidiasis [55].

Choice of Agent and Dose-schedule

All patients with candidemia should receive antifungal therapy. We recommend the administration of fluconazole, 600-800 mg/day IV for three days, particularly if the infecting organism is known to be, or is likely to be,

C. albicans. If the patient responds rapidly to this regimen, the dosage may be decreased to 400 mg/day and administered orally. For patients with hematogenous candidiasis known to be colonized by *C. glabrata, C. krusei,* or *C. lusitaniae*, amphotericin B, 0.5 to 0.7 mg/kg/day, remains the treatment of choice. For patients who are hemodynamically unstable and for those who have high-grade persistent fungemia, we recommend a two-drug antifungal regimen; the combination of fluconazole and flucytosine or that of amphotericin B and flucytosine depending on the infecting strain.

Clinical data on the effects of itraconazole in hematogenous candidiasis are scant. Given that itraconazole has limited bioavailability in the presence of antacids and H_2-receptor blockers, it should not be used to treat hematogenous candidiasis in the critically ill.

Liposomal formulations of amphotericin B offer new therapeutic alternatives. However, their substantial cost limits their routine use, except if the patient has renal failure and is infected with an azole-resistant strain.

Duration of Therapy

Duration of therapy depends on the extent and seriousness of the infection. Therapy can be limited to 7-10 days for patients with catheter-related and low-grade fungemia, without evidence of organ involvement or hemodynamic instability. On the other hand, patients with high-grade fungemia, evidence of organ involvement or hemodynamic instability need to receive antifungal therapy for 10-14 days after resolution of all signs and symptoms of infection.

Antifungal Prophylaxis

Prophylaxis may be considered in surgical patients at high risk for invasive *Candida* infection. Trials of antifungal prophylaxis have shown benefit as part of selective bowel decontamination, or in the form of low-dose amphotericin B, or liposomal formulations of amphotericin B in surgical transplant recipients [56,57]. Recently, a double-blind randomized trial showed that intravenous fluconazole prophylaxis was effective in preventing *Candida*l colonization and infections in surgical patients with recurrent gastrointestinal perforation or those with anastomotic leakage [58].

In burn patients, a retrospective study reported that topical nystatin in the burn wound dressing was associated with significant decrease in overall yeast acquisitions in burn wounds and fungemia but with an increase in colonization and fungemia caused by nystatin-resistant, amphotericin B-susceptible *Candida* rugosa [59].

Invasive fungal infections are one of the most important causes of mortality in transplant patients. Antifungal prophylaxis in organ transplant recipient receiving immunosuppressive treatment has been recommended, but there is controversy about which drug to use that is most effective and with minimal toxicity. Some physicians use fluconazole as a prophylactic treatment in organ transplant [60,61]. Other physicians recommended itraconazole or liposomal amphotericin B.

Systemic Antifungal Agents

Amphotericin B

Amphotericin B is structurally similar to membrane sterols, and its major mechanism of action is believed to be through interaction with membrane sterols and creation of pores in the fungal outer membrane [50,62]. The clinical usefulness of amphotericin B is attributable to the greater affinity of amphotericin B for ergosterol (found in fungal cell membranes) than for cholesterol (the principal sterol found in mammalian cell membranes). Oxidation-dependent amphotericin B-induced stimulation of macrophages is another proposed mechanism of action [63]. Most species of fungi that cause human infections are susceptible to amphotericin B.

The use of amphotericin B is associated with frequent and potentially severe side effects, including infusion-related events such as fever, rigors, and hypotension, as well as metabolic derangements such as hypokalemia and nephrotoxicity [64]. Infusion-related toxicities (e.g., fever, chills, rigors) are likely due to amphotericin B stimulation of cytokine and prostaglandin synthesis. Nephrotoxicity, the primary non-infusion-related toxicity, likely results from the nonselective cytotoxic interaction between Amphotericin B and cholesterol-containing mammalian cells [65]. An acute infusion-related reaction, consisting of fever, hypotension, and tachycardia, occurs in about 20 % of patients [66]. Premeditation regimes with, for example, acetaminophen, or hydrocortisone, are of little if any value. Meperidine (25-50 mg IV), will alleviate fevers and chills if given after they occur [67]. Hypotension, hypertension, hypothermia, and bradycardia are other reported infusion-related toxic effect of amphotericin B. Ventricular arrhythmias have been associated with administration of amphotericin B in patients with severe hypokalemia, renal failure or those in whom the infusion was rapidly given. Amphotericin B suppresses production of red blood cells and causes a normocytic, normochromic anemia.

Common practice is to give a 1-mg test dose and observe the patient for one hour in the hope of identifying patients at risk of severe acute reactions. The full dose of the drug (0.3 –0.7 mg/kg/day) is then infused over a period of 4 to 6 hours, although recent data suggest that much shorter infusion times (e.g., one hour in patients with adequate cardiopulmonary and renal function) may be acceptable [68]. The total dose depends on the extent of the infection and the patient's condition. Patients must be monitored carefully during the first day of therapy. The infusion should be discontinued if the patient becomes hemodynamically unstable.

The ability of the drug to form stable complexes with lipids has allowed the development of new formulations of amphotericin B based on this property. Three new lipid formulations of amphotericin B are approved by the FDA: amphotericin B lipid complex (Abelcet), amphotericin B colloidal dispersion (Amphotec), and liposomal amphotericin B (Ambisome). Another type of amphotericin B preparation can be made by mixing amphotericin B deoxycholate with a fat emulsion usually employed for parenteral nutrition (Intralipid). Clinical experience with these preparations showed that adverse reactions and nephrotoxicity were significantly reduced

Amphotericin B nephrotoxicity may be minimized by avoiding other agents with synergistic nephrotoxicity (e.g., aminoglycosides, vancomycin, cisplatin, and cyclosporin), and by administering sodium supplementation. The latter approach consists of the intravenous infusion of 500 ml of 0.9% saline solution 30 minutes before the administration of amphotericin B and a second infusion of the same amount of saline after the amphotericin B infusion is completed [69].

If the serum creatinine level exceeds 3.5 mg/dl, amphotericin B should be discontinued and the serum creatinine level monitored twice weekly. Administration of amphotericin B may be resumed at 50 to 75 % of the original dosage when the serum creatinine level falls below 3 mg/dl.

Flucytosine

Flucytosine can be useful for the treatment of hematogenous candidiasis; however, a high failure rate and secondary emergence of resistance have been reported when flucytosine was used alone, and serious concerns exist regarding its myelosuppressive potential. A review of the literature on the activity of flucytosine when administered with amphotericin B in acute disseminated candidiasis and candidemia indicates a good response rate.

The standard dosage for flucytosine is 37.5 mg/kg every 6 hours. On the basis of the pharmacokinetics of flucytosine and the *in vitro* susceptibility of *Candida* species to the drug, much lower dosages of flucytosine (e.g., 12.5 mg/kg every 12 hours) would probably maintain serum and tissue levels significantly above the minimal inhibitory concentration (MIC) needed for most susceptible strains throughout therapy. This approach may decrease the myelosuppressive potential that the drug usually exhibits at levels of 100 mg/ml. This adverse reaction may be caused by fluorouracil (which is produced by metabolism of flucytosine by enterobacillary flora in the gut) rather than by the parent compound [70].

Peak serum concentrations should be monitored and the dosage adjusted so as to maintain a peak level of about 25 mg/ml. Flucytosine is removed by hemodialysis and peritoneal dialysis. Patients undergoing hemodialysis should receive a 37.5 mg/kg dose of flucytosine after each dialysis session unless their initial peak serum concentration is higher than 25 mg/ml or their postdialysis concentration is higher than 10 mg/ml. Patients undergoing peritoneal dialysis should receive a single 37.5 mg/kg dose daily.

Fluconazole

The mechanism of action of fluconazole is preferential inhibition of cytochrome P450 enzymes in fungal organisms. Fluconazole is active against several *Candida* species, including C. tropicalis. C. krusei, however, is highly resistant to this agent [4,38,39,50]. Fluconazole is available in either an oral form or an intravenous form, both of which are rapidly and almost completely absorbed from the gastrointestinal tract. The serum concentrations after oral administration are almost identical to those achieved when the drug is administered intravenously. A major advantage of fluconazole over ketoconazole is its high degree of gastrointestinal absorption, which is not affected by gastric acidity or the presence of food. Steady-state serum concentrations of fluconazole are obtained within 5 to 10 days. An initial loading dose that is twice the usual daily dose is recommended. Fluconazole is distributed evenly in body tissues, penetrates into the vitreous humor and the aqueous humor of the eye, and crosses the blood-brain barrier. The drug is excreted largely unchanged in the urine, with only minimal liver metabolism [71,72]. Consequently, dosage schedules must be adjusted in patients with renal impairment. Hemodialysis significantly reduces the serum concentrations, and the drug appears also to be removed by peritoneal dialysis. A standard dose should be given after each course of dialysis.

The toxicities of fluconazole are similar to those of other azoles and include nausea and vomiting in about 2 % of patients; headache, fatigue, abdominal pain, and diarrhea; exfoliative dermatitis also occurs, but very rarely [73]. Transient abnormalities of liver function have been observed in 3% of patients receiving fluconazole. In addition, fatal hepatic necrosis developed in two patients who were receiving fluconazole, but it was unclear whether the agent played a causal role in this event. No significant hormonal abnormalities have been reported after administration of fluconazole.

Itraconazole, and to a lesser extent fluconazole (in high doses) are inhibitors of CYP3A4. Therefore certain agents that are substrates of this enzyme, such as some of the new generation of H1-antihistamines, several HMG-CoA reductase inhibitors and certain benzodiazepines, are contraindicated. Other drugs like cyclosporine and quinidine need careful monitoring if administered concurrently with these triazoles. Because fluconazole interacts with warfarin, phenytoin, and cyclosporine when given in a daily dose of 200 mg or more, serum concentrations of these agents should be monitored.

Itraconazole

Itraconazole is the only available azole that has substantial activity against *Aspergillus* species. It exists in an oral capsule formulation, the bioavailability of which is approximately 55 %. Absorption is enhanced by the presence of food in the stomach but is significantly reduced by the presence of antacids or H_2-receptor blockers. A newly available solution has significantly higher bioavailability but may not be well tolerated by patients. When erratic absorption is of concern, the use of the IV formulation is recommended. The serum elimination half-life is 15 to 25 hr, but increases to 34-42 hr after weeks of administration, and with increasing itraconazole doses.

Itraconazole is metabolized by the liver and excreted primarily in the feces 5 and urine as metabolites. Because itraconazole is metabolized to a large degree in the liver, the dosage must be adjusted in-patients with hepatic failure; however, renal impairment or hemodialysis does not affect its pharmacokinetics [74]. Serum concentrations of itraconazole should be measured in patients with invasive infections.

CONCLUSION

Continued progress in supportive care, including the development of antibiotics with increasingly broad spectra of activity have resulted in an increasing frequency of fugal infections, particularly candidiasis. Because of the inadequacy of the available knowledge base, we do not fully understand the pathophysiology of these infections in surgical patients, nor can we be always certain precisely when prophylaxis and therapy should be administered.

Despite these limitations, there is now sufficient information available to justify an aggressive therapeutic approach to suspected *Candida* infections. Now that less toxic agents are available (the newer triazoles, particularly fluconazole, and the lipid formulations of amphotericin B), the clinical approach to presumed fungal infections in the surgical patients has been made far simpler.

REFERENCES

1. Beck-Sague C, Jarvis WR. Secular trends in the epidemiology of nosocomial fungal infections in the United States, 1980-1990. National Nosocomial Infections Surveillance System. J Infect Dis 1993; 167:1247-1251
2. Wey SB, Mori M , Pfaller MA, et al. Hospital-acquired candidemia. The attributable mortality and excess length of stay. Arch Intern Med 1988; 148:2642-2645
3. Pittet D, Li N , Woolson RF, et al. Microbiological factors influencing the outcome of nosocomial bloodstream infections: a 6-year validated, population-based model. Clin Infect Dis 1997; 24:1068-1078
4. Pfaller MA, Messer SA, Hollis RJ, et al. Trends in species distribution and susceptibility to fluconazole among blood stream isolates of Candida species in the United States. Diagn Microbiol Infect Dis 1999; 33:217-222
5. Raad II, Sabbagh MF, Rand KH, et al. Quantitative tip culture methods and the diagnosis of central venous catheter-related infections. Diagn Microbiol Infect Dis 1992; 15:13-20
6. Widmer AF, Nettleman M, Flint K, et al. The clinical impact of culturing central venous catheters. A prospective study. Arch Intern Med 1992; 152:1299-1302
7. Nguyen MH, Peacock JE Jr, Tanner DC, et al. Therapeutic approaches in patients with candidemia. Evaluation in a multicenter, prospective, observational study. Arch Intern Med 1995; 155:2429-2435
8. Rex JH, Bennett JE, Sugar AM, et al. Intravascular catheter exchange and duration of candidemia. NIAID Mycoses Study Group and the Candidemia Study Group. Clin Infect Dis 1995; 21:994-996
9. Hawser SP, Douglas LJ. Resistance of Candida albicans biofilms to antifungal agents in vitro. Antimicrob Agents Chemother 1995; 39:2128-2131
10. Dato VM, Dajani AS. Candidemia in children with central venous catheters: role of catheter removal and amphotericin B therapy. Pediatr Infect Dis J 1990; 9:309-314
11. Jones GR, Konsler GK, Dunaway RP, et al. Prospective analysis of urokinase in the treatment of catheter sepsis in pediatric hematology-oncology patients. J Pediatr Surg 1993; 28:350-355
12. Parker JC, McCloskey JJ, Knauer KA. Pathobiologic features of human candidiasis. A common deep mycosis of the brain, heart and kidney in the altered host. Am J Clin Pathol 1976; 65:991-1000

13. Krause W, Matheis H, Wulf K. Fungaemia and funguria after oral administration of Candida albicans. Lancet 1969; 1:598-599
14. DeWitt RC, Kudsk KA. The gut's role in metabolism, mucosal barrier function, and gut immunology. Infect Dis Clin North Am 1999; 13:465-481
15. Voss A, Hollis RJ, Pfaller MA, et al. Investigation of the sequence of colonization and candidemia in nonneutropenic patients. J Clin Microbiol 1994; 32:975-980
16. Pfaller M, Cabezudo I, Koontz F, et al. Predictive value of surveillance cultures for systemic infection due to Candida species. Eur J Clin Microbiol 1987; 6:628-633
17. Pittet D, Monod M, Suter PM, et al. Candida colonization and subsequent infections in critically ill surgical patients. Ann Surg 1994; 220:751-758
18. Wey SB, Mori M, Pfaller MA, et al. Risk factors for hospital-acquired candidemia. A matched case- control study. Arch Intern Med 1989; 149:2349-2353
19. Berenguer J, Buck M, Witebsky F, et al. Lysis-centrifugation blood cultures in the detection of tissue- proven invasive candidiasis. Disseminated versus single-organ infection. Diagn Microbiol Infect Dis 1993; 17:103-109
20. Bougnoux ME, Hill C, Moissenet D, et al. Comparison of antibody, antigen, and metabolite assays for hospitalized patients with disseminated or peripheral candidiasis. J Clin Microbiol 1990; 28:905-909
21. Gentry LO, Wilkinson ID, Lea AS, et al. Latex agglutination test for detection of Candida antigen in patients with disseminated disease. Eur J Clin Microbiol 1983; 2:122-128
22. Navarro D, Monzonis E, Lopez-Ribot JL, et al. Diagnosis of systemic candidiasis by enzyme immunoassay detection of specific antibodies to mycelial phase cell wall and cytoplasmic candidal antigens. Eur J Clin Microbiol Infect Dis 1993; 12:839-846
23. van Deventer AJ, van Vliet HJ, Hop WC, et al. Diagnostic value of anti-Candida enolase antibodies. J Clin Microbiol 1994; 32:17-23
24. Fung JC, Donta ST, Tilton RC. Candida detection system (CAND-TEC) to differentiate between Candida albicans colonization and disease. J Clin Microbiol 1986; 24:542-547
25. Burnie JP, Williams JD. Evaluation of the Ramco latex agglutination test in the early diagnosis of systemic candidiasis. Eur J Clin Microbiol 1985; 4:98-101
26. Bailey JW, Sada E, Brass C, et al. Diagnosis of systemic candidiasis by latex agglutination for serum antigen. J Clin Microbiol 1985; 21:749-752
27. Kohno S, Mitsutake K, Maesaki S, et al. An evaluation of serodiagnostic tests in patients with candidemia: beta-glucan, mannan, candida antigen by Cand-Tec and D-arabinitol. Microbiol Immunol 1993; 37:207-212
28. Miyazaki T, Kohno S, Mitsutake K, et al. Plasma (1-->3)-beta-D-glucan and fungal antigenemia in patients with candidemia, aspergillosis, and cryptococcosis. J Clin Microbiol 1995; 33:3115-3118
29. Reiss E, Morrison CJ. Nonculture methods for diagnosis of disseminated candidiasis. Clin Microbiol Rev 1993; 6:311-323
30. Walsh TJ, Merz WG, Lee JW, et al. Diagnosis and therapeutic monitoring of invasive candidiasis by rapid enzymatic detection of serum D-arabinitol. Am J Med 1995; 99:164-172
31. Hauser CJ, Bosco P, Davenport M, et al. Surgical management of fungal peripheral thrombophlebitis. Surgery 1989; 105:510-514
32. Walsh TJ, Bustamente CI, Vlahov D, et al. Candidal suppurative peripheral thrombophlebitis: recognition, prevention, and management. Infect Control 1986; 7:16-22
33. Benoit D, Decruyenaere J, Vandewoude K, et al. Management of candidal thrombophlebitis of the central veins: case report and review. Clin Infect Dis 1998; 26:393-397

34. Nassoura Z, Ivatury RR, Simon RJ, et al. Candiduria as an early marker of disseminated infection in critically ill surgical patients: the role of fluconazole therapy. J Trauma 1993; 35:290-295

35. Edwards JEJ, Bodey GP, Bowden RA, et al. International Conference for the Development of a Consensus on the Management and Prevention of Severe Candidal Infections. Clin Infect Dis 1997; 25:43-59

36. Solomkin JS, Flohr AB, Quie PG, et al. The role of Candida in intraperitoneal infections. Surgery 1980; 88:524-530

37. Pfaller MA, Messer SA, Houston A, et al. National epidemiology of mycoses survey: a multicenter study of strain variation and antifungal susceptibility among isolates of Candida species. Diagn Microbiol Infect Dis 1998; 31:289-296

38. Pfaller MA, Jones RN, Doern GV, et al. International surveillance of bloodstream infections due to Candida species: frequency of occurrence and antifungal susceptibilities of isolates collected in 1997 in the United States, Canada, and South America for the SENTRY Program. The SENTRY Participant Group. J Clin Microbiol 1998; 36:1886-1889

39. Martins MD, Rex JH. Resistance to antifungal agents in the critical care setting: problems and perspectives. New Horiz 1996; 4:338-344

40. Calandra T, Bille J, Schneider R, et al. Clinical significance of Candida isolated from peritoneum in surgical patients. Lancet 1989; 2:1437-1440

41. Rantala A, Lehtonen OP, Kuttila K, et al. Diagnostic factors for postoperative candidosis in abdominal surgery. Ann Chir Gynaecol 1991; 80:323-328

42. Khardori N, Wong E, Carrasco CH, et al. Infections associated with biliary drainage procedures in patients with cancer. Rev Infect Dis 1991; 13:587-591

43. Aloia T, Solomkin J, Fink AS, et al. Candida in pancreatic infection: a clinical experience. Am Surg 1994; 60:793-796

44. Ho HS, Frey CF. The role of antibiotic prophylaxis in severe acute pancreatitis. Arch Surg 1997; 132:487-492

45. Sobel JD, Kauffman CA, McKinsey D, et al. Candiduria: a randomized, double-blind study of treatment with fluconazole and placebo. The National Institute of Allergy and Infectious Diseases (NIAID) Mycoses Study Group. Clin InfectDis 2000; 30:19-24.

46. Dyess DL, Garrison RN, Fry DE. Candida sepsis. Implications of polymicrobial blood-borne infection. Arch Surg 1985; 120:345-348

47. Richards KE, Pierson CL, Bucciarelli L, et al. Monilial sepsis in the surgical patient. Surg Clin North Am 1972; 52:1399-1406

48. Solomkin JS, Flohr AM, Simmons RL. Indications for therapy for fungemia in postoperative patients. Arch Surg 1982; 117:1272-1275

49. Solomkin JS, Flohr A, Simmons RL. Candida infections in surgical patients. Dose requirements and toxicity of amphotericin B. Ann Surg 1982; 195:177-185

50. Bodey GP. Azole antifungal agents. Clin Infect Dis 1992; 14 Suppl 1:S161-S169

51. Rex JH, Bennett JE, Sugar AM, et al. A randomized trial comparing fluconazole with amphotericin B for the treatment of candidemia in patients without neutropenia. Candidemia Study Group and the National Institute. N Engl J Med 1994; 331:1325-1330

52. Anaissie EJ, Vartivarian SE, Abi-Said D, et al. Fluconazole versus amphotericin B in the treatment of hematogenous candidiasis: a matched cohort study. Am J Med 1996; 101:170-176

53. de Marie S, Janknegt R, Bakker-Woudenberg IA. Clinical use of liposomal and lipid-complexed amphotericin B. J Antimicrob Chemother 1994; 33:907-916

54. Brajtburg J, Bolard J. Carrier effects on biological activity of amphotericin B. Clin Microbiol Rev 1996; 9:512-531

55. Walsh TJ, Hiemenz JW, Seibel NL, et al. Amphotericin B lipid complex for invasive fungal infections: analysis of safety and efficacy in 556 cases. Clin Infect Dis 1998; 26:1383-1396

56. Gorensek MJ, Carey WD, Washington JA, et al. Selective bowel decontamination with quinolones and nystatin reduces gram-negative and fungal infections in orthotopic liver transplant recipients. Cleve Clin J Med 1993; 60:139-144

57. Singh N, Mieles L, Yu VL, et al. Invasive aspergillosis in liver transplant recipients: association with candidemia and consumption coagulopathy and failure of prophylaxis with low-dose amphotericin B. Clin Infect Dis 1993; 17:906-908

58. Eggimann P, Francioli P, Bille J, et al. Fluconazole prophylaxis prevents intra-abdominal candidiasis in high-risk surgical patients. Crit Care Med 1999; 27:1066-1072

59. Dube MP, Heseltine PNR, Rinaldi MG, et al. Fungemia and colonization with nystatin-resistant Candida rugosa in a burn unit. Clin Infect Dis 1994; 18:77-82

60. Lumbreras C, Cuervas-Mons V, Jara P, et al. Randomized trial of fluconazole versus nystatin for the prophylaxis of Candida infection following liver transplantation. J Infect Dis 1996; 174:583-588

61. Fisher NC, Cooper MA, Hastings JG, et al. Fungal colonisation and fluconazole therapy in acute liver disease. Liver 1998; 18:320-325

62. Brajtburg J, Powderly WG, Kobayashi GS, et al. Amphotericin B: current understanding of mechanisms of action. Antimicrob Agents Chemother 1990; 34:183-188

63. Sokol-Anderson M, Sligh JEJ, Elberg S, et al. Role of cell defense against oxidative damage in the resistance of Candida albicans to the killing effect of amphotericin B. Antimicrob Agents Chemother 1988; 32:702-705

64. Gallis HA, Drew RH, Pickard WW. Amphotericin B: 30 years of clinical experience. Rev Infect Dis 1990; 12:308-329

65. Sabra R, Branch RA. Amphotericin B nephrotoxicity. Drug Saf 1990; 5:94-108

66. Khoo SH, Bond J, Denning DW. Administering amphotericin B--a practical approach. J Antimicrob Chemother 1994; 33:203-213

67. Goodwin SD, Cleary JD, Walawander CA, et al. Pretreatment regimens for adverse events related to infusion of amphotericin B. Clin Infect Dis 1995; 20:755-761

68. Cleary JD, Weisdorf D, Fletcher CV. Effect of infusion rate on amphotericin B-associated febrile reactions. Drug Intell Clin Pharm 1988; 22:769-772

69. Anderson CM. Sodium chloride treatment of amphotericin B nephrotoxicity. Standard of care? West J Med 1995; 162:313-317

70. Lyman CA, Walsh TJ. Systemically administered antifungal agents. A review of their clinical pharmacology and therapeutic applications. Drugs 1992; 44:9-35

71. Debruyne D. Clinical pharmacokinetics of fluconazole in superficial and systemic mycoses. Clin Pharmacokinet 1997; 33:52-77

72. Rosemurgy AS, Markowsky S, Goode SE, et al. Bioavailability of fluconazole in surgical intensive care unit patients: a study comparing routes of administration. J Trauma 1995; 39:445-447

73. Terrell CL. Antifungal agents. Part II. The azoles. Mayo Clin Proc 1999; 74:78-100

74. Schafer-Korting M. Pharmacokinetic optimisation of oral antifungal therapy. Clin Pharmacokinet 1993; 25:329-341

33

WHY, WHEN, AND HOW TO ISOLATE ICU PATIENTS

Bina Rubinovitch
Philippe Eggimann
Didier Pittet

Transmissible diseases can evoke uncertainty and fear among healthcare workers. The higher the disastrous potential of a disease the more 'precautious anxiety' it stimulates. Examples are certain viral hemorrhagic fevers, notorious for their propensity to cause epidemics, but also the 'flesh-eating bacteria' group A streptococcal infections, or fulminant meningococcemia.

Unfortunately, healthcare workers tend to be indifferent toward the transmission risks of more common infections. This 'benign neglect' has led to numerous well-documented nosocomial outbreaks of influenza, hepatitis A, rotavirus and tuberculosis, many of which could have been prevented if adherence to infection control measures had been optimal [1-4].

The importance of nosocomial transmission in the intensive care unit (ICU) cannot be overemphasized: more than a third of nosocomial infections are acquired in ICUs, accounting for a crude incidence of 15-40 % of ICU admissions, depending on the type of unit [5]. Since more severely ill patients have higher risks for both acquiring nosocomial infection and for mortality, assessment of the mortality attributable to nosocomial infection in ICU patients is not straightforward. Nevertheless, nosocomial infections are definitely associated with substantial excess length of stay and additional hospital costs [6-9]. Although patients' intrinsic risk factors for developing infections can not largely be modified, the risk of microorganism transmission could, and should, be kept to a minimum.

Although only 10 % of nosocomial infections originate from outbreaks, three-quarters of outbreaks occur in ICUs, reflecting the higher likelihood of patient-to-patient spread in these settings. The medical literature abounds with examples of nosocomial outbreaks of typical ICU microorganisms, successfully controlled after the implementation or reinforcement of appropriate infection control measures [5,10].

Finally, ICUs are the epicenters of spread of antibiotic-resistant microorganisms in the hospital. Adherence to appropriate isolation precautions can markedly diminish resistance dissemination.

This chapter discusses concepts of infection transmission in the hospital, emphasizes the high risks for infection transmission and infection acquisition in critically ill patients and, finally, provides practical guidelines to be implemented for appropriate infection control measures.

INFECTION TRANSMISSION

The Chain of Transmission

Infection transmission, or the spread of microorganisms, occurs when a pathogenic source, a susceptible host and a means of transmission are present. The ICU setting particularly favors cross-transmission: highly infection-prone patients are present, readily transmissible nosocomial pathogens are prevalent and hands of healthcare workers, the most significant means of transmission, play a dominant role in patient-care. Regrettably, host susceptibility to infection cannot generally be modified and the presence of microorganisms is unavoidable. Consequently, the prevention of infection dissemination critically depends on eliminating the means of transmission.

More than 50 % of those admitted in ICUs harbor nosocomial microorganisms that may serve as a reservoir for subsequent endemic and epidemic spread [11-13]. Transmission is essentially via the hands of healthcare workers. Direct transmission from one patient to another occurs infrequently. Occasionally, infections originate directly from a contaminated environmental source (e.g., aspergillosis and legionellosis). Table 1 summarizes the risk of infection transmission versus infection acquisition in patients, healthcare workers, and visitors.

Infection control does not equal extinction of microorganisms. For highly virulent pathogens e.g., Mycobacterium tuberculosis, prevention of transmission would theoretically lead to disease eradication, since there is no colonization state. For less pathogenic microorganisms, the goal of minimizing transmission is to reduce the risk of infection and associated morbidity and mortality in high-risk patients. Therefore, efforts to eliminate transmission are required for hospitalized patients colonized with certain microorganisms but may not be justified in the non-hospital setting. For example, coagulase-negative staphylococci are common human commensals, rarely pathogenic in healthy individuals. However, due to their predilection for prosthetic devices, coagulase-negative staphylococci are the leading cause of nosocomial bloodstream infections, accounting for more than 20% of episodes in ICUs and associated with a 5-22 % risk of mortality [6,14,15]. A significant proportion of those episodes would be averted by preventing transmission of coagulase-negative staphylococci to susceptible patients.

Population	Reservoir for infection dissemination	Risk of directly transmitting infection	Risk of acquiring infection [*]
Infected patients	+++ [*]	+/- [†]	+++ [*]
Colonized patients	+++ [*]	+/-	+++ [*]
Non-infected/colonized HCW	-	+++ [‡]	+/- [§]
Infected/colonized HCW [‖]	+	+++	+/- [§]
Visitors	+/-	+/-	+/- [†]

[*] Examples are: methicillin-resistant *Staphylococcus aureus* (MRSA), coagulase-negative staplylococci (CoNS), *Clostridium difficile*
[†] Examples are: pulmonary and laryngeal tuberculosis
[‡] Examples are: hepatitis A, *Clostridium difficile*, Gram-negative bacteria, and staphylococci
[§] Examples are: hepatitis A, varicella, and pulmonary and laryngeal tuberculosis
[‖] Examples are: MRSA colonization, influenza

Table 1. Infection transmission - infection acquisition

Routes of Transmission

The three major routes of infection transmission in hospitals are contact, droplet, and airborne (Table 2). Additional mechanisms such as common vehicle (e.g., contamination of water supply or equipment) and vector-borne (e.g., mosquitoes and ticks) are less significant for the acquisition of NI in critical care.

Contact transmission is the most important route for infection transmission in the hospital. Transmission is via physical contact with skin, commonly from contaminated or colonized hands of health care workers to patients. Physical contact also applies to contact with contaminated surfaces or instruments such as stethoscopes, blood-pressure cuffs, etc.

Route	Infectious unit	Principle	Example of transmitted pathogens	Examples of diseases predisposing to transmission of pathogens
Contact	Direct transfer of micro-organisms	Physical contact Person-to-person or contaminated environment-to-person	*Staphylococcus aureus* Group A *Streptococci* *Clostridium difficile* Multidrug-resistant microorganisms*	Skin infection or enteric infection Colonization/ infection with multidrug-resistant microorganisms*
Droplet	Respiratory droplets >5 μm	Droplets are deposited on mucous membranes; Close contact < 1meter for transmission	*Neisseria meningitidis* Influenza virus	Meningococcemia and meningitis Influenza
Airborne	Droplet nuclei <5 μm or contaminated dust particles	Inhalation of droplet nuclei; Remain suspended in the air for long periods; migrate long distances	*Mycobacterium tuberculosis* Varicella zoster virus	Pulmonary and/or laryngeal tuberculosis Varicella and disseminated zoster;

* Extended-spectrum betalactamase producing enterobacteriae (ESBL); multidrug-resistant *Pseudomonas aeruginosa*; multidrug-resistant *Enterobacter cloacae*

Table 2. *Routes of transmission of infectious pathogens*

Droplet transmission occurs when large respiratory particles containing infecting microorganisms (produced during coughing, sneezing and talking, or during invasive procedures such as bronchoscopy and suctioning) are subsequently deposited on the mucous membranes of the host's eye, nose and mouth. Close contact, less than 1 m, is necessary for transmission to occur since respiratory droplets do not last very long in the air and usually travel short distances.

Airborne transmission occurs when infectious droplet nuclei or contaminated dust particles are inhaled. Droplet nuclei are less than 5 μm in size and can remain suspended in the air for long periods and travel long distances; therefore special air handling and ventilation are required to prevent transmission [16].

It must be recognized that transmission from an infected/colonized patient via the hands of healthcare workers to another susceptible patient is by far the most common route of nosocomial transmission. In the acute care setting, most nursing and medical patient-care activities include significant direct patient contact. Therefore, it is not surprising that pathogens transmitted via direct hand contact with patient skin, mucous membranes, and critical-equipment components are responsible for the most frequent nosocomial infections in ICU patients: vascular catheter-associated infection, late-onset ventilator-associated pneumonia, and wound infection. In addition, bloodstream and urinary catheter-associated fungal infections frequently originate from cross-transmission [17]. Although the risk of developing an infection depends on additional host intrinsic factors, numerous reports clearly demonstrate the role of contact transmission in ICU outbreaks [18]. Moreover, unless an active infection surveillance is carried out, low-grade chronic outbreaks due to common microorganisms may go unnoticed and be regarded as sporadic, unavoidable infections.

The following example illustrates the fact that outbreaks due to unusual or multidrug resistant (MDR) microorganisms are frequently markers for inadequate infection control practices in a unit. In a neonatal ICU, an outbreak due to *Malassezia parachydermatis* (a lipophylic yeast, rarely described as a human pathogen) involved fifteen infants over a 15-month period. Eight had bloodstream infection, one, meningitis, two, urinary tract infection, and four, asymptomatic colonization [13]. An investigation carried out by the Centers for Disease Control and Prevention (CDC) revealed a person-to-person transmission associated with a colonization of healthcare workers' pet dogs. The outbreak was terminated after reinforcement of appropriate hand washing practices.

ISOLATION PRECAUTIONS

Isolation guidelines enable healthcare workers to identify patients who need to be isolated, and to institute the appropriate measures. The first modern isolation system in hospitals was practiced at the beginning of the 20th century and included segregation of infected patients and application of aseptic techniques recommended in nursing textbooks. The CDC first formalized guidelines for isolation in hospitals in 1970. These were subsequently modified several times to address emerging problems in infectious diseases, in particular in hospital infections. Finally, the CDC and the Hospital Infection Control Practice Advisory Committee (HICPAC) has issued new recommendations in 1996 defining two levels of transmission prevention: *standard precautions*, applied to all patients, and *transmission-based precautions,* applied to patients with documented or suspected colonization and infection with specific microorganisms [16].

Standard Precautions

Standard precautions delineate the concept that all patients, irrespective of their diagnosis, should be treated in a way that minimizes the risk of microorganisms' dissemination in the hospital. Standard precautions (Table 3) apply to blood; all body fluids (secretions and excretions except sweat) visibly bloody or not; and non-intact skin and mucous membranes. The recommendations are based on solid rationale and on extensive suggestive evidence that routine adherence to precautions decreases the risk of infection transmission in hospitals.

Transmission-based Precautions

The second level of precautions applies to selected patients having either a suspected or confirmed clinical syndrome or a specific diagnosis that predictably places others at risk of acquiring an infection. These patients are to be isolated accordingly (Table 4) [16]. Of note, many infectious diseases do not warrant specific precautions in the hospital setting. For example, as meningococcal meningitis has the propensity to cause epidemics, hospitalized patients should be placed under droplet isolation and close contacts be given post-exposure prophylaxis. However, bacterial meningitis due to *Streptococcus pneumoniae* is generally a sporadic disease affecting certain individuals with predisposing factors, and specific isolation is not required in those patients.

   The duration of isolation depends on the duration of the transmissible state. For many conditions, specific isolation measures can be safely terminated 24 hrs after initiation of appropriate therapy. Typical examples are meningitis and meningococcemia due to *Neisseria meningitidis* (droplet precautions), scarlet fever due to Group A streptococci (droplet precautions), major skin/soft tissue infection due to Group A streptococci (contact precautions), or scabies (contact precautions). For other infections, patients require specific isolation for the duration of disease. Examples include influenza (droplet precautions), disseminated varicella zoster (airborne and contact precautions), measles (airborne precautions), major draining wound infections (contact precautions). For varicella, airborne isolation is also indicated for the period of suspected incubation. In case of doubt regarding route of transmission or duration of isolation, always consult infection control professionals in the institution.

Component	Field of application
Hand hygiene	After contact with blood, body fluids, secretions, excretions, contaminated items Immediately before gloving and after removing gloves Between patient contacts
Gloves	For anticipated contact with blood, body fluids, secretions, excretions, contaminated items For anticipated contact with mucous membranes, non-intact skin
Mask, eye protection, face shield	To protect mucous membranes of the eyes, nose and mouth during procedures and patient-care activities likely to generate splashes or spray of blood, body fluids, secretions and excretions
Gowns	To protect skin and prevent soiling of clothing during procedures and patient-care activities likely to generate splashes or spray of blood, body fluids, secretions and excretions
Patient-care equipment handling	To ensure that skin, mucous-membranes and cloths are not exposed to equipment soiled with any body fluids To ensure that reusable equipment is not reused until it has been appropriately reprocessed To ensure that single-use items are discarded properly
Sharp object handling	Avoid recapping used needles Place used sharp objects and needles in puncture-resistant containers

Table 3. Standard precautions. Adapted from HICPAC guidelines [16]. Available on-line at: http://www.cdc.gov/ncidod/hip/isolat/isolat.htm

HAND HYGIENE

In the mid-1800s, fifty years before the discovery of microbes, Ignaz Semmelweis, obstetrician in Vienna, demonstrated the role of contaminated hands of healthcare workers in transmitting infections from one patient to another. He notably reduced the mortality associated with puerperal sepsis by the implementation of systematic hand disinfection in chlorinated lime before patient examination [19]. Although numerous epidemics originating from cross-transmission via the hands of healthcare workers have since been reported, it is occasionally argued that the causal link between hand hygiene and nosocomial infection has never been demonstrated [11-13].

Pittet and collaborators recently provided compelling direct and indirect evidence supporting the 150-year old hypothesis that this simple measure has a dominant role in the prevention of nosocomial infection [10].

Microbial Flora

The non-infected skin harbors two types of microorganisms, the resident and the transient or contaminant flora. The resident flora consists mainly of CoNS, *Corynebacterium spp* and *Micrococcus spp*, has a low pathogenic potential unless introduced into the body via invasive devices; and enables intact skin to resist colonization with virulent microorganisms [20,21]. The resident flora is difficult to remove mechanically. The transient flora consists of Gram-negative bacteria, is highly virulent, but is short-lived on skin.

How does patient care affect microbial adherence to the hands of healthcare worksers? In a neonatal ICU, Gram-negative bacilli were found to be on the hands of 75 % of healthcare workers [22]. In a recent US national survey, hands of healthcare workers from 13 ICUs were systematically cultured over an 18-month period. Thirty-three percent (range: 18-58 %) and 29 % (range: 8-62 %) of healthcare workers, in the adult and pediatric ICUs respectively, were positive for *Candida spp* [17]. We have found that bacterial contamination of hands increases linearly with time on ungloved hands during patient care. Higher contamination levels were independently associated with direct patient contact, respiratory care, handling of body fluids, and rupture in the sequence of patient care [23].

Contact precautions	
Apply for patients known or suspected to have diseases transmitted by direct physical contact / contact with items in the patient's environment	
Infection/colonization with multidrug-resistant bacteria[†]	According to infection control policy and guidelines at the hospital
Enteric infections	*Clostridium difficile* *Escherichia coli* O157:H7 *Shigella spp* Hepatitis A virus Rotavirus
Respiratory infections in children	Respiratory syncytial virus Parainfluenza virus Enteroviral infections
Highly contagious skin infections	Neonatal or mucocutaneous Herpes simplex Disseminated zoster[†] Impetigo Staphylococcal furunculosis in infants and children Non-covered abscesses, cellulitis, decubitus Pediculosis and scabies
Viral hemorrhagic conjunctivitis	
Viral hemorrhagic fevers	Lassa, Ebola, Marbug viruses

Droplet precautions	
Apply for patients known or suspected to have diseases transmitted by large droplets	
Systemic syndromes	*Neisseria meningitidis* infections *Haemophilus influenzae* meningitis GAS[§] scarlet fever, toxic shock syndrome
Respiratory infections	*Haemophilus influenzae,* pneumonia, epiglottitis GAS[§] pharyngitis *Mycoplama pneumoniae* Pertussis
Serious viral infections	Adenovirus Influenza Mumps Parvovirus B19 Rubella

Airborne precautions	
Apply for patients known or suspected to have diseases transmitted by airborne particles	
Respiratory infections	Measles Varicella and disseminated zoster Tuberculosis, pulmonary and laryngeal
Viral hemorrhagic fevers	Lassa, Ebola, Marbug viruses

[†] Extended-spectrum betalactamase producing enterobacteriae (ESBL); multi-resistant *Pseudomonas aeruginosa*; multi-resistant *Enterobacter cloacae*
[§] Group A Streptococci

Table 4. *Transmission-based precautions (adapted from the HICPAC guidelines [16])*

Healthcare workers' hands are the principal tools in the course of complete nursing and highly invasive ICU care. Lack of, or inadequate, hand hygiene practice, was the direct cause for cross-transmission in many endemic and epidemic situations. For example, Webster et al. eliminated endemic MRSA in a neonatal ICU in seven months after the introduction of a new disinfectant [24]. Zafar et al. were unable to control an outbreak of MRSA in a neonatal ICU in spite of the implementation of control measures, until another disinfectant was introduced [25].

Hand Hygiene Techniques

Hand hygiene is the term used for hand cleansing methods. These methods includes hand washing with water alone and plain soap, or an antimicrobial soap; handrub with waterless alcohol-based compound; and surgical hand scrub [26]. Hand disinfection refers to any action where an antiseptic solution is used to clean hands, either medicated soap or alcohol. Surgical hand scrub will not be further discussed in this chapter (precise recommendations and scientific basis are available online at http://www.cdc.gov/ncidod/hip/sterile/sterile.htm).

Hand washing procedures mechanically remove dirt (extraneous substances, sweat, skin lipids, epithelial debris, etc.) and adhering skin bacteria, mainly transient flora [16,27]. Hand disinfectant kills the adhering flora, the efficacy depending on the duration of procedure and the type of product used. The efficacy of hand hygiene methods is determined by calculating the difference in $\log_{10}$ colony forming units (cfu) before and after the procedure.

For hand washing with water and soap, the main reduction of transient flora is achieved within the first 30 seconds (0.6 to 1.1 logs at 15 sec and 1.8 to 2.8 logs at 30 sec). Extending the procedure results in reductions of 2.7 to 3.0 logs, 3.3 logs, and 3.7 logs after one, two and four minutes, respectively [28]. Appropriate hand washing is performed as follows: wetting hands with running water; application of 3-5 ml of cleansing agent, thoroughly distributed over hands; vigorously rubbing hands together for 10-15 seconds, covering all surfaces of hands, fingers and fingernails; rinsing to remove residual washing solution; drying hands with a clean, disposable (or single use) towel.

Alcohol-based waterless hand-rub consists of applying a small amount (3-5ml) of a fast-acting antiseptic preparation on both hands; covering all surfaces of the hands and fingers then rubbing hands together for 10-15 seconds; passive drying is obtained in 10-15 sec depending on the alcohol proportion of the solution [26]. This technique allows maximum efficacy in a minimum of time and circumvents the additional need to go to a sink to dry hands. The reduction in transient flora achieved after 30 sec is 3.4 to 3.7 logs for alcohol (1-minute hand-rub: 4.0 to 5.8 logs). Similar reductions are achieved with chlorhexidine gluconate, but this effect is maintained for at least 3 to 4 hours [29].

We investigated colonization on hands of healthcare workers during routine patient-care activities under various clinical situations. In a multivariate analysis, we have found that healthcare workers who washed their hands with plain soap had an excess of 52 cfus on their fingertips compared with those who used a disinfectant solution [23].

Although hand washing with water and soap may be less effective in microbial decontamination, currently, there is no evidence that hand disinfection is superior for preventing nosocomial transmission. However, compliance issues make the handrub-based de-germing technique preferred over hand washing [20].

Guidelines for hand washing and hand disinfection are provided in Table 5. Of note, it is unnecessary and not recommended to perform more than a single hand hygiene practice for a given indication.

Situation or type of activity		Hand washing	Alcohol-based hand disinfection
Macroscopically soiled hands		Yes	No
Contact	Before patient contact	Yes	Yes
	After patient contact	Yes	Yes
	After contact with a source of microorganisms	Yes	Yes
Gloves	Before wearing gloves	Yes	Yes
	After glove removal	Yes	Yes
	Gloved hands	No	No
Before invasive procedure		(Yes)	Yes
To reduce both transient and resident skin flora		Yes	Yes
Inaccessible hand washing facilities		No	Yes

Table 5. Recommendations for healthcare workers regarding handwashing and hand disinfection in hospitals (Adapted from the APIC [26])

Compliance with Hand Hygiene

Despite the large body of evidence supporting the effectiveness of hand hygiene in preventing cross transmission, healthcare workers are reluctant to comply with recommendations. The vast majority of observational studies report compliance rates that are unacceptably low, usually below 50 % [30-32 %]. Possible explanations for low compliance rates include inferior priority compared with other patient needs, insufficient time, inconvenient placement of hand-cleansing facilities, allergy or intolerance to hand-hygiene solutions, lack of role model, and unawareness of recommendations or skepticism towards their effect on nosocomial infection [16,20,33,34].

A theoretical calculation indicates that in ICUs, approximately two-thirds of staff work-time will be required for hand washing if 100 % adherence to guidelines is attempted [35]. Not surprisingly, high demand for hand hygiene practice (i.e., heavy workload) was found to be a risk factor for low-rate compliance, compliance being inversely correlated to the number of opportunities for hand hygiene per hour of patient care [31]. Poor compliance with appropriate infection control measures can also be predicted in crowded ICUs, especially when the nurse-to-patient ratio is decreased and was found to be an independent risk factor for various outbreaks [34].

Compliance was found to be associated with the use of a specific method for hand hygiene, although not consistently. In a medical ICU in France, an improved compliance from 42.4 to 60.9 % was attributed to the availability of an alcohol-based handrub solution [32]. However, the effect was not sustained and compliance decreased over a three-month period to 51.3 %. In a prospective multi-crossover study in three ICUs, Doebbeling et al. demonstrated a decreased rate of nosocomial infection in periods where the hand hygiene method was disinfection with chlorhexidine as compared with periods where hand hygiene was based on alcohol and soap alone. Reduction in the infection rate was attributed to a significantly higher compliance when chlorhexidine was used [36].

A comprehensive discussion on the complex barriers to compliance with hand hygiene recommendations is beyond the scope of this chapter. However, we consider that our experience at the University of Geneva Hospitals illustrates this complexity well. In 1995, a hospital-wide campaign of an alcohol-based handrub disinfection, widely distributed as disposable individual pocket-bottles, was launched [10]. Compliance with hand hygiene constantly improved from 48 to 66 % over a four-year period. During that period, the prevalence of NI and the incidence of hospital-acquired methicillin resistant *Staph. aureus* (MRSA) bacteremia decreased from 16.9 to 9.9 per 100 admissions, and from 0.74 to 0.24 episodes per 10,000 patient-days, respectively. Assuming that only 25 % of the reduction in infection rate were attributed to improved compliance with hand hygiene practice, the intervention averted more than 900 nosocomial infections [10].

The success of this campaign can be ascribed to its multi-modal and multi-disciplinary approach that incorporated communication and education tools such as 'talking-walls' (hospital-wide cartoon posters); active participation of healthcare workers in the creation of the campaign; positive feedback at both individual and institutional levels; and regular involvement of institution directory [20,37-39].

In summary, embarrassing as it is, appropriate hand hygiene is practiced in only 50 % of cases in ICUs at best. Alcohol-based handrubs overcome some of the barriers for compliance with hand hygiene requirements in the busy ICU setting, but, innovative approaches at both institution and ICU level are required to maximize compliance [20].

ISOLATION PRACTICE

Barrier Precautions

Personal protective equipment consists of the application of isolation precautions and includes gloves, gown, mask, eye protection, and face shield (Table 6).

Gloves

Gloves should be worn for anticipated contact with blood, mucous membranes, non-intact skin, secretions, and moist body substance of all patients, in order to limit cross contamination during such contact (standard precautions). Wearing gloves reduces the risk of exposure to blood-borne pathogens, including sharp instrument accidents. Wearing gloves also reduces the likelihood of transmitting microorganisms present on hands during invasive procedures or during contact with mucous membranes and non-intact skin. Gloves are also to be worn as part of contact isolation [40].

Wearing gloves does not obviate the need for hand hygiene for the following reasons: Gloves may have small and/or non-apparent defects and therefore may be responsible for cross-transmission of microorganisms [16,41]. When randomly tested, up to 5.5 % of unused latex gloves had leaks. Leakage rate increased at the end of a surgical procedure and ranged from 52 %, 29 % and 25 % for the surgeon, first assistant, and scrub nurse, respectively, and gloves may be torn during use, hands may become contaminated during their removal [42]. Washing gloved hands is ineffective for decontamination, 5 to 10 % of hands are contaminated after gloves are removed [43]. In addition, heat and moisture favor microorganism proliferation if hands are not correctly washed or disinfected before gloving [44]. Therefore, wearing gloves should always be accompanied by appropriate hand hygiene measures, before wearing and after removing and should always be changed between patient contacts.

Indication	Gloves	Gown	Mask	Eye protection
Anticipated contact with any body fluid* For venipunctures and all invasive procedures	Yes	No	No	No
Contact with mucous membrane or non-intact skin	Yes	No	No	No
During all patient-care activities likely to generate splash or spray of any body fluid*	Yes	Yes	Yes†	Yes
Protection against contact-transmitted pathogens	Yes	Yes	No	No
Protection against droplet-transmitted pathogens	No	No	Yes†	Yes
Protection against airborne-transmitted pathogens	No	No	Yes‡	No

*   Blood, bloody or non-bloody body fluid, excretions and secretions, except sweat
†   Surgical mask
‡   High-efficiency particulate air (HEPA) respiratory systems. N-95 standard mask [45]

Table 6. *Requirements for personal barrier equipment*

Gown

Gowns and other protective apparel are available to prevent soiling and contamination of skin and clothing during patient-care activities likely to generate projections (Table 3) and are also recommended for contact isolation [16]. Many institutions have now switched to disposable gowns that are less expensive and may further reduce the risk of reusing contaminated material.

Mask, Eye Protection, and Face Shield

Various types of masks, goggles, and face shields are available for mucous membrane protection during patient-care activities likely to generate projections of blood, body fluid secretions and excretions (Table 3).

A surgical mask provides an adequate protection against respiratory droplets larger than 5μm. For respiratory care of mechanically-ventilated patients (e.g., mouth-care, suction or endotracheal manipulation), simultaneous use of goggles, or the use of a mask that includes a transparent eye-shield is strongly recommended. It should be remembered that the protection provided by paper masks is of limited duration (30 minutes), especially if they become damp. Masks made of synthetic material, even when wet, preserve their full filtration capacity for several hours. A used mask should not be hung around the neck or kept in a pocket to be used again, but should be discarded immediately after removal.

A surgical mask is definitely an inadequate protection against airborne transmitted pathogens. Individual disposable, high-efficiency particulate air (HEPA) respiratory systems designed to prevent the transmission of 1-5 μm particles have been recommended [46]. However, HEPA systems are expensive and require training and adaptation for use [47]. In addition, their role in preventing transmission of tuberculosis is unknown. Therefore, for protection against airborne infections, any high-efficiency masks (dust-masks) that have been approved by the National Institute for Occupational Safety and Health is appropriate (N-95 standard) [45]. Table 6 summarizes the requirements for personal barrier equipment.

Placement of Patients

ICUs should be equipped with at least one private room. A private room is mandatory for airborne-transmitted pathogens. Patients with pulmonary and laryngeal tuberculosis, varicella and disseminated zoster, acute viral hemorrhagic fever, or measles should be placed in a room with negative air pressure in relation to the surrounding area with at least six air changes per hour and on appropriate discharge of air before it is circulated to other areas in the hospital [46]. The door of the room should be kept closed. An isolation room with an anteroom is sometimes used; however, it is unknown whether it adds to the effectiveness of isolation. Its main role is to allow air pressure differentials to be maintained at time of door opening. When an isolation room with an anteroom is used, the two doors should not be opened at the same time.

A private room with facilities for hand washing and a toilet is recommended for patients requiring contact and droplet transmission precautions. The private room serves as a physical barrier and helps to reinforce hand hygiene before entering and exiting the room. It is particularly important when the source patient has poor hygiene habits or when compliance with precautions cannot be expected (i.e., children and patients with altered mental status) and the patient may contaminate the environment or transmit pathogens directly to others. Private rooms or cubicles may be difficult to obtain in the ICU. In addition, the need for aggressive support for organ failure may overrule requirements for the special placement of patients. Nevertheless, appropriate hand hygiene practices, standard and barrier precautions can and should all be applied regardless of placement in a private room.

When a private room is not available, patients infected or colonized with the same microorganism can share a room (cohorting). Cohorting is useful when there is shortage of private rooms or during an outbreak and is safe, provided that cohorted patients are not infected with other transmissible pathogens and the likelihood of re-infection with the same microorganism is minimal. It is recommended that cohorting also include designated nursing staff to further minimize transmission to patients in the unit.

Frequently however, an infected patient or sometimes a patient colonized with epidemiologically-important microorganisms shares a room with a non-infected patient (s). Under these circumstances, personnel, patients and visitors should be instructed to take appropriate precautions.

Consultation with infection control professionals is advised for selecting minimal risk room-mates.

Transport of Isolated Patients

Movement of patients outside an isolation room should be limited. When indicated:

i)   use appropriate barriers on patients (mask, dressings) to reduce transmission to other patients, healthcare workers, and visitors, and minimize contamination of the environment;

ii)   notify personnel in the area where the patient will arrive to take appropriate precautions and, whenever relevant;

iii) inform patients about the route of potential transmission of microorganisms so they may assist in required measures. Practical recommendations for transmission-based precautions are summarized in Table 7.

Isolation type	Room	Personal barrier	Patient transport
Contact	Private if possible. Cohorting in case of an outbreak. Door can remain open	Skin and clothing protection; gloves, non-sterile and gown, clean, non-sterile should be worn upon entering the room, changed after contact with an infective item (gloves); be removed before exiting the room (gown then gloves), followed by hand washing /disinfection	Should be limited. Patients should be covered appropriately when exiting the room
Droplet	Private if possible. Cohorting in case of an outbreak. Maintain 1 meter distance between infected and other patients if private room / cohorting non-available. Door can remain open	Mucous membrane protection within 1 meter of infected patient; mask (may be easier to remember to put on a mask upon entering)	Should be limited. Patient should wear surgical mask when exiting the room
Airborne	Private; negative-air pressure (6-12 changes/h, adequate air discharge) Door should remain closed	Respiratory protection; appropriate N-95 mask should be worn upon entering the room	Should be strictly limited. Patients should wear appropriate N-95 mask when exiting the room

Table 7. Practices of specific isolation. (Adapted from HICPAC guidelines [16]. Available on-line at: http://www.cdc.gov/ncidod/hip/isolat/isolat.htm)

Cleansing

Patient-care Equipment

Special procedures for the handling or disposal of used patient-care equipment are based on the likelihood of contamination with infective material, the risk of injury (needles, scalpels and other sharp instruments) and environmental stability of pathogens involved [16]. Contaminated materials must be eliminated in a closed bag [48]. Specific guidelines for disposal and reuse of patient-care equipment are available online at http://www.cdc.gov/ncidod/hip/sterile/sterile.htm.

Patient-care equipment in direct contact with intact skin may be colonized with epidemiologically-important microorganisms. Sixty to 85 % of stethoscope membranes were found to be colonized with high counts of pathogenic bacteria and, hence, should be considered as a potential source of cross-transmission [49-51]. Personal stethoscope membranes and alike should be disinfected between patient contacts. Simple alcohol-based disinfection is probably adequate.

The risk of microorganism transmission by linen and eating utensils is negligible if they are handled according to any applicable hospital policy.

Environment

The room, cubicle and bedside equipment of patients on specific isolation is to be cleansed as routinely recommended for hospitals. For microorganisms capable of surviving for long periods in an inanimate environment, such as enterococci or spores of *Clostridium difficile,* special cleansing procedures are required according to hospital policy [52]. Specific guidelines and precise recommendations are also available on the site http://www.cdc.gov/ncidod/hip/guide/guide.htm.

SPECIAL CONSIDERATIONS

Empiric Isolation

Patients are frequently admitted to the hospital without a definitive diagnosis, and may have an infectious disease that places other patients and healthcare workers at risk. Therefore, patients presenting with certain clinical syndromes may warrant the institution of empirical specific isolation pending a definitive diagnosis (Table 8).

Colonization or Infection with Multidrug-Resistant Organisms

The emergence and widespread of drug-resistant organisms are complex processes. However, the two most important steps are the use/overuse of antimicrobials and the cross-transmission of resistant pathogens [53].

The highest prevalence of multidrug-resistance (MDR) among nosocomial microorganisms is found in ICUs. Over 70 % of patients are treated with antimicrobials during their hospitalization [6]. The intense exposure creates both a selective pressure on endogenous flora of the host and on environmental free-living bacteria, such as *Pseudomonas aeruginosa* and *Acinetobacter spp.*, inherently resistant to multiple antibiotics.

ICUs are also the epicenters for hospital-wide and interhospital dissemination of these organisms, since patients harboring MDR microorganisms are rarely discharged home but are rather transferred to other units in the hospital or to other healthcare facilities [54,55].

Infections due to MDR pathogens frequently pose serious therapeutic problems, often respond slowly to therapy (therefore time during which cross-transmission may occur is prolonged), and are associated with significant excess morbidity and additional hospital costs [56-59].

Can we effectively control epidemic and endemic spread of MDR organisms? For the ICU setting the answer is definitely affirmative. Two principles should be considered:

i) in endemic situations, the major reservoir for subsequent spread of MDR organisms may be asymptomatic carriers [55];

ii) barrier precautions significantly reduce the risk of cross-transmission compared with standard precautions [60].

Therefore, a successful control strategy should combine systematic screening of patients and contact precautions. The role of antibiotic restriction in controlling dissemination of MDR microorganisms is not completely understood. However, adherence to published guidelines on the appropriate use of antimicrobials is strongly recommended [61,62].

The following examples illustrate these principles. In a hospital endemic for MRSA, Chaix et al. systematically screened high-risk patients for MRSA colonization on admission to the ICU. MRSA-infected and colonized patients were placed in contact isolation. Consequently, the incidence of nosocomial MRSA has decreased by 75 %, although the prevalence of imported cases remained constant [63]. In an ICU endemic for extended spectrum beta-lactamase (ESBL)-producing enterobacteriaceae, Lucet et al. systematically screened admitted patients, and implemented contact precautions for both carriers and infected patients. Over the study period, the incidence of nosocomial cases decreased by almost 90 % although, as in the previous example, the prevalence of imported cases remained stable. Of note, the incidence of clinical cases of *Acinetobacter baumannii* and MRSA was also reduced markedly, 62 % and 38 %, respectively [55].

Clinical syndrome / condition	Modified circumstances	Potential pathogen	Empiric precautions
Acute diarrhea	Any patient	Enteric pathogens[†]	Contact
	Recent hospitalization/antibiotic exposure	*Clostridium difficile*	Contact
Meningitis	Children and adults < 50 y	*Neisseria meningitidis*	Droplet
Fever and generalized rash	Petechial	*Neisseria meningitidis*	Droplet
	Vesicular, non-immune to VZV[‡]	VZV [‡]	Airborne[+] Contact
	Maculopapular[+] coryza, non-immune to measles	Measles virus	Airborne
Respiratory manifestations (cough; fever; dyspnea)	Patients with upper lobe pulmonary infiltrate	*Mycobacterium tuberculosis*	Airborne
	HIV-infected / at high risk of HIV infection	*Mycobacterium tuberculosis*	Airborne
	Child (bronchiolitis/croup)	RSV[§]	Contact
Risk of MDR[‖]	History of colonization MDR[§]	Resistant bacteria	Contact
	Recent hospital or nursing home stay	Resistant bacteria	Contact
	Suspected GISA[‖] infection / colonization	GISA[¶]	Airborne[+] Droplet[+] Contact
Skin or wound infection	Abscess or draining wound that cannot be covered	*Staphylococcus aureus*; GAS [**]	Contact

[†] *Escherichia coli* O157:H7; *Shigella spp*; hepatitis A virus; rotavirus
[‡] VZV=Varicelle zoster virus
[§] RSV=Respiratory syncytial virus
[‖] MDR=multidrug-resistant microorganisms, including: extended-spectrum betalactamase producing enterobacteriae (ESBL); multi-resistant *P. aeruginosa*; multi-resistant *Enterobacter cloacae*
[¶] GISA=Glycopeptide-intermediate *Staphylococcus aureus*
[**] GAS=Group A *Streptococci*

Table 8. *Examples of states requiring empiric specific isolation in addition to standard precautions. Adapted from HICPAC guidelines [16], non exhaustive list*

The listing of nosocomial microorganisms that warrants special control measures, 'epidemiologically important microorganisms' (Table 9), is subject to epidemic and endemic occurrence of these pathogens in a hospital, and subject to constant update. Scrupulous hand hygiene and adherence to contact precautions are important measures to minimize the dissemination.

Guidelines specifying control measures for glycopeptide intermediate *Staph.* *aureus* (GISA) and vancomycin resistant enterococci (VRE) are available on line at: http://www.cdc.gov/ncidod/hip/guide/guide.htm [64] For other drug resistant pathogens the reader should consult the local infection control professional.

Immunocompromised Patients

Immunocompromised patients differ in their susceptibility to infection, depending on the type, severity and duration of immunosuppression. Generally, patients are at increased risk for infections both from endogenous and exogenous sources. Moreover, those patients are susceptible to oppurtunistic free-living microorganisms, such as *P. aeruginosa*, *Acinetobacter spp* and *Enterobacter spp.*, abundant in the inanimate environment of the ICU. Hand hygiene practice and standard precautions should be meticulously applied in all immunocompromized patients.

Protective or reversed isolation refers to total barrier precautions (wearing mask, gown, and gloves) when entering the room of neutropenic patients. Although widely employed, this approach has not modified the high risk of developing infections in such patients, reflecting the fact that neutropenia-related infections arise primarily from patients' endogenous flora [65,66].

Total protective environment has shown efficacy in preventing infections with prolonged neutropenia. This expensive technique, poorly tolerated by patients, consists of: private room; HEPA filtration; disinfection or sterilization of all objects in contact with the patient; use of sterile gowns, mask, gloves, caps and boots by any person (personnel or visitors) entering the room; use of sterile or filtrated water; use of low-microbial count food; and decontamination of the digestive tract [67]. Total protective environment has been shown to reduce the incidence of infection. Accordingly, the use of HEPA filtration is recommended to protect patients with prolonged and profound neutropenia against invasive aspergillosis, a disease poorly responsive to therapy and with high mortality rate [68].

Organ-transplanted patients have lifelong increased risk of infection. However, bacterial and fungal nosocomial infections during the early post-transplantation period are associated with risk factors shared by other surgical critically-ill patients and the same precautions are required. Protective isolation was not found beneficial in organ transplant patients [45].

Microorganism	Epidemiological significance	Isolation precautions	Additional recommended control measures
Gram-positive bacteria			
MRSA*	Excess LOS and costs; may evolve into GISA	Contact	Screening high-risk ICU patients; decolonization
GISA†	Currently no reliable treatment	Contact and droplet	Control of vancomycin use; staff screening
Multi-resistant CoNS‡	Difficult-to-treat prosthetic devices infections	Not recommended	
VRE§	Difficult-to-treat infections	Contact	Control of glycopeptide use Special cleansing procedures; hand disinfection
Gram-negative bacteria			
ESBL-producing enterobacteriaceae‖	Difficult-to-treat infections	Contact	Control of antibiotic use; usefulness of selective digestive decontamination is debated
Pseudomonas aeuroginosa	No available treatment if multi-drug resistant	Contact	Use of synergistic combination therapy
Acinetobacter baumanii	No available treatment if multi-drug resistant	Contact	Environment disinfection
Burkholderia cepacia	Epidemics in cystic-fibrosis patients	Contact, droplet¶	Negative patients with cystic fibrosis should not be housed with positive patients
Stenotrophomonas maltophilia	Outbreaks of cross-contamination Reservoir of resistance genes	Contact, droplet¶	
Fungi			
Resistant *Candida* spp		Not recommended	

* MRSA=methicillin-resistant *Staphylococcus ureus;* † GISA=glycopeptide intermediate-*Staphylococcus aureus;* ‡ CoNS=coagulase-negative staphylococci; § VRE=vancomycin-resistant enterococci; ‖ ESBL= extended spectrum beta-lactamase; ¶ Droplet precautions if colonization/infection of the respiratory tract

***Table 9**. Epidemiologically-important multidrug-resistant microorganisms in the ICU setting*

Pediatric ICU

Principles of prevention of nosocomial transmission are identical for pediatric and adult patients. Since pediatric hospitalization is often due to communicable diseases, awareness of and adherence to specific isolation guidelines is particularly important in this setting. Infants and children younger than two years are highly vulnerable to nosocomial transmission of respiratory viruses. The CDC guidelines suggest contact precautions for children with acute respiratory infection of unknown etiology, due to respiratory syncytial virus or parainfluenza virus; droplet precautions for influenza and pertussis and both droplet and contact for adenoviral infections. Healthcare workers in pediatric wards or units are at high-risk for nosocomial respiratory viral infections and should take precautions to prevent inoculation of eyes and other mucous membranes with infectious droplets.

Hospitalized children with varicella should be under contact and airborne isolation until all lesions are crusted. Exposed non-immune adults (healthcare workers and visitors) and immunocompromized patients should receive varicella vaccine or varicella-zoster immune globulin (VZIG), within 96 hrs of exposure. (Recommendations available online at: http://www.cdc.gov/ncidod/srp/varicella.htm)

Neonatal ICU

The incidence of nosocomial infection is highest in the neonatal ICU (NICU) [17]. Each unit has a unique endemic flora with colonized infants serving as a reservoir for transmission to newly-admitted infants. NICU strains are frequently antibiotic-resistant. Infection rates increase with overcrowding and understaffing. Haley et al. reported a 16-fold increase in outbreaks of *S. aureus* infection when the infant-to-nurse ratio exceeded 7 and a 7-fold increase when the unit was crowded [69]. More recently, they reported increasing rates of endemic MRSA linked to overcrowding and understating [70]. Others have reported a 70 % decrease in the rate of nosocomial infection after a move to a new ICU with more nurses, more space per infant and more accessible sinks [11]. As already discussed, the conjugation between understaffing and overcrowding and increased infection rates is through poor compliance with infection control measures, mainly hand hygiene practices. We recently experienced a cluster of cross-infections due to *Enterobacter cloacae* related to overcrowding, relative understaffing and documented poor hand hygiene practices in our NICU [34].

When necessary, an isolation area can be defined in a NICU by curtains, partitions or other markers. A closed incubator may be helpful in maintaining barrier precautions but because incubator surfaces and entry ports readily become contaminated with microorganisms carried by the infant, the outside of the incubator should be considered contaminated and the boundaries of isolation should extend beyond the incubator itself. Newborns are unlikely to generate large-droplet aerosols, but aerolization may be a problem with infected infants on respirators. These infants should be ventilated in an area away from other infants; if this is not possible, respirator exhaust filters could be considered.

CONCLUSION

More than 50 % of patients admitted to ICUs are already colonized at the time of admission with organism(s) responsible for subsequent endogenous and exogenous infections.

The CDC has published guidelines on isolation precautions to minimize the risk of transmission of infectious agents from colonized/infected patients to other patients or healthcare workers. These are based on the application of standard precautions among which hand hygiene is the most important measure. In addition, specific precautions based on the mode of spread of the microorganism, i.e., via airborne particles, infectious droplets or direct contact, are also recommended.

Recommended measures are restrictive and unpopular and compliance is difficult to maintain, particularly in busy ICUs. However, they are both effective and cost-effective in the control of serious nosocomial infection such as those due to MRSA or multi-drug resistant Gram-negative bacteria.

The scientific rationale of isolation precautions is discussed in detail and practical guidelines are presented in simplified tables.

It is suggested that local factors be taken into account whenever application of recommendations requires changes of healthcare worker behavior.

REFERENCES

1. Pachucki CT, Pappas SA, Fuller GF, et al. Influenza A among hospital personnel and patients. Implications for recognition, prevention, and control. Arch Intern Med 1989; 149:77-80
2. Doebbeling BN, Li N, Wenzel RP. An outbreak of hepatitis A among health care workers: risk factors for transmission. Am J Public Health 1993; 83:1679-1684

3. Gaggero A, Avendano LF, Fernandez J, et al. Nosocomial transmission of rotavirus from patients admitted with diarrhea. J Clin Microbiol 1992; 30:3294-3297

4. Garret DO, Dooley SW, Snider DE, et al. M. tuberculosis. In: Mayhall G, ed. Hospital Epidemiology and Infection Control. Baltimore: Williams & Wilkins; 1999:477-503

5. Pittet D, Harbarth S. The intensive care unit. In: Bennett JV, Brachman PS, eds. Hospital infections. 4th ed. Boston, MA: Little, Brown and Company; 1998:381-402

6. Vincent JL, Bihari DJ, Suter PM, et al. The prevalence of nosocomial infection in intensive care units in Europe. Results of the European Prevalence of Infection in Intensive Care (EPIC) Study. JAMA 1995; 274:639-644

7. Pittet D, Tarara D, Wenzel RP. Nosocomial bloodstream infection in critically ill patients. Excess length of stay, extra costs, and attributable mortality. JAMA 1994; 271:1598-1601

8. Fagon JY, Chastre J, Vuagnat A, et al. Nosocomial pneumonia and mortality among patients in intensive care units. JAMA 1996; 275:866-869

9. Kollef MH, Sherman G, Ward S, et al. Inadequate antimicrobial treatment of infections: a risk factor for hospital mortality among critically ill patients. Chest 1999; 115:462-474

10. Pittet D, Hugonnet S, Harbarth S, et al. Effectiveness of a hospital-wide programme to improve compliance with hand hygiene. Lancet 2000; 356:1307-1312

11. Vicca AF. Nursing staff workload as a determinant of methicillin-resistant Staphylococcus aureus spread in an adult intensive therapy unit. J Hosp Infect 1999; 43:109-113

12. Finkelstein R, Reinhertz G, Hashman N, et al. Outbreak of Candida tropicalis fungemia in a neonatal intensive care unit. Infect Control Hosp Epidemiol 1993; 14:587-590

13. Chang HJ, Miller HL, Watkins N, et al. An epidemic of Malassezia pachydermatis in an intensive care nursery associated with colonization of health care workers' pet dogs. N Engl J Med 1998; 338:706-711

14. Jarvis WR, Martone W. Predominant pathogens in hospital infections. J Antimicrob Chemother 1992; 29 Suppl A:19-24

15. National Nosocomial Infection surveillance (NNIS) System report. Data summary from January 1990 - May 1999. Am J Infect Control 1999; 27:520-532

16. Garner JS. Guideline for isolation precautions in hospitals. The hospital infection control practices advisory committee. Infect Control Hosp Epidemiol 1996; 17:53-80

17. Rangel-Frausto MS, Wiblin T, Blumberg HM, et al. National epidemiology of mycoses survey (NEMIS): variations in rates of bloodstream infections due to Candida species in seven surgical intensive care units and six neonatal intensive care units. Clin Infect Dis 1999; 29:253-258

18. Harbarth S, Pittet D. Identification and management of infectious outbreaks in the critical care unit. Curr Opin Crit Care 1996; 2:352-60

19. Jarvis WR. Handwashing--the Semmelweis lesson forgotten? Lancet 1994; 344:1311-1312

20. Pittet D. Improving compliance with hand hygiene in hospitals. Infect Control Hosp Epidemiol 2000; 21:381-386

21. Mackowiak PA. The normal microbial flora. N Engl J Med 1982; 307:83-93

22. Goldmann DA, Leclair J, Macone A. Bacterial colonization of neonates admitted to an intensive care environment. J Pediatr 1978; 93:288-293

23. Pittet D, Dharan S, Touveneau S, et al. Bacterial contamination of the hands of hospital staff during routine patient care. Arch Intern Med 1999; 159:821-826

24. Webster J, Faoagali JL, Cartwright D. Elimination of methicillin-resistant Staphylococcus aureus from a neonatal intensive care unit after hand washing with triclosan. J Paediatr Child Health 1994; 30:59-64

25. Zafar AB, Butler RC, Reese DJ, et al. Use of 0.3% triclosan (Bacti-Stat) to eradicate an outbreak of methicillin-resistant Staphylococcus aureus in a neonatal nursery. Am J Infect Control 1995; 23:200-208

26. Larson EL. APIC guideline for handwashing and hand antisepsis in health care settings. Am J Infect Control 1995; 23:251-269

27. Albert RK, Condie F. Hand-washing patterns in medical intensive-care units. N Engl J Med 1981; 304:1465-1466
28. Larson E, McGinley KJ, Grove GL, et al. Physiologic, microbiologic, and seasonal effects of handwashing on the skin of health care personnel. Am J Infect Control 1986; 14:51-59
29. Rotter ML, Simpson RA, Koller W. Surgical hand disinfection with alcohols at various concentrations: parallel experiments using the new proposed European standards method. Infect Control Hosp Epidemiol 1998; 19:778-781
30. Sproat LJ, Inglis TJ. A multicentre survey of hand hygiene practice in intensive care units. J Hosp Infect 1994; 26:137-148
31. Pittet D, Mourouga P, Perneger TV, et al. Compliance with handwashing in a teaching hospital. Ann Intern Med 1999; 130:126-130
32. Maury E, Alzieu M, Baudel JL, et al. Availability of an alcohol solution can improve hand disinfection compliance in an intensive care unit. Am J Respir Crit Care Med 2000; 162:324-327
33. Larson E, Killien M. Factors influencing handwashing behavior of patient care personnel. Am J Infect Control 1982; 10:93-99
34. Harbarth S, Sudre P, Dharan S, et al. Outbreak of Enterobacter cloacae related to understaffing, overcrowding, and poor hygiene practices. Infect Control Hosp Epidemiol 1999; 20:598-603
35. Voss A, Widmer AF. No time for handwashing ? Handwashing versus alcoholic rub: can we afford 100% compliance ? Infect Control Hosp Epidemiol 1997; 18:205-208
36. Doebbeling BN, Stanley GL, Sheetz CT, et al. Comparative efficacy of alternative hand-washing agents in reducing nosocomial infections in intensive care units. N Engl J Med 1992; 327:88-93
37. Kretzer EK, Larson EL. Behavioral interventions to improve infection control practices. Am J Infect Control 1998; 26:245-253
38. Larson EL, Bryan JL, Adler LM, et al. A multifaceted approach to changing handwashing behavior. Am J Infect Control 1997; 25:3-10
39. Greco PJ, Eisenberg JM. Changing physicians' practices. N Engl J Med 1993; 329:1271-3.
40. Patterson JE. Isolation of patients with communicable diseases. In: Mayhall G, ed. Hospital epidemiology and infection control. Williams & Wilkins, Baltimore, 1996 pp:1032-1051
41. Olsen RJ, Lynch P, Coyle MB, et al. Examination gloves as barriers to hand contamination in clinical practice. JAMA 1993; 270:350-353
42. Albin MS, Bunegin L, Duke ES, et al. Anatomy of a defective barrier: sequential glove leak detection in a surgical and dental environment. Crit Care Med 1992; 20:170-184
43. Doebbeling BN, Pfaller MA, Houston AK, et al. Removal of nosocomial pathogens from the contaminated glove. Implications for glove reuse and handwashing. Ann Intern Med 1988; 109:394-398
44. Hannigan P, Shields JW. Handwashing and use of examination gloves. Lancet 1998; 351:571
45. Edmond M. Isolation. Infect Control Hosp Epidemiol 1997; 18:58-64
46. Guidelines for preventing the transmission of Mycobacterium tuberculosis in health-care facilities, 1994. Centers for Disease Control and Prevention. Morb Mortal Wkly Rep 1994; 43:1-132
47. Jarvis WR, Bolyard EA, Bozzi CJ, et al. Respirators, recommendations, and regulations: the controversy surrounding protection of health care workers from tuberculosis. Ann Intern Med 1995; 122:142-146
48. Maki DG, Alvarado C, Hassemer C. Double-bagging of items from isolation rooms is unnecessary as an infection control measure: a comparative study of surface contamination with single- and double-bagging. Infect Control 1986; 7:535-537
49. Smith MA, Mathewson JJ, Ulert IA, et al. Contaminated stethoscopes revisited. Arch Intern Med 1996; 156:82-84

50. Bernard L, Kereveur A, Durand D, et al. Bacterial contamination of hospital physicians' stethoscopes. Infect Control Hosp Epidemiol 1999; 20:626-628
51. Wright IM, Orr H, Porter C. Stethoscope contamination in the neonatal intensive care unit. J Hosp Infect 1995; 29:65-68
52. Recommendations for preventing the spread of vancomycin resistance. Recommendations of the Hospital Infection Control Practices Advisory Committee (HICPAC). Morb Mortal Wkly Rep 1995; 44:1-13
53. Gordts B, Van Landuyt H, Ieven M, et al. Vancomycin-resistant enterococci colonizing the intestinal tracts of hospitalized patients. J Clin Microbiol 1995; 33:2842-2846
54. Monnet DL, Archibald LK, Phillips L, et al. Antimicrobial use and resistance in eight US hospitals: complexities of analysis and modeling. Intensive Care Antimicrobial Resistance Epidemiology Project and National Nosocomial Infections Surveillance System Hospitals. Infect Control Hosp Epidemiol 1998; 19:388-394
55. Lucet JC, Decre D, Fichelle A, et al. Control of a prolonged outbreak of extended-spectrum beta- lactamase-producing enterobacteriaceae in a university hospital. Clin Infect Dis 1999; 29:1411-1418
56. Edmond MB, Ober JF, Weinbaum DL, et al. Vancomycin-resistant enterococcus faecium bacteremia: risk factors for infection. Clin Infect Dis 1995; 20:1126-1133
57. Hershow RC, Khayr WF, Smith NL. A comparison of clinical virulence of nosocomially acquired methicillin-resistant and methicillin-sensitive Staphylococcus aureus infections in a university hospital. Infect Control Hosp Epidemiol 1992; 13:587-593
58. Bonten MJ, Bergmans DC, Speijer H, et al. Characteristics of polyclonal endemicity of Pseudomonas aeruginosa colonization in intensive care units. Implications for infection control. Am J Respir Crit Care Med 1999; 160:1212-1219
59. Hanberger H, Garcia-Rodriguez JA, Gobernado M, et al. Antibiotic susceptibility among aerobic gram-negative bacilli in intensive care units in 5 European countries. French and Portuguese ICU Study Groups. JAMA 1999; 281:67-71
60. Jernigan JA, Titus MG, Groschel DH, et al. Effectiveness of contact isolation during a hospital outbreak of methicillin-resistant Staphylococcus aureus. Am J Epidemiol 1996; 143:496-504
61. Quale J, Landman D, Saurina G, et al. Manipulation of a hospital antimicrobial formulary to control an outbreak of vancomycin-resistant enterococci. Clin Infect Dis 1996; 23:1020-1025
62. De Champs C, Sauvant MP, Chanal C, et al. Prospective survey of colonization and infection caused by expanded-spectrum-beta-lactamase-producing members of the family enterobacteriaceae in an intensive care unit. J Clin Microbiol 1989; 27:2887-2890
63. Chaix C, Durand-Zaleski I, Alberti C, et al. Control of endemic methicillin-resistant Staphylococcus aureus: a cost-benefit analysis in an intensive care unit. JAMA 1999; 282:1745-1751
64. Goldmann DA, the subcommittee on Prevention and Control of Antimicrobial-resistant Microorganisms in Hospitals. Recommendations for preventing the spread of vancomycin resistance - Recommendations of the Hospital Infection Control Practice Advisory Committee (HICPAC). Morb Mortal Wkly Rep 1995; 44:1-13
65. Nauseef WM, Maki DG. A study of the value of simple protective isolation in patients with granulocytopenia. N Engl J Med 1981; 304:448-453
66. Walsh TR, Guttendorf J, Dummer S, et al. The value of protective isolation procedures in cardiac allograft recipients. Ann Thorac Surg 1989; 47:539-544
67. Pizzo PA. The value of protective isolation in preventing nosocomial infections in high risk patients. Am J Med 1981; 70:631-637
68. Denning DW. Therapeutic outcome in invasive aspergillosis. Clin Infect Dis 1996; 23:608-615

69. Haley RW, Bregman DA. The role of understaffing and overcrowding in recurrent outbreaks of staphylococcal infection in a neonatal special-care unit. J Infect Dis 1982; 145:875-885

70. Haley RW, Cushion NB, Tenover FC, et al. Eradication of endemic methicillin-resistant Staphylococcus aureus infections from a neonatal intensive care unit. J Infect Dis 1995; 171:614-624

34

THE LUNG IN SEPSIS

Peter M. Suter

Severe infection and sepsis are frequently complicated by some form of respiratory dysfunction. There are several reasons for this association:

1) pulmonary infection such as pneumonia is a frequent cause of sepsis, and this is particularly important in the hospitalized patient;
2) infection in other areas and organs of the body can lead to distinct alterations in morphology and function of lung parenchyma, alveolar space and airways;
3) cardiovascular changes secondary to sepsis such as a hyperdynamic circulation and disturbances in microvascular permeability can have major influences on pulmonary hemodynamics and gas exchange.

All these changes can exist to different degrees and intensities, depending on a number of factors, such as :

- type of infection
- the microbial agents involved
- host response to infection, including intensity of immunological defense mechanisms and susceptibility to vital organ dysfunction
- preexisting morbidities involving the respiratory system
- respiratory reserves related to muscle function and lung parenchymal integrity.

The purpose of the present chapter is to review briefly respiratory symptoms of sepsis involving lung, chest wall and airways, to summarize the mechanisms and mediators involved in these changes, and finally to present a few principles of management in these patients.

The respiratory complications of sepsis most frequently present as acute lung injury (ALI) or acute respiratory distress syndrome (ARDS). These syndromes are characterized by acute onset, more or less marked systemic hypoxemia and a typical chest X-ray appearance (Table 1) [1].

Criteria	Timing	Oxygenation	Chest radiograph	Pulmonary artery wedge pressure
ALI	Acute onset	$PaO_2/FiO_2 \leq$ 300 mm Hg (regardless of PEEP level)	Bilateral infiltrates seen on frontal chest radiograph	≤ 18 mm Hg when measured or no clinical evidence of left atrial hypertension
ARDS	Acute onset	$PaO_2/FiO_2 \leq$ 200 mm Hg (regardless of PEEP level)	Bilateral infiltrates seen on frontal chest radiograph	≤ 18 mm Hg when measured or no clinical evidence of left atrial hyper-tension

Table 1. The American-European consensus committee recommended criteria for acute lung injury (ALI) and acute respiratory distress syndrome (ARDS) [1]

The frequency of the severe form of respiratory failure, i.e., ARDS, in sepsis varies widely in published studies. Reported incidences range between 18 and 41 % (Table 2) [2-11].

The reasons for these differences are not clear. However, more severe forms of sepsis, and, in particular, the presence of septic shock and its duration appear to be associated with a higher incidence of ARDS [1].

RESPIRATORY SIGNS AND SYMPTOMS

The first symptoms of respiratory involvement in sepsis are frequently related to the increased body temperature and hyperdynamic state, e.g.,
- increased respiratory frequency (tachypnea)
- increased minute ventilation (polypnea).

In more severe forms of septic lung disease, signs of respiratory failure/dysfunction can appear, including
- dyspnea
- cyanosis of skin and mucosa
- respiratory distress - use of accessory muscles.

In up to one third of patients with sepsis, the early clinical manifestations include severe respiratory distress of the ARDS type [3,9]. The symptoms are usually impressive for the patient, his family and the team. Rapid and aggressive management is mandatory, including oxygen administration, as well as considering invasive or non-invasive mechanical ventilation.

In addition to the respiratory signs mentioned, cardiovascular and neurologic alterations can be present, confounding respiratory dysfunction. These symptoms can include a hyperdynamic circulation with marked tachycardia, early hypertension or hypotension or shock, and altered mental status with agitation, confusion or (rarely) a comatose state.

Investigations such as chest x-ray, cardiac echocardiography, hemodynamic evaluation using a pulmonary artery catheter, etc. are frequently helpful to better understand and monitor cardiovascular changes, as well as to assess the effect of therapy and to follow the clinical course.

Study	Incidence of ARDS in sepsis/septic shock (%)
Pepe et al, 1982 [2]	5 / 13 (38)
Fein et al, 1983 [3]	21 / 116 (18)
Weinberg et al, 1984 [4]	10 / 40 (25)
Luce et al, 1988 [5]	27 / 75 (36)
Langlois et al, 1988 [6]	22 / 87 (25)
Bone et al, 1989 [7]	38 / 152 (25)
Danner et al, 1991 [8]	37 / 100 (37)
Hudson et al 1995 [9]	56 / 136 (41)
Rangel-Frausto, 1995 [10]	20 / 110* (18)
Rangel-Frausto, 1995 [10]	15 / 84 + (18)

* culture-positive septic shock, + culture-negative septic shock

Table 2. *Frequency of ARDS in sepsis [11]*

ELEMENTS OF RESPIRATORY DYSFUNCTION

Pulmonary gas exchange is altered in sepsis, secondary to combined changes in alveolar ventilation and in ventilation/perfusion (V/Q) distribution. An increased microvascular permeability causes interstitial edema producing alveolar collapse and closure of small airways, thereby creating low V/Q areas predominating in dependent lung regions.

This type of regional difference in aerated versus collapsed lung regions is seen in ARDS and ALI of other origins, and the respiratory management of these problems is similar.

The consequences of these changes are systemic hypoxemia due to massive venous admixture [13], and a discreet increase in deadspace ventilation, but also a fall in respiratory compliance, particularly at low positive end-expiratory pressure (PEEP) levels, i.e., low lung volumes.

Increased systemic oxygen consumption and carbon dioxide production are observed in severe infections or sepsis. These patients are in general also hyperthermic. This is thought to be a consequence of increased local - in the area of active infection - and systemic metabolic demands. This hyperdynamic situation has respiratory consequences: minute ventilation is increased, and cyanosis can be present secondary to a high oxygen extraction and marked venous oxygen desaturation. As mentioned earlier, consecutive polypnea, tachypnea and respiratory distress can be observed - the latter however rarely in the absence of some pathologic changes of the respiratory system.

Besides the respiratory compensation for the increased metabolic demands, a substantially higher than normal cardiac output will allow an increased oxygen availability for the systemic circulation and peripheral organs, as well as adequate CO_2 transport from systemic tissues to the lungs, for appropriate elimination.

PATHOPHYSIOLOGY AND MECHANISMS OF SEPSIS-INDUCED LUNG INJURY (ALI AND ARDS)

Both ALI and ARDS are now recognized as an expression of an intense inflammatory reaction of the pulmonary parenchyma to an insult of infectious or non-infectious origin, that can be local or systemic [12]. It has been shown that a certain compartimentalization of this inflammatory response exists [14,15]. For instance, during significant pneumonia or after endotracheal endotoxin administration [15,16] the local intrapulmonary concentration of polymorphonuclear leukocytes (PMN) and cytokines is markedly higher than in the systemic circulation. The same observations have been made in severe human ARDS of septic or non-septic origin [14] and in ventilator-induced lung injury [17].

The pathomechanism of development of ALI and ARDS in sepsis involves mainly inflammatory mediators including lipopolysaccharide (LPS) and cytokines, as well as circulating leukocytes, pulmonary endothelial and epithelial cells (Figure 1). Other factors may also play important roles, such as macrophages and oxygen radicals producing lipid peroxidation. Persisting increased levels of proinflammatory cytokines in plasma and or bronchoalveolar lavage (BAL) fluid correlate with a protracted course of respiratory failure and reduced survival [18].

Tissue repair mechanisms are initiated early on in sepsis-related lung dysfunction. However, their duration and the final result can vary widely. After the acute, exudative phase, a fibroproliferative stage can be observed, followed by a fibrotic phase. Each of these stages has a duration of a few days but this also is variable. The resolution of the underlying sepsis is one of the key elements for restoration of normal lung function.

MORPHOLOGIC CHANGES

Due to the increased capillary permeability, both lung parenchyma and chest wall show marked edema in sepsis-related respiratory dysfunction. This leads, for the chest wall, to an increased stiffness, i.e. a higher elastance and a lower compliance. The lung tissue becomes edematous and due to the gravitational forces, interstitial water is much more abundant in dependent area, i.e. the dorsal regions of the lung. Concomitantly the higher interstitial pressure causes collapse of distal alveoli and airways by compression. This results in very low V/Q ratios in dependent areas and a marked increase in intrapulmonary shunting.

Histologically, edema and inflammation dominate in early phases (Figure 2) [19]. After a few days, hyaline membranes can be seen in the alveoli, corresponding to fibrin deposition. In the interstitium fibroblasts and collagen deposition appear. The normal pulmonary architecture may disappear to a large extent, and later a profound remodelling of tissue structure can occur. This repair process is parallelled by a decrease in the number of PMNs, and a replacement by mononuclear cells within the parenchyma. Alveolar epithelial type I cells disappear progressively, type II cells proliferate and cover the (new) alveolar structures, finally differentiating into type I cells.

Important transformations occur in the vascular system too. Microvascular obstruction and capillary damage are hallmarks of early and intermediate phases of ARDS. Eventually vascular remodeling and possibly neovascularization take place in the most involved tissue areas, restoring the possibility of gas exchange between alveolar spaces and new microvessels. This remodeling process does not really result in a normal lung parenchyma, and a certain number of these patients have long term sequellae in their respiratory function [20,21].

SEPSIS
↓
Release of inflammatory mediators
LPS, cytokines (TNF-α, IL-1β, IL-8)

• ACUTE SYSTEMIC INFLAMMATORY RESPONSE
↓

• NEUTROPHIL SEQUESTRATION
More immature, less deformable, less motile PMNs
↓
Increased adhesiveness of PMNs to endothelium
↓

• NEUTROPHIL ACTIVATION/ADHESION
Expression of neutrophil adhesion molecules
E-, P-, L- selections and integrins (CD11b/CD18)
↓
Initial loose adhesion ('rolling' effect)
↓
Expression of ICAM by endothelium
↓
'Firm' adhesion of neutrophils to endothelium
↓

• NEUTROPHIL MIGRATION (CHEMOTAXIS)
from vascular space into the pulmonary interstitium
or alveolar space
Expression of IL-8
↓

• NEUTROPHIL ACTIVATION/RELEASE OF OXIDATIVE
METABOLITES AND PROTEOLYTIC ENZYMES
↓

• EPITHELIAL & ENDOTHELIAL INJURY
↓
Loss of barrier function, increased capillary permeability,
impaired gas exchange

● ALI/ARDS ●

Figure 1. *Pathophysiological mechanisms of ALI and ARDS in sepsis. From [11] with permission*

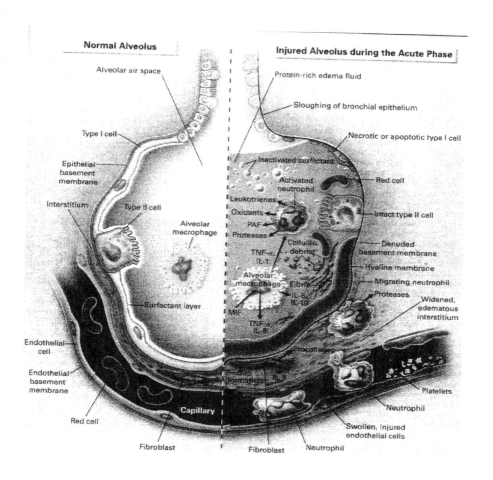

Figure 2: Schematic representation of the morphology of a normal alveolo-capillary space, and the changes involved in the acute phase of ARDS. Reproduced from [19] with permission.

MANAGEMENT

Acute lung failure in sepsis has to be managed by supportive care, i.e., supplemental oxygen administration, intubation and mechanical ventilatory support when respiratory fatigue is a potential danger or is present. All these means together have decreased the mortality of ARDS from different causes over the last 10 or 15 years [22].

Of outmost importance for the clinical course and outcome of sepsis-related acute pulmonary failure is the successful treatment of infection. Adequate antibiotics, surgical drainage if necessary and close microbiologic monitoring are part of an appropriate strategy.

Ventilatory support must be given by an invasive approach in most patients - non-invasive mechanical ventilation by mask has not been clearly shown to be effective in this situation. Further investigations in this area are warranted. The main pulmonary changes, i.e., interstitial edema and collapse of basal lung regions can be counteracted by PEEP and adequate tidal volumes. Both contribute to recruitment of non or hypo-ventilated areas [23,24], and consecutive improvement of gas exchange.

Indications for intubation and mechanical ventilation in sepsis include marked hypoxemia despite supplemental oxygen, severe tachypnea (respiratory rate above 40/min), muscular fatigue or failure, and altered mental status.

Important elements of mechanical ventilatory support [25] include
- a low tidal volume, about 6 ml/kg ideal body weight;
- an end-inspiratory plateau pressure as low as possible, preferably below 30 cm H_2O;
- a PEEP level of 10-18 cm H_2O, depending on the resulting increase in arterial oxygenation and hemodynamic tolerance;
- after an initial stabilization period, daily trials of spontaneous breathing should be made to achieve extubation as early as possible.

Permissive hypercapnia may be acceptable in this situation, allowing a decrease in high inspiratory pressure and thereby the risk of barotrauma [26].

Position changes and prone positioning may be considered in severe ARDS not improving over a few days. This maneuver can be associated with an improvement in systemic oxygenation [27].

Appropriate fluid therapy is essential to support cardiovascular function in sepsis, but efforts have to be made to decrease or limit the extent of pulmonary edema. It has been recognized that the capacity of resorption of alveolar fluid is decreased in ARDS compared to normal lung [28]. Therefore, it is of major importance to maintain an adequate fluid balance in this situation.

Anti-inflammatory agents have not been shown to be of any benefit in early phases of ALI or ARDS. In late phases (i.e., after one week of evolution) when gas exchange disturbance remains severe, requiring high FiO_2 and PEEP levels, and signs of pulmonary inflammation persist, intravenous corticosteroids can be considered [29].

Other treatments such as inhaled vasodilators (nitric oxide, prostacyclins) can be options for salvage therapy.

CONCLUSION

Despite increasing knowledge about the pathophysiology and mediators involved in acute lung failure complicating sepsis, large areas of the biological and physiological response and repair mechanisms require further investigation [19].

The management of these patients remains essentially supportive. The use of modern monitoring and ventilatory techniques together with good general ICU care has improved outcome substantially over the last years [30]. However, much remains to be done in the area of therapeutic and outcome research, to know more about long term results, and to improve treatment modalities further.

REFERENCES

1. Bernard GR, Artigas A, Brigham KL, et al. The American-European consensus conference on ARDS. Definitions, mechanisms, relevant outcomes, and clinical trial coordination. Am J Respir Crit Care Med 1994; 149:818-824
2. Pepe PE, Potkin RT, Holtman Reus D, et al. Clinical predictors of the adult respiratory distress syndrome. Am J Surg 1982; 144:24-30
3. Fein AM, Lippmann M, Holzman H, et al. The risk factors, incidence, and prognosis of ARDS following septicemia. Chest 1983; 83:40-42
4. Weinberg PF, Matthay MA, Webster RO, et al. Biologically active products of complement and acute lung injury in patients with the sepsis syndrome. Am Rev Respir Dis 1984; 130:791-796
5. Luce JM, Montgomery B, Marks JD, et al. Ineffectiveness of high-dose methylprednisolone in preventing parenchymal lung injury and improving mortality in patients with septic shock. Am Rev Respir Dis 1988; 138:62-68
6. Langlois PF, Gawryl MS. Accentuated formation of the terminal C5b-9 complement complex in patient plasma precedes development of the adult respiratory distress syndrome. Am Rev Respir Dis 1988; 138:368-375
7. Bone RC, Fisher CJ, Clemmer TP, et al. Sepsis syndrome : A valid clinical entity. Crit Care Med 1989; 17:389-393
8. Danner RL, Elin EJ, Hosseini JM, et al. Endotoxemia in human septic shock. Chest 1991; 99:169-175
9. Hudson LD, Milberg JA, Anardi D, Maunder RJ. Clinical risks for development of the acute respiratory distress syndrome.Am J Respir Crit Care Med 1995; 151:293-301
10. Rangel-Frausto MS, Pittet D, Costigan M, et al. The natural history of the systemic inflammatory response syndrome (SIRS). A prospective study. JAMA 1995; 273:117-123
11. Fein AM, Calalang-Colucci MG. Acute lung injury and acute respiratory distress syndrome in sepsis and septic shock. Crit Care Clin 2000; 16:289-317
12. The ACCP/SCCM consensus conference committee : Bone RC, Balk RA, Cerra FB,

Dellinger RP, et al. Definitions for sepsis and organ failure and guidelines for the use of innovative therapies in sepsis. Chest 1992; 101:1644-1655

13. Martin GS, Bernard GR. Airway and lung in sepsis. Intensive Care Med 2001; 27:S63-S79

14. Suter PM, Suter S, Girardin E, et al. High broncho-alveolar levels of tumor necrosis factor and its inhibitors, interleukin-1, interferon and elastase in patients with ARDS after trauma, shock or sepsis. Am Rev Respir Dis 1992; 145:1016-1022

15. O'Grady NP, Preas HL, Puhin J, et al. Local inflammatory responses following bronchial endotoxin instillation in humans. Am J Respir Crit Care Med 2001; 163:1591-1598

16. Tutor JD, Mason CM, Dobard E, et al. Loss of compartmentalization of alveolar tumor necrosis factor after lung inuury. Am J Respir Crit Care Med 1994; 149:1107-1111

17. Ranieri VM, Suter PM, Tortorella C, et al. Effect of mechanical ventilation on inflammatory mediators in patients with acute respiratory distress syndrome. A randomized controlled trial. JAMA 1999; 282:54-61

18. Meduri GU, Headley S, Tolley E, et al. Plasma and BAL cytokine response to corticosteroid rescue treatment in late ARDS. Chest 1995; 108:1315-1325

19. Ware LB, Matthay MA. The acute respiratory distress syndrome. N Engl J Med 2000; 342:1334-1349

20. Angus DC, Musthafa AA, Clermont G, et al. Quality-adjusted survival in the first year after the acute respiratory distress syndrome. Am J Respir Crit Care Med 2001; 163:1389-1394

21. Davidson TA, Caldwell ES, Curtis JR, et al. Reduced quality of life in survivors of acute respiratory distress syndrome compared with critically ill control patients. JAMA 1999; 281:354-360

22. Milberg JA, Davis DR, Steiberg KP, Hudson LD. Improved Survival of Patients With Acute Respiratory Distress Syndrome (ARDS): 1983-1993. JAMA 1995; 273:306-309

23. Gattinoni L, D'Andrea L, Pelosi P, et al. Regional effects and mechanism of positive end expiratory pressure in early adult respiratory distress syndrome. JAMA 1993; 269:2122-2127

24. Gattinoni L, Bombino M, Pelosi P, et al. Lung structure and function in different stages of severe adult respiratory distress syndrome. JAMA 1994; 271:1772-1779

25. Tobin MJ. Advances in mechanical ventilation. Review article. N Engl J Med 2001; 344: 1986-1996

26. Bidani A, Tzouanakis AE, Cardenas VJ Jr, Zwischenberger JB. :Permissive hypercapnia in acute respiratory failure. JAMA 1994; 272: 957-962

27. Gattinoni L, Tognoni G, Pesenti A, et al. Effect of prone position on the survival of patients with acute respiratory failure. N Engl J Med 2001; 345:568-73

28. Ware LB, Matthay MA. Alveolar fluid clearance is impaired in the majority of patients with acute lung injury and the acute respiratory distress syndrome. Am J Respir Crit Care Med 2001; 163:1376-1831

29. Meduri GU, Headley AS, Golden E, et al. Effect of prolonged methylprednisolone therapy in unresolving acute respiratory distress syndrome: A randomized controlled trial. JAMA 1998; 280:159-165

30. The acute respiratory distress syndrome network. Ventilation with lower tidal volumes as compared with traditional tidal volumes for acute lung injury and the acute respiratory distress syndrome. N Engl J Med 2000; 342:1302-1308

35

THE HEART IN SEPSIS

Benoit Tavernier
Alexandre Mebazaa

Myocardial dysfunction in sepsis is now well established [1,2]. It starts a couple of hours or days after the onset of sepsis and involves both right and left ventricles. In patients who survive, myocardial function recovers within 5-7 days *ad integrum*. Although myocardial depressing factors have been suggested to be involved in the reduction in myocardial contractility in septic animals and patients [3,4], they appear to exert short-acting 'reversible' effects that usually last less than an hour [5-7]. The main mechanism of the long lasting myocardial dysfunction appears therefore to be intrinsic myocardial alterations [8-13]. Indeed, hearts, papillary muscles or single cardiomyocytes isolated from septic animals showed depression in contractile function that lasts several hours with no signs of recovery.

We will focus our chapter on four topics, the knowledge of which has improved greatly in recent years:

1. The diagnosis of myocardial depression in septic patients. Cardiac echocardiography is now a usual tool in intensive care units (ICUs) and many intensivists are very familiar with measurements of ventricular contractility, surface area and relaxation.

2. Great improvements have been made in our understanding of the underlying mechanisms of myocardial dysfunction in sepsis. We, and others, have clearly established that sepsis-related reduction in myocardial contractility is due to a reduction of cardiac myofilament response to intracellular calcium.

3. The acute effect of a sepsis-related overproduction of nitric oxide (NO) has been suggested to be a major player in the reduction of myocardial contractility. This could not be demonstrated in animals or in humans *in vivo* [8, 9, 13, 14]. In contrast, several authors have suggested recently

that NO could rather play a role in the inactivation of cardiac proteins via the production of peroxynitrite [15,16]. This may participate to the long lasting effect of sepsis on cardiac contractile function.

4. Any clinician would like to be able to treat myocardial alteration during sepsis. However, few agents are really specific. A recent publication from the American Society of Critical Care Medicine emphasized the role of volume loading as a first choice associated with dobutamine and/or norepinephrine when needed [17].

CARDIAC FUNCTION IN HUMAN SEPTIC SHOCK

According to a series of clinical and experimental studies by Parrillo's group using radionucleide gated blood-pool scanning and simultaneous thermodilution hemodynamic measurements [18,19], the typical pattern of cardiac function in septic shock includes:
1. a reduced biventricular ejection fraction
2. increased left and right ventricular end-diastolic volumes
3. an elevated heart rate and cardiac output
4. a decreased systemic vascular resistance.

Cardiac dysfunction occurs 24 to 48 hours after the onset of sepsis and is reversible in patients who survive 5 to 10 days after its onset [18]. However, this typical pattern of cardiac depression may not be present in a number of patients with septic shock, and it is likely that pre-existing cardiac disease, fluid loading, inotropic support, as well as the severity of septic shock itself may alter the pattern of cardiac dysfunction in septic patients.

The occurrence of acute biventricular dilatation in human septic shock has remained the most controversial issue since its initial description. In contrast with the studies by Parrillo's group showing a 40-50 % increase in left ventricular (LV) end-diastolic volume (EDV) in 33 survivors [20], Jardin and colleagues were unable to observe such an acute dilatation in septic patients studied with transthoracic echocardiography [21-23]. Despite the increasing routine use of echocardiography in many ICU, this controversy has not yet been resolved, but several recent studies may help to understand better the pattern of septic cardiac dysfunction in humans. In 1999, Jardin et al. reported a longitudinal transthoracic echocardiographic study in 90 septic shock patients without prior cardiopulmonary disease [23]. They confirmed some results from Parrillo's group such as depressed LV systolic function at the initial phase of septic shock, with an even lower ejection fraction in their patients that ultimately recovered. In accordance with their previous studies, Jardin et al. found LVEDVs within the normal range (day 1: 75.3 ± 20.1 ml/m^2 in survivors, and 64.9 ± 25.0 ml/m^2 in nonsurvivors, versus 68.5 ±

14.7 ml/m^2 in a control group of volunteers). Interestingly, in their patients who survived, LVEDV increased by approximately 15 % (80.3 ± 20.9 ml/m^2) at day 2, whereas volumes in nonsurvivors tended to decrease and were significantly smaller than in survivors. Thus, a trend for a reversible increase in LV end-diastolic dimensions was also found by Jardin et al., although to a smaller extent than that described by Parrillo's group. Because no attempt was made to maximize cardiac output by Jardin et al., optimal conditions to observe LV dilatation were probably not met in all patients. Given the large standard deviations reported in the results of LVEDV, it is likely that some survivors still had relative hypovolemia, while others might have been 'better' resuscitated and had clearly increased LVEDVs.

The crucial role of fluid loading in the occurrence of LV dilatation appears in another recent study by Tavernier et al. [24]. In this study, LV end-diastolic area (obtained by transesophageal echocardiography [TEE]) was measured along with other preload parameters in 15 patients with sepsis-induced hypotension. In each patient, successive volume loading steps (VLSs) were performed until a nonresponder VLS was obtained. Fluid loading increased LV end-diastolic area from 9.6 ± 3.6 cm^2/m^2 (baseline measurements) to 12.8 ± 3.7 cm^2/m^2 (cardiac output maximized). In the literature, the values reported in nonseptic patients without previous cardiac disease in similar conditions were approximately 7.0-9.0 ± 3.0 cm^2/m^2, which suggests a ~ 30-40 % increase in LV end-diastolic surface when cardiac output was maximized in septic patients.

Heterogeneity of myocardial dysfunction has also been shown with the combination of hemodynamic monitoring and transesophageal Doppler echocardiography in 25 patients with persistent, vasopressor-dependent septic shock [25]. In fact, these data suggested that cardiac dysfunction in septic shock could be described as a *continuum* from isolated diastolic dysfunction to both diastolic and systolic ventricular failure. In this group of septic shock patients, LV end-diastolic area was in the upper values of the normal range (~ 9 cm^2/m^2), which could be expected at this stage of septic shock (evaluation was performed 10 ± 8 days after ICU admission, with many patients without systolic depression).

CALCIUM HOMEOSTASIS IN THE SEPTIC HEART

In experimental studies, contraction of heart, papillary muscles as well as single cardiac myocytes isolated from septic animals has been shown to be persistently impaired *ex vivo*. These observations have led to the concept of *intrinsic* myocardial dysfunction in sepsis. Studies have then attempted to establish the subcellular basis of intrinsic contractile depression in *in vivo* models, for example with correlation of contractile dysfunction and subcellular processes in tissues studied *ex vivo*. In intact myocardial cells, the amplitude and rate of tension development and relaxation are primarily determined by the rate of Ca^{2+} mobilization and deprivation, by the crossbridge cycling rate, or by the contribution of both [26]. From this perspective, changes in myocardial contractility may theoretically result from alterations in three general types of mechanisms:

1. regulation of the Ca^{2+} mobilizing process ('upstream' mechanism)
2. binding of Ca^{2+} to troponin C ('central' mechanism), and
3. response of the myofilaments to a given level of occupancy of Ca^{2+} binding sites on troponin C ('downstream' mechanism) [26].

While it is well known that the 'upstream' mechanism, via alterations in sarcolemmal ion flux and/or in sarcoplasmic reticulum (SR) function, is involved in several cardiac diseases and inotropic interventions, there is now a growing body of evidence for the existence of 'central' or 'downstream' mechanisms as well. In particular, alterations in troponin I function, leading to changes in myofilament Ca^{2+} sensitivity, have been implicated in the pathophysiology of failing human myocardium (decrease in troponin I phosphorylation) and myocardial stunning (proteolysis of troponin I) [27-29].

In sepsis, the relative roles of changes in intracellular Ca^{2+} transient versus alterations in myofilament response to Ca^{2+} as determinants of myocardial depression have only recently been studied. The results may have potential therapeutic implications (see below).

Early data have suggested that myocyte cytoplasmic Ca^{2+} transient was altered in hearts removed from endotoxemic animals. In a series of experimental studies in a canine model, endotoxic shock impaired ATP-dependent Ca^{2+} uptake by SR, leading to a reduction in the Ca^{2+}-induced Ca^{2+} release mechanism [30]. Endotoxin administration in dogs also impaired the ATP-dependent Ca^{2+} transport by the sarcolemma as well as the Na^+-Ca^{2+} exchanger in some studies [31], whereas others found a normal Na^+-Ca^{2+} exchange and sarcolemmal Ca^{2+} transport [32]. More recently, Hung and Lew used a model of endotoxemia in rabbits where normal arterial blood pressures, pH and PO_2 were maintained to avoid ischemia, acidosis or hypoxia as causes for cardiac depression [12]. They showed a decrease in the action potential duration in left ventricular myocytes, with little or no endotoxin-induced alteration in SR function or resting membrane potential. They subsequently attributed this effect to a decrease in functional L-type Ca^{2+} channels, as reflected by the number of dihydropyridine receptors [33]. Consistent with these findings, the density of cardiac L-type Ca^{2+} current was reduced in myocytes isolated from animals treated with endotoxin [13, 34]. Interestingly, in a model of endotoxemia in rat, the time-course of L-type Ca^{2+} current reduction was shown to parallel the severity of cardiac dysfunction assessed *in vivo* [13].

More recently, the sensitivity of cardiac myofilament to Ca^{2+} (studied in 'skinned' ventricular fibers) was reported to be decreased during endotoxin shock in conscious rabbit. This effect was dose- and time-dependent, and reversible with time [10]. The reduction in myofilament Ca^{2+} sensitivity was subsequently confirmed in left ventricular 'skinned' fibers taken from rabbit hearts in a non-lethal model of endotoxemia without shock [9]. The latter study also found that cross-bridge properties were preserved. The precise mechanism of reduction in the myofilament Ca^{2+} response in the septic heart has not yet been elucidated, but a phosphorylation of contractile proteins was shown to be involved [9]. Moreover, we have recently found in intact cardiac myocytes isolated 12 hours after induction of endotoxemia in conscious rats (when, in this model, *in vivo* hemodynamic alterations reproduce the 'hyperdynamic' profile of septic shock) that myofilament response to Ca^{2+} was the major determinant of intrinsic cardiac depression in systemic endotoxemia (Figures 1 and 2) This effect appeared to be unrelated to changes in intracellular pH (acidosis reduces myofilament response to Ca^{2+}), but associated with an increase in myocardial troponin I phosphorylation [8]. Although *in vitro* studies have suggested that NO, *via* phosphorylation of troponin I by cGMP-dependent protein kinase, reduces myofilament responses to Ca^{2+} [9,35], the decrease in myofilament sensitivity to Ca^{2+} in the septic heart does not seem to be the direct effect of activation of the NO-cGMP pathway since NO synthase (NOS) inhibitors had no effect on myocardial dysfunction in several *ex vivo* studies. An alternative to increased protein kinase activity as an explanation for the increased troponin I phosphorylation could be an inhibition of specific phosphatase activity, since the phosphorylation level of most proteins depends upon the balance between protein kinase and phosphatase activities. Nevertheless, these alterations in myofilament properties may constitute the cellular basis of the acute ventricular dilatation frequently observed in septic shock patients in response to fluid loading. Indeed, a reduction in myofilament responsiveness to Ca^{2+} is associated with an increased length in single cardiac myocytes and an increased ventricular distensibility [36]. Moreover, phosphorylation of myofilaments has been shown to amplify the length-dependent change in the Ca^{2+}-tension relationship of myocardium [37]. Since this relationship is the dominant theory for the cellular basis of Starling's law [38], the phosphorylation-dependent decrease in Ca^{2+} sensitivity of septic myocardium may contribute to the positive fluid responsiveness usually observed in septic patients despite myocardial depression. In addition, the finding that a reduced myofilament sensitivity to Ca^{2+} is a determinant of intrinsic myocardial depression in septic shock raises the possibility that Ca^{2+}-sensitizing agents might be appropriate treatment to improve heart function in sepsis.

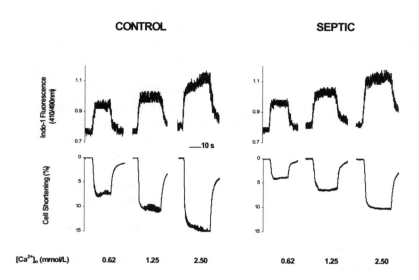

Figure 1. *Representative examples of assessement of myofilament response to Ca²⁺ in tetanized cardiac myocytes. Figure shows indo- 1 fluoresence ratio (top) and simultaneously measured cell shortening (bottom) during repetitive tetanization of a control cell (left panel) and a septic myocyte (right panel); Ca²⁺]₀ varied between 0.62 and 2.5 mmol/L in both cells. Tetanic shortening at equivalent tetanic fluorescence transients is reduced markedly in the septic cell. From [8] with permission.*

Finally, the relative importance of the reduced myofilament Ca^{2+} responsiveness compared with altered myoplasmic Ca^{2+} availability has not yet been determined. Conflicting results have been found and may be partly explained by the use of different sepsis models and/or methods of assessment of contractile function [8,35,39]. In addition, it is likely that some of the discrepancies found in the literature are due to the fact that the preparations were engaged at different stages of the septic process. Accordingly, in a model of mild endotoxemia without shock in rats, we found that during the first few hours of endotoxemia, the predominant alteration was a reduced myofilament response to Ca^{2+} [8]. In more severe forms of endotoxemia, alterations leading to reduced Ca^{2+} transient and alterations in myofilament properties seem to be involved. In these cases, the decrease in myofilament response to Ca^{2+} may aggravate further the consequences of a reduced Ca^{2+} influx in cardiac myocytes during sepsis.

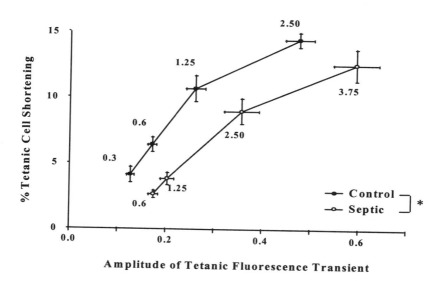

Figure 2. *Relationship between amplitude of indo-1 fluoresence ratio transient (an index of intracellular calcium concentration) and percent cell shortering (an index of contractility) in intact rat cardiac myocytes. Cells were stimulated at varying $Ca^2+]_0$ from 0.3 - 3.75 mmol/l, this is indicated next to each point. Control group comprised 41 myocytes and septic group 40 myocytes. This figure shows that sepsis caused a rightward shift of the relationship between intracellular calcium concentration and shortening in single cardiac myocytes. This indicates a reduction in myofilament response to calcium in the septic heart; *: $p<0.001$. From [8] with permission.*

ROLE OF NO IN MYOCARDIAL ALTERATIONS IN SEPSIS

Role of NO in the Normal Heart

Since the first report showing a direct effect of NO on myocardial contractility in the early 1990s, numerous studies have been published to describe its effects on the heart (review in [40,41]). It is now established that NO has effects on both myocardial contraction and relaxation.

Several studies indicate that low doses of NO (< 1 μM/l) may exert a positive inotropic effect in cardiac myocytes from rat and humans, potentially by an adenylyl cyclase stimulation [42]. However, similar effects could not be seen in human ventricular strips nor in human patients *in vivo* [43]. Higher doses of NO (> 1 μM/l) have been reported to exert negative inotropic effects via the activation of protein kinase G.

More interestingly, it is well established that NO has a great effect on myocardial relaxation. In isolated ferret papillary muscles and in isolated guinea pig hearts, NO caused an earlier onset of isometric twitch and a premature left ventricular relaxation respectively. This is associated with an increase in length and a reduction in active diastolic tone in isolated cardiac myocytes. Analogous changes have been described with NO donors in clinical studies. Paulus et al. published a series of papers showing that both sodium nitroprusside (an NO donor) and substance P (that stimulates endogenous NO release from coronary endothelium) induced an earlier onset of LV relaxation, no changes in LV dP/dt max, and an increase in LV diastolic distensibility [44, 45].

Shah and collegues further demonstrated that endogenous NO facilitates the Frank-Starling response in the whole heart, probably by increasing diastolic distensibility [46]. Thus, the release and/or action of NO might be better at higher LVEDVs. This is in accordance with data published by Pinsky et al. showing that increasing preload in beating hearts induced a parallel increase in myocardial NO release, measured by a porphyrinic NO sensor [47]. Shah and MacCarthy recently suggested that increased LV chamber stretch may augment the intracardiac release of NO, which in turn facilitates an increase in cardiac output by increasing diastolic distensibility and LV filling [40].

Role of NO in the Septic Heart

The effects of NO described in the normal heart could also be applied in the septic heart. But the expression of a Ca^{2+}-independent inducible isoform of NOS (namely NOS2) markedly enhances myocardial NO production that may exert more 'toxic' than beneficial effects. Thus, authors have suggested that myocardial NO overproduction may explain the sepsis-related myocardial dysfunction based on the following unrelated items:
1. the time course of NO overproduction appeared to parallel the alteration in myocardial function
2. the effects of NO donors in normal hearts were said to mimic sepsis-related myocardial alteration, and
3. it is well established that sepsis-related vascular dysfunction is related to an NOS2-related NO overproduction.

Increased expression of NOS2 is well established in septic hearts [15, 41]. Lipopolysaccharide (LPS) and numerous cytokines including interleukin (IL)-1β, tumor necrosis factor (TNF)-α, interferon (IFN)-γ, IL-6 have been shown to induce NOS2 mRNA and activity in cardiac myocytes [48]. NOS2 has also been detected in other cellular constituents of cardiac muscle including endocardial and coronary endothelial cells, fibroblasts and macrophages (review in [15]). Myocardial NOS2 overexpression induces NO hyperproduction in septic hearts. The physiological role and pathological consequences of sepsis-related myocardial NO overproduction are however still unclear. In an *in vitro* model, Balligand and colleagues showed that NOS2-related overproduction of NO may reduce isoproterenol-induced increased contractility ˙in cardiac myocytes exposed to LPS and various cytokines [41]. Brady et al. suggested that NOS2 expression in cardiac myocytes contributed to the LPS-induced reduction in contractility [49]. No direct evidence of NOS2 expression was however provided. Several subsequent studies failed to reproduce this result neither in cardiac myocytes nor in more integrated models. We recently showed in models of LPS-induced myocardial depression in rats and rabbits that various NOS inhibitors could not restore contractility in cardiac myocytes, papillary muscles or isolated hearts [8,9]. This is in accordance with data recently published in human septic shock in which the unspecific inhibitor L-NMMA increased mean arterial pressure but reduced cardiac output [14]. Thus, increasing evidence shows that sepsis is associated with myocardial NOS2 expression and myocardial NO overproduction. However, myocardial depression is unrelated to a direct 'negative' inotropic (potentially reversible) effect of NO.

In contrast, NO may react with superoxide to generate peroxynitrite, a powerful oxidant and an important mediator of cell damage under conditions of inflammation and oxidant stress [8,9]. We and others hypothesized that NO-derived peroxynitrite may act at the early phase of sepsis to alter the structure of some proteins such as cardiac myofilaments via nitration or hydroxylation of aromatic compounds including tyrosine and tryptophan. We recently showed a reduction in the force generated by biopsies of skeletal muscles taken from septic patients compared to normal patients. Despite an important expression of NOS2, the reduction in muscle force could not be restored by the addition of various NOS inhibitors in electrically stimulated biopsies of septic patients [16]. However, reduction in muscle force was associated with peroxynitrite formation [16]. This suggests for the first time that muscular force alteration and potentially organ dysfunction are related to a deleterious effect of NO-derived peroxynitrite rather than a direct effect of NO overproduction in septic patients.

TREATMENT OF MYOCARDIAL DYSFUNCTION IN SEPTIC PATIENTS

The Society of Critical Care Medicine (SCCM) recently gave recommendations on the hemodynamic support of sepsis in adult patients

[17]. Clinicians should first restore organ perfusion pressure mostly with fluid administration alone. However, when fluid therapy fails to restore adequate arterial pressure and organ perfusion, vasopressor agents are recommended. Norepinephrine appears to be the first choice to restore mean arterial pressure (MAP) in septic patients. It successfully increases blood pressure with no reduction in organ perfusion in adequately volume-resuscitated patients. It should be used as early as possible, even at low doses ~ 0.01 µg/kg/min. Although effective to increase MAP, dopamine frequently increases heart rate and reduces arterial oxygenation. Because of its potentially harmful effects on the splanchnic circulation, epinephrine should be limited to the patients who are failing to respond to dopamine and/or to norepinephrine.

The use of inotropic therapy is still debatable in sepsis. In accordance with the recent recommendations of the SCCM, we believe that the large number of septic patients that have an increased cardiac output do not need inotropic agents. In contrast, some septic patients, especially those with prior heart disease may benefit from inotropic support when cardiac output is inadequate. Dobutamine is currently the most used inotropic agent in septic patients and inotropic support usually lasts a couple of days.

Beta-adrenergic receptor agonists should be used with caution in sepsis since their inotropic effects depend on the stage of sepsis. Indeed, we recently showed that a potentiation in the positive inotropic effect of isoproterenol is seen in the early phase of sepsis [13]. This potentiation of β-adrenergic receptor agonist effects disappeared 36 hours after LPS administration. In a further step, especially in non-survivors, dobutamine had effect on myocardial contractile function in severe septic shock [50].

Since there is increasing evidence that a reduction in cardiac myofilament response to calcium is a major mechanism of myocardial dysfunction in sepsis, one may suggest that a calcium sensitizing agent may have interesting actions. This is now under investigation.

REFERENCES

1.   Parrillo J. Pathogenetic mechanisms of septic shock. N Engl J Med 1993; 328: 1471-1477.
2.   Wheeler A, Bernard G. Treating patients with severe sepsis. N Engl J Med 1999; 340: 207-214
3.   Parrillo J, Burch C, Shelhamer J, et al. A circulating myocardial depressant substance in humans with septic shock. J Clin Invest 1985; 76:1539-1553
4.   Parrillo J. The cardiovascular pathophysiology of sepsis. Ann Rev Med 1989; 40:469-485
5.   Finkel M, Oddis C, Jacob T, et al. Negative inotropic effect of cytokines on the heart mediated by Nitric Oxide. Science 1992; 257:387-389

6. Oral H, Dorn GW, Mann DL. Sphingosin mediates the immediate negative inotropic effects of tumor necrosis factor-α in the adult mammalian cardiac myocyte. J Biol Chem 1997; 272:4836 (Abst)
7. Yokoyama T, Vaca L, Rossen RD, et al. Cellular basis for the negative inotropic effects of tumor necrosis factor-α in the adult mammalian heart. J Clin Invest 1993; 92:2303-2312
8. Tavernier B, Li J-M, El-Omar MM, et al. Cardiac contractile impairment associated with increased phosphorylation of troponin I in endotoxemic rats. FASEB J 2001; 15:294-296
9. Tavernier B, Mebazaa A, Mateo P, et al. Phosphorylation-dependent alteration in myofilament calcium sensitivity but normal mitochondrial function in septic heart. Am J Respir Crit Care Med 2001; 163:362-367
10. Tavernier B, Garrigue D, Boulle C, et al. Myofilament calcium sensitivity is decreased in skinned cardiac fibres of endotoxin-treated rabbits. Cardiovasc Res 1998; 38:472-479
11. Hung J, Lew WYW. Temporal sequence of endotoxin-induced systolic and diastolic myocardial depression in rabbits. Am J Physiol 1993; 265: H810-819
12. Hung J, Lew WYW. Cellular mechanisms of endotoxin-induced myocardial depression in rabbits. Circ Res 1993; 73:125-134
13. Abi Gerges N, Tavernier B, Mebazaa A, et al. Sequential changes in autonomic regulation of cardiac myocytes after in vivo endotoxin injection in rat. Am J Respir Crit Care Med 1999; 160:1196-1204
14. Grover R, Zaccardelli D, Colice G, et al. An open-label dose escalation study of the nitric oxide synthase inhibitor, N(G)-methyl-L-arginine hypochloride (546C88), in patients with septic shock. Glaxo Wellcome International Septic Shock Study Group. Crit Care Med 1999; 27:913-922
15. Shah A. Inducible nitric oxide synthase and cardiovascular disease. Cardiovasc Res 2000; 31:847-867
16. Lanone S, Mebazaa A, Heymes C, et al. Muscular contractile failure in septic patients: role of the inducible nitric oxide synthase pathway. Am J Respir Crit Care Med; 2001 (in press)
17. Task force of the American College of Critical Care Medicine SCCM. Practice parameters for hemodynamic support of sepsis in adult patients in sepsis. Crit Care Med 1999; 27:639-660
18. Parrillo J. Myocardial depression during septic shock in humans. Crit Care Med 1990; 18: 1183-1184
19. Ognibene F, Parker M, Natanson C, et al. Depressed left ventricular performance. Response to volume infusion in patients with sepsis and septic shock. Chest 1988; 93:903-910
20. Parker MM, Suffredini AF, Natanson C, et al. Responses of left ventricular function in survivors and nonsurvivors of septic shock. J Crit Care 1989; 4: 19-25
21. Jardin F, Brun-Ney D, Auvert B, et al. Sepsis-related cardiogenic shock. Crit Care Med 1990; 18: 1055-1060
22. Jardin F, Valtier B, Beauchet A, et al. Invasive monitoring combined with two-dimensional echocardiographic study in septic shock. Intensive Care Med 1994; 20:550-554
23. Jardin F, Fourme T, Page B, et al. Persistent preload defect in severe sepsis despite fluid loading: a longitudinal echocardiographic study in patients with septic shock. Chest 1999; 116: 1354-1359
24. Tavernier B, Makhotine O, Lebuffe G, et al. Systolic pressure variation as a guide to fluid therapy in patients with sepsis-induced hypotension. Anesthesiology 1998; 89:1313-1321
25. Poelaert J, Declerck C, Vogelaers D, et al. Left ventricular systolic and diastolic function in septic shock. Intensive Care Med. 1997; 23:553-560

26. Endoh M. Regulation of myocardial contractility by a downstream mechanism. Circ. Res. 1998; 83:230-232
27. Gao W, Atar D, Liu Y, et al. Role of troponin I proteolysis in the pathogenesis of stunned myocardium. Circ Res 1997; 80:393-399
28. Bodor G, Oakeley A, Allen P, et al. Troponin I phosphorylation in the normal and failing adult human heart. Circulation 1997; 96:1495-1500
29. Zakhary D, Moravec C, Stewart R, et al. Protein kinase A (PKA)-dependent troponin-I phosphorylation and PKA regulatory subunits are decreased in human dilated cardiomyopathy. Circulation 1999; 99:505-510
30. Liu M, Wu L. Reduction in the calcium-induced calcium release from canine cardiac sarcoplasmic reticulum following endotoxin administration. Biochem Biophys Res Commun 1991; 174:1248-1254
31. Wu L, Liu M. Heart sarcolemmal calcium transport in endotoxonic shock: I. Impairment of ATP-dependent calcium transport. Mol Cell Biochem 1992; 112:125-133
32. Kutsky P, Parker J. Calcium fluxes in cardiac sarcolemma and sarcoplasmic reticulum isolated from endotoxin-shocked guinea-pigs. Circ Shock 1990; 30:349-364
33. Lew W, Yasuda S, Yuan T, et al. Endotoxin-induced cardiac depression is associated with decreased cardiac dihydropyridine receptors in rabbits. J Mol Cell Cardiol 1996; 28:1367-1371
34. Zhong J, Hwang T, Adams H, et al. Reduced L-type calcium current in ventricular myocytes from endotoxemic guinea pigs. Am J Physiol 1997; 273:H2312-2324
35. Powers F, Farias S, Minami H, et al. Cardiac myofilament protein function is altered during sepsis. J Mol Cell Cardiol 1998; 30: 967-978
36. Shah A. Paracrine modulation of heart cell function by endothelial cells. Cardiovasc Res 1998; 31:847-867
37. Komukai K, Kurihara S. Length-dependence of calcium-tension relationship in aequorin-injected ferret papillary muscles. Am J Physiol 1997; 273:H1068-1074
38. Solaro R, Rarick H. Troponin and tropomyosin. Proteins that switch on and tune in the activity of cardiac myofilaments. Circ Res 1998; 83:471-480
39. Rigby S, Hofmann P, Zhong J, et al. Endotoxemia-induced myocardial dysfunction is not associated with changes in myofilament calcium responsiveness. Am J Physiol 1998; 274: H580-H590
40. Shah A, MacCarthy P. Paracrine and autocrine effects of nitric oxide on myocardial function. Pharmacol Therapeutics 2000; 86: 49-86
41. Kelly R, Balligand J, Smith T. Nitric oxide and cardiac function. Circ Res 1996; 79:363-380
42. Kirstein M, Rivet-Bastide M, Hatem S, et al. Nitric oxide regulates the calcium current in isolated human atrial myocytes. J Clin Invest 1995; 95:794-802
43. Flesh M, Kilter H, Cremers B, et al. Acute effect of nitric oxide and cyclic GMP on human myocardial contractility. J Pharmacol Exp Ther 1997; 281:1340-1349
44. Paulus WJ, Vantrimpont PJ, Shah AM. Acute effects of nitric oxide on left ventricular relaxation and diastolic distensibility in man. Circulation 1994; 89:2070-2078
45. Paulus W, Vantrimpont PJ, Shah AM. Paracrine coronary endothelial control of left ventricular function in humans. Circulation 1995; 92:2119-2126
46. Prendergast BD, Sagach VF, Shah AM. Basal release of nitric oxide augments the Frank-Starling response in the isolated heart. Circulation 1997; 96:1320-1329
47. Pinsky DJ, Patton S, Mesaros S, et al. Mechanical transduction of nitric oxide synthesis in the beating heart. Circ Res 1997; 81:372-379
48. Corda S, Mebazaa A, Tavernier B, et al. Paracrine regulation of cardiac myocytes in normal and septic heart. J Crit Care 1998; 13:39-47

49. Brady AJB, Poole-Wilson PA, Harding SE, et al. Nitric oxide production within cardiac myocytes reduces their contractility in endotoxemia. Am J Physiol 1992; 263:H1963-H1966

50. Silverman HJ, Penaranda R, Orens JB et al. Impaired β-adrenergic receptor stimulation of cyclic adenosine monophosphate in human septic shock: association with myocardial hyporesponsiveness to catecholamines. Crit Care Med 1993; 21:31-39

36

THE BRAIN IN SEPSIS

Barbara Philips
David Bennett

Confusion and decreased awareness are among the earliest signs of developing sepsis and yet very little is understood about brain dysfunction in systemic sepsis. A number of authors have tried to define septic encephalopathy but as the quoted incidence of between 9 and 71% of all patients with sepsis illustrates [1-4], the exact definition remains vague.

It was Hippocrates (460-370 B.C.), over 2 000 years ago, who first described the relationship between systemic illnesses and brain dysfunction. He wrote of liver dysfunction and personality changes, "those who are mad on account of phlegm are quiet, but those on account of bile are vociferous, viscous and do not keep quiet" [5]. For septic encephalopathy he described "phrenitis" as a complication of fever, abscesses or spreading redness and swelling of the limbs [6]. Galen (131-200 A.D.) too, observed these relationships [7,8], stating that inflammation affected the mind "sympathetically" causing delirium. Yellow bile was thought to induce acute diseases running a rapid course and accompanied by a high temperature and black bile was believed to cause disease such as mental derangement, apoplexy and convulsions [5].

Sepsis and its sequelae is the leading cause of death in intensive care units (ICUs), accounting for 10 -50% of all deaths [1]. Mortality increases as the number of organs failing increases, reaching almost 100% with six organ failure [9]. Brain failure or septic encephalopathy is included in this analysis and its individual effect on mortality verified by the Veterans Administration systemic sepsis study [2] which found that hypothermia, hypotension, thrombocytopenia and the absence of shaking chills plus an altered mental status were predictive of mortality.

CLINICAL FEATURES

The exact definition of septic encephalopathy remains elusive, primarily because it is usually considered after the patient has been sedated for treatments such as mechanical ventilation. In a prospective study, prior to such interventions, of 69 patients with fever and a positive blood culture, Young and colleagues [3] found 49 (71 %) had evidence of brain dysfunction on detailed clinical testing. Seventeen had a mild encephalopathy and 32 had severe brain dysfunction and it is this study that provides us with one of the better clinical descriptions of septic encephalopathy.

The diagnosis requires evidence of extra-cranial infection and an impaired mental state. Patients behave inappropriately becoming, agitated, disorientated and confused and as severity worsens they become increasingly less responsive. Paratonic rigidity (a velocity dependent resistance to passive movement of the limbs) is said to be typical but focal signs, seizures and cranial nerve palsies are rare and warrant careful search for an alternative explanation. Asterixis, tremor and multifocal myoclonus, found in hepatic and uraemic encephalopathies are not typical of septic encephalopathy. Table 1 lists some of the alternative diagnoses that might be considered in a patient with fever and an altered mental state. Most will be obvious from the presenting history or associated signs and symptoms.

Other clinical indices of sepsis or septic shock have been suggested to correlate with the severity of the septic encephalopathy. Eidelman and colleagues [4] in a prospective study of 50 patients with altered mental status found that a deteriorating Glasgow Coma Score was the best measure of encephalopathy and predictive of mortality. They also found a correlation with blood urea concentrations and bilirubin but not with other metabolic or physiological indices. In contrast, Young and colleagues [3] found a variety of abnormalities correlated with the severity of brain dysfunction, including, axonal neuropathies, increased white cell count, increased blood concentrations of alkaline phosphatase, bilirubin, creatinine, urea, phosphate and potassium and decreased blood pressure and serum albumin levels. However, none of the markers of other organ damage were severely enough deranged to account for the encephalopathy independently.

INVESTIGATIONS

In septic encephalopathy, lumbar puncture may reveal a mild elevation in protein content in the cerebrospinal fluid (CSF), but cell counts and glucose concentrations are unaffected. The value of performing lumbar punctures in all patients with fever and an altered mental state is disputed but they may be useful for excluding central nervous system (CNS) infection, subarachnoid hemorrhage or CNS malignancy for patients in whom the diagnosis is in doubt.

CNS Infections	Meningitis
	Hemophilus influenzae
	Streptococcus pneumoniae
	Neisseria meningitidis
	Listeria monocytogenes
	Meningoencephalitis
	Viral (e.g. arboviruses, coxsackie)
	Fungal (e.g. cryptococcus neoformans)
	Leptospirosis (Weils disease)
	Rickettsial diseases
	Brain abscess
	e.g. staphylococcus spp, streptococcus spp, gram negative bacteria)
	Subdural empyema
	Usually polymicrobial
Intracranial vascular events	Vertebrobasilar stroke
	Intracranial hemorrhage
Neurotrauma	Cerebral injury (particularly hypothalamic injury)
	Fat embolism
Metabolic Encephalopathies (those associated with fever)	Acute adrenal insufficiency
	Thyrotoxicosis
	Porphyria
	Reye's syndrome
Systemic Inflammatory Response	Acute pancreatitis
	Trauma (e.g. pelvic trauma)
	Burns
Hyperthermia	Heatstroke
	Salicylate poisoning
	3,4-methylenedioxymethamphetamine (MDMA) poisoning
	Status epilepticus
	Neuroleptic malignant syndrome
	Malignant hyperpyrexia
Malignancy	Leukemia
	Some brain tumors

Table 1. *Differential diagnosis of reduced consciousness with fever in the ICU patient*

Adelson-Mitty and colleagues [10] found in a retrospective analysis of treatment of 70 patients with non-neurosurgical problems, that routine lumbar puncture for investigation of fever and altered mental status alone was not useful in the diagnosis and management of such patients. The use of lumbar punctures therefore should be based on the index of suspicion for a primary neurological condition (e.g. meningitis) and the balance of risks, e.g. contraindicated for patients with sepsis and a coagulopathy.

Computed tomography (CT) scans are unremarkable in septic encephalopathy [11] and are only useful if required to exclude other pathology, e.g., ischemic events or the presence of cerebral edema prior to performing a lumbar puncture.

The electroencephalogram (EEG) can be useful in septic encephalopathy. In mild encephalopathy, generalized delta activity is observed and as severity worsens, triphasic waves then appear followed by burst suppression or generalised suppression in severe encephalopathy [12]. Although these changes are said to be typical for septic encephalopathy, they are not specific to the condition but serial recordings may be useful for assessing the progression of the brain dysfunction [13].

PATHOGENESIS OF SEPTIC ENCEPHALOPATHY

The pathogenesis of septic encephalopathy is not known. Investigators have failed to find evidence of direct infection of the brain or a constant association with hepatic or renal failure [14]. It is likely that the cause of the metabolic encephalopathy is multi-factorial and the most likely factors will be discussed here.

Consciousness is multifaceted. It is a state requiring the capacity for self-awareness and alertness. The ways in which these can be disrupted are numerous and occur at every level within the central nervous system. Since focal signs are absent and neuro-imaging unhelpful in septic encephalopathy consideration will be made on how global insults may impair consciousness in sepsis.

Cerebral Hypoperfusion

Sepsis is normally associated with a high cardiac output and low systemic vascular resistance but its effects on perfusion of individual organs is variable. Regional blood flow to the myocardium and to the liver has been reported as increased, whereas blood flow to the spleen, gastrointestinal tract and kidney is reportedly decreased [15-17]. The effect of sepsis on cerebral perfusion is uncertain. Cerebral blood flow (CBF) has variously been reported as decreased [18-21], unchanged [22], and increased [23,24]. Overall the consensus in the literature would suggest that CBF is decreased in sepsis. Values as low as 25 ml/100g/min have been suggested [21] but whether the decrease is sufficient to be the cause of a reduction in conscious level remains in doubt. Flow thresholds have been established for the loss of cell function; EEG slowing is first observed at CBF of less than 24 ml/100g/min and electrical stand still, i.e. cell death, occurs at flow rates of 10-18 ml/100g/min, but these are under experimental conditions. The normal value for CBF in a patient sedated on an ICU is not certain. CBF as low as 28 ml/100g/min have been reported in healthy individuals anesthetized with oxygen, nitrous oxide, isoflurane and a Fentanyl infusion [25]. Intravenous agents such as propofol, midazolam, barbiturates and opiates, all decrease CBF and the cerebral metabolic rate for oxygen [26-28]. The mechanisms which normally protect the brain from circulatory fluctuations, i.e., autoregulation and cerebral vascular reactivity to carbon dioxide, have been variously reported as maintained during sepsis [19, 29-32] and disrupted [24]. Most of the studies involving direct measurement of the CBF would suggest that autoregulation remains intact. This has implications for the likely role of the vascular endothelium in the pathogenesis of the brain dysfunction.

Direct Infection of the Brain.

It has been suggested that septic encephalopathy is a consequence of direct cerebral infection seeded during systemic infection [11,33]. Certainly, the development of cerebral micro-abscesses have been described as a complication of sepsis; Parker and colleagues [34] observed cerebral candidal infections in 19 of 45 patients all of whom had verified tissue invasive *Candida* infections elsewhere. All 19 had proven or suspected Gram-negative sepsis and had received antibiotics. Pendlebury and colleagues identified 92 patients with evidence of CNS infection. Most had a primary chest infection and on examination at post-mortem, 35 had multiple micro-abscesses. The predominant organisms were *Staphylococcus aureus* and *Candida albicans*. However, in a more recent study of the brains from four patients who died from sepsis and who had septic encephalopathy, no evidence of direct cerebral infection could be found [14].

The natural evolution of septic encephalopathy, the apparent full neurological recovery as the patients recovers from the sepsis and the absence of focal signs, all imply a metabolic cause for the brain dysfunction. The questions therefore are what is the mediator or mediators, and how is the brain affected? A number of suggestions have been made. Firstly, the brain dysfunction may be a consequence of a circulating metabolite or toxin, perhaps secondary to liver or renal failure, having direct effect on neurones. Secondly it may be due to an inflammatory process set up within the brain. Endothelial cells, leukocytes and glial cells, could all potentially be involved.

Neurones

Papadopoulos and colleagues [35] observed dark shrunken neurones in the frontal cortices of hemodynamically controlled septic pigs after only 8 hours of experimental peritonitis. These were not evident in sham operated pigs, and such changes, if these occur in humans, are likely to cause irreversible sequelae of septic encephalopathy. Unfortunately, detailed neuropsychiatric follow up of patients surviving sepsis has not been reported. Analysis of rabbit brains after infusions of endotoxin failed to find any obvious neuronal damage and it remains to be seen whether these occur in humans or not [36].

A metabolic cause is likely for septic encephalopathy and septic encephalopathy has been likened to hepatic encephalopathy. However, patients do not need to be in overt liver failure to become encephalopathic during sepsis. Nevertheless, investigators have looked to hepatic encephalopathy for clues to the pathogenesis of septic encephalopathy. Amino acid imbalance within the brain and enhanced gaberminergic neurotransmission are plausible metabolic derangements, which may affect the functioning of neurones.

A characteristic amino acid pattern in the blood occurs in hepatic encephalopathy and has been reported in animal models and in patients with septic encephalopathy [37-40]. Aromatic amino acids (i.e. phenylalanine, tyrosine and tryptophan) increase secondary to decreased hepatic breakdown. Combined with normal concentrations of branch chain amino acids (valine, leucine and isoleucine), there is an increase in the aromatic amino acid to branch chain amino acid ratio. The aromatic amino acids compete directly with branch chain amino acids for the same transport system in to the brain causing an increase in the aromatic amino acid concentration within the brain. There, they may have direct effects or act as substrates for serotonin and false neurotransmitters such as octopamine. Increased serotonin levels and increased serotonin turnover have been observed in animal models of sepsis [37,41]. Soejima and colleagues [42] mapped the utilization of cerebral glucose in septic rats to discrete brain regions related to the serotonergic and noradrenergic systems. Nevertheless, a good correlation between the degree of amino acid imbalance and the degree of encephalopathy has never been shown for either hepatic or septic brain dysfunction.

Several reports have suggested that an increase in the CNS inhibitory neurotransmitter, γ-aminobutyric acid (GABA), or its receptors, may be involved in the pathogenesis of hepatic encephalopathy [43-47]. Sprung and colleagues [39] found γ-aminobutyric acid increased in the plasma of patients with septic encephalopathy, but this finding has not been repeated. Kadoi and colleagues [48] observed an increased density of receptors in the forebrains of septic rats but could not detect an actual increase in GABA, either in blood or brain. In hepatic encephalopathy, efforts to decrease GABA have failed to reverse the condition [49,50]. Increased sensitivity to exogenous benzodiazepines has been reported in animal studies [51] and if true, may have significance for the clinical use of benzodiazepines for septic patients, particularly if the sepsis is complicated by hepatic and renal impairment.

Glutamate, is the excitatory neurotransmitter in 40% of synapses within the brain [52] and in hepatic encephalopathy its cerebral concentrations decrease and the glutamate binding sites on the post-synaptic membrane of neurones down regulate. One contributing factor may be increased circulating ammonia concentrations. Ammonia inhibits glutamate re-uptake in to neurones and enhances the conversion of glutamate to glutamine within astrocytes (part of the normal control of this neurotransmitter). Glutamine has osmotic activity and its accumulation can lead to excess water in the brain parenchyma. Congenital urea cycle disorders, Reyes syndrome and hepatic encephalopathy share some common pathological changes (e.g., cerebral edema, type II astrocytosis) which have been, at least in part, attributed to hyperammonemia. Furthermore, ammonia activates benzodiazepine receptors and facilitates the uptake of tryptophan in to the brain (a precursor for neurotransmitters including serotonin). However, the one study directly considering these possibilities found that raised ammonia concentrations were a feature of hepatic but not septic encephalopathy [40].

Leukocytes

During the systemic inflammatory response syndrome (SIRS) and sepsis, a systemic release of inflammatory mediators has marked effect on the lung, liver, kidney, gastrointestinal tract and heart. The resulting pan-endothelial injury causes obliteration of some vessels and increased leakage of intravascular contents into the interstitial tissues surrounding. Leukocytes accumulate in these tissues setting up inflammatory reactions in the process. The brain however, appears to be resistant to the accumulation of leukocytes, a unique feature thought to have developed to protect the brain from the acute damage caused by inflammation [35,53,54]. The blood brain barrier is probably the main mechanism of protection and although its integrity is functionally damaged during sepsis, the tight junctions appear to remain intact preventing the passage of cells [35,36]. In addition the cerebrovascular endothelium expresses very low concentrations of the leukocyte adhesion molecules vascular cell adhesion molecule (VCAM)-1 and intercellular adhesion molecule (ICAM)-1.

Cerebrovascular Endothelium

The integrity of the blood brain barrier is in part dependent on the integrity of the cerebrovascular endothelium. The cerebrovascular endothelium has unique features. It has intercellular tight junctions, few pinocytotic vesicles and no fenestration. However, despite evidence from electron microscopy that the tight junctions remaining intact during sepsis [35,36] functional breach of the blood brain barrier has been illustrated. Clinically, it accounts for the increase in CSF protein observed in some patients. In animal studies the breach has been illustrated by the passage of a number of markers from the circulation into the brain parenchyma, including ^{125}I-albumin, ^{14}C-amino acids and colloidal iron oxide [36,55,56]. The postulated mechanisms are either a breach in the tight junctions, not visible by electron microscopy, or an increase in the number and frequency of pinocytic vesicles forming within the cerebrovascular endothelial cells. These mechanisms might render the brain susceptible to circulating cytokines or toxins.

A notable feature of cerebral damage in animal models of sepsis is perimicrovessel edema [35,36]. Significant swelling could cause intracranial hypertension and this has been produced in an endotoxin model of sepsis in pigs [57]. Whether raised intracranial pressure ever occurs in human sepsis remains uncertain. Many animal models of sepsis do not truly reflect the human condition, however cerebral edema has been reported as a mode of death in the toxic shock syndrome [58-60] and cannot be discounted in other forms of sepsis. Even if the degree of swelling is insufficient to cause intracranial hypertension, perimicrovascular edema could have effect on local utilization of oxygen, nutrients and the removal of cellular waste.

Astrocytes

In conjunction with the perimicrovessel oedema observed in the brains of a pig model of fecal peritonitis, the end feet of astrocytes were grossly swollen and their perimicrovessel walls disrupted [35]. Astrocytes make up over 50% of the cell mass within the brain [61] and may play a significant role in the generation of septic encephalopathy. These cells serve numerous functions in the control of the local environment for neurones. First, they provide nutritional support [62], containing large glycogen stores and the facility to convert the glycogen to both lactate and glucose. Second, they are essential in the control of glutamate [63]. Third, their integrity is essential to the functioning of the blood brain barrier [61] and finally they are immunocompetent cells, capable of responding to, and producing cytokines [64,65]. One possible mode of injury to neurones in sepsis is the generation of inducible nitric oxide (NO) by astrocytes in response to circulating cytokines that penetrate the blood brain barrier. Neurones are exquisitely sensitive to NO and its metabolites and mitochondrial damage through this from of injury has been suggested for a number of neurological disorders; Parkinson's disease, Alzheimer's disease, multiple sclerosis and stroke, to name a few. If disruption of the mitochondrial electron transport chain is an integral part of the pathogenesis of septic shock, septic encephalopathy could conceivably be cause by the direct action of NO on neurones, generated by astrocytes. In addition, TNF-α has been shown to markedly alter ionic exchange mechanisms within astrocytes [66] and alter calcium homeostasis [65]. Not only would this lead to the generation of NO, but it is shown to directly alter the electrical excitability of astrocytes and indirectly affect the neighboring neurones.

CONCLUSION

Septic encephalopathy is an early manifestation of sepsis. At times it can be profound and patients with septic encephalopathy have a higher mortality than those without. Its pathogenesis is uncertain but it has the hallmarks of a global metabolic brain injury and even if severe it appears to be reversible. Nevertheless some preliminary animal work suggests that neuronal injury does occur but it remains to be seen if significant damage occurs in humans. Studies considering long term neurological or neuro-psychiatric sequelae are required.

REFERENCES

1. Pine RW, Wertz MJ, Lennard ES, Dellinger EP, Carrico CJ, Minshew BH. Determinants of organ malfunction or death in patients with intra-abdominal sepsis. A discriminant analysis. Arch Surg, 1983; 118:242-249
2. Sprung CL, Peduzzi PN, Shatney CH, et al. Impact of encephalopathy on mortality in the sepsis syndrome. The Veterans Administration Systemic Sepsis Cooperative Study Group. Crit Care Med 1990; 18:801-806
3. Young GB, Bolton CF, Austin TW, Archibald YM, Gonder J, Wells GA. The encephalopathy associated with septic illness. Clin Invest Med 1990; 13:297-304
4. Eidelman LA, Putterman D, Putterman C, Sprung CL. The spectrum of septic encephalopathy. Definitions, etiologies, and mortalities. JAMA 1996; 275:470-473
5. Frerichs FT, Murchison C. A Clinical Treatise on Diseases of the Liver. New Sydenham Society, London, 1860
6. Chadwick J, Mann WN. The Medical Work of Hippocrates. Chadwick J, Mann WN (eds) Blackwell, Oxford, 1950. pp: 50-223
7. Walsh JM. Observations on the symptomatology and pathogensis of hepatic coma. Q J Med 1951; 20:421 - 438

8. Mendez MF. Delerium. Neurology in Clinical Practice. In: Bradley WG, Daroff RB, Fenichel GM (Eds) Butterworth-Heinemann, Boston 1996, pp: 29-38
9. Moreno R, Vincent JL, Matos R, et al., The use of maximum SOFA score to quantify organ dysfunction/failure in intensive care. Results of a prospective, multicentre study. Working Group on Sepsis related Problems of the ESICM. Intensive Care Med 1999; 25: 686-696
10. Adelson-Mitty J, Fink MP, Lisbon A. The value of lumbar puncture in the evaluation of critically ill, non-immunosuppressed, surgical patients: a retrospective analysis of 70 cases. Intensive Care Med 1997; 23:749-752
11. Jackson AC, Gilbert JJ, Young GB, Bolton CF. The encephalopathy of sepsis. Can J Neurol Sci 1985; 12:303-307
12. Young GB, Kreeft JH, McLachlan RS, Demelo J. EEG and clinical associations with mortality in comatose patients in a general intensive care unit. J Clin Neurophysiol 1999; 16:354-360
13. Young GB. Metabolic and inflammatory cerebral diseases: electrophysiological aspects. Can J Neurol Sci 1998; 25:S16-S20
14. Bleck TP, Smith MC, Pierre-Louis SJ, Jares JJ, Murray J, Hansen CA. Neurologic complications of critical medical illnesses. Crit Care Med 1993; 21:98-103
15. Creteur J, De Backer D, Vincent JL, A dobutamine test can disclose hepatosplanchnic hypoperfusion in septic patients. Am J Respir Crit Care Med 1999; 160:839-845
16. De Backer D, Creteur J, Zhang H, Norrenberg M, Vincent JL. Lactate production by the lungs in acute lung injury. Am J Respir Crit Care Med 1997; 156:1099-1104
17. Bellomo R, Kellum JA, Wisniewski SR, Pinsky MR. Effects of norepinephrine on the renal vasculature in normal and endotoxemic dogs. Am J Respir Crit Care Med 1999; 159:1186-1192
18. Ekstrom-Jodal B, Haggendal J, Larsson LE, Westerlind A. Cerebral hemodynamics, oxygen uptake and cerebral arteriovenous differences of catecholamines following E. coli endotoxin in dogs. Acta Anaesthesiol Scand 1982; 26:446-452
19. Ekstrom-Jodal B, Haggendal E, Larsson LE. Cerebral blood flow and oxygen uptake in endotoxic shock. An experimental study in dogs. Acta Anaesthesiol Scand 1982; 26:163-170
20. Ekstrom-Jodal B, Larsson LE. The effects of high dose methylprednisolone or fluid volume expansion on cerebral haemodynamics and oxygen uptake in endotoxic shock. An experimental study in dogs. Acta Anaesthesiol Scand 1982; 26:175-179
21. Bowton DL, Bertels NH, Prough DS, Stump DA. Cerebral blood flow is reduced in patients with sepsis syndrome. Crit Care Med 1989; 17:399-403
22. Kreimeier U, Ruiz-Morales M, Messmer K. Comparison of the effects of volume resuscitation with Dextran 60 vs. Ringer's lactate on central hemodynamics, regional blood flow, pulmonary function, and blood composition during hyperdynamic endotoxemia. Circ Shock 1993; 39:89-99
23. Kreimeier U, Hammersen F, Ruiz-Morales M, Yang Z, Messmer K. Redistribution of intraorgan blood flow in acute, hyperdynamic porcine endotoxemia. Eur Surg Res 1991; 23:85-99
24. Smith SM, Padayachee S, Modaresi KB, Smithies MN, Bihari DJ. Cerebral blood flow is proportional to cardiac index in patients with septic shock. J Crit Care 1998; 13:104-109
25. Newman B, Gelb AW, Lam AM. The effect of isoflurane-induced hypotension on cerebral blood flow and cerebral metabolic rate for oxygen in humans. Anesthesiology 1986; 64:307-310
26. Van Hemelrijck J, Fitch W, Mattheussen M, Van Aken H, Plets C, Lauwers T. Effect of propofol on cerebral circulation and autoregulation in the baboon. Anesth Analg 1990; 71:49-54

27. Ostapkovich ND, Baker KZ, Fogarty-Mack P, Sisti MB, Young WL. Cerebral blood flow and CO2 reactivity is similar during remifentanil/N2O and fentanyl/N2O anesthesia. Anesthesiology 1998; 89:358-363
28. Cheng MA, Hoffman WE, Baughman VL, Albrecht RF. The effects of midazolam and sufentanil sedation on middle cerebral artery blood flow velocity in awake patients. J Neurosurg Anesthesiol 1993; 5:232-236
29. Parker JL, TE Emerson Jr. Cerebral hemodynamics, vascular reactivity, and metabolism during canine endotoxin shock. Circ Shock 1977; 4:41-53
30. Sari A, Yamashita S, Ohosita S, et al. Cerebrovascular reactivity to CO2 in patients with hepatic or septic encephalopathy. Resuscitation 1990; 19:125-134
31. Straver JS, Keunen RW, Stam CJ, et al. Transcranial Doppler and systemic hemodynamic studies in septic shock. Neurol Res 1996; 18:313-318
32. Matta BF, Stow PJ. Sepsis-induced vasoparalysis does not involve the cerebral vasculature: indirect evidence from autoregulation and carbon dioxide reactivity studies. Br J Anaesth 1996; 76:790-794
33. Pendlebury WW, Perl DP, Munoz DG. Multiple microabscesses in the central nervous system: a clinicopathologic study. J Neuropathol Exp Neurol 1989; 48:290-300
34. Parker JC Jr, McCloskey JJ, Lee RS. Human cerebral candidosis--a postmortem evaluation of 19 patients. Hum Pathol 1981; 12:23-28
35. Papadopoulos MC, Lamb FJ, Moss RF, Davies DC, Tighe D, Bennett ED. Faecal peritonitis causes oedema and neuronal injury in pig cerebral cortex. Clin Sci (Colch) 1999; 96:461-466
36. Clawson CC, Hartmann JF, Vernier RL. Electron microscopy of the effect of gram-negative endotoxin on the blood-brain barrier. J Comp Neurol 1966; 127:183-198
37. Freund HR, Muggia-Sullam M, LaFrance R, Holroyde J, Fischer JE. Regional brain amino acid and neurotransmitter derangements during abdominal sepsis and septic encephalopathy in the rat. The effect of amino acid infusions. Arch Surg 1986; 121:209-216
38. Freund HR, Muggia-Sullam M, Peiser J, Melamed E. Brain neurotransmitter profile is deranged during sepsis and septic encephalopathy in the rat. J Surg Res 1985; 38:267-271
39. Sprung CL, Cerra FB, Freund HR, et al. Amino acid alterations and encephalopathy in the sepsis syndrome. Crit Care Med 1991; 19:753-757
40. Mizock BA, Sabelli HC, Dubin A, Javaid JI, Poulos A, Rackow EC. Septic encephalopathy. Evidence for altered phenylalanine metabolism and comparison with hepatic encephalopathy. Arch Intern Med 1990; 150:443-449
41. Shimizu I, Adachi N, Liu K, Lei B, Nagaro T, Arai T. Sepsis facilitates brain serotonin activity and impairs learning ability in rats. Brain Res 1999; 830:94-100
42. Soejima Y, Fujii Y, Ishikawa T, Takeshita H, Maekawa T. Local cerebral glucose utilization in septic rats. Crit Care Med 1990; 18:423-427
43. Albrecht J, Jones EA. Hepatic encephalopathy: molecular mechanisms underlying the clinical syndrome. J Neurol Sci 1999; 170:138-146
44. Rothuizen J, de Kok Y, Slob A, Mol JA. GABAergic inhibition of the pituitary release of adrenocorticotropin and alpha-melanotropin is impaired in dogs with hepatic encephalopathy. Domest Anim Endocrinol 1996; 13:59-68
45. Mousseau DD, Butterworth RF. Current theories on the pathogenesis of hepatic encephalopathy. Proc Soc Exp Biol Med 1994; 206:329-344
46. Basile AS. The contribution of endogenous benzodiazepine receptor ligands to the pathogenesis of hepatic encephalopathy. Synapse 1991; 7:141-150
47. Levy LJ, Losowsky MS. Plasma gamma aminobutyric acid concentrations provide evidence of different mechanisms in the pathogenesis of hepatic encephalopathy in acute and chronic liver disease. Hepatogastroenterology 1989; 36:494-498

48. Kadoi Y, Saito S. An alteration in the gamma-aminobutyric acid receptor system in experimentally induced septic shock in rats. Crit Care Med 1996; 24:298-305

49. Loscher W, Kretz FJ, Tung LC, Dillinger U. Reduction of highly elevated plasma levels of gamma-aminobutyric acid does not reverse hepatic coma. Hepatogastroenterology 1989; 36:504-505

50. Thirlby RC, Fenster LF, Coatsworth JJ, Petty F. Reversal of chronic hepatic encephalopathy by colonic exclusion: poor correlation with blood GABA levels. Am J Gastroenterol 1990; 85:1637-1641

51. Komatsubara T, Kadoi Y, Saito S. Augmented sensitivity to benzodiazepine in septic shock rats. Can J Anaesth 1995; 42:937-943

52. Coyle JT, Puttfarcken P. Oxidative stress, glutamate, and neurodegenerative disorders. Science 1993; 262:689-695

53. Perry VH, Brown MC, Andersson PB. Macrophage responses to central and peripheral nerve injury. Adv Neurol 1993; 59:309-314

54. Andersson PB, Perry VH, Gordon S. The CNS acute inflammatory response to excitotoxic neuronal cell death. Immunol Lett 1991; 30:177-181

55. Jeppsson B, Freund HR, Gimmon Z, James JH, von Meyenfeldt MF, Fischer JE. Blood-brain barrier derangement in sepsis: cause of septic encephalopathy? Am J Surg 1981; 141:136-142

56. Deng X, Wang X, Andersson R. Endothelial barrier resistance in multiple organs after septic and nonseptic challenges in the rat. J Appl Physiol 1995; 78:2052-2061

57. Hariri RJ, Ghajar JB, Bahramian K, Sharif S, Barie PS. Alterations in intracranial pressure and cerebral blood volume in endotoxemia. Surg Gynecol Obstet 1993; 176:155-166

58. Pehrson PO, Lofgren A, Gaines H, Toikkanen S. Brain edema in toxic shock syndrome. The first fatal case in Sweden? Lakartidningen 1985; 82:1593-1594

59. Ambrose RE, Cheung H. Case report: fatal non-menstrual toxic shock in a Chinese woman. Clin Radiol 1992; 45:355-357

60. Smith DB, Gulinson J. Fatal cerebral edema complicating toxic shock syndrome. Neurosurgery 1988; 22:598-599

61. Fillenz M, Lowry JP, Boutelle MG, Fray AE. The role of astrocytes and noradrenaline in neuronal glucose metabolism. Acta Physiol Scand 1999; 167:275-284

62. Wiesinger H, Hamprecht B, Dringen R. Metabolic pathways for glucose in astrocytes. Glia 1997; 21:22-34

63. Bezzi P, Vesce S, Panzarasa P, Volterra A. Astrocytes as active participants of glutamatergic function and regulators of its homeostasis. Adv Exp Med Biol 1999; 468:69-80

64. Aschner M. Immune and inflammatory responses in the CNS: modulation by astrocytes. Toxicol Lett 1998; 102-103:283-287

65. Koller H, Thiem K, Siebler M. Tumour necrosis factor-alpha increases intracellular Ca2+ and induces a depolarization in cultured astroglial cells. Brain 1996; 119:2021-2027

66. Benos DJ, Hahn BH, Bubien JK, Ghosh SK, et al. Envelope glycoprotein gp120 of human immunodeficiency virus type 1 alters ion transport in astrocytes: implications for AIDS dementia complex. Proc Natl Acad Sci USA 1994; 91:494-498

37

THE GUT IN SEPSIS

Benoit Vallet

In the sixties, Evans and Darin [1] demonstrated that a 90 % distal enterectomy protected dogs from endotoxic shock: survival was improved from 13 % in control animals to 52 % in enterectomy treated animals. Accordingly, the authors suggested the gastrointestinal tract has an important role in the pathogenesis of organ failure and death in septic shock. Based on a growing body of evidence, Meakins and Marshall [2] later proposed in a review article that the gut may act as a 'motor' of the multiple organ dysfunction syndrome (MODS). Their original proposition was that gut mucosal dysoxia (i.e., oxygen supply insufficient to meet oxygen requirements) occurs during shock states as a consequence of an inadequate splanchnic oxygen delivery (DO_2) to oxygen uptake (VO_2) and as a cause of loss in gut mucosal barrier. Hyperpermeability would then result in bacterial or endotoxin translocation leading, ultimately, to remote organ injury and MODS. This hypothesis could explain the clinical paradoxes observed in septic MODS:

1. organs that fail frequently are not initially directly injured
2. there is a lag period of time between the initial insult and the development of MODS
3. not all patients with clinical sepsis and MODS have microbiologic evidence of infection
4. no septic focus can be identified clinically or at autopsy in more than 30 % of bacteremic patients dying of clinical sepsis and MODS
5. identification and treatment of suppurative infections in patients with MODS may not improve survival.

However to date, there is no demonstrated causal relationship between increased intestinal permeability and the severity of splanchnic ischemia, infectious complications or MODS score [3]. Bacterial translocation and changes in intestinal permeability may be independent process, and the correlation between survival and bacterial translocation is certainly related to the magnitude of the inflammatory insult [4], but the potential relationship between gut barrier failure function or injury and MODS may be more complex than initially assumed.

Experimental and clinical evidence [5-7] suggests that, during septic shock, altered blood flow distribution within the gut wall may contribute to the generation of mucosal hypoxia and hyperpermeability, despite normal or increased overall splanchnic blood flow. However, other reports [8-10] suggest that gut mucosal hyperpermeability in sepsis might not be solely due to the decrease in mucosal perfusion. Abnormal or decreased utilization of oxygen by epithelial cells has been advocated to explain observed abnormalities [11]. This chapter will review how both hypotheses are currently presented.

CIRCULATORY SHOCK AND GUT MUCOSAL HYPOPERFUSION

The intact mucosal barrier is thought to play an important role in defending the host from translocation of intact microorganisms or their breakdown products and toxins [12]. The mucosa is the mucous membrane that lines the digestive tract. It consists of three layers: an epithelial layer, the lamina propria, and the muscularis mucosa. The submucosa contains blood vessels, lymphatics, nerves, and in some regions glands. Mucosal blood flow in the intestine originates from the submucosal arterioles that arborise into a dense network of capillaries. These capillaries pass through the mucosa, supply the crypts and extend into the mucosal villi [13]. Venous blood from mucosal capillaries drains into the mucosal venules, which eventually re-enter the submucosa.

The mucosa vascular architecture creates a situation where the oxygenation of cells at the tips of the villi are relatively susceptible to conditions that reduce the overall oxygen supply to the mucosa. The capillaries supplying blood flow to the intestinal villi form a 'hairpin loop' arrangement, with arteriolar and venular ends coursing in parallel along the villus which has the potential to create a countercurrent exchange of oxygen from the inflow vessels to the outflow vessels with a base-to-tip gradient in the partial pressure of oxygen. The extensive length of the capillaries supplying the villi magnifies this gradient between the base and tips of the villi, with lower oxygen tensions at the apex of the hairpin loop [5, 14]. This architecture is crucial for maintaining the vital functions of secretion and absorption of the alimentary tract cells.

The gut has a relative overperfusion as related to the needs of the tissue [15], and the intestinal vascular bed can compensate for a reduced blood flow by increasing oxygen extraction. In studies of isolated intestine segments autoperfused with blood from the femoral artery, graded hemorrhage of the animal induced a progressive increase in gut vascular resistance that was caused by systemic baroreflex vasoconstriction. This was responsible for a progressive decrease in gut blood flow and DO_2. When gut oxygen extraction reached a value of approximately 65 %, gut VO_2 became supply limited and gut VO_2 fell with further reductions in gut flow [16]. In later experiments where an isolated gut segment was perfused with blood using a roller pump, it was possible to locally reduce gut blood flow while keeping the animal systematically normotensive. This experiment allowed a separation of the local effects of hypoperfusion from the integrated response seen when the baroreflex vasoconstriction was activated [17]. Interestingly, the local ability of the gut to increase oxygen extraction in response to a decrease in pump speed and DO_2 was significantly improved when the animal was progressively hemorrhaged, but was found to be only 45 % when the animal was kept normotensive. While holding gut DO_2 constant, subsequent hemorrhage of the animal caused an increase in local gut oxygen extraction. These results show that the extraction ability may be improved by augmenting baroreflex vasoconstriction.

Peripheral vasoconstriction is a major compensatory mechanism of hypovolemia that participates in redistribution of whole body DO_2 among organs with diversion of unnecessary flow from organs such as the gut to the heart and the brain. When vasoconstriction is prolonged and/or severe, it may lead to mucosal dysoxia and morphologic injury. If tissue hypoperfusion duration is short enough, intestinal VO_2 is restored with correction of DO_2. If hypoperfusion lasts longer, reperfusion does not insure DO_2 correction and might even favor increased production of reactive oxygen metabolites and related tissue injury [18]. After a two-hour period of mesenteric ischemia, the apical villi are severely denuded, with evidence of an exposed basement membrane [19].

In a situation like septic shock, the gut mucosa is at even higher risks of dysoxia. Indeed, alteration of normal microcirculatory control mechanisms rends gut oxygen consumption unable to recover with fluid resuscitation after a short period of hypodynamic shock [5]. In this situation, it has been suggested that blood flow-controlling sites in the gut microcirculation are inadequate to maintain mucosal perfusion and oxygenation despite more than adequate blood flow to the whole gastrointestinal tract. Interestingly enough,

Xu et al. [20] demonstrated that reactive oxygen metabolites are likely to be involved in these microcirculatory abnormalities. Their activity might be reinforced by sepsis-induced changes in local scavengers.

ALTERED GUT PERFUSION AND OXYGENATION IN SEPSIS

The local ability of the gut to adjust its oxygen extraction in response to changes in gut DO_2 is impaired in experimental models of sepsis [21, 22]. The oxygen extraction dysfunction could be due to a dysregulation of perfusion distribution within or between the gut layers, leading to existence of tissue regions that receive excess flow with respect to their metabolic needs while other tissue regions are not supplied adequately. In a study with pump-perfused canine intestine, Connolly et al. [23] found that the redistribution of blood flow toward mucosa that normally occurs when systemic baroreflex vasoconstriction is activated was abolished during endotoxemia. Drazenovic et al. [24] found evidence of impaired regulation of intestinal mucosal capillary recruitment in a canine model of endotoxemia. Moreover, gut adjustments in perfused capillary density in response to a decrease in local DO_2 were impaired after endotoxin (lipopolysaccharide, LPS) administration, with a strong correlation between loss of capillary recruitment capabilities and loss of oxygen extraction capabilities. Whithworth et al. [25] showed an imbalance in vasoactive tone between intestinal small arterioles in a hyperdynamic model of sepsis in rats. Third-order arterioles, which terminate as central villous arterioles, were more constricted than first- or second-order arterioles, leading specifically to compromised mucosal blood flow.

If sepsis or endotoxemia renders microvessels in the mucosa incapable of regulating perfusion, some cells in the more poorly perfused regions could be supply-limited while other cells enjoy luxury perfusion. Detecting such a defect is technically difficult even under carefully controlled experimental conditions, because the tissue as a whole would still exhibit a bilinear relationship between DO_2 and VO_2. The problem becomes even larger if the regions of relative hypoperfusion change over time, a state referred to temporal heterogeneity. In that case, different regions of cells could be ischemic at different times, leading to widespread tissue hypoxic injury that would not necessarily be apparent at the level of overall organ DO_2 and VO_2. Vallet et al. [5] found that LPS infusion caused an acute decrease in cardiac output, blood pressure, and gut perfusion with a decrease in mean tissue PO_2 ($PtiO_2$), as determined using polarographic electrode arrays, both in muscularis and mucosa. During fluid resuscitation, the tissue PO_2 in the muscularis returned to baseline levels but tissue PO_2 in the mucosa remained almost anoxic (Figure 1). This was consistent with an increased intramucosal PCO_2 and a low intramucosal pH (pHi) as assessed by ileal tonometry. Increase in mucosal PCO_2 and decrease in pHi are indirectly indicative of a decrease in mucosal flow [26]. Thus, despite a short period of hypodynamic shock, short enough to be theoretically associated with oxygenation recovery during pure hypovolemia, mucosal perfusion and oxygenation did not recover during resuscitation to the same extent as the muscularis in this septic shock model.

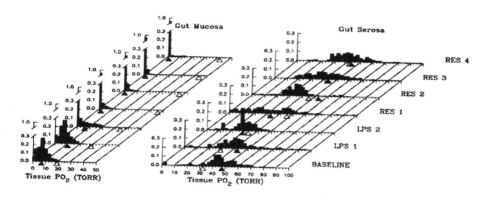

Figure 1. *Combined tissue PO_2 (PtiO$_2$) distributions obtained during baseline; 30 and 60 min of endotoxin infusion (LPS1 and LPS2); and 30, 60, 90, and 120 min of dextran infusion (RES1, RES2, RES3, and RES4). Closed triangle: mean PtiO$_2$; open triangle: mean venous PO_2. From [5] with permission*

Similarily, Hasibeder et al. [27] recently found a decrease in mucosal HbO_2 (HbO$_2$i) and PO_2 in a porcine model of endotoxin shock despite fluid resuscitation. By comparison with control animals, the presence of sustained tissue hypoxia suggested for the authors the existence of septic microvascular injury. More recently, Mayer et al. [6] investigated the impact of *E. coli* hemolysin (HlyA), a medically relevant pore-forming bacterial toxin, on the mucosal microvasculature in a constant-flow blood-perfused rabbit ileum model. Spatial distribution of HbO$_2$i, relative mucosal Hb content, and mucosal-arterial PCO_2 gap, an indirect marker of mucosal hypoperfusion [26], were assessed with microsensor techniques. Administration of low-doses of HlyA (0.005 to 0.1 hemolytic units/ml) into the mesenteric artery provoked a transient vasoconstrictor response. Whereas physiological mucosal oxygenation was homogeneous, severe heterogeneity in capillary blood flow distribution appeared, paralleled by a marked increase in the mucosal-arterial PCO_2 gap. In addition, HlyA provoked a dose-dependent increase in relative Hb concentration values and edema formation, suggesting postcapillary vasoconstriction and capillary leakage. Very importantly, the observed changes occurred while fully maintaining mesenteric DO_2. The authors concluded that low doses of pore-forming bacterial toxins are contributors to severe mucosal microcirculatory disturbances in the rabbit ileum under maintenance of global hemodynamics, reminiscent of septic perfusion abnormalities (Figure 2).

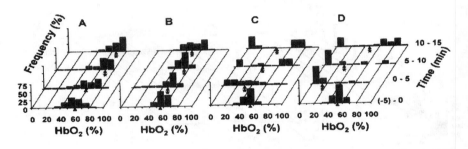

Figure 2. Distribution of HbO_2i values before (-5 to 0 min) and after different E. coli hemolysin concentrations administered at time zero. For each toxin dose, data are pooled. Each histogram depicts a time period of 5 min (approximately 1,600 individual HbO_2i measurements). (A) 0.005 hemolytic units [HU]/ml; (B) 0.015 HU/ml; (C) 0.05 HU/ml; (D) 0.1 HU/ml. Closed triangle, mean HbO_2i; asterisk, p<0.05 compared with baseline. From [6] with permission

Stehr et al [28] investigated whether ileal mucosal acidosis during hyperdynamic porcine endotoxemia is associated with impaired villus microcirculation. Anesthetized and ventilated pigs received continuous IV LPS for 24 hours or placebo. Intravital video records of the ileal microcirculation were assessed together with ileal mucosal-arterial PCO_2 gap and bowel wall capillary HbO_2. At 12 and 24 hours LPS infusion, about half of the evaluated villi were not, or were heterogeneously, perfused which was paralleled by a progressive significant increase of the PCO_2 gap whereas capillary HbO_2 distribution remained unchanged. The unchanged capillary HbO_2 distribution suggested for the authors the existence of microvascular shunting in the intestinal mucosa during endotoxemia. It was also noticed that in the Mayer et al. study only the largest exotoxin doses [6] were capable of inducing pronounced heterogeneity of the intracapillary oxygenation.

Measurement of gut microvascular PO_2 in pigs has shown the development of a PO_2 gap betwen microvascular PO_2 and venous PO_2 during hemorrhage and endotoxemia, with a larger gap occurring in sepsis than in hemorrhage [29]. Similar observations were made by Vallet et al. [5] in dogs receiving endotoxin, with a widening between mean mucosal $PtiO_2$ and venous PO_2 as shock progressed, and this despite resuscitation and increased global gut O_2 delivery (Figure 1).

Mucosal HbO_2 was also found recently to be decreased in patients with septic shock [7], with tailing of the histogram of distribution of HbO_2i values and increased dispersion. This was observed in association with intramucosal acidosis (low tonometered intramucosal pH) and in spite of high whole-body O_2 delivery (Figure 3).

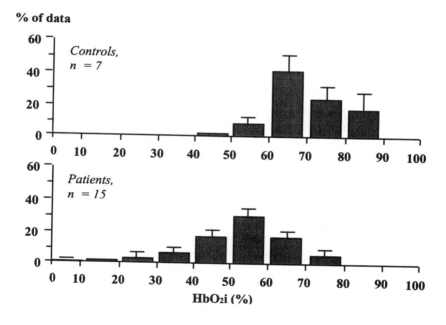

Figure 3. Gastric mucosal HbO_2 (HbO_2i) histograms in normal controls (upper panel) and septic patients (lower panel). Data are given as mean ± SEM. In normal control subjects, values for skewness and kurtosis were -0.04 ± 0.05 and -0.76 ± 0.1, respectively. These values were significantly different from the corresponding data in the septic patients (0.823 ± 0.04 and 0.88 ± 0.09, respectively). From [7] with permission

Experimental and clinical evidence point to the susceptibility of the gastro-intestinal tract to microvascular dysfunction in sepsis, which may relate to the emerging utility of the gut as a sentinel organ and may shed light on the relationship between the function of the gut and the pathogenesis of MODS in sepsis [30].

Several studies have described evidence of microvascular gut ischemia during endotoxic shock utilizing techniques of *in vivo* videomicroscopy, radioactive microspheres, real time measurement of microvascular blood flow by laser Doppler flowmetry [25,30-33], mucosal transmembrane potential differences [34], lactate flux and measurements of intramucosal pH [35]. These studies underscore the importance of the vascular architecture and its consequences for villus oxygenation in states of microvascular regulatory dysfunction.

Numerous studies have presented convincing evidence of impaired contractile responses to adrenergic agonists in vessels from endotoxemic animals [36,37]. Impaired tissue oxygen extraction ability is logically observed in the situation which resembles that of animals with α-adrenergic blockade [38] or with lowered baroreflex vasoconstriction in the study previously discussed [17]. However, treatment that increases vasoconstrictor tone during septic shock is not sufficient to fully restore oxygen extraction [39]. Because oxygen extraction is supposed to be the result of an adequate balance between vasoconstrictor and vasodilator tones, impaired oxygen extraction during septic shock may be related not only to impaired vasoconstrictor, but also to impaired vasodilator, tone [40].

Following *in vivo* endotoxemia, numerous investigations have demonstrated attenuated endothelium-dependent relaxation in *in vitro* vascular rings isolated from large arteries. Such studies suggest that this defect is due to impaired release of nitric oxide (NO) by the endothelial constitutive NO synthase (NOS) isoform or secondary to induction of smooth muscle NOS [36,37] and enhanced basal activation of guanylated cyclase which limits further relaxation in response to the acetylcholine-stimulated release of NO. Similar mechanisms were observed in the small intestine microvasculature. Wang et al. [41] demonstrated that acetylcholine-induced endothelium-dependent relaxation was decreased in an animal model of peritonitis.

'CYTOPATHIC HYPOXIA': A POTENTIAL MECHANISM OF GUT FAILURE IN SEPSIS ?

During sepsis, growing evidence suggests that blood flow distribution within the gut wall may contribute to the generation of mucosal hypoxia, despite normal global gut blood flow. However, Fink et al. [42] concluded that the increase in gut mucosal permeability in a porcine model of endotoxemia was not solely due to the decrease in mucosal perfusion. They advocated a role for 'cytopathic hypoxia', a term used to indicate impaired production of adenosine triphosphate (ATP) despite adequate availability of oxygen in the vicinity of mitochondria within cells [43]. In experimental sepsis, this group showed that tissue acidosis can occur even in the absence of hypoperfusion or hypoxia (Figure 4) [8].

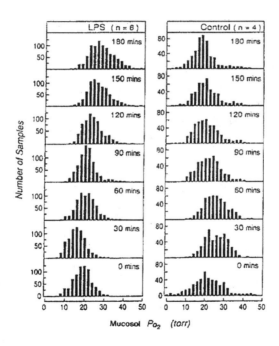

Figure 4. Mucosal PO₂ histograms in normal controls (right panel) and septic pigs (left panel) 0 to 180 minutes after endotoxin (LPS) infusion. From [8] with permission

A strong correlation was demonstrated between the degree of ileal mucosal acidosis and the degree of ileal mucosal hyperpermeability induced by either systemic endotoxemia or partial mechanical occlusion of the mesenteric artery [19]. To the authors, these findings suggested that the adverse effects of endotoxemia or ischemia on intestinal epithelial permeability were related to the resultant derangements in tissue pH rather than simply to the changes in tissue oxygenation *per se*. This notion was further supported by the observation that ileal epithelial permeability was increased in pigs when mucosal acidosis was induced by an acute increase in arterial CO_2 tension even in the absence of tissue hypoxia [44].

Interestingly, NO, which is produced at an accelerated rate by the inducible isoform of NOS during sepsis, appears to be capable of modulating intestinal permeability. Support for the notion that NO has a deleterious effect on enterocytes comes from work by Tepperman et al. [45] who showed that administration of LPS to rats decreased the viability of freshly isolated gut epithelial cells and increased the activity of NOS. In their system, pretreatment with the NOS inhibitor, L-nitroarginine methyl ester (L-NAME), significantly ameliorated the adverse effect of LPS on enterocyte function and viability. In a model of intestinal epithelium (Caco-2$_{BBe}$ monolayers), Salzman et al. [44] reported that incubation with the NO donors sodium nitroprusside (SNP), S-nitroso-N-acetylpenicillamine, or 1 % NO gas reduced ATP levels and reversibly increased the permeability of tight junctions. High concentrations of NO can interfere with cellular respiration by competing with oxygen at the cytochrome oxidase site in the electron transport chain [46]. However, the authors argued that this hyperpermeability was not due to the loss of cellular viability, since the monolayers rendered hyperpermeable by exposure to SNP were capable of restoring their original permeability after incubation in medium devoid of an NO donor. In support of this maintained cell viability despite impaired mitochondrial respiration due to increased production of NO, aminoguanidine, a selective inhibitor of inducible NOS was able to return gut VO_2 to normal in LPS-treated rats [47].

These results disagree, however, with those reported by some other groups working with various models. Kubes [48] has shown in contrast that infusion of the NOS blocker L-NAME into the mesenteric artery of cats leads to a sixfold increase in epithelial permeability, without obvious manifestation of mucosal ischemia. Payne and Kubes [49] also documented that infusion of an NO donor ameliorates gut mucosal hyperpermeability induced by ischemia and reperfusion. Moreover, treatment with NOS inhibitors has been shown to exacerbate gut epithelial hyperpermeability induced by ischemia-reperfusion [50] and macroscopic mucosal damage induced by LPS [51]. These apparent controversial results can be reconciled if one considers time elapsed since the beginning of sepsis. Indeed, it has been demonstrated that the early phase of endotoxic shock is a state of NO deficiency, or nitrosopenia, when the late phase represents a high output NO state [52]. Nitrosopenia is associated with loss of endothelium-derived relaxation, increased leukocyte and platelet adhesion, and increased tissue factor expression with coagulation activation, all of these features contributing to impaired tissue perfusion [53]. Administration of the NO donor SNP could be of interest during this early phase, while blocking inducible NOS by L-NAME, or a more selective agent, might be more favorable during the late one. In contrast, use of L-NAME during the early phase, and use of SNP during the late would be catastrophic.

With this in mind, it is very important to determine the temporal sequence of alterations with relative contribution of nitrosopenia and tissue hypoperfusion, NO overproduction and inflammation. Crouser et al. [54] recently tested the hypothesis that epithelial necrosis and/or apoptosis correlate with NO dysregulation in a presumably non-ischemic model of sepsis-induced ileal injury. To do so they used an *in situ* autoperfused feline ileal preparation in which global blood flow and DO_2 can be sustained. Two and four hours after LPS or saline injection, ileal segments were obtained for simultaneous evaluations of cellular and mitochondrial ultrastructure, immunoprevalence of inducible NOS and 3-nitrotyrosine (a stable marker of peroxynitrite), and histochemical evidence of apoptosis. Epithelial necrosis was prominent by 2 hours post-LPS, while apoptosis and increases in inducible NOS and 3-nitrotyrosine were not evident before 4 hours suggesting that the early ileal mucosal necrosis may be due to LPS-induced activation of inflammatory pathways and/or microcirculatory disturbances, whereas NO dysregulation participates in later events.

The hypothesis that the vascular and tissue oxygenation defect during sepsis is due entirely to excessive NO synthesis appears too simplistic. Indeed, inhibition of NOS using the nonspecific inhibitor L-NAME *in vivo* failed to restore a normal oxygen extraction response in canine intestine segments during endotoxemia [22]. Administration of this compound during endotoxemia produced a partial restoration of systemic blood pressure, but cardiac output decreased significantly, even though left atrial pressures were maintained. It is conceivable however that an inhibitor which acts selectively on the inducible isoform of NOS might be more beneficial, since physiological NO synthesis by the constitutive isoform in endothelial cells would be preserved.

A THERAPEUTIC GOAL: TO IMPROVE GUT MUCOSAL BLOOD FLOW AND OXYGENATION IN SEPSIS

Animal Models

In the acute situation, specific pharmacologic interventions aimed at restoring blood flow toward the mucosa may help to lessen the possibility of mucosal ischemia. Also, pharmacologic interventions with adrenergic agents combined with fluid resuscitation may improve the distribution of perfusion while also increasing overall flow to the gut. On the other hand, it is possible that α-adrenergic agents could decrease mesenteric flow, a response that is seen in the absence of sepsis. However, after administration of endotoxin or live bacteria, or in cecal ligation-puncture models [55,56], infusion of α-adrenergic agents failed to redistribute total body volume and flow from non-vital organs, i.e., the gut, to vital organs such as the heart and brain.

Interestingly, the effects of β-adrenergic agonists in promoting blood flow to the mucosa were explored by Shepherd et al. [57]. Using radioactive microspheres and laser Doppler flowmetry, they observed that the β_1-β_2-adrenergic agonist isoproterenol was able to increase gut blood flow and to favor mucosal flow at the expense of muscularis in anesthetized animals. More specifically, Cain and Curtis [58] showed in endotoxic dogs that dextran plus dopexamine, a potent β_2-adrenergic agonist, supported gut VO_2 at higher levels than did dextran alone. The authors postulated that the β_2-adrenergic agonist activity of dopexamine would preferentially promote blood flow to the gut mucosa and attenuate the regional production of lactate by correcting the tissue hypoxia within the gut wall. This hypothesis was supported by observation of lower lactate efflux and higher VO_2 in dopexamine-treated animals indicating a treatment beneficial effect which was not achieved by dextran alone.

Another report described the effects of a low dose of the β_1-β_2-adrenergic agonist dobutamine (5 µg/kg.min) on gastric and intestinal mucosal blood flow in a fluid resuscitated porcine model of endotoxic shock [33]. Hemodynamics, oxygen transport and gastrointestinal mucosal perfusion assessed by laser Doppler flowmetry and pHi were compared in a saline-treated group and in saline plus dobutamine-treated animals. Endotoxin plus saline treatment maintained systemic blood flow, but produced a decrease of gastric and intestinal microvascular blood flow along with a decrease in gastric and intestinal pHi. By constrast, the saline plus dobutamine treatment group demonstrated a return of gut microvascular blood flow and a normalization of gut pHi at the end of treatment. The authors related these findings to the dobutamine β_2-adrenergic stimulation on mucosal blood flow. Although the decrease in pHi was not reversed entirely, saline plus dobutamine resuscitation did appear to limit the decrease in gut pHi.

In another porcine model of acute endotoxemia [59], high doses of dobutamine were used to maintain mesenteric blood flow. Fluid resuscitation was used in a control group to create a normodynamic model of acute endotoxemia. Additional resuscitation in form of either hetastarch or hetastarch plus dobutamine converted this into a hyperdynamic, hypotensive model. Permeability was measured in the plasma-to-lumen direction in this study, which allowed to quantify the derangement in the permeability barrier. The six-fold increase in transmucosal permeability seen in control animals was prevented in the hetastarch-dobutamine regimen. In this study, ileal pHi was measured using the tonometric technique. This technique provided results that imply similar conclusions as those obtained with quantification of barrier permeability. Infusion of LPS caused a marked degree of mucosal acidosis. This mucosal acidosis was partly ameliorated by resuscitation with hetastarch and completely ameliorated with hetastarch plus dobutamine.

Clinical Studies

Experimental studies described earlier have shown that gut pHi and/or ileal mucosal-arterial PCO_2 gap measurements may be useful in detecting gut mucosal ischemia. Clinical studies suggest that gastric tonometry may be useful in identifying alternative therapeutic options in patients with mucosal ischemia and critical illness. For example, Silverman et al. [60] demonstrated that dobutamine increased gastric tonometric pHi values in septic patients, suggesting that this agent may improve splanchnic tissue oxygenation. By contrast, packed red blood cell transfusions administered to increase systemic DO_2 failed to improve gastric pHi [61]. The adverse effects of blood transfusion were related to the age of packed red blood cells (RBCs) and loss of red cell deformability. Therefore, the failure of packed RBC transfusions to improve pHi could have been related to a decrease in mucosal blood flow secondary to the abnormal rheologic properties of the red cells.

In septic patients, a variety of pharmacological agents have been shown to reverse the intramucosal acidosis that was refractory to increases in systemic DO_2 [62, 63]. These drugs may act by redistributing blood flow and DO_2 within the gut wall, thereby improving or redistributing DO_2 preferentially to or within the mucosa. For example, Smithies et al. [64] demonstrated that dopexamine was able to increase gastric pHi in septic patients. Splanchnic blood flow, which was assessed by indocyanine green (ICG) clearance, tended to increase but the trend did not reach statistical significance. The improvements in gastric pHi were therefore unrelated to changes in splanchnic blood flow, cardiac output or systemic DO_2. These findings suggest that the distribution of oxygen supply within the gut wall was improved by the drug, most likely representing an improvement in mucosal flow at the expense of the muscularis layer.

The beneficial effect of dobutamine on gastric intramucosal acidosis has also been tested by Gutierrez et al. [65] in septic patients with and without elevated arterial lactate. These investigators found that dobutamine increased gastric pHi when infused at 5 μg/kg.min and 10 μg/kg.min. It was speculated that dobutamine may reverse gastric intramucosal acidosis by increasing splanchnic blood flow and/or mucosal perfusion. The effects of low dose dobutamine on mucosal perfusion and pHi were recently assessed using laser Doppler flow measurements [33]. In the septic patients studied, dobutamine at 5 μg/kg.min produced increases in systemic DO_2 and a significant increase in gastric pHi. At the same time, gastric mucosal blood flow increased out of proportion to the systemic DO_2.

In 36 hemodynamically stable septic patients, Creteur et al. [66] explored whether changes in gastric mucosal-arterial PCO_2 gap induced by a short-term dobutamine infusion may reveal hepatosplanchnic hypoperfusion. Hepatosplanchnic blood flow (HSBF) was determined by the continuous ICG infusion technique and gastric mucosal ($PgCO_2$) by saline tonometry. In each patient, hemodynamic measurements, blood samples, and $PgCO_2$ determinations were performed three times: first at baseline (DOB 0), second during a dobutamine infusion at a dose of 5 μg/kg.min (DOB 5), and third at a dose of 10 μg/kg.min (DOB 10). The PCO_2 gap decreased preferentially in groups of patients with inadequate hepatosplanchnic perfusion, i.e., with a low fractional HSBF, defined as the ratio of the HSBF to the simultaneous cardiac index (HSBF/CI), or a high gradient between the mixed venous blood and the suprahepatic blood O_2 saturations ($DSvhO_2$). In the 11 patients with a $DSvhO_2$ above 20 % at baseline, PCO_2 gap decreased from 12.1 mm Hg at DOB 0 to 6.2 mm Hg at DOB 5, and to 4.2 mm Hg at DOB 10, whereas in the 25 patients with a $DSvhO_2$ below 20% at baseline, PCO_2 gap did not change significantly. At no time was the PCO_2 gap correlated with HSBF/CI or $DSvhO_2$. The authors concluded that although the PCO_2 gap does not correlate well with global indexes of gut oxygenation, a simple dobutamine infusion test could identify patients with inadequate hepatosplanchnic perfusion.

Treatment with a selective vasodilator in addition to conventional resuscitation (fluids and inotropic drugs) may help to increase gastointestinal mucosal flow even after perfusion pressure is restored. In dopamine resistant septic shock, Levy et al. [67, 68] presented evidence that a low-dose dobutamine infusion in association with epinephrine or norepinephrine improved pHi faster than did epinephrine alone. To compare respective effects of epinephrine, norepinephrine, and the combination of norepinephrine and dobutamine (5 μg/kg.min) on systemic hemodynamic parameters and gastric mucosal perfusion, Duranteau et al. [69] used gastric tonometry and laser-Doppler flowmetry techniques in a prospective, controlled, randomized, crossover study in twelve patients with septic shock.

Each patient received in a random succession epinephrine, norepinephrine, and norepinephrine plus dobutamine. Dosages of epinephrine and norepinephrine were adjusted to achieve a MAP between 70 and 80 mm Hg. The increase in gastric mucosal perfusion detected by laser-Doppler flowmetry was higher with epinephrine and the combination of norepinephrine and dobutamine than with norepinephrine alone. In addition, the ratio of gastric mucosal perfusion (local DO_2) to systemic DO_2 was increased after norepinephrine plus dobutamine as compared with norepinephrine alone and epinephrine. Although values of pHi and gastro-to-arterial PCO_2 tended to be higher with norepinephrine plus dobutamine compared with those obtained with norepinephrine and epinephrine, differences were not statistically significant. The authors concluded that for the same MAP in patients with septic shock, administration of epinephrine increased gastric mucosal perfusion more than norepinephrine administration alone. Addition of dobutamine to norepinephrine improved gastric mucosal perfusion.

In summary, improvements in blood flow to the gastric mucosa, and possibly to the intestinal mucosa, may become an appropriate goal for the treatment of critically ill patients with sepsis. Such therapeutic approaches have the potential to prevent mucosal ischemia, local inflammatory activation and the risk for remote organ injury and MODS. Gutierrez et al. [70] showed in a large controlled randomized study (n = 260) that patients monitored and treated for low pHi had lower mortality than those monitored only for conventional endpoints of resuscitation such as blood pressure and urine output. These findings suggest that gut-directed therapies may have the potential to improve the outcome of critically ill patients. There is a great need for further confirmation of these results in large scale studies.

CONCLUSION

As demonstrated in a variety of experimental shock models, perfusion of the splanchnic circulation is especially susceptible to decreases in systemic blood flow. Factors that decrease cardiac output elicit neurohumoral reflex vasoconstriction in the gut, causing a disproportional decrease in its local perfusion. The mechanisms underlying splanchnic hypoperfusion in low-flow states have been extensively studied using experimental models of cardiogenic and hemorrhagic shock. Adrenergic activity is a major determinant of this acute vascular response to cardiogenic and hemorrhagic shock [71] and the local intestinal response to systemic hemorrhage provides an example of the competition for blood flow between mucosa and muscularis.

Evidence of regional hypoperfusion, especially at the level of the gut, resulting from dysregulation of vascular tone in arterial and venous vessels has been reported in sepsis. Dissimilar effects may occur among different vascular beds, resulting in abnormalities in the distribution of capillary blood flow and blood volume [72]. Large differences among species have been noted regarding the effects of endotoxemia on the responsiveness of isolated blood vessels [73]. Also, widely divergent results have been obtained among studies looking at the effects of sepsis on mesenteric or splanchnic blood flow, depending on factors such as adequacy of resuscitation and characteristics of septic model [74]. In these models, administration of endotoxin causes a decrease in gut mucosal pH and an increase in gut permeability, despite fluid resuscitation. Within the gut wall, the mucosa has been identified as an important target of injury during sepsis. This observation may help to explain why the gut is increasingly regarded as a sentinel organ in septic patients [14] and why tonometric estimates of mucosal perfusion [65] appear to provide a reliable prognostic indication in patients with sepsis [70]. However, the cellular mechanisms underlying the special sensitivity of the gut mucosal microcirculation to sepsis or endotoxemia are still not clear.

Clinical and experimental evidence suggests that β-adrenergic agonists may be useful in promoting a redistribution of blood flow toward the gastrointestinal mucosa, which may help to correct local limitations in its oxygenation. For the patient as a whole, it is important to remember that the gut mucosa is one of many tissues whose local oxygen supply may be at risk during critical illness, even though systemic DO_2 and VO_2 appear to be within normal limits. Although evidence of pathological oxygen supply dependency at the whole body level is usually not detectable, local perfusion abnormalities may exist at the microcirculatory level in selective tissues, rendering them liable to encounter cellular injury even when all appears adequate at the systemic level.

REFERENCES

1. Evans WE, Darin JC. Effect of enterectomy in endotoxin shock. Surgery 1966; 60:1026-1029
2. Meakins JL, Marshall JC. The gastrointestinal tract: the 'motor' of multiple organ failure. Arch Surg 1986; 121:197-201
3. Vallet B, Lebuffe G. The role of the gut in multiple organ failure. In Vincent JL (ed) Yearbook of intensive care and emergency medicine. Springer, Berlin, 1999 pp 539-546
4. Nieuwenhuijzen GA, Deitch EA, Goris RJ. Infection, the gut and the development of the

multiple organ dysfunction syndrome. Eur J Surg 1996; 162:259-273
5. Vallet B, Lund N, Curtis SE, et al. Gut and muscle tissue PO$_2$ in endotoxemic dogs during shock and resuscitation. J Appl Physiol 1994; 76:793-800
6. Mayer K, Temmesfeld-Wollbrück B, Friedland A, et al. Severe microcirculatory abnormalities elicited by E. coli hemolysin in the rabbit ileum mucosa. Am J Respir Crit Care Med 1999; 160:1171-1178
7. Temmesfeld-Wollbrück B, Szalay A, Mayer K, et al. Abnormalities of gastric mucosal oxygenation in septic shock. Am J Respir Crit Care Med 1998;1586-1592
8. VanderMeer TJ, Wang H, Fink MP. Endotoxemia causes ileal mucosal acidosis in the absence of mucosal hypoxia in a normodynamic porcine model of septic shock. Crit Care Med 1995, 23:1217-1226
9. Unno N, Menconi MJ, Smith M, et al. Hyperpermeability of intestinal epithelial monolayers is induced by NO: effect of low extracellular pH. Am J Physiol 1997; 272:G923-34
10. Unno N, Wang H, Menconi MJ, et al. Inhibition of inducible nitric oxide synthase ameliorates endotoxin-induced gut mucosal barrier dysfunction in rats. Gastroenterology 1997; 113:1246-1257
11. Crouser ED, Julian MW, Dorinsky P. Ileal VO$_2$-DO$_2$ alterations induced by endotoxin correlate with severity of mitochondrial injury. Am J Respir Crit Care Med 1999; 160:1347-1353
12. Wells CL, Maddaus M, Simmons RL. Proposed mechanisms for the translocation of intestinal bacteria. Rev Infectious Dis 1988; 10:958-979
13. Gannon B, Browning J, O'Brien P, Rogers P. Mucosal microvascular architecture of the fundus and body of human stomach. Gastroenterology 1984; 86:866-875
14. Landow L, Andersen LW. Splanchnic ischemia and its role in multiple organ failure. Acta Anaesthesiol Scand 1994; 38:626-639
15. Lundgren O. Physiology of the intestinal circulation. In: Marston A, Bulkley GB, Fiddian-Green RG, Haglund U (eds) Splanchnic Ischemia and Multiple Organ Failure. Edward Arnold, London, 1989 pp 29-40
16. Nelson DP, King CE, Dodd SL, et al. Systemic and intestinal limits of O$_2$ extraction in the dog. J Appl Physiol 1987; 63:387-394
17. Samsel RW, Schumacker PT. Systemic hemorrhage augments local O$_2$ extraction in canine intestine. J Appl Physiol 1994; 77:2291-2298
18. Salzman A, Wollert PS, Wang H, et al. Intraluminal oxygenation ameliorates ischemia/reperfusion-induced gut mucosal hyperpermeability in pigs. Circ Shock 1993; 40:37-46
19. Salzman AL, Wang H, Wollert PS, et al. Endotoxin-induced ileal mucosal hyperpermeability in pigs: role of tissue acidosis. Am J Physiol 1994; 266:G633-G646
20. Xu D, Qi L, Guillory D, et al. Mechanisms of endotoxin-induced intestinal injury in a hyperdynamic model of sepsis. J Trauma 1993; 34:676-683
21. Nelson DP, Samsel RW, Wood LDH, et al. Pathological supply dependence of systemic and intestinal O$_2$ uptake during endotoxemia. J Appl Physiol 1988; 64:2410-2419
22. Schumacker PT, Kazaglis J, Connolly HV, et al. Systemic and gut oxygen extraction during endotoxemia: role of nitric oxide synthesis. Am J Respir Crit Care Med 1995; 151:107-115
23. Connolly HV, Maginniss LA, Schumacker PT. Transit time heterogeneity in canine small intestine: significance for oxygen transport. J Clin Invest 1997; 99:228-238
24. Drazenovic R, Samsel RW, Wylam ME, et al. Regulation of perfused capillary density in canine intestinal mucosa during endotoxemia. J Appl Physiol 1992; 72:259-265
25. Whithworth PW, Cryer HM, Garrisson RN, et al. Hypoperfusion of the intestinal microcirculation without decreased cardiac output during live Escherichia coli in rats.

Circ Shock 1989; 27:111-122

26. Vallet B. Regional capnometry. In Vincent JL (ed) Yearbook on Intensive Care and Emergency Medicine. Springer, Berlin, 1997 pp 669-676

27. Hasibeder W, Germann R, Wolf et al. Effects of short-term endotoxemia and dopamne on mucosal oxygenation in porcine jejunum. Am J Physiol 1996; 270:G667-G675

28. Stehr A, Tugtekin IF, Matejovic M, et al. Effect of endotoxemia on microcirculation of the small bowel mucosa in pigs. Chir Forum 2000; 29:505-508

29. Ince C, Sinaasappel M. Microcirculatory oxygenation and shunting in sepsis and shock. Crit Care Med 1999; 27:1369-1377

30. Navaratman RL, Morris SE, Traber DL, et al. Endotoxin (LPS) increases mesenteric vascular resistance (MVR) and bacterial translocation (BT). J Trauma 1990; 30:1104-1113

31. Theuer CJ, Wilson MA, Steeb GD, et al. Microvascular vasoconstriction and mucosal hypoperfusion of the rat small intestine during bacteremia. Circ Shock 1993; 40:61-68

32. Nevière R, Mathieu D, Chagnon JL, et al. The contrasting effects of dobutamine and dopamine on gastric mucosal perfusion in septic patients. Am J Respir Crit Care Med 1996; 154:1684-1688

33. Nevière R, Chagnon LJ, Vallet B, et al. Dobutamine improves gastro-intestinal mucosal blood flow in a porcine model of endotoxic shock. Crit Care Med 1997; 25:1371-1377

34. Jutabha R, Poa L, Jensen DM. Stress ulceration in the critically ill. Curr Opin Crit Care 1995, 1:125-129

35. Nash J, Lambert L, Deakin M. Histamine H2-receptor antagonists in peptic ulcer disease. Evidence for a prophylactic use. Drugs 1994; 47:862-871

36. Julou-Schaeffer G, Gray GA, Fleming I, Schott C, Parratt JR, Stoclet JC. Loss of vascular responsiveness induced by endotoxin involves L-arginine pathway. Am J Physiol 1990; 259:H1038-H1043

37. Parker JL, Keller RS, DeFily DV, et al. Coronary vascular smooth muscle function in E. coli endotoxemia in dogs. Am J Physiol 1991; 260:H832-H842

38. Maginiss LA, Connolly H, Samsel RW, Schumacker PT. Adrenergic vasoconstriction augments tissue O_2 extraction during reductions in O_2 delivery. J Appl Physiol 1994; 76:1454-1461

39. Zhang H, Spapen H, Vincent JL. Effects of dobutamine and norepinephrine on oxygen availability in tamponade-induced stagnant hypoxia: a prospective, randomized, controlled study. Crit Care Med 1994; 22:299-305

40. Vallet B. Vascular reactivity and tissue oxygenation. Intensive Care Med 1998; 24:3-11

41. Wang P, Ba ZF, Chaudry IH. Endothelium-dependent relaxation is depressed at the macro- and microcirculatory levels during sepsis. Am J Physiol 1995; 269:R988-R994

42. Fink MP, Antonsson JB, Wang HL, et al. Increased intestinal permeability in endotoxic pigs. Mesenteric hypoperfusion as an etiologic factor. Arch Surg 1991; 126:211-218

43. Fink MP. Cytopathic hypoxia: mitochondrial dysfunction as a potential mechanism contributing to organ failure in sepsis. In Sibbald WJ, Messmer K, Fink MP (eds) Tissue Oxygenation in Acute Medicine. Springer, Berlin, 1998 pp 128-137

44. Salzman AL, Menconi MJ, Unno N, et al. Nitric oxide dilates tight junctions and depletes ATP in cultured Caco-2BBe intestinal epithelial monolayers. Am J Physiol 1995; 268:G361-G373

45. Tepperman BL, Brown JF, Whittle BJR. Nitric oxide synthase induction and intestinal viability in rats. Am J Physiol 1993; 265:G214-G218

46. Brown GC, Cooper CE. Nanomolar concentrations of nitric oxide reversibly inhibit synaptosomal respiration by competing with oxygen at cytochrome oxidase. FEBS Letters 1994; 356:295-298

47. King CJ, Tytgat S, Delude RL, et al. Ileal mucosal oxygen consumption is decreased in

endotoxemic rats but is restored toward normal by treatment with aminoguanidine. Crit Care Med 1999; 27:2518-2524

48. Kubes P. Nitric oxide modulates epithelial permeability in the feline small intestine. Am J Physiol 1992; 262:G1138-G1142

49. Payne D, Kubes P. Nitric oxide donors reduce the rise in reperfusion-induced intestinal mucosal permeability. Am J Physiol 1994; 265:G189-G195

50. Kubes P. Ischemia-reperfusion in the feline small intestine: a role for nitric oxide. Am J Physiol 1993; 264:G143-G149

51. Hutcheson IR, Whittle BJ, Bouhton-Smith NK. Role of nitric oxide in maintaining vascular integrity in endotoxin-induced intestinal damage in the rat. Br J Pharmacol 1990; 101:815-820

52. Salzman AL. Endotoxic nitrosopenia. Intensive Care Med 1998; 24:1239-1241

53. Vallet B, Leclerc J. Endothelial cell dysfunction in septic shock. In Vincent JL (ed) Yearbook of Intensive Care and Emergency Medicine. Springer, Berlin, 1998 pp 133-142

54. Crouser ED, Julian MW, Weinstein DM, et al. Endotoxin-induced ileal mucosal injury and nitric oxide dysregulation are temporally dissociated. Am J Respir Crit Care Med 2000; 161:1705-1712

55. Bersten AD, Hersch M, Cheung H, et al. The effect of various sympathomimetics on the regional circulations in hyperdynamic sepsis. Surgery 1992; 112:549-561

56. Breslow MJ, Miller CF, Parker SD, Walman AT, Traystman RJ. Effect of vasopressors on organ blood flow during endotoxin shock in pigs. Am J Physiol 1987; 252:H291-H300

57. Shepherd AP, Riedel GL, Maxwell LC, et al. Selective vasodilators redistribute intestinal blood flow and depress oxygen uptake. Am J Physiol 1984; 247:G377-G384

58. Cain SM, Curtis SE. Systemic and regional oxygen uptake and lactate flux in endotoxic dogs resuscitated with dextran and dopexamine or dextran alone. Circ Shock 1992; 38:173-181

59. Fink MP, Kaups KL, Wang H, et al. Maintenance of superior mesenteric arterial perfusion prevents increased intestinal mucosal permeablity in endotoxic pigs. Surgery 1991; 110:154-161

60. Silverman HJ, Tuma P. Gastric tonometry in patients with sepsis: effects of dobutamine infusion and packed red blood cell transfusions. Chest 1992; 102:184-188

61. Marik PE, Sibbald WJ. The effect of stored blood transfusion on oxygen delivery in patients with sepsis. JAMA 1993; 269:3024-3029

62. Silva E, DeBacker D, Creteur J, Vincent JL. Effects of vasoactive drugs on gastric intramucosal pH. Crit Care Med 1998; 26:1749-1758

63. Reinhart K, Sakka SG, Meier-Hellmann A. Hemodynamic management of a patient with septic shock. Eur J Anaesthesiol 2000; 17:6-17

64. Smithies M, Yee TH, Jackson L et al. Protecting the gut and the liver in the critically ill: effects of dopexamine. Crit Care Med 1994; 22:789-795

65. Gutierrez G, Clark C, Brown SD, et al. Effect of dobutamine on oxygen consumption and gastric mucosal pH in septic patients. Am J Respir Crit Care Med 1994; 150:324-329

66. Creteur J, De Backer D, Vincent JL. A dobutamine test can disclose hepatosplanchnic hypoperfusion in septic patients. Am J Respir Crit Care Med 1999; 160:839-45

67. Levy B, Bollaert PE, Lucchelli JP, et al. Dobutamine improves the adequacy of gastric mucosal perfusion in epinephrine-treated septic shock. Crit Care Med 1997; 25:1649-1654

68. Levy B, Bollaert PE, Nace L, Charpentier C, Bauer PH, Larcan A. Comparison of norepinephrine and dobutamine to epinephrine for hemodynamics, lactate metabolism and gastric tonometric variables in septic shock. A prospective randomized study.

Intensive Care Med 1997; 23:282-287
69. Duranteau J, Sitbon P, Teboul JL, et al. Effects of epinephrine, norepinephrine, or the combination of norepinephrine and dobutamine on gastric mucosa in septic shock. Crit Care Med 1999; 27:893-900
70. Gutierrez G, Palizas F, Doglio G, et al. Gastric intramucosal pH as a therapeutic index of tissue oxygenation in critically ill patients. Lancet 1992; 339:195-199
71. Porter JM, Sussman MS, Bulkley GB. Splanchnic vasospasm in circulatory shock in splanchnic ischemia and multiple organ failure. Marston A, Bulkley GB, Fiddian-Green RG et al. (eds) Splanchnic Ischemia and Multiple Organ Failure. CV Mosby, St Louis, 1989, pp 73-88
72. Carrol G, Synder J. Hyperdynamic severe intravascular sepsis depends on fluid administration in cyonomolgus monkey. Am J Physiol 1982; 243:R131-R141
73. Umans JG, Wylam ME, Samsel RW, et al. Effects of endotoxin in vivo on endothelial and smooth-muscle function in rabbit and rat aorta. Am Rev Repir Dis 1993; 148: 1638-1645
74. Fink MP. Systemic and splanchnic hemodynamic derangements in the sepsis syndrome. In: Marston A, Bulkley GB, Fiddian-Green RG, Haglund U (eds) Splanchnic Ischemia and Multiple Organ Failure. CV Mosby, St Louis, 1989 pp: 101-106

38

THE KIDNEY IN SEPSIS

Marc G Vervloet
Harro A Piepot
AB Johan Groeneveld

The majority of critically ill patients with multiple organ failure (MOF) associated with sepsis have acute renal failure (ARF) [1,2]. Conversely, the frequency of ARF in severe sepsis ranges from 20 to 50 % [1,2]. The chances of survival once ARF has developed in the course of sepsis are poor, despite of appropriate supporting therapy, since the mortality rate exceeds 60 % [1,2].

The kidney may be either directly or indirectly affected by sepsis. Haematologic spread of sepsis may lead to interstitial micro-abscess formation in the kidney. In animals, renal dysfunction is common after the infusion of endotoxin derived from Gram-negative bacteria or induction of bacterial sepsis [3-30]. However, not only endotoxin but other components of Gram-negative and Gram-positive bacteria may be capable of inducing ARF, and compounds differ in their renal toxicity [9,27,28,31,32].

MANIFESTATIONS AND PATHOPHYSIOLOGY

Impending ARF is heralded by oliguria progressing to anuria, and a rise in circulating creatinine and urea, as evidence of a fall in the glomerular filtration rate [33,34]. Hypovolemia and prerenal renal failure usually result in avid sodium resorption so that the sodium concentration and the fractional excretion of sodium into the urine is low [33]. The glomerular filtration rate (GFR) can be estimated from the steady state creatinine (inulin) clearance rate [33,34]. Sophisticated (radionuclide) techniques to estimate the GFR in man are primarily applied for research purposes [13,14,17,27,28,33,35,36].

Progressive tubular dysfunction in the progression of prerenal failure to ARF usually leads to sodium losses into the urine, that may also contain casts and tubular enzymes and proteins, but oliguria usually persists [11,17,33]. Nevertheless, non- or even poly-uric forms of ARF may occur. In the course of sepsis, a filtration rate and blood flow-independent early rise in natriuresis and diuresis is sometimes observed [35,37]. In endotoxin or bacterial shock in rats, this 'inappropriate' diuresis develops in the course of hours after the challenge, even when renal blood flow and gomerular filtration have diminished [28]. Increased water and sodium excretion may indeed aggravate hypovolaemia and ultimately contribute to non-oliguric ARF [34]. The interstitial hypertonicity in the medulla may be diminished following preferential blood flow distribution to the medulla, mediated by nitric oxide (NO), and this may reduce the maximal concentration and sodium resorption ability [36-39]. The 'inappropriate' diuresis may also be caused by hyporesponsiveness of the collecting duct cells to antidiuretic hormone (ADH), rather than by blood flow redistribution or diminished ADH secretion, since ADH may be released following non-osmotic stimuli during endotoxaemia and sepsis [35]. Finally, increased atrial natriuretic peptide (α-ANP), and a less active Na^+-K^+ ATPase by a reduced energy charge in the tubular cell can lead to a diminished sodium resorption [6,23,40].

Histopathological studies showed that shock can lead to ischemic necrosis of tubular cells [41], the so called tubulorrhexis or acute tubular necrosis (ATN). However, ARF in the course of sepsis may occur even in the absence of overt histopathological changes [17]. The consequence of ATN can be tubular obstruction, and backleak of ultrafiltrate proximal from the obstruction by a rise of intratubular pressure and loss of part of the anatomical barrier between the tubular lumen and the postglomerular, efferent capillaries, surrounding the tubules [33]. It has been shown that the relative clearance of dextrans of high molecular weight exceeded that of inulin in ARF [33]. This suggests a high ratio of inulin backleak compared to dextrans with molecular sizes exceeding the diameter of pores in the tubular basement membrane. In addition, the pressure in Bowman's capsule will rise, thereby reducing net hydraulic pressure for ultrafiltration across the glomerular membrane [33].

PATHOGENESIS OF ARF IN SEPSIS

In contrast to the limited variation in the clinical presentation of ARF, i.e., an oliguric or non-oliguric decline in GFR with varying degrees of proteinuria, the underlying pathogenesis is complicated. The present knowledge on the pathogenesis is largely based on animal models or *in vitro* experiments. The host inflammatory response evoked by sepsis may affect the kidney directly and indirectly. Hemodynamic and inflammatory factors may synergize in injuring the cell, leading to Ca^{2+} overload, apoptosis or cell death, resulting in tubular and glomerular dysfunction [42].

Hemodynamic Changes

The association between cardiopulmonary failure and the development of ARF suggests that hemodynamic factors play a central role in ARF development following sepsis [1]. A fall in renal blood flow is considered the predominant factor involved in ARF development, resulting from the global circulatory changes associated with sepsis, and/or from local factors, affecting the renal (micro)circulation [33,43]. However, estimation of renal blood flow is difficult at the bedside. Authors have tried to measure renal blood flow with invasive renal vein thermodilution techniques or with duplex Doppler ultrasound measurements [35,36,43-45]. Measurements of effective renal blood flow with help of plasma clearance of substances that are excreted by the tubules, may be unreliable, since in sepsis-induced ARF the normal 90 % or greater extraction by the kidney of hippurate may decline, in an unpredictable manner, to less than 50 %, so that the hippurate clearance can underestimate true renal blood flow. Nevertheless, hippurate clearance is widely used in animal and human experiments [3-5,9,12,13,17,18,22,27,28, 35,36,45]. In experimental studies, renal blood flow has also been assessed with help of microspheres and flow probes around the renal artery [7,8,10, 13-15,20,37,45]. Videomicroscopy and laser Doppler have been used to study the renal microcirculation [16,19,24-26].

Septic shock in man is usually characterized by hypotension and a normal to supranormal cardiac output, particularly after fluid loading. Most studies in which renal blood flow was assessed indicate a decline in renal perfusion, despite a hyperdynamic state, but some studies suggest an elevated renal blood flow [4,8,12,35,36,43,46]. Hypoperfusion of the kidneys usually occurs in experimental models of endotoxin or septic shock, even if a hyperdynamic state prevails [4,7-9,15-17,19,20,22-25,37,46-48]. Hence, the kidney may not participate in the general vasodilated state, particularly during hypotension, associated with selective renal vasoconstriction. Nevertheless, renal hypoperfusion and (prerenal) failure may occur during endotoxaemia/sepsis, even in the absence of a severe fall in blood pressure [4,6,9,17,19,26,31]. Intrarenal hemodynamic changes may include preferential preglomerular afferent arteriolar vasoconstriction, tubular hypoperfusion and cortical to medullary blood flow redistribution [9,16,19, 24,25,26,37].

Glomerular Hemodynamics

Glomeruli need an adequate supply of plasma for ultrafiltration and an adequate blood pressure, which is the principal driving force for ultrafiltration across the glomerular membrane. Both renal plasma flow and glomerular blood pressure can fluctuate during arterial pressure changes within the margins of renal autoregulation [33,49]. At some point during progressive global hypoperfusion, however, renal vasodilation to preserve renal blood flow in face of a fall in perfusion pressure, is reversed into vasoconstriction, because vasoconstrictor override vasodilator influences [50]. During sepsis and shock also, renal blood flow may become more dependent on perfusion pressure than normal [20,25,49]. Locally applied endotoxin in the renal artery caused vasoconstriction, but left autoregulatory pressure-responsiveness intact, provided that the endothelium was intact, whereas systemically administered endotoxin caused both renal vasoconstriction and exaggerated pressure-dependency [25].

During a progressive fall in renal perfusion,the GFR is better autoregulated than renal blood flow, thereby resulting in a rise in the filtration fraction [13]. A rise in tone of the efferent versus the afferent glomerular arterioles may help to maintain ultrafiltration. Both the function of the glomerular membrane and the area available for ultrafiltration, which can be regulated by the mesangium, affect the GFR and can change in the course of sepsis [33]. The often observed lack of rise in the filtration fraction, or a greater decrease in GFR than in renal blood flow, during sepsis may thus indicate diminished filtration autoregulation and relate to the afferent vasoconstriction, mesangial contraction and non-hemodynamic inflammatory factors affecting the glomerular membrane [4,9,11,15-17,19,20,24-28,36]. In fact, glomeruli and tubular interstitium may contain increased numbers of (activated) neutrophils in the course of experimental endotoxaemia, independently of hypoperfusion, although some time may be needed for this phenomenon to develop [13,14,21,28,30,51]. Micropuncture studies in animals have shown that the GFR may decline during endotoxemia, despite a preservation of perfusion pressure to the kidney and a normal proximal tubular pressure [9].

Tubular Hypoperfusion and Medullary Redistribution

Tubular resorption requires energy and thereby oxygen, so that tubular hypoperfusion may lead to an oxygen deficit and thereby to ATN and ARF [8]. Indeed, renal oxygen uptake may decrease during endotoxaemia/sepsis-induced hypoperfusion, although this does not necessarily imply a tubular oxygen deficit if energy-consuming tubular resorption declines following a fall in filtered load [8,15]. Moreover, some investigators found that renal oxygen uptake did not decrease concomitantly with increased renal oxygen extraction during a reduced oxygen delivery (DO_2), following endotoxemia or bacteremia [15,27,28]. If the latter does not match increased metabolic needs during sepsis, for instance as a consequence of metabolic inefficiency or an increase in energy-consuming metabolic processes such as gluconeogenesis, an oxygen deficit may still develop, in spite of a decline in energy-consuming tubular resorption [15,27,28]. In studies on energy metabolism and ATP levels, the renal cells showed a reduction of energy charge following experimental sepsis, arguing in favor of an oxygen deficit [4,6,13]. Nevertheless, a normal energy status has been reported as well, predominantly in models of reversible (prerenal) ARF, during endotoxaemia or bacterial sepsis [27,28].

During a progressive decline in global renal perfusion during sepsis or endotoxemia in animals, blood is intrarenally redistributed in favor of the medulla, since the vasodilator reserve in the cortex is less than in the medulla, thereby limiting DO_2 to the cortex [9,19,24,26,37]. Nevertheless cortical-medullary redistribution may also occur during hyperdynamic septic shock with augmented renal blood flow [37]. The medulla contains nephrons more capable of concentrating urine and to preserve circulating volume than the cortex does [9,37,38]. The renal medulla normally faces a critical oxygen supply, following a countercurrent blood flow mechanism in peritubular blood vessels, causing a low oxygen tension [38]. The relative rise in metabolic demands following enhanced filtration and energy-consuming resorption in juxtaglomerular nephrons adds to the dysbalance between metabolic needs and actual delivery of oxygen to medullary tubules during hypoperfusion and blood flow redistribution [38].

Cascades involved in Renal Hemodynamics during Sepsis

The substances involved in ARF during sepsis can be divided into two groups. In the first group, constitutive systems are involved, having a physiological role in regulating renal hemodynamics and trying to correct the influence of global hemodynamic changes on renal perfusion, or being deranged by the septic process. In the second group are sepsis-induced mediators or substances with vasoactive properties, without an apparent intended role in regulating renal hemodynamics (Table 1).

Altered physiological systems	Sepsis-induced factors
Sympathetic nervous system Renin-angiotensin-aldosterone system Arachidonic acid metabolites Kinin-kallikrein system α-Atrial natriuretic peptide Antidiuretic hormone	**Primary mediators:** TNF-α, IL-1ß, IL-6, IL-8, chemokines Platelet activating factor **Vessel wall factors:** decreased cNOS, increased iNOS, endothelin **Adhesion molecules:** ECAM, ICAM-1, selectins **Neutrophil-derived:** proteases, oxygen radicals

Table 1. Factors involved in renal hemodynamics and filtration during sepsis.

Finally, the kidney may be challenged by the direct (cyto-)toxic effects of inflammatory cellular and humoral factors, e.g., activated monocytes and neutrophils, releasing cytokines, proteases and oxygen radicals [30]. Conversely, the injury evoked during reperfusion after an episode of ischemia (I/R injury) may involve a renal inflammatory response. Many of the mechanisms and factors mentioned may influence each other.

The Sympathetic Nervous System

There is evidence that the sympathetic nervous system is activated early during endotoxemia/sepsis [3,10,17]. The renal α-receptors of the sympathetic nervous system can be activated by nerve endings as well as by circulating catecholamines and activation may contribute to selective renal vasoconstriction, intrarenal cortical to medullary blood flow redistribution and hypofiltration during endotoxaemia, sepsis and shock [3,47]. Activation of the sympathetic nervous system may involve the sensitive baroreceptors in the proximal arterial system, the renal chemoreceptors, or the brain, where endotoxin passes the blood-brain barrier [17,47]. Besides the interactions between the sympathetic nervous system, the RAAS and arachidonic acid metabolites, the renal sympathetic nervous system also downregulates the vasodilating products of the kinin-kallikrein system, thereby further contributing to renal vasoconstriction [3,17]. Moreover, direct involvement in regulating renal vascular tone is likely, since constriction of the afferent arteriole during sepsis can be prevented by α-blockade [3,16,17]. However, in a model of mild sepsis, the innervated kidney was protected from hypoperfusion at the end of the experiment, as compared to the denervated kidney [10].

The Renin-angiotensin-aldosterone System (RAAS)

The RAAS is activated during sepsis and hypotension [3,9,16,17,20,33]. Animal studies have demonstrated that, even shortly after an insult with bacteria or endotoxins, hyperplasia of the juxtaglomerular apparatus is a frequent finding [17]. The adrenals, however, may fail to increase aldosterone excretion following activation of the RAAS in the critically ill and this may be attributed to shock and adrenal damage and could contribute to renal water and sodium losses and hypovolaemia [52]. Under physiological circumstances, the RAAS is important in volume homeostasis. Angiotensin II liberates various factors. It may increase local noradrenaline release via angiotensin II receptors on terminal nervous ends of the sympathetic nervous system of the kidneys. Angiotensin II also stimulates local production of vasodilating prostaglandins, interacts with NO, and activates the kallikrein system, the latter probably indirectly via a rise in aldosterone [16,53]. In turn, renin release is, apart from being controlled by the afferent blood pressure and distal tubular sodium (or chloride) content, influenced by the sympathetic nervous system, prostaglandins and the kallikrein system [3,9]. Angiotensin II constricts efferent arterioles in particular, thereby reducing renal blood flow but increasing the ultrafiltration coefficient and thereby the filtration fraction. Besides its effects on arteriolae, angiotensin II is nevertheless also capable to contract mesangial cells, reducing the surface area in the glomeruli available for ultrafiltration. In sepsis, angiotensin II appears to have also vasoconstrictive properties on the afferent arteriole, partly because of high circulating levels, upregulated receptors, or both [9,16]. Angiotensin converting enzyme inhibition indeed improved glomerular hemodynamics after endotoxin challenge in animals, but this can lead to severe hypotension in septic individuals [9,17].

Metabolites of Arachidonic Acid

During endotoxemia/sepsis, the concentrations of products of arachidonic acid metabolism are generally elevated in blood (and urine) [3,12,17,18,20,54,55]. Arachidonic acid can be metabolized via three major metabolic pathways, each yielding distinct products. These are the cyclooxygenase pathway generating prostaglandins and thromboxane, the lipoxygenase pathway generating leukotrienes, and the cytochrome P450 system [55]. The production depends on the availability of arachidonic acid, stored in cell membranes, and on phospholipase A_2. Activation of phospholipase A_2 and increased production of arachidonic acid metabolites can be triggered by endotoxin, cytokines, platelet activating factor (PAF), tissue hypoxia and changes in intracellular Ca^{2+} content, oxygen radicals, angiotensin II, ADH, catecholamines and bradykinin [12,16-18,54-56]. The oxygen radicals may catalyze or non-enzymatically induce the production of several metabolites of arachidonic acid, that have vasoconstrictive properties on afferent arterioles, probably via the thromboxane A_2 receptor [24,54,55, 57]. The prostaglandins interfere with other regulatory systems, since they may mediate renin secretion, may reduce catecholamine actions and may increase the release but antagonise the actions of ADH [9,17,55].

Particularly, the role of prostaglandin E_2 (PGE_2), prostaglandin I_2 (prostacyclin, PGI_2) and thromboxane A_2 in (septic) ARF has been the subject of study, as assessed, among others, from circulating or urinary concentrations of stable breakdown products of the latter two, such as 6-keto-$PGF_{1\alpha}$ and thromboxane B_2, respectively [3,12,17,20,50,55]. PGE_2 and PGI_2 are potent vasodilators, whereas thromboxane A_2 is a vasoconstrictive agent, particularly in the afferent arteriole, so that the balance between the two may be critical [12,54,55,58]. Furthermore, thromboxane A_2 can contract mesangial cells, thereby reducing glomerular surface area and the ultrafiltration coefficient, whereas PGE_2 and PGI_2 can relax the mesangium [17]. PGE_2 infusion may protect against haemodynamically mediated (and toxin mediated) ARF [59]. Finally, PGE_2, PGI_2 and P450 arachidonic acid derivates may inhibit tubular sodium and water resorption.

Normal renal hemodynamics do not depend on the vasoactive substances produced by the cyclooxygenase pathway of arachidonic acid [3,16,50,55]. During a fall in cardiac output, as occurring after endotoxemia in dogs, however, renal release of vasodilating prostaglandins defends renal blood flow, until vasoconstricting factors overwhelm defending vasodilatory ones and renal blood flow and filtration fall [3,12,50]. Inhibition of the cyclooxygenase-derived compounds by non-steroidal antiinflammatory drugs (NSAID's) increases renal vascular resistance and reduces renal blood flow during experimental sepsis, suggesting a predominantly renal vasodilating effect of renal prostaglandins released during sepsis [3,12,16,20,55]. This may be explained by a greater release of PGE_2 and PGI_2 than of thromboxane A_2 [3,12]. Some studies, however, failed to demonstrate a deleterious effect of non-steroidal anti-inflammatory drugs (NSAIDs) [3,7,9,18,20,54,55]. This may relate to a detrimental role of prostaglandins in the global circulatory response to endotoxin/sepsis [3]. Conversely, (selective) inhibition of thromboxane A_2 synthetase protected from renal hypoperfusion during endotoxaemia, sepsis or mediator infusion in some studies [17,18,54,55].

Activation of the lipoxygenase pathway during sepsis yields leukotrienes [54,55,60]. Some compounds have vasoconstrictive properties, adversely interfering with the ultrafiltration coefficient, causing capillary leak, and acting chemotactically and favoring coagulation, so that blockade may be beneficial for renal perfusion and function during endotoxaemia [54,55,60].

Other physiological systems

The renal kallikrein system, converting kininogens into the vasodilating kinin, is considered to interact with the RAAS system and to antagonise the local vasoconstrictive effects of angiotensin II, so that urinary excretion of the compounds rises during sodium restriction or hypovolemia [17]. Despite increased levels of angiotensin II during sepsis, urinary kallikrein declines, but rises again prior to recovery from oliguria [17]. The decrease seems to be mediated by the renal sympathetic nervous system [17]. The vasodilating properties of the renal kinins are partly dependent on NO and prostaglandins [17].

α-ANP has renal hemodynamic and tubular effects, via actions on particulate gyanylate cyclase and induction of cyclic guanosine monophosphate (cGMP), so that the compound may synergize with NO in cGMP-dependent effects [40]. α-ANP inhibits release of endothelin, while endothelin may induce α-ANP release [23,34,40]. It is considered to selectively dilate the renal artery, causing afferent vasodilation and efferent constriction, thereby increasing GFR [34]. The compound decreases tubular oxygen demand by decreasing sodium reabsorption and has a renal protective role during sepsis, during which circulating levels increase, probably as a consequence of cardiorespiratory changes and cardiac distension [23,34,40]. Only denervated kidneys (less sympathetic vasoconstriction) may benefit from α-ANP following experimental endotoxemia [61].

Adenosine might play a role in the pathophysiology of sepsis-associated ARF [14]. Adenosine may have (mainly medullary and efferent) vasodilating properties, but may also ameliorate neutrophil activation and endothelium interaction. It may increase diuresis by inhibiting ADH action [38]. The local adenosine concentration may rise due to interleukin (IL)-1β and, to a lesser extent, tumor necrosis factor (TNF)-α induced upregulation of enzymes involved in adenosine generation. However, prevention of adenosine production and action do not aggravate but protect against endotoxin-induced ARF, presumably by amelioration of afferent vasoconstriction and efferent vasodilation [5].

Sepsis-induced Substances

Several inflammatory factors can interfere with renal hemodynamics and may modulate the above mentioned systems. Local renal inflammation may amplify deteriorating hemodynamcis.

The Cytokine Cascade and Others

Endotoxin may not directly harm the kidney but may induce a variety of mediators, including TNF-α, IL-1β and IL-8, in various organs including the kidneys, and in a variety of cells, including neutrophils [30,62-64]. In the kidneys, the cytokines can also be secreted by mesangial cells, glomerular endothelium or tubular epithelium, following a challenge by endotoxin [51, 62-64]. The relative importance of cytokines derived from renal cells or resident macrophages and acting in a autocrine or paracrine fashion, to those delivered by the blood stream to the kidney, is unclear [51].

Endotoxin-stimulated TNF-α, IL-1β and IL-8 are neutrophil chemoat-tractants, promote neutrophil adhesion by upregulating adhesion molecules like intercellular adhesion molecule (ICAM)-1, and may contribute to neutrophil sequestration in glomeruli [21,51,62-64]. During sepsis-associated ARF in humans, neutrophils indeed appear to be activated, as judged from circulating degranulation products [65]. The cytokines may also stimulate renal cells to produce prostaglandins and oxygen radicals and may thereby induce mesangial contraction and mesangiolysis, which may contribute to a decrease of the ultrafiltration coefficient and filtration fraction [62,64]. The effects of TNF-α and IL-1β on renal hemodynamics are probably mediated in part by (released) prostaglandins, PAF, endothelin, NO and adenosine, resulting, among others, in complex alterations in vascular tone [18,51,56,62,64]. TNF-α may release prostaglandins that in turn may downregulate cytokine release. Tubulointerstitial effects of the cytokines such as TNF-α and IL-1β may include alterations in tubular transport with increased diuresis and natriuresis, partly mediated by prostaglandins [64].

Another important mediator of ARF in sepsis is PAF, since some of the actions of endotoxin in animals, including renal changes, can be ameliorated by PAF antagonists [32,56]. Specific antagonists of PAF in animals not only prevented or ameliorated the global hemodynamic derangements of sepsis but also protected renal function and structure [32,56]. The primary source of PAF in sepsis appears to be the circulating monocytes and the renal endothelium and mesangium, upon stimulation by cytokines, complement products, thrombin, angiotensin II or ADH [56]. Activated complement may also release PAF from neutrophils. When infused in animals, PAF may mimic endotoxin-induced septic shock and PAF can have deleterious effects on the kidneys, including a decline in renal blood flow and perhaps an even greater decline in GFR, possibly associated with mesangial contraction [56]. PAF may induce renal vasoconstriction in conjunction with thromboxane A_2 and endothelin, may stimulate oxygen radical release from mesangial cells, and may contribute to aggregation of platelets and neutrophils in glomeruli [54,56]. Renal PAF release is accompanied by release of PGE_2 antagonizing PAF production and action, but release of vasoconstricting may predominate over that of vasodilating prostaglandins [56]. In humans with sepsis-associated ARF, circulating PAF is elevated and may relate to circulating levels and urinary secretion of cytokines [66].

Activation of the complement system, either via the classic or alternative pathway, is believed to contribute to the pathophysiology of sepsis and shock. Complement activation may play a role in ARF, via the neutrophil chemoattractant properties of activation products.

Endothelin

There is evidence that an increased local endothelin to NO balance plays a critical role in renal hypoperfusion and ARF development during sepsis [48]. Endothelin is a potent vasoconstrictive peptide and the kidney is very sensitive to its effects, probably because of a high density of endothelin receptors, which may become expressed after challenges [38,54,62]. Both afferent and efferent vessels constrict to endothelin, but the preglomerular effects may be more pronounced, which, together with contraction of the mesangium, will lead to decrease of renal blood flow and an even greater decrease of GFR, whereas endothelin also decreases tubular resorption [38,54,62]. α-ANP and NO may inhibit endothelin release [62]. Endothelin may induce release of α-ANP, vasodilating prostaglandins, PAF and NO, possibly by activating phospholipases [40,62].

Circulating endothelin levels steeply rise following sepsis, endotoxin or TNF-α administration, and this interacts with concomitantly released compounds such as IL-1β, transforming growth factor β, thrombin, angiotensin II, epinephrine, ADH and α-ANP [40,54,62,67]. In fact, the kidney can produce relatively large amounts of endothelin, in renal (glomerular) endothelium and in mesangial and tubular epithelial cells, upon stimuli including endotoxin and TNF-α [54,62,67]. Locally produced endothelin exerts its effects mainly in an autocrine or paracrine fashion [62]. Treatment with anti-endothelin antibodies ameliorated the fall in renal perfusion and function during endotoxemia in rats [48].

Nitric oxide

NO is derived by enzymatic cleavage from L-arginine by the NO synthases (NOS). Otherwise, L-arginine can also be broken down by decarboxylase to agmatine, a new bioactive metabolite, shown to regulate renal filtration and absorption [68]. NO diffuses to vascular muscle cells where it induces soluble guanylate cyclase yielding intracellular cGMP. This, in turn, influences Ca^{2+} handling and leads to relaxation of cellular contractile elements. Constitutive (endothelial) NOS-derived NO regulates vascular tone, influences the ultrafiltration coefficient by relaxing glomerular mesangial cells, mediates the effects of macula densa stimulation, defends medullary oxygen supply and mediates (pressure-induced) sodium excretion [38,39,53]. Under normal conditions, NO primarily dilates afferent vessels in a paracrine fashion, in response to shear stress and pulsatile flow and angiotensin II-mediated vasoconstriction, and inhibits tubuloglomerular feedback, so that release of NO via cNOS activation by acetylcholine may increase renal blood flow but decrease GFR, at least in animals [16,19,39,53]. In experimental studies, there may be also an effect of NO on efferent (less than on afferent) vessel tone, if blood-free perfusion precludes NO scavenging by hemoglobin passing through glomerular vessels [38,53]. The diminishing diuresis and natriuresis following a decreased perfusion (pressure) of the kidney can be intensified by L-arginine blockers, suggesting that NO serves to preserve filtration and sodium excretion [39,53]. In fact, infusion of L-arginine to generate NO in healthy volunteers may increase and blockade of NO may decrease diuresis and natriuresis, while the former was associated with a rise in renal blood flow but unchanged GFR, thereby suggesting a tubular effect of NO, medullary blood flow redistribution, or both [39,53]. NO antagonizes many vascular, glomerular and tubular effects of angiotensin II [39,53].

During sepsis and shock in man, increased vessel wall synthesis of NO by inducible NOS (iNOS) may be partly responsible for increased nitrate/nitrite plasma levels, a globally diminished vascular tone [69]. In the kidneys, iNOS can be expressed in glomeruli and tubuli and NO breakdown products can be secreted via the urine during sepsis; the former is mediated by TNF-α and IL-1β, among others [32,70]. In the kidneys, the sources of iNOS-derived NO can be vascular smooth muscle cells, endothelial, mesangial and tubular cells, and (circulating and resident) neutrophils and macrophages [70]. Increased iNOS, however, may not preserve renal perfusion during sepsis and shock, when predominated by vasoconstrictive influences [29]. Moreover, increased iNOS-derived NO may downregulate endothelial cNOS-derived NO and thereby prevent (endothelium-mediated) vasodilation [29,71,72]. Moreover, selectively diminished vasodilator responses of renal vessels after endotoxin exposure, both *in vitro* as well as *in vivo*, have been described, even before expression of iNOS [71,72]. The phenomenon may increase the propensity for vasoconstriction and may contribute to abnormal dependency of renal perfusion and function on pressure [19,71,72]. For instance, Figure 1 shows the diminished vasodilator responses and NO production (direct measurement by electrode) upon acetylcholine (Ach) or calcium ionophore A23187 stimulation of isolated rat renal arteries (left column) incubated for 2 h with endotoxin (LPS) versus saline controls. Superior mesenteric arteries (right column) did not show such cNOS impairment. Excessive NO may be cytotoxic and may, together with liberated oxygen radicals, form the even more cytotoxic peroxynitrite thereby limiting vasodilation. On the other hand, NO inhibits neutrophil and platelet aggregation, so that release of iNOS-derived NO may be a two-edged sword, independently of hemodynamics. The idea prevails that iNOS-derived NO is deleterious and cNOS-derived NO is beneficial for the kidney [29]. In humans, increased levels of NO breakdown products have been suggested to relate to organ dysfunction, including ARF, and ultimate demise, but conclusions on cause/effect relations are hard to draw [69].

The effects on the kidney of (non-selective) inhibition of NOS, using inactive L-arginine analogues, are contradictory, with some authors reporting improved renal perfusion and function [23,26,73], while others observed a deterioration [19,29,38,70]. This discrepancy can be partly explained by an improved renal perfusion pressure, due to a rise in global blood pressure when iNOS is blocked in face of global vasodilation and by less NO cytotoxicity on the one hand, and by a disturbed renal microperfusion on the other hand, when renal vasoconstriction outweighs a rise in perfusion pressure [23,26,38,73]. In fact, blocking cNOS by non-selective NOS

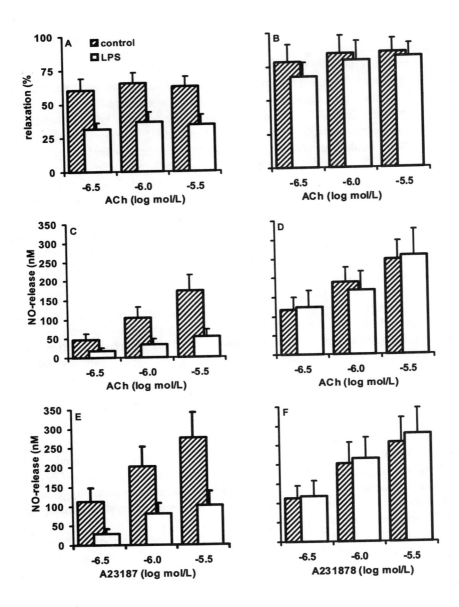

Figure 1. *Left: rat renal arteries incubated for 2 h with lipopolysaccharide (LPS) or saline; right: rat superior mesenteric arteries. Shown are relaxation responses and NO production (NO sensitive electrode) to submaximal doses of endothelial cNOS-dependent acetylcholine (Ach) and calcium ionophore A23187. The differences between LPS and control were statistically significant for the renal artery (mean/SD, p<0.05). From [72] with permission*

blockers may be deleterious for the kidney [19,29,70,72]. In contrast, selective iNOS inhibition would partly prevent adverse effects [29,74].

Neutrophil- and Oxygen Radical-mediated Renal Injury in Sepsis

The evidence is increasing that neutrophils and oxygen radicals are involved in septic ARF [21,22,24,30]. Renal injury by neutrophil is caused by both neutrophil-derived oxygen radicals and proteases [30]. Mesangial cells can also be a source of oxygen radicals, after stimulation by cytokines or PAF [62]. Oxygen radicals may contribute to afferent vasoconstriction and ARF during bacteremia, at least in rats [24]. Oxygen radicals may activate latent proteases and inactivate protease inhibitors. This may underlie the damaging effect of activated neutrophils on the glomerular basement membrane. Otherwise, oxygen radicals cause peroxidation of lipids, interfering with cellular membrane integrity, downregulating the vasodilating prostaglandins and cNOS, scavenging NO and producing vasoconstrictive compounds from non-enzymatic oxidation of arachidonic acid [24,57]. Antioxidants may protect against endotoxin-induced ARF [22,24,57].

Role of Coagulation and Platelets

Diffuse intravascular coagulation (DIC) might contribute to ARF during sepsis and shock, although glomerular fibrin/platelet deposits could not be found in some studies [5,17,51,54,60]. Glomerular thrombosis and ARF is a frequent feature of the Shwartzmann phenomenon, i.e., the development of widespread intravascular coagulation and necrosis following a rechallenge with endotoxin after prior sensitization [5,17,60,75]. This may mimic the occurrence of bilateral cortical necrosis during postpartum sepsis or meningococcal sepsis in man. In fact, cytokines may be involved in the intraglomerular expression of coagulation-promoting tissue factor and of fibrinolysis inhibitors [62,64,75]. TNF-α, PAF and leukotrienes may promote, and NO may inhibit, intraglomerular thrombosis, since PAF antagonists or leukotrienes blockade partly prevented and NO blockade aggravated intraglomerular fibrin deposition, thrombosis and thereby ARF following endotoxemia [29,60,55,64,70,75].

Ischemia and Reperfusion

Resuscitation following hypoperfusion may be aggravated by reperfusion injury and this can explain why renal blood flow may be (near) normal while glomerular filtration and thus the filtration fraction are still depressed in the course of sepsis [15,20,36,43]. I/R injury of the kidney may involve release of inflammatory factors such as oxygen radicals, cytokines, PAF, complement and arachidonic acid activation, adhesion molecule expression, and thereby accumulation of activated neutrophils, and this may contribute to cell apoptosis, death and ARF during sepsis, shock and resuscitation, since blocking of some of these compounds may prevent in part or ameliorate experimental I/R injury [30,56,61]. The I/R injury, otherwise, includes vascular changes, with diminished capability to autoregulate vascular tone following endothelial dysfunction and diminished dilator responses, even in the presence of active cNOS [58].

After mild I/R of the kidneys, endotoxin exposure and neutrophil priming can contribute to ARF, probably by an oxygen radical-induced upregulation of ICAM-1 and, as a consequence, retention of activated neutrophils and further release of proteases and oxygen radicals [30]. For neutrophils to directly injure normal kidneys, a high state of activation is required [30,76]. Prior endotoxin exposure or hyperthermia can also augment I/R renal injury, independently from hemodynamics. Primed and particularly activated neutrophils during clinical sepsis could contribute to ARF following transient or mild hypoperfusion [30,65].

THERAPEUTIC IMPLICATIONS

Therapies intervening in the inflammatory process have generally failed to beneficially affect morbidity and mortality during sepsis, even in the presence of some positive animal studies [56,63]. Global measures include optimization of hemodynamics and renal replacement therapy when complications of ARF are impending. For renal salvage, MAP should be probably at least 75-80 mmHg [49]. Administration of norepinephrine during septic shock (after appropriate fluid loading) may increase arterial blood pressure without a detrimental fall in cardiac output, and this may increase renal function and diuresis, possible as a consequence of improved renal blood flow [49,77]. Conversely, α-receptor blockers or angiotensin converting enzyme inhibitors may alleviate renal hypoperfusion in some endotoxin/bacterial shock models [9,16,47], but the clinial application of these drugs may be hampered by their hypotensive effect.

The preventive effect of fluid loading is unclear, even if promoting renal blood flow and filtration [5,17,23,27]. Nephrotoxic substances should be avoided [31]. There is insufficient evidence that drugs like dopamine and loop diuretics have specific renal protective properties in septic patients with (impending) ARF, even though the former drug may increase renal blood flow, GFR and diuresis in experimental models of endotoxin shock [14,49,78]. Low dose dopamine may only transiently increase renal blood flow and may act as a diuretic rather than prevent or ameliorate ARF and increase GFR in septic patients [43,49]. The idea behind the potential protective effect of diuretics is a fall in energy-consuming sodium and water absorption and less tubular obstruction, while mannitol may also have oxygen radical scavenging effects. Kallikrein inhibitors such as aprotinin may increase arterial blood pressure and thereby renal function, in spite of a potential deleterious effect on the renal kallikrein system [17].

Future studies will clarify the role of $ATP-MgCl_2$, Ca^{2+} channel blockers, endothelin receptor antagonists, antioxidants/scavengers, anti-cytokine/PAF therapies including the monocyte inhibitor pentoxifylline, PGE_2, inhibitors of neutrophil adhesion molecules, selective iNOS inhibitors or NO donors, and other substances applied in animal models of ARF [5,17,22-24,26,30,32,48,54,56,59,73]. α-ANP analogs may have a beneficial role in animal models of ARF and may increase dialysis-free survival in critically ill patients with oliguric ARF [34,61].

REFERENCES

1. Groeneveld ABJ, Tran DD, Van der Meulen J, et al. Acute renal failure in the medical intensive care unit: predisposing, complicating factors and outcome. Nephron 1991; 59:602-610
2. Brivet FG, Kleinknecht DJ, Loirat P, et al. Acute renal failure in intensive care units - causes, outcome, and prognostic factors of hospital mortality: a prospective multicenter study. Crit Care Med 1996; 24:192-198
3. Henrich WL, Hamasaki Y, Said SI, et al. Dissociation of systemic and renal effects in endotoxemia. J Clin Invest 1982; 69:691-699
4. Haybron DM, Townsend MC, Hampton WW, et al. Effective renal blood flow and renal energy charge in murine peritonitis. Arch Surg 1986; 52:625-629
5. Churchill PC, Bidani AK, Schwartz MM. Renal effects of endotoxin in the male rat. Am J Physiol 1987; 253:F244-F250
6. Shimahara Y, Kono Y, Tanaka J, et al. Pathophysiology of acute renal failure following living Escherichia Coli injections in the rat: high-energy metabolism and renal functions. Circ Shock 1987; 21:197-205
7. Beck RR, Abel FL, Papadakis E. Influence of ibuprofen on renal function in acutely endotoxemic dogs. Circ Shock 1989; 28:37-47
8. Gullichsen E, Nelimarkka O, Halkola L, et al. Renal oxygenation in endotoxin shock in

dogs. Crit Care Med 1989; 17:547-50

9. Lugon JR, Boim MA, Ramos OL, et al. Renal function and glomerular hemodynamics in male endotoxic rats. Kidney Int 1989; 36:570-575

10. O'Hair DP, Adams MB, Tunberg TC, et al. Relationships among endotoxemia, arterial pressure, and renal function in dogs. Circ Shock 1989; 27:199-210

11. Rao PS, Cavanagh DM, Fiorica JV, et al. Endotoxin-induced alterations in renal function with particular reference to tubular enzyme activity. Circ Shock 1990; 31:333-342

12. Schaer GL, Fink MP, Chernow B, et al. Renal hemodynamics and prostaglandin E_2 excretion in a nonhuman primate model of septic shock. Crit Care Med 1990; 18:52-59

13. Van Lambalgen AA, Van Kraats AA, Van den Bos GC, et al. Renal function and metabolism during endotoxemia in rats: role of hypoperfusion. Shock 1991; 35:164-173

14. Van Lambalgen AA, Kraats AA van, Van de Vaart-Mulder MF, et al. Systemic and renal actions of dopexamine and dobutamine during endotoxin shock in the rat. J Crit Care 1991; 6:61-70

15. Weber A, Schwieger IM, Poinsot O, et al. Sequential changes in renal oxygen consumption and sodium transport during hyperdynamic sepsis in sheep. Am J Physiol 1992; 262:F965-F971

16. Cryer HG, Bloom ITM, Unger LS, et al. Factors affecting renal microvascular blood flow in rat hyperdynamic bacteremia. Am J Physiol 1993; 264:H1988-H1997

17. Cumming AD. Acute renal failure and sepsis: therapeutic approaches. Nephrol Dial Transplant 1994; 9:Suppl 4:159-163

18. Girardin E, Grau GE, Paunier L, et al. Early hemodynamic and renal effects of tumor necrosis factor alpha: role of thromboxane. Circ Shock 1994; 42:20-26

19. Spain DA, Wilson MA, Bloom ITM, et al. Renal microvascular responses to sepsis are dependent on nitric oxide. J Surg Res 1994; 56:524-529

20. Weber A, Schwieger IM, Poinsot O, et al. Time course of systemic and renal plasma prostanoid concentrations and renal function in ovine hyperdynamic sepsis. Clin Sci 1994; 86:599-610

21. Kang Y-H, Falk MC, Bentley TB, et al. Distribution and role of lipopolysaccharide in the pathogenesis of acute renal proximal tubule injury. Shock 1995; 4:441-449

22. Zuvrosky Y, Gispaan I. Antioxidants attenuate endotoxin-induced acute renal failure in rats. Am J Kidney Dis 1995; 25:51-57

23. Hinder F, Brooke m, Traber LD, et al. Nitric oxide synthase inhibition during experimental sepsis improves renal excretory function in the presence of chronically increased atrial natriuretic peptide. Crit Care Med 1996; 24:131-136

24. Krysztopik RJ, Bentley FR, Spain DA, et al. Free radical scavenging by lazaroids improves renal blood flow during sepsis. Surgery 1996; 120:657-662

25. Van Lambalgen AA, Bouriquet N, Casellas D. Effects of endotoxin on tone and pressure-responsiveness of preglomerular juxtamedullary vessels. Eur J Physiol 1996; 432:574-577

26. Millar CGM, Thiemermann C. Intrarenal haemodynamics and renal dysfunction in endotoxaemia: effects of nitric oxide synthase inhibition. Br J Pharmacol 1997; 121:1824-1830

27. Heemskerk AEJ, Huisman E, Van Lambalgen AA, et al. Influence of fluid resuscitation on renal function in bacteremic and endotoxemic rats. J Crit Care 1997; 12:120-131

28. Heemskerk AE, Huisman E, Van Lambalgen AA, et al. Renal function and oxygen consumption during bacteraemia and endotoxaemia in rats. Nephrol Dial Transplant 1997; 12:1586-1594

29. Schwartz D, Mendonca M, Schwartz I, et al. Inhibition of constitutive nitric oxide synthase (NOS) by nitric oxide generated by inducible NOS after lipopolysaccharide administration provokes renal dysfunction in rats. J Clin Invest 1997; 100:439-448

30. Lauriat S, Linas SL. The role of neutrophils in acute renal failure. Semin Nephrol 1998; 18:498-504

31. Zager RA, Prior RB. Gentamicin and Gram-negative bacteremia. A synergism for the development of experimental nephrotoxic acute renal failure. J Clin Invest 1986; 78:196-204

32. De Kimpe SJ, Thiemermann C, Vane JR. Role for intracellular platelet-activating factor in tne circulatory failure in a model of Gram-positive shock. Br J Pharmacol 1995; 116:3191-3198

33. Myers BD, Moran SM. Hemodynamically mediated acute renal failure. N Engl J Med 1986; 314:97-105

34. Rahman SN, Kim GE, Mathew AS, et al. Effects of atrial natriuretic peptide in clinical acute renal failure. Kidney Int 1994; 45:1731-1738

35. Cortez A, Zito J, Lucas CE, et al. Mechanism of inappropriate polyuria in septic patients. Arch Surg 1977; 112:471-476

36. Brenner M, Schaer Gl, Mallory DL, et al. Detection of renal blood flow in septic and critically ill patients using a newly developed indwelling thermodilution renal vein catheter. Chest 1990; 98:170-179

37. Cronenwett JL, Lindenauer SM. Distribution of intrarenal blood flow during bacterial sepsis. J Surg Res 1978; 24:132-141

38. Brezis M, Rosen S. Hypoxia of the renal medulla-its implications for disease. N Engl J Med 1995; 332:647-655

39. Kone BC, Baylis C. Biosynthesis and homeostatic roles of nitric oxide in the normal kidney. Am J Physiol 1997; 272:F561-F578

40. Hartemink KJ, Groeneveld ABJ, De Groot MCM, et al. α-atrial natriuretic peptide, cyclic guanosine monophosphate and endothelin in plasma as markers of myocardial depression in human septic shock. Crit Care Med 2001; 29:80-87

41. Jones DB. Ultrastructure of human acute renal failure. Lab Invest 1982; 46:254-264

42. Messmer UK, Briner VA, Pfeilschifter J. Tumor necrosis factor-α and lipopolysaccharide induce apoptotic cell death in bovine glomerular endothelial cells. Kidney Int 1999; 55:2322-2337

43. Stevens PE, Gwyther SJ, Hanson ME, et al. Noninvasive monitoring of renal blood flow characteristics during acute renal failure in man. Intensive Care Med 1990; 16:153-158

44. Platt JF, Rubin JM, Ellis JH. Acute renal failure: possible role of Duplex Doppler US in distinction between acute prerenal failure and acute tubular necrosis. Radiology 1991; 179:419-423

45. Haywood GA, Stewart JT, Counihan PJ, et al. Validation of bedside measurements of absolute human renal blood flow by a continuous thermodilution technique. Crit Care Med 1992; 20:659-664

46. Groeneveld ABJ. Redistribution of blood flow in hypovolemic and septic shock. Réan Urgen 1996; 5:224-237

47. Koyama S. Participation of central of central α-receptors on hemodynamic response to E. Coli endotoxin. Am J Physiol 1984; 247:R655-R662

48. Mitaka C, Hirata Y, Yokoyama K, et al. Improvement of renal dysfunction in dogs with endotoxemia by a nonselective endothelin receptor antagonist. Crit Care Med 1999; 27:146-153

49. Bersten AD, Holt AW. Vasoactive drugs and the importance of renal perfusion pressure.

New Horiz 1995; 3:650-661

50. Oliver JA, Sciacca RR, Pinto J, et al. Participation of the prostaglandins in the control of renal blood flow during acute reductions of cardiac output in the dog. J Clin Invest 1981; 67:229-237

51. Laszik Z, Nadasdy T, Johnson LD, et al. Renal interleukin-1 expression during endotoxemia and gram-negative septicemia in conscious rats. Circ Shock 1994; 43:115-121

52. Davenport MW, Zipser RD. Association of hypotension with hyperreninemic hypoaldosteronism in the critically ill. Arch Intern Med 1983; 143:735-737

53. Ito S, Carretero OA, Abe K. Nitric oxide in the regulation of renal blood flow. New Horizons 1995; 3:615-623

54. Badr KF. Sepsis-associated renal vasoconstriction: potential targets for future therapy. Am J Kidney Dis 1992; 20:207-213

55. Klahr R. Role of arachidonic acid metabolites in acute renal failure and sepsis. Nephrol Dial Transplant 1994; 9:Suppl 4:52-56

56. López-Novoa JM. Potential role of platelet activating factor in acute renal failure. Kidney Int 1999; 55:1672-1682

57. Baud L, Ardaillou R. Involvement of reactive oxygen species in kidney damage. Br Med Bull 1993; 49:621-629

58. Conger J, Robinette J, Villar A, et al. Increased nitric oxide synthase activity despite lack of response to endothelium-dependent vasodilators in postischemic acute renal failure in rats. J Clin Invest 1995; 96:631-638

59. Mauk RH, Patak RV, Fadem SZ, et al. Effects of prostaglandin E_2 administration in a nephrotoxic and a vasoconstrictor model of acute renal failure. Kidney Int 1977; 12:122-130

60. Schaub RG, Ochoa R, Simmons CA, et al. Renal microthrombosis following endotoxin infusion may be mediated by lipoxygenase products. Circ Shock 1987; 21:261-270

61. Hiki N, Mimura Y. Atrial natriuretic peptide has no potential to protect against endotoxin induced acute renal failure in the absence of renal nerves. Endocrin J 1998; 45:75-81

62. Kohan DE. Role of endothelin and tumour necrosis factor in the renal response to sepsis. Nephrol Dial Transplant 1994; 9:Suppl 4:73-77

63. Von Asmuth EJU, Dentener MA, Ceska M, et al. IL-6, IL-8 and TNF production by cytokine and lipopolysaccharide-stimulated human renal cortical epithelial cells in vitro. Eur Cytokine Netw 1994; 5:301-310

64. Baud L, Ardaillou R. Tumor necrosis factor in renal injury. Miner Electrolyte Metab 1995; 21:336-341

65. Hörl WH, Schäfer RM, Hörl M, et al. Neutrophil activation in acute renal failure and sepsis. Arch Surg 1990; 125:651-654

66. Mariano F, Guida D, Donati D, et al. Production of platelet-activating factor in patients with sepsis-associated acute renal failure. Nephrol Dial Transplant 1999; 14:1150-1157

67. Kaddoura S, Curzen NP, Evans TW, et al. Tissue expression of endothelin-1 mRNA in endotoxaemia. Biochem Biophys Res Comm 1996; 218:641-647

68. Lortie MJ, Novotny WF, Peterson OW, et al. Agmatine, a bioactive metabolite of arginine. Production, degradation, and functional effects in the kidney of the rat. J Clin Invest 1996; 97:413-420

69. Groeneveld PHP, Kwappenberg KMC, Langermans JAM, et al. Nitric oxide production correlates with renal insufficiency and multiple organ dysfunction syndrome in severe sepsis. Intensive Care Med 1996; 22:1197-1202

70. Shultz PJ, Raij L. Endogenously synthesized nitric oxide prevents endotoxin-induced glomerular thrombosis. J Clin Invest 1992; 90:1718-1725
71. Pastor CM. Vascular hyporesponsiveness of the renal circulation during endotoxemia in anesthetized pigs. Crit Care Med 1999; 27:2735-2740
72. Piepot HA, Boer C, Groeneveld ABJ, et al. Lipopolysaccharide impairs endothelial nitric oxide synthesis in rat renal arteries. Kidney Intern 2000; 57:2502-2510
73. Grover R, Zaccardelli D, Colice G, et al. An open-label dose escalation study of the nitric oxide synthase inhibitor, N^G-methyl-L-arginine hydrochloride (546C88), in patients with septic shock. Crit Care Med 1999; 27:913-922
74. Mitaka C, Hirata Y, Masaki Y, et al. S-methylisothiourea sulfate improves renal, but not hepatic dysfunction in canine entotoxic shock model. Intensive Care Med 2000; 26:117-124
75. Ueada Y, Hoon Lee K, Ito S, et al. In vivo neutralization of tumor necrosis factor attenuates the generalized Shwartzman reaction in the rabbit. J Endotoxin Res 1996; 3:67-75
76. Zager RA. Escherichia coli endotoxin injections potentiate experimental ischemic renal injury. Am J Physiol 1986; 251:F988-F994
77. Redl-Wenzl EM, Armbruster C, Edelmann G, et al. The effects of norepinephrine on hemodynamics and renal function in severe septic shock states. Intensive Care Med 1993; 19:151-154
78. Kellum JA. The use of diuretics and dopamine in acute renal failure: a systematic review of the evidence. Crit Care 1997; 1:53-59

39

THE COAGULATION SYSTEM IN SEPSIS

C. Erik Hack

Sepsis/septic shock results from the excessive activation of various inflammatory systems and mediators. The release of various cytokines, hormone-like proteins that interact upon specific receptors on cells, is presumably a key event during sepsis inducing in their turn the release and activation of a number of secondary and tertiary mediators [1]. The main cytokines involved in the pathogenesis of sepsis are tumor necrosis factor-α (TNF), interleukin-1α/β, (IL-1) and interleukin-1-receptor antagonist (IL-1ra), IL-6, IL-8 and other chemokines, IL-10, IL-12, and interferon-gamma (IFN-γ). Among the secondary mediators activated by cytokines is the coagulation system, which belongs to the so-called plasma cascade systems. These also include the contact, fibrinolytic, protein C and complement systems. A typical feature of plasma cascade systems is that their proteins circulate as inactive precursor molecules, for example pro-enzymes, which are activated in a waterfall or 'cascade'-like fashion into active molecules, for example serine proteinases.

Inappropriate, mostly excessive, activation of the coagulation system frequently, if not always, occurs in animal models for sepsis, and to some extent also in humans with sepsis. In this chapter the role of coagulation in sepsis will be discussed. It is not the aim to give a comprehensive overview of clotting abnormalities in sepsis, since reviews on this topic have appeared elsewhere (see for example [2]). Rather we will focus on studies providing mechanistic insight in the role of coagulation in sepsis. As a consequence, the emphasis will be on experimental studies in animals. The contact system, which also is known as the intrinsic pathway of coagulation, will also be summarized here. Two anti-coagulant systems, the fibrinolytic and protein C system, will also be discussed. First, a short summary of the biochemistry and the biology of these systems will be given, thereafter their role in animal models for sepsis as well as in human sepsis will be discussed. Intervention studies on the efficacy of clotting inhibitors in sepsis will be discussed in another chapter.

THE COAGULATION SYSTEM

The Common Pathway

Thrombin is the key enzyme of the coagulation system. It catalyzes the conversion of fibrinogen into fibrin, and hence has procoagulant properties. Notably, it also has anti-coagulant activities via its interaction with protein C, which is known as the thrombin paradox [3]. Thus, low concentrations of thrombin do not necessarily induce fibrin formation, but rather protect against thromboembolic events by activating protein C (Figure 1).

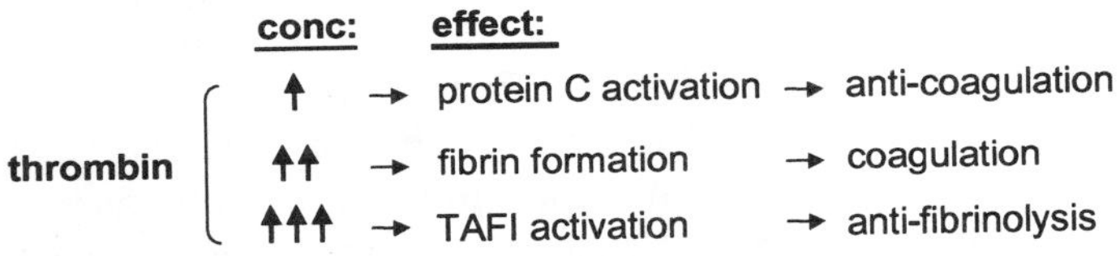

Figure 1. *The thrombin paradox. See text for further explanation.*

Thrombin is generated from prothrombin by activated factor X (FXa) in the presence of a various cofactors, i.e., factor Va (FVa), phospholipids (which serve as a surface to assemble the clotting factors), and calcium ions. Activation of factor X is considered to occur either via an extrinsic pathway (one of the components of this pathway, tissue factor [TF], is not present in plasma) or an intrinsic pathway (all components are present in plasma). The activity of the common pathway is regulated by the serine proteinase inhibitor antithrombin III (ATIII), and, to a lesser extent, by the multispecific proteinase inhibitor α2-macroglobulin (α2M). In experimental sepsis models either inhibitor indeed has been found to inhibit thrombin [4,5].

The Extrinsic Pathway

This consists of factor VII and the transmembrane protein TF. Normally, TF is not exposed on peripheral blood or endothelial cells, but is abundantly present on extravascular cells [6]. Activation of this pathway occurs either upon disruption of the continuous layer of the endothelium inducing blood to be exposed to these extravascular cells, or because endothelial or circulating neutrophils and monocytes are triggered to expose TF on their membranes. Activation of the extrinsic coagulation pathway in sepsis mainly results from TF exposure by blood mononuclear cells or the endothelium, rather than from endothelial lesions. Also phospholipid microparticles shed from cells may contain TF [7]. Agonists for TF expression during sepsis include endotoxin, cytokines (TNF or IL-1), activated complement [8-14], and presumably others. Once exposed to blood, TF binds and activates factor VII, which then activates factor X. In turn, FXa then converts prothrombin. Extrinsic pathway activation is tightly regulated by tissue factor pathway inhibitor (TFPI) [15], which rapidly shuts down the activity of the initial TF/FVIIa/FXa complexes. To circumvent the inhibitory activity of TFPI at low concentrations of TF/FVIIa/FXa concentrations [16], the activation of factor IX by TF/FVIIa (see below) is needed to propagate further thrombin generation.

The Intrinsic Pathway

Contact of blood with glass results in the rapid formation of a blood clot. This formation is dependent on the common pathway (thrombin and FXa), which, however, in this case is not activated by TF/FVIIa, but rather by a number of clotting factors together termed the intrinsic pathway. Activation of this pathway is triggered by the binding and activation of factor XII (FXII, formerly Hageman factor) on an activator. The nature of the activating surface *in vivo* is unknown. FXIIa converts prekallikrein, assembled onto the surface as a complex with high molecular weight kininogen (HK), into kallikrein. Kallikrein in its turn further activates FXII bound to the surface ('reciprocal activation'; the two proteins activate each other), resulting in a burst of FXIIa activity. FXIIa can activate factor XI, which is also assembled onto the surface as a complex with HK. FXIa in its turn activates factor IX to generate FIXa. Finally, FIXa, in the presence of FVIIIa (generated from factor VIII by thrombin), converts factor X into FXa thereby activating the common pathway. As activation of factor XII, prekallikrein, HK and factor XI requires contact of these proteins with the activating surface, these proteins are also known as the contact system. The main inhibitor of this system is C1-inhibitor (C1-Inh), which also is the main inhibitor of activated C1 of the classical pathway of complement.

Integration of Extrinsic and Intrinsic Pathways

The concept of two different pathways leading to activation of FX is based on *in vitro* studies. Clinical syndromes resulting from congenital deficiencies, however, do not support this concept, and in particular challenge that of the intrinsic pathway: persons with factor VIII or IX deficiency have an overt bleeding tendency, those with factor XI deficiency a mild bleeding disorder, whereas those with factor XII deficiency rather have thrombo-embolic problems. Thus deficiencies of factors supposedly participating in the same pathway lead to opposite hemostatic problems. Further research has identified that the TF/factor VIIa complex not only activates factor X, but also factor IX, which in the presence of FVIIIa can generate FXa (see figure 2). This amplifcation loop at the level of factor VII is necessary for proper hemostasis under normal conditions, as is dramatically illustrated by the clinical picture of hemofilia. More recently a second thrombin-generating amplification loop involving factor XI [17-20], has been identified (see figure 2). FXIa generated by thrombin activates factor IX, which via factor X induces further thrombin generation.

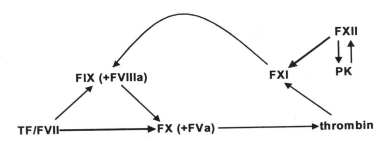

Figure 2. Simplified scheme of the coagulation cascade. Thrombin formation occurs mainly via tissue factor (TF) pathway. Note the 2 amplification loops, one involving factor VII-dependent activation of factor IX, the other thrombin-dependent activation of FXI. Initial activation occurs by interaction of FVII with TF, or by activation of FXII. Under normal and most pathophysiological conditions TF-induced activation predominates.

Factor XI-mediated bursts of thrombin will activate TAFI (thrombin-activatable fibrinolysis inhibitor), which cleaves off binding sites for plasminogen on fibrin thereby inhibiting fibrinolysis [21-23]. Thus, via these two ampification loops, sufficient amounts of thrombin may be generated to allow blood clotting, even when induced by limiting amounts of TF.

Notably, the activity of the cofactors FVIIIa and FVa is regulated by activated protein C (APC), which degrades these cofactors to inactive species. This is the main anti-coagulant function of APC. APC is generated from protein C by thrombin bound to the membrane protein thrombomodulin (TM). Under normal conditions TM is expressed by endothelial cells and contributes to the anti-coagulant properties of the endothelium. During inflammation, cytokines like TNF and IL-1 down-regulate the synthesis of TM, and inflammatory proteases cleave off this membrane-protein from the endothelium Together with the expression of TF, this will convert the endothelium into a clot-promoting surface [9-12]. In local infections this phenomenon helps to localize micro-organisms, but in septic conditions it may lead to widespread fibrin formation and contribute to the development of organ dysfunction.

PRECLINICAL MODELS FOR SEPSIS

Coagulation has been studied in animals challenged with endotoxin (or other bacterial constituents), or bacteria (live or killed). The septic challenge is given intravenously or locally, for example by implantation of infected fibrin clots in the peritoneal cavity or cecal puncture and ligation. Studies of coagulation in animal models are hampered since most of the sophisticated assays for activated clotting factors were developed for humans and do not perform well in animals due to poor cross-reactivity of the antibodies used in the assays. Therefore, detailed studies of coagulation in animals is only possible in primates. An experimental endotoxemia model in humans has also been developed. The challenge in this model is very mild, inducing a flu-like illness. Activation patterns of the coagulation system in this model may greatly differ from those in (sub)lethal models. Hence, results obtained in human endotoxemia should only be extrapolated to actual septic shock with great care.

To precisely identify the mechanism of coagulation and the implications for clinical symptoms, clotting inhibitors have been used in sepsis models. For the common pathway active site-blocked FXa (DEGR-Xa) and ATIII have been used; for the extrinsic pathway TFPI (see above), anti-TF monoclonal antibody (mAb), anti-FVII mAb and active site-blocked FVIIa (DEGR-FVIIa). Also low molecular weight inhibitors such as nafamostat have been tested in sepsis models [24,25], but these will not be discussed here further. For the intrinsic pathway, and in particular the contact system, mAb against factor XII and C1-Inh have been used. Finally, a number of studies with APC have been done in sepsis models.

ACTIVATION OF COAGULATION BY CYTOKINES

Agonists for TF expression which may play a role in the pathogenesis of clotting abnormalities in sepsis include endotoxin, the cytokines TNF and IL-1, and activated complement. Histological studies in animals injected with TNF or IL-1 demonstrate the activation of neutrophils and the deposition of fibrin at the site of injection [26-28], supporting the procoagulant properties of either cytokine. Systemic injection of TNF in healthy volunteers also induces activation of coagulation and fibrinolysis; typically, coagulation proceeds for hours after injection of the cytokine, whereas fibrinolysis is only shortly (approximately 60 minutes) activated to become increasingly inhibited thereafter, resulting in a net procoagulant state [29,30]. A similar procoagulant state is induced by a low dose (3 ng/kg of body weight) of IL-1β (AC Ogilvie, CE Hack, unpublished observations).

Activation of coagulation (and fibrinolysis) by TNF or IL-1 has also been studied in non-human primates. In baboons challenged with 100 µg of TNF per kg of body weight a significant rise in thrombin-antithrombin III (TAT) complexes was not observed unless a monoclonal antibody that blocks protein C, was co-administered [31]. In this model, TNF-induced activation of clotting was enhanced by injection of phospholipid microvesicles. IL-1α at a concentration of 10 µg per kg also induced rises in TAT complexes in baboons, even in the absence of protein C inhibition [32]. IL-6 has also been found to induce thrombin generation [33]. The mechanism of this generation is unknown, but may involve the acute phase protein C-reactive protein (CRP) [34]. Finally, the cytokines IL-2 and IL-12 are also able to stimulate thrombin generation in primates; that induced by IL-2 strongly resembles that observed after low doses TNF or endotoxin [35]. In contrast, that by IL-12 is more variable and more sustained, continuing for over 24 hours [36]. Likely, thrombin generation by either cytokine is mediated by the release of TNF and IL-1.

Notably, the claim that some cytokines may induce a procoagulant state must be considered with caution: the low doses of thrombin observed in these studies may only have stimulated protein C activation resulting in an anti-coagulant state (see above). Furthermore, it is assumed that the generation of thrombin by cytokines largely occurs via the extrinsic pathway. Yet cytokines, for example high doses of IL-2, may induce significant activation of the contact system [37]. This raises the possibility that not all thrombin generated resulted from extrinsic pathway activation. In spite of these considerations, the studies discussed in this paragraph have clearly shown that cytokines, key mediators of the septic cascade, are able to induce activation of coagulation.

ACTIVATION OF COAGULATION IN SEPSIS MODELS

Extrinsic and Common Pathway Activation

A challenge with endotoxin or live bacteria in animals elicits the release of TNF, IL-1, IL-6, and other cytokines, as well as a transient activation of the coagulation system. Depending on the model, this is accompanied by significant fibrin formation. In humans a low dose of endotoxin does nor induce significant fibrin formation. In this mode, coagulation exclusively occurs via the extrinsic pathway as became clear from studies with anti-factor VII or anti-TF antibodies [38,39]. Notably, these interventions had no effect on cytokine responses. Studies with anti-TNF antibodies, soluble TNF-receptors or IL-1ra, revealed that thrombin generation in this experimental human model occurs independently of cytokines (in contrast to fibrinolysis which is driven by TNF), and likely results from direct triggering of peripheral blood mononuclear cells or endothelial cells by endotoxin [40]. Plasmin generation, reflecting activation of the fibrinolytic system, during experimental endotoxemia is already shut down (due to increasing levels of plasminogen activator inhibitor-1 [PAI-1]) when coagulation activation is maximal (at about 3-4 hours after the challenge) [41,42], which situation is referred to as a procoagulant state. As stated earlier, this interpretation may not be correct since at low concentrations thrombin exerts anti-coagulant effects by activating protein C (the 'thrombin paradox', see above). In the analogous model in chimpanzees similar findings have been made [39]. Surprisingly, intervention with anti-IL-6 mAb has revealed a role for IL-6 in the activation of coagulation by low dose endotoxin, although the mechanism is not known [43].

Peak levels of TNF occur approximately 1 to 2 hours after a lethal or sublethal challenge with endotoxin or live bacteria, whereas those of IL-1β occur somewhat later. In these models, both the fibrinolytic as well as the clotting system are activated, again fibrinolysis being inhibited a few hours after the challenge whereas coagulation proceeds for a longer period [4]. Notably, this activation is accompanied by moderate too marked fibrinogen consumption and fibrin formation. In contrast to low grade endotoxemia, in the more severe models for sepsis, inhibition of TNF reduces activation of coagulation, but has hardly any effect on fibrinolysis [44]. Similarly, IL-1ra attenuates activation of coagulation in these models without affecting plasmin formation [32]. Thus, in the severe models of sepsis (strong) activation of coagulation largely depends on the release of inflammatory cytokines. Finally, inhibitors of coagulation reduce the formation of plasmin in these models. Thus, in contrast to experimental low grade endotoxemia, fibrin greatly enhances the formation of plasmin in (sub)lethal sepsis models.

The site(s) of TF expression during sepsis have been studied in the severe models for sepsis. TF has been found on peripheral blood leukocytes, on leukocytes infiltrating in the various organs [45,46], on endothelial cells from the spleen or aorta, [47-49], and in the lungs and kidneys [47,50-52]. An additional source of TF may be phospholipid microparticles originating from monocytes stimulated with endotoxin [7]. Indeed, TF-positive, thrombin-generating microparticles may circulate in patients with meningococcal sepsis [53].

Anti-TF treatment in a lethal endotoxin model in mice reduced mortality and consumption of clotting factors, whereas it had no effect on TNF release [54]. Similarly, anti-TF mAb attenuated the coagulopathic response and improved survival in a lethal *E. coli* model in baboons [55]. Also active site-inhibited FVIIa (DEGR-factor VIIa) improved outcome, and reduced coagulopathic and, remarkably, also inflammatory responses [56]. A number of studies have been done with TFPI. Creasey et al. showed in baboons challenged with a lethal dose of *E. coli* that TFPI given shortly after the challenge could prevent mortality completely [57]. This effect was accompanied by a significant attenuation of clotting and a reduced inflammatory response as evidenced by decreased IL-6 responses [57]. Even when given 4 hours after the challenge, TFPI yielded a 40% survival rate. Remarkably, no effect of TFPI on clinical or hemodynamic parameters during the first 12 hours were found. Similar results were found in subsequent studies [58-62]. TFPI also improved outcome in a Gram-negative peritonitis model in rabbits, protecting against mortality [63].

As discussed in the previous paragraph, clotting inhibitors such as TFPI, DEGR-VIIa and anti-TF mAb can favorably influence outcome in sepsis models. Similar beneficial effects were observed with APC [64], and high doses of ATIII [65,66]. In all these studies, not only significant inhibition of coagulation was observed, but also attenuation of the inflammatory response, for example as reflected by reduced IL-6 and IL-8 release. Clotting proteases, as thrombin, FVIIa and FXa, can trigger cells by interacting with protease-activated receptors [67], and possibly other receptors [68,69]. Hence, one may speculate that inhibition of clotting improves mortality in sepsis by reducing other cellular, presumably inflammatory, responses (the effects on inflammation are secondary to those on coagulation). Yet, inhibition of coagulation itself is not sufficient to improve outcome in sepsis, as was shown in a study with DEGR-Xa [70]. Apparently, some clotting inhibitors have unique effects on inflammatory responses that are not secondary to effects on coagulation. Ongoing research should identify the molecular mechanisms of these anti-inflammatory effects of clotting inhibitors. Suggested possibilities include cell signaling effects of FVIIa, prostacyclin production by endothelial cells triggered by clotting inhibitors, and stimulation of the recently discovered APC-receptor, which is able to shut down inflammatory responses [69,71,72].

Contact Activation

Discrepancies between clinical manifestations of genetic deficiencies and the supposed role of intrinsic pathway clotting factors, have led to a revised concept of the coagulation system postulating that the main clotting function of factors VIII, IX and XI is to amplify extrinsic pathway activation (see above). As a consequence, the precise role of XII in hemostasis *in vivo* has become less clear. The structure of factor XII suggests a role in fibrinolysis. Indeed, some fibrinolytic responses in patients with factor XII deficiency are impaired [73], which may explain the association between low factor XII levels and thrombo-embolic disease. In addition these activities, the contact system is notorious for its capacity to generate bradykinin from HK (by kallikrein). This nonapeptide induces vasodilation, hypotension, an increase in vasopermeability and bronchoconstriction at low concentrations [74]. Some of these effects are due to the induction of the formation of nitric oxide (NO). Moreover, other activation products of the contact system can attract neutrophils and activate complement [75-77]. Thus, the contact system is a potent inflammatory system which may contribute to the pathogenesis of sepsis.

Circulating levels of activation products such as bradykinin are increased in experimental sepsis models, whereas the concentrations of factor XII, prekallikrein or HK are decreased [78,79], indicative for activation of the contact system. These changes are most pronounced in lethal sepsis, and were accompanied by a protracted decline in mean arterial pressure in a baboon model suggesting that bradykinin is involved in the hemodynamic alterations during lethal sepsis [79]. Pretreatment of baboons with a mAb blocks factor XII activation, reduced irreversible hypotension, and prolonged survival of baboons challenged intravenously with a lethal dose of *E. coli* [80]. MAb treatment also led to less complement activation, reduced fibrinolytic activation, and attenuated release of cytokines and neutrophil elastase, demonstrating the multiple pro-inflammatory effects of factor XII [81]. This raises the possibility that the hypotensive effect of contact activation during sepsis is mediated by the cross talk with other inflammatory systems, the more since bradykinin receptor antagonists have no effect on the hypotensive response following endotoxemia [82]. Favorable effects of other less specific inhibitors of the contact system have also been described in animal models: α1-antitrypsin-Pittsburgh (α1-antitrypsin mutated at the so-called P1-position of the reactive center to yield a potent factor XIIa/kallikrein/thrombin inhibitor) was shown to delay the drop of contact system proteins and to prolong survival of pigs challenged with a lethal dose of *P. aeruginosa* (in this model 90 % of the animals have deceased within 6 hours), although ultimate mortality was not influenced [83]. However, in a follow up study in septic baboons the "Pittsburgh" mutant appeared to exacerbate coagulopathy presumably due to accumulation of a proteolytically cleaved form [84]. Hence, this inhibitor likely will not be evaluated in clinical sepsis.

In another study in dogs, high doses of C1-Inh were shown to improve the early pulmonary dysfunction following a challenge with *E. coli* endotoxin, which was accompanied by less consumption of prekallikrein and factor XI, whereas the decrease in factor XII was unaffected.[85]. Favorable effects of C1-inhibitor were also seen in a baboon model for sepsis (animals observed for up to 7 days), which was accompanied by reduced contact activation but also reduced complement activation [86]. Taken together, these studies demonstrate that administration of contact system inhibitors may have beneficial, though mild, effects in experimental sepsis.

Bacterial products such as endotoxin can activate the contact system *in vitro* [87,88]. Hence, it can be postulated that the direct interaction of contact system proteins with bacteria or their products triggers the activation during sepsis. However, in the lethal baboon model, contact activation was more pronounced later in the course, i.e., hours after the challenge [79]. Moreover, following a challenge with low dose of endotoxin in healthy volunteers, contact activation was not observed until after 3 to 5 hours following intravenous injection of endotoxin [89]. This time-course suggests that the observed activation did not result from direct activation of the system by bacteria or the injected endotoxin, but points to another mechanism (via activation of the endothelium?). Notably, contact activation during experimental endotoxemia in humans is not consistently found [41]. Also, injection with TNF-α, which produces most of the effects of endotoxin *in vivo*, does not induce contact activation in humans [29]. Thus, whether or not contact activation occurs following a mild inflammatory (endotoxin) stimulus, is still not clear.

ACTIVATION OF COAGULATION IN CLINICAL SEPSIS

In this chapter we focus on the mechanistic aspects of coagulation activation in sepsis. Hence, clinical studies of coagulation in sepsis can only be briefly touched. Activation of coagulation in patients with sepsis is established based on clinical criteria such as the occurrence of pupura in patients with meningococcal sepsis, or, more often, by performing coagulation assays on blood samples. These assays include assessment of platelet numbers, clotting times, antigenic levels of clotting factors and of levels of specific activation products.

In the authors view, the results of clotting assays are often misinterpreted in patients with sepsis:

1) Platelet numbers are often decreased in patients with sepsis. This is generally considered to reflect activation of coagulation, since thrombin is a potent agonist for platelets. Similar decreases of platelet numbers occur in many animal models. Surprisingly, no clotting inhibitor has been shown to reduce the drop in platelets in sepsis models in spite of efficient inhibition of thrombin formation. Hence, the decrease in platelets during sepsis may result from, and be independent of, activation of coagulation, and result from other processes. Correlation analysis in patients points to a mechanism involving complement and cytokines [90], although the precise nature of this mechanism is far from clear.

2) Decreased levels of clotting factors result in prolongation of clotting times, and are often considered as a sign for activation of coagulation *in vivo*. In cases of full blown diffuse intravascular coagulation (DIC) intense consumption of clotting factors indeed may explain such changes. However, it should be realized that decreased synthesis of clotting proteins may yield similar changes. Decreased synthesis likely occurs during sepsis, for example because of liver failure or underlying liver disease, or because of an ongoing acute phase reaction. In primates injected with IL-6, the main inducer of acute phase reactions, circulating levels of clotting factors decrease and clotting times prolong 24 hours after injection, i.e., at the time CRP levels were high [91]. Although in this study it was concluded that IL-6 was able to activate coagulation *in vivo*, circulating TAT complexes remained normal, whereas the assay used is suitable for studies in primates [4]. Hence, these data should be interpreted that during acute phase reactions levels of some clotting proteins decrease due to reduced synthesis. Clotting proteins such as factor XII and ATIII, indeed have been shown to be negative acute phase proteins [92,93].

3) Increased levels of activation products such as TAT are nowadys used to assess activation of coagulation in patients. Most septic patients indeed have elevated levels of these parameters pointing to activation of coagulation. However, increase is moderate in the majority of the patients and often not accompanied by decreased fibrinogen levels. In contrast, in most animal models TAT levels are often sky high, and accompanied by markedly decreased fibrinogen levels, which in humans mostly occurs in children with meningococcal sepsis and in a minority (10-15%) of adult patients with sepsis. Moreover, the moderate increase in activation parameters, as occurring in the majority of septic patients, may also result from clinical manipulations such as the use of indwelling catheters.

4) Finally, it remains to be established whether moderate generation of thrombin in the absence of significant fibrinogen conversion, is detrimental. Via its effect on protein C such a generation may actually be beneficial (see discussion of 'thrombin paradox' above), although on the other hand septic patients in general have low levels of protein C, which may counteract such a beneficial effect of thrombin.

CONCLUSION

Extrinsic and intrinsic pathways of the coagulation system should no longer be considered as distinct entities, but rather as an integrated system providing optimal thrombin generation via the TF/factor VII complex. The role of factor XII and other contact system proteins in coagulation is less clear, and presumably is more important for fibrinolysis and inflammation.

There is no doubt that activation of coagulation, predominantly, if not exclusively, via the TF/factor VII pathway, occurs in animal and human models for sepsis. In the more severe sepsis animal models, this activation is associated with full-blown DIC. In these latter models inhibitors of TF/FVIIa improve mortality, even when given after the challenge. Surprisingly, all the evidence so far does not support that the beneficial effects of these inhibitors are due to their effects on clotting, but rather seem to be related to their effects on the inflammatory cascade. Identification of the molecular pathways of these anti-inflammatory effects is of critical importance since they seem to be key processes in the events leading to mortality in sepsis.

The interpretation of prolonged clotting times and decreased platelet numbers in patients with sepsis needs further study regarding their clinical implications since they may result from other processes than activation of coagulation.

The implications of moderately increased generation of thrombin in the absence of significant fibrinogen consumption, as occurs in the majority of septic patients, also needs a critical evaluation since such a generation actually may be beneficial by activating protein C.

Intervention studies with clotting inhibitors in patients should reveal the importance and the biological consequences of activation of the coagulation system in the pathogenesis of human sepsis.

REFERENCES

1. Hack CE, Aarden LA, Thijs LG. Role of cytokines in sepsis. Adv Immunol 1997; 66:101-195
2. Vervloet MG, Thijs LG, Hack CE. Derangements of coagulation and fibrinolysis in critically ill patients with sepsis and septic shock. Semin Thromb Hemost 1998; 24:33-44
3. Griffin JH. Blood coagulation. The thrombin paradox. Nature 1995; 378:337-338
4. de Boer JP, Creasy AA, Chang A, et al. Activation patterns of coagulation and fibrinolysis in baboons following infusion with lethal or sublethal dose of Escherichia coli. Circ Shock 1993; 39:59-67
5. de Boer JP, Creasey AA, Chang A, et al. Alpha-2-macroglobulin functions as an inhibitor of fibrinolytic, clotting, and neutrophilic proteinases in sepsis: studies using a baboon model. Infect Immun 1993; 61:5035-5043
6. Semeraro N, Colucci M. Tissue factor in health and disease. Thromb Haemost 1997; 78:759-764
7. Satta N, Toti F, Feugeas O, et al. Monocyte vesiculation is a possible mechanism for dissemination of membrane-associated procoagulant activities and adhesion molecules after stimulation by lipopolysaccharide. J Immunol 1994; 153:3245-3255
8. Osterud B. Tissue factor expression by monocytes: regulation and pathophysiological roles. Blood Coagul Fibrinolysis 1998; 9 Suppl 1:S9-S14
9. Saadi S, Holzknecht RA, Patte CP, et al. Complement-mediated regulation of tissue factor activity in endothelium. J Exp Med 1995; 182:1807-1814
10. Bevilacqua MP, Pober JS, Majeau GR, et al. Recombinant tumor necrosis factor induces procoagulant activity in cultured human vascular endothelium: characterization and comparison with the actions of interleukin 1. Proc Natl Acad Sci USA 1986; 83:4533-4537
11. Nawroth PP, Handley DA, Esmon CT, et al. Interleukin 1 induces endothelial cell procoagulant while suppressing cell-surface anticoagulant activity. Proc Natl Acad Sci USA 1986; 83:3460-3464
12. Bevilacqua MP, Pober JS, Majeau GR, et al. Interleukin 1 (IL-1) induces biosynthesis and cell surface expression of procoagulant activity in human vascular endothelial cells. J Exp Med 1984; 160:618-623
13. Colucci M, Balconi G, Lorenzet R, et al. Cultured human endothelial cells generate tissue factor in response to endotoxin. J Clin Invest 1983; 71:1893-1896
14. Moore KL, Andreoli SP, Esmon NL, et al. Endotoxin enhances tissue factor and suppresses thrombomodulin expression of human vascular endothelium in vitro. J Clin Invest 1987; 79:124-130
15. Sandset PM. Tissue factor pathway inhibitor (TFPI)--an update. Haemostasis 1996; 26 Suppl 4:154-165

16. Veer van 't C, V, Mann KG. Regulation of tissue factor initiated thrombin generation by the stoichiometric inhibitors tissue factor pathway inhibitor, antithrombin- III, and heparin cofactor-II. J Biol Chem 1997; 272:4367-4377
17. Gailani D, Broze GJJ. Factor XI activation in a revised model of blood coagulation. Science 1991; 253:909-912
18. Naito K, Fujikawa K. Activation of human blood coagulation factor XI independent of factor XII. Factor XI is activated by thrombin and factor XIa in the presence of negatively charged surfaces. J Biol Chem 1991; 266:7353-7358
19. Minnema MC, Pajkrt D, Wuillemin WA, et al. Activation of clotting factor XI without detectable contact activation in experimental human endotoxemia. Blood 1998; 92:3294-3301
20. Minnema MC, ten Cate H, Hack CE. The role of factor XI in coagulation. A matter of revision. Semin Thromb Hemost 1999; 25:419-428
21. Bornne von dem P, Bajzar L, Meijers JC, et al. Thrombin-mediated activation of factor XI results in a thrombin-activatable fibrinolysis inhibitor-dependent inhibition of fibrinolysis. J Clin Invest 1997; 99:2323-2327
22. Borne von dem P, Meijers JC, Bouma BN. Feedback activation of factor XI by thrombin in plasma results in additional formation of thrombin that protects fibrin clots from fibrinolysis. Blood 1995; 86:3035-3042
23. Minnema MC, Friederich PW, Levi M, et al. Enhancement of rabbit jugular vein thrombolysis by neutralization of factor XI. In vivo evidence for a role of factor XI as an anti-fibrinolytic factor. J Clin Invest 1998; 101:10-14
24. Uchiba M, Okajima K, Murakami K, et al. Effects of plasma kallikrein specific inhibitor and active-site blocked factor VIIa on the pulmonary vascular injury induced by endotoxin in rats. Thromb Haemost 1997; 78:1209-1214
25. Uchiba M, Okajima K, Murakami K, et al. Effect of nafamostat mesilate on pulmonary vascular injury induced by lipopolysaccharide in rats. Am J Respir Crit Care Med 1997; 155:711-718
26. Butler LD, Layman NK, Cain RL, et al. Interleukin 1-induced pathophysiology: induction of cytokines, development of histopathologic changes, and immunopharmacologic intervention. Clin Immunol Immunopathol 1989; 53:400-421
27. Remick DG, Strieter RM, Eskandari MK, et al. Role of tumor necrosis factor-alpha in lipopolysaccharide-induced pathologic alterations. Am J Pathol 1990; 136:49-60
28. Movat HZ, Burrowes CE, Cybulsky MI, et al. Acute inflammation and a Shwartzman-like reaction induced by interleukin-1 and tumor necrosis factor. Synergistic action of the cytokines in the induction of inflammation and microvascular injury. Am J Pathol 1987; 129:463-476
29. van der Poll T, Buller HR, ten Cate H, et al. Activation of coagulation after administration of tumor necrosis factor to normal subjects. N Engl J Med 1990; 322:1622-1627
30. van der Poll T, Levi M, Buller HR, et al. Fibrinolytic response to tumor necrosis factor in healthy subjects. J Exp Med 1991; 174:729-732
31. Taylor FBJ, He SE, Chang AC, et al. Infusion of phospholipid vesicles amplifies the local thrombotic response to TNF and anti-protein C into a consumptive response. Thromb Haemost 1996; 75:578-584
32. Jansen PM, Boermeester MA, Fischer E, et al. Contribution of interleukin-1 to activation of coagulation and fibrinolysis, neutrophil degranulation, and the release of secretory-type phospholipase A2 in sepsis: studies in nonhuman primates after interleukin-1 alpha administration and during lethal bacteremia. Blood 1995; 86:1027-1034
33. Stouthard JM, Levi M, Hack CE, et al. Interleukin-6 stimulates coagulation, not fibrinolysis, in humans. Thromb Haemost 1996; 76:738-742

34. Cermak J, Key NS, Bach RR, et al. C-reactive protein induces human peripheral blood monocytes to synthesize tissue factor. Blood 1993; 82:513-520
35. Baars JW, de Boer JP, Wagstaff J, et al. Interleukin-2 induces activation of coagulation and fibrinolysis: resemblance to the changes seen during experimental endotoxaemia. Br J Haematol 1992; 82:295-301
36. Lauw FN, Dekkers PE, te VA, et al. Interleukin-12 induces sustained activation of multiple host inflammatory mediator systems in chimpanzees. J Infect Dis 1999; 179:646-652
37. Hack CE, Wagstaff J, Strack vSR, et al. Studies on the contact system of coagulation during therapy with high doses of recombinant IL-2: implications for septic shock. Thromb Haemost 1991; 65:497-503
38. Biemond BJ, Levi M, ten Cate H, et al. Complete inhibition of endotoxin-induced coagulation activation in chimpanzees with a monoclonal Fab fragment against factor VII/VIIa. Thromb Haemost 1995; 73:223-230
39. Levi M, ten Cate H, Bauer KA, et al. Inhibition of endotoxin-induced activation of coagulation and fibrinolysis by pentoxifylline or by a monoclonal anti-tissue factor antibody in chimpanzees. J Clin Invest 1994; 93:114-120
40. van der Poll T, Levi M, van Deventer SJ, et al. Differential effects of anti-tumor necrosis factor monoclonal antibodies on systemic inflammatory responses in experimental endotoxemia in chimpanzees. Blood 1994; 83:446-451
41. van Deventer SJ, Buller HR, ten Cate JW, et al. Experimental endotoxemia in humans: analysis of cytokine release and coagulation, fibrinolytic, and complement pathways. Blood 1990; 76:2520-2526
42. Suffredini AF, Harpel PC, Parrillo JE. Promotion and subsequent inhibition of plasminogen activation after administration of intravenous endotoxin to normal subjects. N Engl J Med 1989; 320:1165-1172
43. van der Poll T, Levi M, Hack CE, et al. Elimination of interleukin 6 attenuates coagulation activation in experimental endotoxemia in chimpanzees. J Exp Med 1994; 179:1253-1259
44. van der Poll T, Jansen PM, Van Zee KJ, et al. Pretreatment with a 55-kDa tumor necrosis factor receptor- immunoglobulin fusion protein attenuates activation of coagulation, but not of fibrinolysis, during lethal bacteremia in baboons. J Infect Dis 1997; 176:296-299
45. Higure A, Okamoto K, Hirata K, et al. Macrophages and neutrophils infiltrating into the liver are responsible for tissue factor expression in a rabbit model of acute obstructive cholangitis. Thromb Haemost 1996; 75:791-795
46. Todoroki H, Higure A, Okamoto K, et al. Possible role of platelet-activating factor in the in vivo expression of tissue factor in neutrophils. J Surg Res 1998; 80:149-155
47. Drake TA, Cheng J, Chang A, et al. Expression of tissue factor, thrombomodulin, and E-selectin in baboons with lethal Escherichia coli sepsis. Am J Pathol 1993; 142:1458-1470
48. Semeraro N, Triggiani R, Montemurro P, et al. Enhanced endothelial tissue factor but normal thrombomodulin in endotoxin-treated rabbits. Thromb Res 1993; 71:479-486
49. Semeraro N, Triggiani R, Montemurro P, et al. Enhanced endothelial tissue factor but normal thrombomodulin in endotoxin-treated rabbits. Thromb Res 1993; 71:479-486
50. Mackman N, Sawdey MS, Keeton MR, et al. Murine tissue factor gene expression in vivo. Tissue and cell specificity and regulation by lipopolysaccharide. Am J Pathol 1993; 143:76-84
51. Erlich J, Fearns C, Mathison J, et al. Lipopolysaccharide induction of tissue factor expression in rabbits. Infect Immun 1999; 67:2540-2546
52. Hara S, Asada Y, Hatakeyama K, et al. Expression of tissue factor and tissue factor pathway inhibitor in rats lungs with lipopolysaccharide-induced disseminated intravascular coagulation. Lab Invest 1997; 77:581-589

53. Nieuwland R, Berckmans RJ, McGregor S, et al. Cellular origin and procoagulant properties of microparticles in meningococcal sepsis. Blood 2000; 95:930-935
54. Dackiw AP, McGilvray ID, Woodside M, et al. Prevention of endotoxin-induced mortality by antitissue factor immunization. Arch Surg 1996; 131:1273-1278
55. Taylor FBJ, Chang A, Ruf W, et al. Lethal E. coli septic shock is prevented by blocking tissue factor with monoclonal antibody. Circ Shock 1991; 33:127-134
56. Taylor FB, Chang AC, Peer G, et al. Active site inhibited factor VIIa (DEGR VIIa) attenuates the coagulant and interleukin-6 and -8, but not tumor necrosis factor, responses of the baboon to LD100 Escherichia coli. Blood 1998; 91:1609-1615
57. Creasey AA, Chang AC, Feigen L, et al. Tissue factor pathway inhibitor reduces mortality from Escherichia coli septic shock. J Clin Invest 1993; 91:2850-2856
58. Carr C, Bild GS, Chang AC, et al. Recombinant E. coli-derived tissue factor pathway inhibitor reduces coagulopathic and lethal effects in the baboon gram-negative model of septic shock. Circ Shock 1994; 44:126-137
59. Randolph MM, White GL, Kosanke SD, et al. Attenuation of tissue thrombosis and hemorrhage by ala-TFPI does not account for its protection against E. coli--a comparative study of treated and untreated non-surviving baboons challenged with LD100 E. coli. Thromb Haemost 1998; 79:1048-1053
60. Bregengard C, Nordfang O, Wildgoose P, et al. The effect of two-domain tissue factor pathway inhibitor on endotoxin- induced disseminated intravascular coagulation in rabbits. Blood Coagul Fibrinolysis 1993; 4:699-706
61. Elsayed YA, Nakagawa K, Kamikubo YI, et al. Effects of recombinant human tissue factor pathway inhibitor on thrombus formation and its in vivo distribution in a rat DIC model. Am J Clin Pathol 1996; 106:574-583
62. Warr TA, Rao LV, Rapaport SI. Disseminated intravascular coagulation in rabbits induced by administration of endotoxin or tissue factor: effect of anti-tissue factor antibodies and measurement of plasma extrinsic pathway inhibitor activity. Blood 1990; 75:1481-1489
63. Camerota AJ, Creasey AA, Patla V, et al. Delayed treatment with recombinant human tissue factor pathway inhibitor improves survival in rabbits with gram-negative peritonitis. J Infect Dis 1998; 177:668-676
64. Taylor FBJ, Chang A, Esmon CT, et al: Protein C prevents the coagulopathic and lethal effects of Escherichia coli infusion in the baboon. J Clin Invest 1987; 79:918-925
65. Taylor FBJ, Emerson TEJ, Jordan R, et al. Antithrombin-III prevents the lethal effects of Escherichia coli infusion in baboons. Circ Shock 1988; 26:227-235
66. Bleeker WK, Teeling JL, Verhoeven AJ, et al. Vasoactive side effects of intravenous immunoglobulin preparations in a rat model and their treatment with recombinant platelet-activating factor acetylhydrolase. Blood 2000; 95:1856-1861
67. Camerer E, Huang W, Coughlin SR. Tissue factor- and factor X-dependent activation of protease-activated receptor 2 by factor VIIa. Proc Natl Acad Sci USA 2000; 97:5255-5260
68. Petersen LC, Thastrup O, Hagel G, et al. Exclusion of known protease-activated receptors in factor VIIa-induced signal transduction. Thromb Haemost 2000; 83:571-576
69. Cunningham MA, Romas P, Hutchinson P, et al. Tissue factor and factor VIIa receptor/ligand interactions induce proinflammatory effects in macrophages. Blood 1999; 94:3413-3420
70. Taylor FBJ, Chang AC, Peer GT, et al. DEGR-factor Xa blocks disseminated intravascular coagulation initiated by Escherichia coli without preventing shock or organ damage. Blood 1991; 78:364-368
71. Harada N, Okajima K, Kushimoto S, et al. Antithrombin reduces ischemia/reperfusion injury of rat liver by increasing the hepatic level of prostacyclin. Blood 1999; 93:157-164

72. Taylor FBJ, Stearns-Kurosawa DJ, Kurosawa S, et al. The endothelial cell protein C receptor aids in host defense against Escherichia coli sepsis. Blood 2000; 95:1680-1686
73. Levi M, Hack CE, de Boer JP, et al. Reduction of contact activation related fibrinolytic activity in factor XII deficient patients. Further evidence for the role of the contact system in fibrinolysis in vivo. J Clin Invest 1991; 88:1155-1160
74. Ichinose M, Barnes PJ. Bradykinin-induced airway microvascular leakage and bronchoconstriction are mediated via a bradykinin B2 receptor. Am Rev Respir Dis 1990; 142:1104-1107
75. Wachtfogel YT, Pixley RA, Kucich U, et al. Purified plasma factor XIIa aggregates human neutrophils and causes degranulation. Blood 1986; 67:1731-1737
76. Wachtfogel YT, Kucich U, James HL, et al. Human plasma kallikrein releases neutrophil elastase during blood coagulation. J Clin Invest 1983; 72:1672-1677
77. Schapira M, Despland E, Scott CF, et al. Purified human plasma kallikrein aggregates human blood neutrophils. J Clin Invest 1982; 69:1199-1202
78. Nies AS, Forsyth RP, Williams HE, et al. Contribution of kinins to endotoxin shock in unanesthetized Rhesus monkeys. Circ Res 1968; 22:155-164
79. Pixley RA, DeLa CR, Page JD, et al. Activation of the contact system in lethal hypotensive bacteremia in a baboon model. Am J Pathol 1992; 140:897-906
80. Pixley RA, De La Cadena R, Page JD, et al. The contact system contributes to hypotension but not disseminated intravascular coagulation in lethal bacteremia. In vivo use of a monoclonal anti-factor XII antibody to block contact activation in baboons. J Clin Invest 1993; 91:61-68
81. Jansen PM, Pixley RA, Brouwer M, et al. Inhibition of factor XII in septic baboons attenuates the activation of complement and fibrinolytic systems and reduces the release of interleukin-6 and neutrophil elastase. Blood 1996; 87:2337-2344
82. Berg T, Schlichting E, Ishida H, et al. Kinin antagonist does not protect against the hypotensive response to endotoxin, anaphylaxis or acute pancreatitis. J Pharmacol Exp Ther 1989; 251:731-734
83. Colman RW, Flores DN, De La Cadena RA, et al. Recombinant alpha 1-antitrypsin Pittsburgh attenuates experimental gram-negative septicemia. Am J Pathol 1988; 130:418-426
84. Harper PL, Taylor FB, DeLa CR, et al. Recombinant antitrypsin Pittsburgh undergoes proteolytic cleavage during E. coli sepsis and fails to prevent the associated coagulopathy in a primate model. Thromb Haemost 1998; 80:816-821
85. Guerrero R, Velasco F, Rodriguez M, et al. Endotoxin-induced pulmonary dysfunction is prevented by C1-esterase inhibitor. J Clin Invest 1993; 91:2754-2760
86. Jansen PM, Eisele B, de J, I, et al. Effect of C1 inhibitor on inflammatory and physiologic response patterns in primates suffering from lethal septic shock. J Immunol 1998; 160:475-484
87. Morrison DC, Cochrane CG. Direct evidence for Hageman factor (factor XII) activation by bacterial lipopolysaccharides (endotoxins). J Exp Med 1974; 140:797-811
88. Herwald H, Morgelin M, Olsen A, et al. Activation of the contact-phase system on bacterial surfaces--a clue to serious complications in infectious diseases. Nat Med 1998; 4:298-302
89. DeLa CR, Suffredini AF, Page JD, et al. Activation of the kallikrein-kinin system after endotoxin administration to normal human volunteers. Blood 1993; 81:3313-3317
90. Hack CE, Nuijens JH, Strack vSR, et al. A model for the interplay of inflammatory mediators in sepsis--a study in 48 patients. Intensive Care Med 1990; 16 Suppl 3:S187-S191
91. Mestries JC, Kruithof EK, Gascon MP, et al. In vivo modulation of coagulation and fibrinolysis by recombinant glycosylated human interleukin-6 in baboons. Eur Cytokine Netw 1994; 5:275-281

92. Citarella F, Felici A, Brouwer M, et al. Interleukin-6 downregulates factor XII production
     by human hepatoma cell line (HepG2). Blood 1997; 90:1501-1507
93. Niessen RW, Lamping RJ, Jansen PM, et al. Antithrombin acts as a negative acute phase
     protein as established with studies on HepG2 cells and in baboons. Thromb Haemost
     1997; 78:1088-1092

40

SHOULD FEVER BE TREATED IN SEPSIS?

Burke A. Cunha

> *"Why, the fever itself is Nature's instrument."*
>
> Sydenham

> *"Fever is the great engine that nature brings to the field to fight disease."*
>
> Hutchinson

> *"While acetylsalicylic acid decreases the temperature in fever, we are not convinced that this has any beneficial effect."*
>
> Hoffmann & Dreser

Patients who are septic are acutely ill with a life-threatening infection due to pathogenic microorganisms. To become septic, host defenses must be overwhelmed at least temporarily, to tip the balance in the favor of the invading microbial pathogens. Local and systemic host defenses are normally so efficient and redundant that sepsis is a relatively uncommon event given the fact that we all live in a microbially dense milieu. For these reasons, sepsis usually occurs as the release of a large inoculum of bacteria from the distal gastrointestinal tract, e.g., colon, genitourinary tract, or by direct intravenous infusion, e.g., central line infections. Certain defects in host defense mechanisms may also rarely result in overwhelming sepsis. Examples include pneumococcal sepsis in patients with impaired splenic function and meningococcal sepsis in patients with defects in the terminal components of complement. These examples illustrate the point that for sepsis to occur, there must be a critical defect in the patient's host defenses. This usually involves a defect in a complement component or impaired splenic function in order to cause sepsis in such individuals [1].

The robustness of our host defenses is attested to by the fact that overwhelming pneumococcal and meningococcal sepsis are such rare events and require specific immune defects which can occasionally overwhelm the host. Normal hosts can be overwhelmed by failing to contain a large inoculum of pathogenic bacteria, (e.g., perforation of the colon). Leukopenic compromised hosts are not infrequently bacteremic, but are rarely septic in their clinical presentation. Non-leukopenic compromised hosts, (e.g., diabetes mellitus, systemic lupus erythematosus, and alcoholics), have partial defects in some components of their host defense array. Because of this, urosepsis is not uncommon in patients with diabetes, lupus, or systemic lupus erythematosis (SLE) with urinary tract infections [2]. Finally, patients with severely impaired hepatic function have impaired hepatic bacterial filtration function as well as a decrease in the reticuloendothelial cell component of a fully functional liver.

In summary, sepsis is not a random event and host defenses either need to be impaired or overwhelmed for clinical sepsis to occur. Since patients are, by definition, acutely ill with sepsis; they need every host defense mechanism in order to ensure survival of the host. The febrile response is primordial in terms of its evolutionary persistence and primary in terms of its host defense importance [3,4]. To diminish or take away fever in a septic patient denies the patient a fundamental and critical host defense mechanism necessary in surviving the septic episode [5].

FEVER AS A PRIMARY HOST MECHANISM

The febrile response is the earliest and most pervasive defense system deployed against microorganisms. Fever is the primary host defense mechanism of many animals as well as humans, and has persisted over millions of years [5]. Fever is the primary host defense mechanism of higher forms of animal life from fish to lizards to mammals to humans. The coordinated febrile response has not changed in its evolution or in its manifestations in different species. For these reasons, we must assume that any biological activity that has such evolutionary survivability and stability, not to mention its commonality in many species, attests to its biological importance in the protection of a species against infection. While it is easy to demonstrate that fever has a beneficial effect on the outcome of infection, it is also clear from such experimental studies that hypothermia has the opposite effect; (i.e., if fever is good, then hypothermia is decidedly bad). This is an observation that has been made in humans for many years. It is well known that patients with pneumococcal pneumonia and fever, all other factors being equal, do much better clinically than alcoholic patients with pneumonia and hypothermia. The same is true of patients with chronic renal failure where hypothermia is not only a sign of sepsis but a negative prognostic factor. Because of confounding variables, it is difficult to use temperature elevations as a predictor of survival in humans. Confounding variables related to the complexity of sepsis in humans obscure the relationship between fever and overall outcome. While there are abundant data in animals, there are limited data in humans attesting to the beneficial effects of fever on outcome [5-7]. Equally true is the fact that there is no data in animals or humans suggesting that lowering the temperature has any benefit whatsoever in the septic patient.

THE BENEFICIAL EFFECTS OF FEVER AND SEPSIS

Host Factors

The beneficial effects of fever on the host are legion. Every host defense parameter that can be measured is enhanced in the presence of fever. Fever enhances phagocytosis of extracellular organisms, as well as the intracellular destruction of ingested intracellular bacteria. Chemotaxis is enhanced by increased temperature. Lysosomal membranes are thermal labile and are lysed in the presence of fever, which assists in destroying intracellular pathogens. Phagolysosomal fusion and destruction of bacteria within the phagolysosome are enhanced in the presence of elevated temperature. In addition, antibody production and activity are increased in the presence of fever. Complement activation is enhanced in the presence of fever via both the classical and alternate pathways. Serum iron is decreased in the presence of fever that denies iron, an important virulence factor in pathogenic bacteria. While there is no question that every aspect of measurable host defense is enhanced in the presence of fever, clinical studies showing outcome is enhanced by fever remain limited, but should increase as investigators recognize the importance of fever as a critical host defense determinant in sepsis [7-11].

Host Factors
- Enhanced chemotaxis
- Enhanced neutrophil migration
- Increase production of neutrophilic antibacterial substances (superoxide anions)
- Promotes heart shock protein synthesis that stabilizes intracellular proteins
- Enhanced phagocytosis
- Increased production/activity of antibody
- Enhanced T-cell proliferation
- Decreases serum iron levels

Microbial Factors
- Fever causes lysis of many bacterial pathogens
- Fever decreases the replication rates of most bacterial pathogens
- Fever increases susceptibility of most pathogens to antibiotics
- Fever decreases antibiotic protein binding and increases volume of distribution which increases antibiotic tissue concentrations
- Decreased microbial virulence with decreased serum iron
- Antibacterial effect of fever is potentiated by acidosis, which frequently accompanies sepsis

Antipyretic Factors
- Acetylsalicylic acid decreases capsule production in some encapsulated bacteria

Bottom Line
- There is no theoretical or clinical benefit to decreasing the temperature in sepsis
- Patients should not be denied the benefits of a fever (unless the temperature elevation threatens brain, heart, or lung function)

Table 1. Beneficial effects of fever in sepsis

Microbial Factors

Fever has adverse effects on many pathogenic organisms. Increased temperature decreases the replication rates of many pathogenic microorganisms. As mentioned previously, the decrease in serum iron adversely affects the virulence of many pathogenic bacteria. Fever also exerts a direct effect on microorganisms if sufficiently elevated [5-7]. Syphilitic spirochetes will lyse in the presence of fever. Microbial thermolysis is an important factor adversely affecting the infecting pathogenic organisms [12-14]. The susceptibility of pathogenic microorganisms to antimicrobial agents is increased, (i.e., decreased mean inhibitory concentrations [MICs] with fever). Acidosis, that usually accompanies sepsis, potentiates the antibacterial effects of fever (Cheston B. Cunha, personal communication).

Antipyretic Factors

There are no theoretical or proven benefits for the host of lowering the temperature in sepsis (Table 1).

THE ADVERSE EFFECTS OF FEVER

Host Factors

Extreme hyperpyrexia, e.g., temperatures ≥106°F (≥41.1°C) may cause central nervous system (CNS) damage or cause death from cellular enzyme protein denaturation. However, there are no infectious diseases that cause temperatures ≥106°F (≥41.1°C), rendering this extreme level of temperature elevation irrelevant in a discussion of sepsis. Temperatures ≥102°F (≥38.8°C) may result in acute myocardial infarction or an exacerbation of congestive heart failure in patients with severe valvular or coronary artery disease. Most patients tolerate temperature elevations of ≥102°F (≥38.8°C) to ≥104°F (≥40.0°C) without much difficulty. In addition, fever may have an adverse effect on patients with advanced pulmonary disease who cannot adequately oxygenate their tissues because of the increased needs due to the elevated temperature. For every degree of temperature elevation in degrees Fahrenheit, there is a commensurate increase in the pulse rate of 10 beats/minute to meet the increased metabolic and cooling needs of the body. Patients with severe cardiopulmonary disease have a limited ability to respond to temperatures ≥102°F (≥38.8°C) often having evidence of diminished clinical capacity of the heart and lungs [15-18].

Microbial Factors

The adverse effects of fever on the microbe are multiple. The activity and efficiency of humoral and cellular immune mechanisms are greatly enhanced in the presence of fever to the detriment of the infecting microbe. Except for selected organisms, primarily non-pathogens for humans, elevated temperature gives the microbe no advantage against the host. All host defense mechanisms are optimized in the presence of fever and collectively work to the detriment of the invading pathogen [12-14,19,20].

Antipyretic Factors

Antipyretics may have an adverse effect with certain antimicrobials. The activity of certain antibiotics is enhanced in the presence of an elevated temperature, and conversely lowering the temperature may have an adverse effect and reaction on certain antimicrobials [14]. Depending upon the antipyretic method used, there may be secondary effects that favor the microbe. For example, salicylate may have a positive effect on reducing capsular expression in certain species, (e.g., *Klebsiella, Strep. pneumoniae)*, but may be antagonistic to certain antibiotics, minimizing or negating their effect, (e.g., doxycycline). Decreasing temperature by whatever antipyretic means can only favor the microbe to the detriment of the host [4,5] (Table 2).

Host Factors
• Because an increase of 1°F (.56°C) results in an increase in the pulse of 10 beats/minute, temperatures ≥102°F (38.8°C) may precipitate an acute myocardial infarction or congestive heart failure in patients with severe valvular or coronary artery disease due to increased oxygen demand.
• Extreme hyperthermia ≥ 106°F (41.1°C) may cause central nervous system damage or protein denaturation of vital enzyme system resulting in death.
• Temperatures ≥106°F (41.1°C) are not infections and do not occur in sepsis
• Fever in neurosurgical patients has adverse effects on brain function
Microbial Factors
• Mild increases in temperature have no effect on the replication rates of most pathogens
• Fever is disadvantageous to the microbe in every way
Antipyretic Factors
• Acetylsalicylic acid decreases/antagonizes the antibacterial activity of some antibiotics
Bottom Line
• Adverse effects of fever are related to physiologic host factors, not microbial or host defense factors

Table 2. Adverse effects of fever in sepsis

CLINICAL RATIONALE FOR AVOIDING ANTI-PYRETICS IN SEPSIS

While there is no benefit in treating the normal adult host except in patients with severe cardiopulmonary disease, fever has never been shown to have any detrimental effect on the host, but the question becomes, how has such a process of lowering fever become so widespread? There are no data, experimental evidence, or clinical experience that suggests that lowering the temperature has any benefit whatsoever, yet nurses and physicians continue to routinely employ temperature lowering modalities when the patient has fever. While no nursing or medical textbook advocates using antipyretics, except in certain situations, it remains a common practice in spite of its potentially deleterious effects [21-23] (Table 3).

<u>Diagnostic Rationale</u>
- Fever patterns are useful in differentiating infectious from non-infectious causes of fever, (e.g., '102°F (38.8°C) rule')
- Pulse-temperature relationships have important differential diagnostic implications, (e.g., the finding of relative bradycardia has important diagnostic implications).
- Antipyretic therapy destroys diagnostic utility of fever patterns and pulse-temperature relationships

<u>Therapeutic Rationale</u>
- Febrile response to antimicrobial therapy is often the only practical way to therapeutically differentiate bacterial from non-bacterial pathogens or between inflammation and bacterial infection.

<u>Bottom Line</u>
- Temperature decrease is the earliest and best indicator of the effectiveness of antimicrobial therapy in sepsis. This key therapeutic indicator is eliminated by antipyretics

Table 3. Clinical rationale for avoiding antipyretics in sepsis

Diagnostic Rationale

There are diagnostic as well as therapeutic reasons for not lowering the septic patient's temperature. The diagnostic rationale for not treating fever in the septic patient is powerful. Firstly, fever has important diagnostic possibilities, both in terms of its elevation and relationship to the pulse. Temperature characteristics can help the astute clinician differentiate bacterial from nonbacterial infections, or infections from non-infections when used in concert with pulse temperature relationships, (e.g., pulse-temperature deficits/relative bradycardia). This has critical implications diagnostically [24-28] (Table 4).

Fever *without* relative bradycardia	Fever *with* relative bradycardia

• **Pneumonias**
  Typical
    Bacterial community acquired
    Aspiration
    Nosocomial
 	
  Atypical
    Mycoplasma pneumoniae
    Chlamydia pneumoniae
	• **Pneumonias**
	  Atypical
	    Legionella
	    Q fever
	    Psittacosis

• **Most infectious diseases**	• **Some Important Infectious Diseases**
	  Malaria
	  Typhoid fever
	  Typhus
	  Babesiosis
	  Rocky Mountain spotted fever
	  Viral hemorrhagic fevers

• **Sepsis**	• **Mimics of sepsis**
	  Drug fevers
	  Central fevers
	  Lymphomas

Table 4. Diagnostic usefulness of relative bradycardia

While infectious diseases may present with low or high-grade fevers, it is equally true that non-infectious diseases commonly occurring in the septic patient, do not result in temperatures $\geq 102°F$ $(\geq 38.8°C)$. The use of the '102°F (38.8°C) rule' has great diagnostic utility in the intensive care setting. Since fever is a nonspecific manifestation that may indicate inflammation or infection, it is critical that the clinician appreciates when the febrile patient is septic, or simply has a fever.

Fever should not be decreased because it denies the clinician from utilizing temperature/pulse relationships in the differential diagnosis of the febrile patient. Ignorance of the '102°F (38.8°C) rule' and the importance of pulse-temperature relationships will lead the unwary clinician to treat many

febrile patients with antibiotics, that have noninfectious disease disorders
causing the patient's temperature elevation [1,27,29] (Table 5).

The 102°F (38.8°C) Rule	
Temperature ≤102°F (38.8°C)	**Temperature ≥102°F(38°C**
Acute pancreatitis	Pancreatic abscess/ infected pseudocyst
Acute myocardial infarction/ congestive heart failure	Myocardial abscess
Post-pericardiotomy syndrome (Dressler's Syndrome)	Acute viral/bacterial pericarditis
Acute respiratory distress syndrome (ARDS)	Nosocomial pneumonia
Gastrointestinal hemorrhage	Bowel infarction/peritonitis
Phlebitis (chemical)	IV-line associated bacteremia
Catheter-associated bacteremia	Urosepsis (only in non-leukopenic compromised hosts, with partial/ total urinary tract obstruction or pre-existing renal disease)
Pulmonary emboli/infarction	Septic pulmonary emboli
Uncomplicated wound infections	Severe/complicated wound infections (invasive group A streptococci, *Vibrio vulnificus*, etc.)
Abdominal/pelvic hematoma/non-infected fluid collection	Intra-abdominal abscess
Cystitis	Acute pyelonephritis
C. difficile diarrhea	*C. difficile* colitis
• Most non-infectious diseases likely to be confused with sepsis have temperatures *≤102°F(38.8°C)* **except** Malignant hyperthermia Drug fevers Lymphomas Acute adrenal insufficiency	• Most acute infectious diseases with the potential for presenting as sepsis usually have temperatures *≥102°F(38.8°)* **except** Elderly Immunosuppressed Renal insufficiency Alcoholics IV drug abusers

Table 5. *Diagnostic importance of fever patterns*

Therapeutic Rationale

As the temperature characteristics are critical diagnostically, they are important therapeutically as well. After treatment with an antimicrobial, the decrease in temperature helps the clinician in assessing the efficacy of the therapeutic agent employed. It also helps the physician differentiate between non-infectious diseases and non-bacterial infections that will not respond to a challenge of appropriate antimicrobials. Many times in clinical cases, the hypothermia blanket or antipyretics have caused clinicians to continue treating a patient, assuming that the decrease in temperature has been due to the antibiotic when in fact the patient has responded to the antipyretics while the infection has continued unabated. Because the therapeutic response has both diagnostic and therapeutic implications, it should not be dampened or eliminated [1,25,27].

WHEN AND HOW TO TREAT FEVER IN THE SEPTIC PATIENT

When to Treat Fever

Extreme hyperpyrexia, i.e., temperatures $\geq106°F$ ($\geq41.1°C$) should always be treated because of the potential for permanent central nervous system damage. Fortunately, hyperpyrexia is uncommon and is never due to sepsis. In any event, such temperatures should be decreased to minimize permanent CNS damage. Temperatures $\geq102°F$ ($\geq38.8°C$) should be treated in children to avoid the possibility of febrile seizures. Adult patients, even with a history of seizure history, do not experience febrile seizures. Patients with severe cardiopulmonary disease, as mentioned previously, should not be permitted to have temperatures $\geq102°F$ ($\geq38.8°C$) for extended periods of time. Most patients tolerate temperature elevations very well, but some have excessive reactions to even modest elevations in temperature, and such patients may demand lowering their temperature [30-32].

How to Treat Fever

Acetaminophen rather than aspirin (acetylsalicylic acid) should be used to lower the temperature. Salicylic acid in aspirin may interfere with the action of certain antimicrobials, and for this reason should not be used. Acetaminophen has the same antipyretic properties as aspirin without anti-inflammatory action, and should be the preferred antipyretic in the septic patient [33]. In selected patients with temperatures of 102°F-106°F (38.8°C-41.1°C) that should be lowered, *vida supra*, then the temperatures should be lowered to achieve an end point in the 102°F (38.8°C) range.

When to Treat Fever
- Patients with severe cardio-pulmonary disease with temperatures ≥ 102°F (≥38.8°C) to prevent cardiopulmonary decompensation
- Children with temperatures ≥ 102°F (≥38.8°C) to possibly prevent febrile seizures
- Adults do not have febrile seizures (even with seizure disorders)
- Patients with extreme hyperpyrexia i.e., temperatures ≥ 106°F (≥41.1°C) (never due to sepsis) to prevent CNS damage

How to Treat Fever
- Decrease temperatures to ~102°F (38.8°C). Do not try to make the patient afebrile
- Rapid changes in temperature will induce shaking chills and a rebound increase in temperature resulting in an iatrogenic "hectic-septic" fever pattern mimicking sepsis
- Rapid decreases in temperature will make the patient feel miserable/worse
- Antipyretic induced "hectic/septic fever patterns will mislead the physician that the patient is clinically worse

What to Use
- Use acetaminophen in preference to acetylsalicylic acid
- Acetaminophen has greater anti-endotoxin effects than acetylsalicyclic acid
- Use hypothermia blankets only for extreme hyperpyrexia, not for infectious fevers

Bottom Line
- Don't treat fever without having a very good physiologic reason. Most fevers are of short duration and pose no threat the host
- Fever is the only known defense mechanism that coordinates and optimizes all known host defense mechanisms and maximizes antibiotic activity
- The benefits of fever should not be denied to septic patients (unless the temperature elevation represents a threat to the host's CNS or cardio-pulmonary function)

Table 6. When and how should fever be treated in sepsis?

The aim of antipyretic therapy is not to render the patient afebrile, but to reduce the temperature into a lower range. If antipyretic devices are used to rapidly decrease the temperature to normal, (i.e., 98°F (37°C), then this induces rapid and wide temperature swings in the patient. This results in the induction of shaking chills, (i.e., rigors), and a rebound hyperthermia. Subsequently, the patient develops an antipyretic-induced "hectic septic fever" and the clinician makes the patient miserable because of the wide fluctuations in temperature and the induction of shaking chills. The induction of a hectic septic fever pattern gives the physician the mistaken impression that the infection is worse and requires more aggressive antipyretic and/or antimicrobial therapy. Relatively very few patients should have their temperatures lowered, as explained previously, and acetaminophen is the most humane way to do this. The use of the hypothermia blanket should be discouraged. It is most uncomfortable for the patient and may result in coronary artery spasm in patients with coronary artery disease secondary to the cold reflex induced by the blanket [1,25,27] (Table 6).

CONCLUSION

The febrile response is a critical host defense mechanism that favors the host and is only detrimental to the infecting pathogen. The height of the fever elevation, the fever pattern, and pulse-temperature relationships have important diagnostic implications which are eliminated if antipyretics are employed. Similarly, in many cases, the only way to assess the efficacy of antimicrobial therapy in a septic patient is the febrile response to appropriate antimicrobial therapy. If a febrile response is removed by antipyretics, the clinician has no way to assess the adequacy or inadequacy of antimicrobial therapy. Because there are no data or reason to employ antipyretics, this practice should be eliminated. Fever has survival value to the host, and confers great advantages to the host, and should not be blunted or eliminated except under relatively few circumstances. The many benefits of fever should not be denied to the septic patient by administering antipyretics [1,34,35].

REFERENCES

1. Cunha BA. Fever in the critical care unit. In: Cunha BA (ed) Infectious Diseases in Critical Care Medicine. Marcel Dekker, New York, 1999
2. Cunha BA. Infections in acutely ill non-leukopenic compromised hosts with diabetes mellitus, SLE, asplenia, or on steroids. Crit Care Clin 1998; 8:263-282
3. Atkins E. Fever: the old and the new. J Infect Dis 1984; 149:339-348
4. Kluger MJ, Ringler DH, Anver MR. Fever and survival. Science 1975; 188:166-168
5. Kluger MJ. Is fever beneficial? Yale J Biol Med 1986; 59:89-95
6. Duff GW. Is fever beneficial to the host: a clinical perspective. Yale J Biol Med 1986; 59:125-130
7. Roberts NJ Jr. Temperature and host defense. Microbiol Rev 1979; 43:241-259
8. Roberts NJ Jr, Sandberg K. Hyperthermia and human leukocyte function II: Enhanced production and response to leukocyte migration inhibition factor (LIF). J Immunol 1979; 122:1990-1993
9. Roszkowski W, Szmigielski S, Janiak M, et al. Effect of hyperthermia on rabbit macrophages. Immunobiology 1980; 157:122-131

10. Jampel HD, Duff GW, Gershon RK, et al. Fever and immunoregulation. III: Fever augments the primary in vitro humoral response. J Exp Med 1983;157:1229-38

11. Van Oss CJ, Absolom DR, Moore LL, et al. Effect of temperature on the chemotaxis, phagocytic engulfment, digestion and O_2 consumption of human polymorphonuclear leukocytes. J Reticuloendothel Soc 1980; 27:561-565

12. Kuhn LR. Effect of elevated body temperature on Cryptococcus in mice. Proc Soc Exp Biol Med 1949; 71:341

13. Mackowiak PA. Direct effects of hyperthermia on pathogenic micro-organisms: teleologic implications with regard to fever. Rev Infect Dis 1981; 3:508-520

14. Mackowiak PA, Marling-Cason M, Cohen RL. Effects of temperature on antimicrobial susceptibility of bacteria. J Infect Dis 1982; 145:550-553

15. Sugimura T, Fujimoto T, Motoyama H, et al. Risks of antipyretics in young children with fever due to infectious disease. Acta Paediatr Jpn 1994; 36:375-378

16. Mackowiak PA, Plaisance KI. Benefits and risks of antipyretic therapy. Ann NY Acad Sci 1989; 856:214-223

17. Mackowiak PA. Assaulting a physiological response. Antibiotics for Clinicians 1998; 4:82-84.

18. Mackowiak PA. Fever: blessing or curse? Ann Intern Med 1994; 120:1037-1040

19. Graham MH, Burrell CJ, Douglas RM, et al. Adverse effects of aspirin, acetaminophen, and ibuprofen on immune function, viral shedding, and clinical status in rhinovirus-infected volunteers. J Infect Dis 1990; 162:1277-82

20. Sawari AR, Mackowiak PA. The pharmacologic consequences of fever. Infect Dis Clin North Am 1996; 10:21-32

21. Shann F. Antipyretics in severe sepsis. Lancet 1995; 345:338

22. Styrt B, Sugarman B. Antipyresis and fever. Arch Intern Med 1990; 150:1589-1597

23. Plaisance KI, Mackowiak PA. Antipyretic therapy: physiologic rationale, diagnostic implications, and clinical consequences. Arch Intern Med 2000; 160:449-456

24. Cunha BA, Shea KW. Fever in the intensive care unit. Infect Dis Clin North Am 1996; 10:185-209

25. Cunha BA. Fever in the intensive care unit. Intensive Care Med 1999; 25:648-651

26. Cunha BA. The diagnostic approach to rash and fever in the CCU. Crit Care Clin 1998; 8:35-54

27. Cunha BA. Clinical approach to fever in the CCU. Crit Care Clin 1998; 8:1-14

28. Cunha BA. The diagnostic significance of relative bradycardia. Intern Med 1999; 20:42-46

29. Cunha BA. The clinical significance of fever patterns. Infect Dis Clin North Am 1996; 10:33-44

30. Albrecht RF 2nd, Wass CT, Lanier WL. Occurrence of potentially detrimental temperature alterations in hospitalized patients at risk for brain injury. Mayo Clin Proc 1998; 73:629-635

31. Done AK. Treatment of fever in 1982: a review. Am J Med 1983; 74:27-35

32. Klein NC, Cunha BA. Treatment of fever. Infect Dis Clin North Am 1996; 10:211-216

33. Pernerstorfer T, Schmid R, Bieglmayer C, et al. Acetaminophen has greater antipyretic efficacy than aspirin in endotoxemia: a randomized, double-blind, placebo-controlled trial. Clin Pharmacol Ther 1999; 66:51-57

34. Mackowiak PA, Browne RH, Southern PM Jr, et al. Polymicrobial sepsis: analysis of 184 cases using log linear models. Am J Med Sci 1980; 280:73-80

35. Bryant RE, Hood AF, Hood CE, et al. Factors affecting mortality of gram-negative rod bacteremia. Arch Intern Med 1971; 127:120-128

41

ANTI-CYTOKINE THERAPY

Edward Abraham

Multiple cytokines have been identified as playing a role in the response to endotoxin, bacterermia, exposure to gram positive cell wall products, such as peptidoglycans, or other infectious challenges. However, the role of only two of these cytokines, interleukin (IL)-1 and tumor necrosis factor (TNF)-α, in contributing to sepsis associated mortality has been directly investigated in clinical studies (Table 1).

AGENT	NUMBER OF PATIENTS ENROLLED IN EACH TRIAL OF THE AGENT [ref]
IL-1ra	99 [22], 893 [23], 696 [24]
Anti-TNF-α monoclonal antibodies	
Murine anti-TNF	971 [28], 564 [29], 1879 [30]
Murine anti-TNF-α Fab₂' fragments	122 [31], 39 [32], 446 [33]
Humanized chimeric anti-TNF	42 [27], 56 [35]
TNF receptor fusion proteins	
p75 TNF receptor fusion protein	141 [34]
p55 TNF receptor fusion protein	498 [17], 1340 (Abraham, unpublished data)

Table 1. Anti-cytokine therapies examined in sepsis

In part, the focus on IL-1 and TNF-α occurred because of the central role that these cytokines were thought to play in endotoxemia-induced organ system dysfunction. Compared to IL-1 and TNF, no other cytokine produced dramatic decreases in blood pressure and organ dysfunction, similar to the pathophysiologic parameters of septic shock in animals or in humans. Additionally, the impressive improvements in survival that occurred in preclinical models of endotoxemia and Gram-negative bacteremia when these cytokines were blocked motivated the initiation of clinical trials to explore anti-IL-1 and anti-TNF-α therapies.

In the absence of infection, high doses of TNF administered to animals induces circulatory collapse and organ dysfunction similar to those observed in humans with septic shock [1]. Infusion of large amounts of IL-1 also causes hypotension, increases cardiac output, and decreases peripheral vascular resistance [1]. Injecting a combination of low doses of IL-1 plus TNF shows synergistic effects of the two cytokines in inducing shock [1]. The findings in animal models were confirmed when humans were injected with either IL-1 or TNF as cancer chemotherapy [2-4], the most impressive physiologic consequence of which was the fall in blood pressure. The hypotension was dose-dependent and, despite a short plasma half-life of less than 10 minutes, the biological consequences could be observed for days.

The biological basis for the development of organ dysfunction or hypotension as a response to increased release of IL-1 or TNF has been established at the molecular level. Both cytokines activate the transcription of genes that increase the production of small, potent, proinflammatory mediator molecules. For example, IL-1 and TNF increase gene expression and synthesis for phospholipase A_2 leading to increased platelet activating factor (PAF) synthesis [5]. Similarly, an increase in cyclooxygenase type II (COX-2) by IL-1 or TNF results in elevated levels of prostaglandin E_2 (PGE_2) [6-8]. Nitric oxide (NO) is a potent vasodilator and thought to be primarily responsible for the hypotension and myocardial suppression in septic shock [9]. IL-1 or TNF activate gene expression and synthesis of inducible NO synthase (iNOS) [1, 10-13]. Interaction of IL-1 or TNF-α with their membrane associated receptors results in increased activation of the transcriptional regulatory factor nuclear factor-kappa B (NF-κB), leading to increased transcription of multiple proinflammatory and immunomodulatory genes.

Neutralizing TNF activity with antibodies [14-16] or soluble receptor fusion constructs [17], or blocking IL-1 receptors [18,19] was effective in preventing death in animal models of lethal bacteremia or endotoxemia. The logical clinical conclusion from these data was that reducing the biological effects of systemic TNF or IL-1 would reduce the risk of dying from septic shock since these cytokines appeared to be essential for the manifestation of the disease.

INTERLEUKIN-1 RECEPTOR ANTAGONIST (IL-1ra)

IL-1ra is a naturally occurring inhibitor of IL-1, which competitively binds to the IL-1 receptor [18,19]. In pre-clinical studies, primarily involving rabbits and mice, infusion of IL-1ra starting before or shortly after the onset of endotoxemia or bacteremia improve survival [18,19]. Interestingly, in baboon studies [20,21], IL-1ra therapy appears to have a minimal effect in blunting endotoxemia-induced increases in IL-6, TNF-α, or circulating levels of TNF receptors, suggesting that, in primates, IL-1 may not have a central role in the sepsis induced inflammatory response.

The initial Phase II study examining IL-1ra in sepsis was an unblinded, dose-ranging trial in patients with sepsis-induced organ failure [22]. In that clinical trial, in which 99 patients were enrolled, a dramatic decrease in mortality was found in patients treated with the highest dose of IL-1ra examined, 133 mg/hr. There also appeared to be a statistically significant relationship between IL-1ra dose and outcome. Mortality at day 28 in the placebo group was 44% and decreased to 16% in patients treated with the highest dose of IL-1ra. Additionally, there were decreases in APACHE II scores and IL-6 levels that appeared to be related to the dose of IL-1ra administered. The study has been criticized since it was unblinded and also because of imbalances between patient groups, with the placebo group being older and with higher APACHE II scores than the patients receiving high dose IL-1ra.

A subsequent Phase III study of IL-1ra enrolled 893 patients into three groups, placebo, 1 mg/kg/hr, and 2 mg/kg/hr [23]. There was no significant increase in survival time in septic patients receiving IL-1ra compared to placebo. Similarly, there was no significant improvement in survival associated with IL-1ra treatment in patients with shock at study entry. In a secondary analysis, there appeared to be improvement in survival time with IL-1ra treatment among patients with an APACHE III predicted risk of mortality of 24% or greater, or dysfunction of one or more organs, defined as ARDS, DIC, renal dysfunction, or hepatobiliary dysfunction.

A third clinical trial with IL-1ra was designed to investigate the utility of such therapy (2 mg/kg/hr IL-1ra versus placebo) in patients with organ dysfunction or high predicted risk of mortality at study entry [24]. The study was stopped for lack of efficacy at the interim analysis, after 696 patients were enrolled. The 28-day, all-cause mortality rate was 33.1% in the IL-1ra treatment group and 36.4% in the placebo group, a 9% relative reduction with IL-1ra (p = 0.36). There were no significant differences between the IL-1ra and placebo groups when analyzed on the basis of shock, organ dysfunction, or predicted risk of mortality at study entry.

The inability of IL-1ra to provide benefit to septic patients may be because

IL-1 does not occupy a central, pivotal role in perpetuating the inflammatory response and producing organ system dysfunction in human sepsis, as was suggested by the baboon endotoxemia studies [20,21] reviewed above. Additionally, the failure of IL-1ra to reduce mortality may reflect a timing issue, generic in sepsis studies. In particular, even if IL-1 is important in initiating a proinflammatory response, its role may be minimal by the time the patients are recognized and entered into a clinical trial. Indeed, very few septic patients have elevated plasma levels of IL-1, so the number of patients who truly had increased IL-1 tissue expression at the time of enrollment into the IL-1ra studies is unknown. Such information is of obvious importance because therapies inhibiting IL-1 would be expected to have a beneficial effect only in patients with increased expression of this cytokine.

ANTI-TUMOR NECROSIS FACTOR THERAPIES

The two major approaches taken to neutralizing TNF have involved either monoclonal anti-TNF antibodies or fusion protein constructs in which the extramembrane portion of the p55 (Type I) or p75 (Type II) TNF receptor is joined to the Fc fragment of a human IgG1 antibody. Pretreatment of animals with anti-TNF-α antibodies or TNF receptor fusion protein constructs before administration of endotoxin, Gram-negative, or Gram-positive bacteria generally results in improvement in survival and amelioration of organ system dysfunction [14-16,25]. However, there is lack of efficacy of anti-TNF antibodies noted in some, but not all, models of peritonitis. There is limited evidence that administration of anti-TNF-α antibodies at the time of initiation of the Gram-negative or -positive bacteremic insult or even shortly thereafter (i.e., within the first hour) is still associated with a significant survival benefit [25]. However, the use of such antibodies at later time points in endotoxemic or bacteremic models does not appear to be associated with any clear benefit.

Small human studies [26,27] suggested that anti-TNF-α antibody therapy improved certain physiologic parameters, such as cardiac output. Additionally, there was evidence that the administration of anti-TNF-α antibodies resulted in more rapid decreases in plasma concentrations of cytokines, such as IL-6, in septic patients. However, these studies were too small to detect any survival benefit.

The initial study powered to examine day 28 survival with monoclonal anti-TNF-α antibodies was the North American Sepsis Trial (NORASEPT I), which used a murine IgG1 monoclonal antibody and separate randomization lists for patients with severe sepsis without hypotension and for those with septic shock [28]. A total of 994 patients were enrolled, of which approximately half were in shock at the time of randomization. Overall, there was no statistically significant benefit associated with anti-TNF therapy. However, in the prospectively defined subgroup of patients with septic shock, a statistically significant reduction in mortality was present during the first 2 weeks after administration of monoclonal anti-TNF-α antibody compared to placebo. At day 28 after anti-TNF-α therapy, the reduction in mortality among septic shock patients was 17% compared to those receiving placebo. By contrast, no benefit was found with anti-TNF-α therapy in patients not in shock at study entry.

In the NORASEPT I shock patients, the beneficial effect of anti-TNF-α antibodies on survival appeared within the first 24 hours after enrollment; the greatest separation between the survival curves for placebo and anti-TNF antibody-treated patients occurred during this time. Approximately 60% of the placebo deaths occurred within the first 3 days of the study. Treatment with 7.5 mg/kg monoclonal anti-TNF-α antibodies was associated with a 49% reduction in mortality versus placebo at day 3 after study enrollment.

A second study, the International Sepsis Trial (INTERSEPT), using the same murine monoclonal anti-TNF-α antibody as NORASEPT I, was undertaken in 14 primarily European countries [29]. Although the INTERSEPT study initially enrolled septic patients with and without shock, after the results of NORASEPT I were available, only shock patients were entered into INTERSEPT. A total of 564 patients, of which 420 were in septic shock, were enrolled. Day 28 mortality was reduced by 14.5% in patients who received 3 mg/kg monoclonal anti-TNF-α antibody, with no reduction in mortality found in those receiving 15 mg/kg. There was no evidence of early survival benefit (i.e. within the first 3 days after anti-TNF antibody infusion), a finding that was different from that seen in NORASEPT I. Additionally, whereas 60% of the placebo deaths among patients in shock occurred within the first 3 study days in NORASEPT I, fewer than 45% of placebo deaths occurred within this period in the INTERSEPT study.

A third study (NORASEPT II) was designed to test the hypothesis that therapy with 7.5 mg/kg of the murine monoclonal anti-TNF-α antibody used in NORASEPT I and INTERSEPT was beneficial in patients with septic shock [30]. NORASEPT II enrolled 1879 patients in 105 hospitals in the USA and Canada that were randomized to 7.5 mg/kg of anti-TNF-α antibody or placebo. No improvement in survival was found in the actively treated group, all-cause mortality at day 28 being 40.3% in monoclonal anti-TNF-α antibody treated patients compared to 42.8% in those receiving placebo. Approximately 40% of the patients had detectable circulating TNF-α concentrations at enrollment, and in this group 41.3% of the anti-TNF-α treated patients died as compared to 45.6% of the placebo treated patients ($p = 0.20$).

Even though the APACHE II scores, day 28 mortality rates, gender ratio, and percentage of patients with one or more organ failures present at baseline were similar in NORASEPT I and NORASEPT II, there did appear to be substantial differences in patient survival patterns. Whereas more than 60% of the deaths in the placebo arm of NORASEPT I occurred in the first 3 days after study entry, the mean time to death in the placebo group of NORASEPT II was delayed, averaging 6.8 days. There are many reasons for the disparity in early mortality rates in NORASEPT I and II. It is possible that there were subtle differences in the patient populations that affected mortality in the two studies, without affecting APACHE II score or organ failures at baseline. However, another explanation is that the differences in survival between the two studies may reflect improvements in supportive care, resulting in better survival from the initial hypotensive episode, a period where proinflammatory cytokine release, including that for TNF-α, may be greatest. If advances in management have permitted critically ill septic patients to better survive the initial state of accelerated cytokine expression, this would diminish the efficacy of therapies aimed at modulating the early proinflammatory response.

An additional concern in interpreting the NORASEPT II data revolves about the efficacy of the anti-TNF antibody used. Even though only a minority of patients had detectable levels of circulating TNF-α at baseline and post-treatment time points, review of post-treatment plasma TNF-α levels showed continued presence of circulating TNF-α in the antibody treated group. Therefore, a question remains as to the ability of the anti-TNF antibody employed in the doses used in NORASEPT I, INTERSEPT, and NORASEPT II to actually block cytokine activity.

The utility of administering $F(ab')_2$ fragments of a murine IgG3 monoclonal antibody to TNF-α has been examined in patients with severe sepsis or septic shock [31,32]. In the initial clinical trial [31], 122 septic patients were enrolled, and no improvement in survival was detected in the overall group of patients receiving anti-TNF treatment. However, a retrospective stratification of patients according to their plasma IL-6 concentrations suggested beneficial effects for the drug in patients (n = 37) with baseline levels greater than 1000 pg/ml. In patients with IL-6 levels greater than 1000 pg/ml, mortality decreased from 80% in the placebo group to 35% in patients who received the highest dose (1 mg/kg) of the anti-TNF-α therapy. Two larger unpublished studies in Europe and North America have shown an aggregate reduction of mortality of approximately 3.5% for patients receiving anti-TNF-α antibody fragments. Interestingly, in the recently completed study, which enrolled more than 2200 patients and stratified the patients dependent on baseline IL-6 levels of less or greater than 1000 pg/ml, similar reductions in mortality were found irrespective of IL-6 levels. Such data, indicating that IL-6 level does not predict response to anti-TNF therapy, is consistent with results from NORASEPT II and studies examining the p55 TNF receptor fusion protein complex [17].

Three clinical studies have reported results using soluble TNF receptor constructs as anti-TNF agents. In the first of these [34], the molecule used consisted of the extramembrane components of the human type II (p75) receptor joined to the Fc portion of a human IgG1 antibody molecule. Patients (n = 141) with septic shock, with or without associated organ system dysfunction, were entered into the study. A significant dose dependent increase in mortality was found in patients treated with this p75 soluble TNF receptor construct, with mortality rising from 30% in the placebo group to 53% in the patients treated with the highest dose (1.5 mg/kg) of the TNF receptor fusion protein. There was no evidence that baseline differences in the severity of illness contributed to the increased mortality in the groups receiving the higher doses of the p75 receptor complex.

The enhanced mortality associated with treatment with the p75 TNF receptor molecule may be related to the extremely high doses used in the study. Although potency estimates are difficult to quantitate, soluble TNF receptor fusion proteins appear to inactivate TNF-α more than fifty times as effectively as the monoclonal antibodies [17], so that therapy with a dose of 1.5 mg/kg of the p75 TNF receptor fusion protein would be expected to completely neutralize TNF-α for a prolonged period, especially given the long half life of the compound (> 60 hours). TNF-α participates in normal inflammatory responses, and prolonged neutralization of its activity may have potent immunosuppressive effects leading to increased mortality. However, an additional issue with the p75 TNF receptor fusion protein complex is the ability of this construct to act as a carrier protein, releasing bioactive TNF. In particular, whereas interaction of TNF-α with monoclonal antibodies or the p55 TNF receptor fusion protein complex appears to be essentially irreversible, such is not the case with the p75 complex, where bioactive TNF apparently can be released after association with this fusion protein. Although late release of TNF was not specifically examined in the study using the p75 fusion protein complex, there was no late increase in plasma IL-6 levels after administration of the p75 TNF receptor fusion protein, indicating that therapy with this molecule did not produce an excessively potentiated or prolonged inflammatory response.

Two clinical trials have examined the role of a p55 TNF receptor fusion protein construct in septic patients [17,34]. In the initial 498 patient study, separate randomization lists were used for patients with severe sepsis with or without early shock, and for those with refractory septic shock (defined as hypotension unresponsive to fluids and requiring vasopressors for at least 2 hours) [11]. The doses of the p55 TNF receptor complex used, 0.008 mg/kg, 0.042 mg/kg, and 0.08 mg/kg, were all lower than the lowest dose of the p75 TNF receptor fusion protein administered [34]. Therapy with 0.08 mg/kg of the p55 TNF receptor fusion protein complex, but not other doses, was associated with a 36% reduction (p = 0.07) in day 28 mortality in the prospectively defined patient group with severe sepsis with or without early septic shock. By contrast, no beneficial effects were apparent with any dose of the p55 receptor complex in patients with refractory septic shock.

Because of the apparent benefit of the p55 TNF receptor fusion protein in severe sepsis with or without early septic shock, a 1340 patient, Phase III study was undertaken in this patient population (Abraham, unpublished data). No improvement in day 28 all cause mortality or in surrogate endpoints, such as organ failure scores, was found in patients treated with the p55 TNF receptor construct compared to placebo. The p55 TNF receptor fusion protein used in the Phase III study was from a different batch than the Phase II study, with differences in glycosylation, and had slightly lower TNF neutralizing ability, so that higher doses (approximately 0.125 mg/kg) were used. It is unknown what role, if any, these alterations in molecular structure or binding potency played in the different outcomes between the Phase II and Phase III clinical trials.

CONCLUSION

Agents able to neutralize the effects of IL-1 or TNF have impressive effects in preclinical models of endotoxemia or sepsis. However, the ability of such therapies to reduce mortality or morbidity in critically ill septic patients appears to be, at best, very limited. Although it is simply possible that neither TNF-α nor IL-1 play an important role in clinical sepsis, it is more likely that the disappointing results of clinical trials reflects the heterogeneity of patient populations recruited into such studies. Both IL-1 and TNF-α are likely to be elevated early in proinflammatory cascades initiated by infection. These cytokines may be less important in perpetuating inflammatory processes once organ system dysfunction develops. In no study were patients identified and enrolled based on documented elevations in tissue or circulating levels of IL-1 or TNF-α. Therefore, it is difficult to know if the patients enrolled actually had excessive production of the cytokines being blocked. However, in the NORASEPT II study [30], a retrospective analysis of patients with detectable circulating TNF-α levels only showed a relative decrease in mortality of 9% in patients treated with anti-TNF-α antibodies. These results would suggest that even if septic patients with elevated TNF-α could be identified, the impact of anti-TNF-α therapies would be relatively modest.

REFERENCES

1. Okusawa S, Gelfand JA, Ikejima T, et al. Interleukin 1 induces a shock-like state in rabbits. Synergism with tumor necrosis factor and the effect of cyclooxygenase inhibition. J Clin Invest 1988; 81:1162-1172
2. Chapman PB, Lester TJ, Casper ES, et al . Clinical pharmacology of recombinant human tumor necrosis factor in patients with advanced cancer. J Clin Oncol 1987;5:1942-1951
3. Smith JW, Urba WJ, Curti BD, et al. The toxic and hematologic effects of interleukin-1 alpha administered in a phase I trial to patients with advanced malignancies. J Clin Oncol 1992;10:1141-1152
4. Van der Poll T, Buller HR, ten Cate HT. Activation of coagulation after administration of TNF to normal subjects. N Engl J Med 1990;322: 1622-1627
5. Endo S, Inada K, Nakae H, et al. Plasma levels of type II phospholipase A2 and cytokines in patients with sepsis. Res Comm Mol Path Pharmacol 1995;90:413-421
6. Diaz A, Chepenik KP, Korn JH, et al. Differential regulation of cyclooxygenases 1 and 2 by interleukin-1β, tumor necrosis factor-α, and transforming growth factor-β1 in human lung fibroblasts. Exp Cell Res 1998; 241:222-229.
7. Newton R, Stevens DA, Hart LA, et al. Superinduction of COX-2 mRNA by cycloheximide and interleukin-1β involves increased transcription and correlates with increased NF-κB and JNK activation. FEBS Letters 1997; 418:135-138
8. Guan Z, Baier LD, Morrison AR. p38 mitogen-activated protein kinase down-regulates nitric oxide and up-regulates prostaglandin E2 biosynthesis stimulated by interleukin-1β. J Biol Chem 1997; 272:8083-8089
9. Moncada S, Palmer RMJ, Higgs EA. Nitric oxide: physiology, pathophysiology, and pharmacology. Pharmacol Rev 1991; 43:109-142
10. Dinarello CA. Biological basis for interleukin-1 in disease. Blood 1996; 87:2095-2147
11. Heremans H, van Damme J, Dillen C, et al. Interferon-γ, a mediator of lethal lipopolysaccharide-induced Shwartzman-like shock in mice. J Exp Med 1990; 171:1853-1861
12. Huang S, Hendriks W, Althage A, et al. Immune response in mice that lack the interferon-gamma receptor. Science 1993; 259:1742-1745
13. Car BD, Eng VM, Schnyder B, Ozmen L, et al. Interferon gamma receptor deficient mice are resistant to endotoxic shock. J Exp Med 1994; 179: 1437-1444
14. Tracey KJ, Fong Y, Hesse DG, et al. Anti-cachectin/TNF monoclonal antibodies prevent septic shock during lethal bacteremia. Nature 1987; 330: 662-664
15. Fong Y, Tracey KJ, Moldawer LL, et al. Antibodies to cachectin/TNF reduce interleukin-1 and interleukin-6 appearance during lethal bacteremia. J Exp Med 1989; 170:1627-1633
16. Hinshaw LB, Tekamp-Olson P, Chang AC, et al. Survival of primates in LD_{100} septic shock following therapy with antibody to tumor necrosis factor (TNF). Circ Shock 1990; 30:279-292
17. Abraham E, Glauser MP, Butler T, et al. p55 tumor necrosis factor receptor fusion protein in the treatment of patients with severe sepsis and septic shock. JAMA 1997; 277: 1531-1534
18. Ohlsson K, Bjork P, Bergenfeldt M, et al. Interleukin-1 receptor antagonist reduces mortality from endotoxin shock. Nature 1990; 348:550-552
19. Wakabayashi G, Gelfand JA, Burke JF, et al. A specific receptor antagonist for interleukin-1 prevents Escherichia coli-induced shock. FASEB J 1991; 5:338-343
20. Hawes AS, Fischer E, Marano MA, et al. Comparison of peripheral blood leukocyte kinetics after live Escherichia coli, endotoxin, or interleukin-1 alpha administration. Studies using a novel interleukin-1 receptor antagonist. Ann Surg 1993; 218:79-90

21. Fischer E, Marano MA, Van Zee KJ, et al. Interleukin-1 receptor blockade improves survival and hemodynamic performance in Escherichia coli septic shock, but fails to alter host responses to sublethal endotoxemia. J Clin Invest 1992; 89:1551-1557

22. Fisher CJ Jr., Slotman GJ, Opal SM, et al. Initial evaluation of human recombinant interleukin-1 receptor antagonist in the treatment of sepsis syndrome: a randomized, open-label, placebo-controlled multicenter trial. The IL-1RA Sepsis Syndrome Study Group. Crit Care Med 1994; 22:12-21

23. Fisher CJ Jr., Dhainaut JF, Opal SM, et al. Recombinant human interleukin 1 receptor antagonist in the treatment of patients with sepsis syndrome. Results from a randomized, double-blind, placebo-controlled trial. Phase III rhIL-1ra Sepsis Syndrome Study Group. JAMA 1994; 271:1836-1843

24. Opal SM, Fisher CJ, Pribble JP, et al. The confirmatory interleukin-1 receptor antagonist trial in severe sepsis: a phase III randomized, double-blind, placebo-controlled, multicenter trial. Crit Care Med 1997; 25:1115-1124

25. Hinshaw LB, Emerson TE Jr., Taylor FB Jr, et al. Lethal S. aureus shock in primates: prevention of death with anti-TNF antibody. J Trauma 1992; 33:568-573

26. Vincent JL, Bakker J, Marecaux G, et al. Administration of anti-TNF antibody improves left ventricular function in septic shock patients. Results of a pilot study. Chest 1992; 101: 810-815

27. Dhainaut J-F A, Vincent J-L, Richard C, et al. CDP571, a humanized antibody to human tumor necrosis factor-α: Safety, pharmacokinetics, immune response, and influence of the antibody on cytokine concentrations in patients with septic shock Crit Care Med 1995; 23:1461-1469

28. Abraham E, Wunderink R, Silverman H, et al. Monoclonal antibody to human tumor necrosis factor alpha (TNF MAb): Efficacy and safety in patients with the sepsis syndrome. JAMA 1995; 273:934-941

29. Cohen J, Carlet J. INTERSEPT: An international, multicenter, placebo-controlled trial of monoclonal antibody to human tumor necrosis factor-α in patients with sepsis. Crit Care Med 1996; 24:1431-1440

30. Abraham E, Anzueto A, Gutierrez G, et al. Monoclonal antibody to human tumor necrosis factor alpha (TNF Mab) in the treatment of patients with septic shock: A multi-center, placebo controlled, randomized, double-blind clinical trial. Lancet 1998; 351:929-933

31. Reinhart K, Wiegand-Lohnert C, Grimminger F, et al. Assessment of the safety and efficacy of the monoclonal anti-tumor necrosis factor antibody-fragment, MAK 195F, in patients with sepsis and septic shock: A multicenter, randomized, placebo-controlled, dose-ranging study. Crit Care Med 1996; 24: 733-742

32. Zeni F, Freeman B, Natanson C. Anti-inflammatory therapies to treat sepsis and septic shock: a reassessment. Crit Care Med 1997; 25:1095-1100

33. Natanson C, Esposito CJ, Banks SM. The sirens' songs of confirmatory sepsis trials: selection bias and sampling error. Crit Care Med 1998; 26:1927-1931

34. Fisher CJ Jr., Agosti JM, Opal SM, et al. Treatment of septic shock with the tumor necrosis factor receptor Fc fusion protein. N Engl J Med 1996; 334:1697-1702

35. Clark MA, Plank LD, Connolly AB, et al. Effect of a chimeric antibody to tumor necrosis factor-α on cytokine and physiologic responses in patients with severe sepsis – a randomized, clinical trial. Crit Care Med 1998; 26:1650-1659

42

HEAT SHOCK PROTEINS AND SEPSIS: A HOT STORY

Jesús Villar
Arthur S. Slutsky

Sepsis represents one of the most challenging problems in the field of intensive care medicine. Even with the use of powerful anti-microbial agents, sepsis continues to represent the most common cause of multiple system organ dysfunction and death in most patients admitted to intensive care units. Cumulative experimental and clinical evidence indicates a major role for cytokine production and systemic effects of sepsis-induced inflammatory responses. Thus, blocking cytokine activation and/or pharmacological effects with specific cytokine-receptor antagonists represents a logical strategy for the treatment or attenuation of sepsis-related inflammation [1-3]. While strategies which make it possible to selectively down-regulate the effects of specific cytokines would be particularly attractive from the therapeutic perspective, achieving this objective is far from straightforward since the effects of specific cytokine inhibition *in vivo* has been demonstrated to be extremely unpredictable. For example, despite data from animal studies showing the dramatic efficacy of antibodies against endotoxin and tumor necrosis factor (TNF)-α, and interleukin (IL)-1 receptor antagonist (IL-1ra) in the treatment of sepsis, corresponding beneficial effects have not been observed in recent human trials [4,5]. Accordingly, it appears that information concerning cytokine biology will need to be considerably enhanced before the development of a 'magic bullet' that attenuates inflammatory responses during organ injury and prevents organ dysfunction.

In previous chapters of this book the cellular events involved in organ inflammation have been extensively discussed; damage and repair are ultimately controlled at the molecular level and cannot be fully understood without consideration of the functions of the relevant genes and their products. It is now widely recognized that various cellular stimuli mediate physiologic effects by the induction of complex intracellular signalling cascades which culminate in the activation or induction of a particular gene or subset of genes. As a result, activation leads to the synthesis of particular sets of proteins and a consequent change in cellular behavior. Cytokines are a critical set of proteins involved in directing the inflammatory response with a direct or indirect influence on tissue damage or repair. Depending on the nature of the pathological perturbation, these steps represent potential targets for intervention and potentially novel therapeutic strategies.

THE UNIVERSAL HEAT SHOCK OR STRESS RESPONSE

During their life span, all living organisms are exposed to environmental stresses to which they must adapt with varying degrees of structural and functional changes in order to survive. All forms of life on Earth, from bacteria to man, have evolved mechanisms of response to maintain homeostasis in the face of diverse and complex environmental stresses which can jeopardise their survival. The oldest response is the heat shock or stress response. The heat shock response is a complex, transient reprogramming of cellular activities which: i) protects essential cell components from irreversible stress injury; ii) helps to ensure survival during the stress period; and iii) allows a rapid and complete resumption of normal cellular activities in the recovery period [6]. The general theme of the stress response is the rapid and almost exclusive transcription and translation of a set of highly conserved proteins known as the heat shock or stress proteins (HSP); concomitantly, there is a corresponding decrease in the production of most other cellular polypeptides [6,7].

The heat shock response was originally described in 1962 by Ritossa, an Italian scientist, as a phenomenon of inducible gene expression after brief heat treatment of *Drosophila* larvae, as judged by the changes in puffing patterns observed in the salivary gland polytene chromosomes [8]. These observations, although initially considered to be experimental tricks, opened the way to the description of a general stress response system in eukaryotic cells with the discovery of the HSP in 1974 by Tissières et al. [9]. Almost two dozen proteins are induced in response to a range of different stresses. The best studied of these stresses is heat shock. Mammalian cells have been shown to synthesize HSPs after a brief period of hyperthermia at temperatures 3-5°C above normal body temperature. HSP induction is observed both *in vivo* and *in vitro*. Besides heat shock, the induction of the heat stress response can be achieved by hypoxia, glucose starvation followed by refeeding, ethanol, sodium arsenite, cadmium, dexamethasone, heavy exercise, viral infection and agents which affect cell cycle [6]. HSPs may be induced directly by such agents or indirectly, by virtue of increased expression of other proteins which in turn provoke HSP gene expression. Thus for example, increases in HSP expression in injured cardiac muscle cells have been linked to increases in TNF-α and IL-1 production [10]. Synthesis of almost all HSPs can be detected in normal, unstressed cells, thereby implicating their probable participation in cellular processes distinct from physiological stress. The formation of induced HSP is usually dependent on a concomitant formation of new cytoplasmic mRNA. This finding is supported by the observation that HSP synthesis is inhibited by actinomycin D [6].

HSPs are classified into five protein families based on molecular mass in SDS (sodium dodecyl sulfate) polyacrylamide gels. These include the large molecular weight HSPs (100 kD), the HSP90 family, the highly conserved HSP70 family which represents the most prominent eukaryotic group of HSPs, the HSP 60 family which is found in bacteria, chloroplasts, and mitochondria, and the small HSP family, expressed predominantly in plants. Comparison of the sequences of the respective heat shock genes from bacteria, plants, flies, and man, have indicated these genes to be among the most highly conserved proteins in nature. All major HSP genes have been cloned and investigated by restriction mapping and sequence analysis. Pairwise comparisons of HSP sequences from almost any two organisms reveals that about half of the amino acids residues are identical and that many of the remaining residues are similar. The ancestors of humans and mycobacteria diverged about 1500 million years ago but their HSP65 have identical amino acids in about 50% of the protein sequence and the similarity approaches 65% when conservative substitutes are included. The HSP70 of drosophila and yeast have a 72% amino acid identity and their HSP 84 have a 63% identity. The derived protein sequence of a human HSP70 gene is found to be 73% homologous with *drosophila* HSP70 and that from maize is 68% homologous[11].

With few exceptions, HSP70 is a constitutive protein of eukaryotic cells, part of it being closely associated with the microtubular and intermediate filament cytoskeletal systems and with the plasma membrane. Four members of the human HSP70 protein family have been identified: HSP70, HSP72, HSP73, and grp78 [12]. At least ten HSP70 related genes have been found in human cells, some of which map between the complement and TNF-α and β genes on chromosome 6. HSP70 is both the major heat-inducible protein and a cell cycle regulated protein. HSP72 is a protein expressed only after heat shock. HSP73 is constitutively expressed at high levels in growing cells.

Grp78 is a glucose-regulated protein located in the endoplasmic reticulum. HSP have been identified as components of the plasma membrane, the Golgi apparatus, cytoplasmic mRNP, the nucleus and the nucleolus. Moreover, HSP70 is an integral component of the cytoskeleton which may be a primary target of heat stress or shock treatments.

HEAT SHOCK PROTEINS ARE RESPONSIBLE FOR ACQUISITION OF STRESS TOLERANCE AND SURVIVAL

The HSPs appear to manifest many diverse functions. HSP genes have been implicated in a variety of cellular processes which include DNA replication, the transport of proteins across membranes, the assembly or disassembly of protein complexes, the binding of proteins in the endoplasmic reticulum, and the uncoating of coated vesicles. The finding that HSP70-related proteins reside in the endoplasmic reticulum and in mitochondria and that HSP70 is translocated into the nucleus upon heat shock suggests that 70 kDa proteins perform important functions in all cellular compartments. The induction of the HSP genes, particularly the HSP70 gene, appears to be necessary for cell division even in the absence of stress. It has been suggested for example that members of the HSP70 family act in the protection of cellular damage by binding to denatured or abnormal proteins following heat shock and thereby preventing protein aggregation.

Heat shock and other stress proteins are almost certainly involved in protecting cells from the deleterious effects of heat and other stresses. Perhaps the most compelling argument that HSPs have protective functions is the phenomenon of thermotolerance [13]. Thermotolerance represents a property of all living cells and refers to the capacity of cells to survive or recover from normally lethal exposures to abrupt, severe heat shock or stress conditions if prior to the lethal stress, the cells are exposed to a more mild or shorter period of heat/stress. It is well known that to function optimally under cellular conditions of increased temperature, proteins must retain a degree of structural flexibility that allows rapid and reversible changes in conformation and assembly [14]. By being only marginally stable at physiological temperatures, proteins clearly face the risk of significant thermal damage. Body temperatures in vertebrates span in a range from -2°C (in the case of a Antarctic notothenioid fish) to 47°C (for the desert iguana). HSP are induced at temperatures near the upper range of an organism's normal body temperature as part of an adaptative response. The basic observation is that a group of cells or organisms die rapidly when shifted directly from their normal growing temperature to a much higher temperature. However, a matched group that is given a mild preheat treatment to induce HSP dies much more slowly. For example, this approach to cellular stress has been shown to markedly reduce the extent of heat-induced central nervous system (CNS) injury [15].

Moreover, treatment with heat as the stressor can induce tolerance to other forms of stress. Accordingly, recent studies [16,17] have addressed the question as to whether the induction of the stress response might protect animals against subsequent injury. In this context, following their demonstration that a brief period of warming induced HSP72 gene and protein expression in a time-related fashion in the rat lungs (Figure 1), Villar et al. [16] examined the effects of the induction of HSP in attenuating lung damage and outcome in an animal model of acute lung injury (ALI) induced by intratracheal instillation of phospholipase A_2, a phospholipid-degrading enzyme and a potent mediator of inflammation. These authors reported that a brief exposure of experimental animals to transient hyperthermia, resulting in HSP72 protein accumulation in the rat lung, attenuated lung damage and significantly decreased mortality. Under control conditions, 27% of the unheated animals died by 48 hours after intratracheal instillation of phospholipase A_2, compared to zero mortality in the heat-treated group.

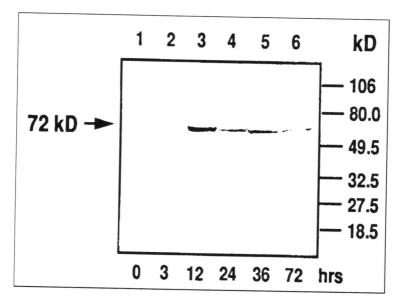

Figure 1. *Time course of HSP72 protein accumulation in rat lungs by Western analysis. HSP72 peaks between 12 and 24 hours after heating and remains at high levels up to 72 h (from [16] with permission).*

In an experimental model of hyperoxia-induced ALI, Winston et al [17] were also able to reduce mortality rate after exposing pre-heated animals to 100% oxygen for 60 hours.

An interesting clinical observation of the implications for the HSP response resulted from the potential benefits and the observed problems of localized hyperthermia as a means of cancer therapy [18]. Human and other mammalian tumor cells die after a modest degree of hypothermia of 4-8°C above normal. To be successful, this procedure will require a basic understanding of the biology of fractionated heating procedures as well as the development of the thermotolerance that will ensue. Unfortunately, the development of thermotolerance is a major impediment to the effective application of clinical hyperthermia. Chemical agents are being developed for clinical use which will increase the cell-killing powers of hyperthermia and eliminate the development of thermotolerance. Besides hyperthermia, the expression of HSP70 can be induced by oncogene products of the DNA tumor virus adenovirus 5 as well as by the rearranged c-*myc* mouse oncogene [19]. Such oncogenes are implicated in the immortalization of primary cells in culture and it may be that HSP70 has a critical role to play in animal cell growth. Irrespective of the mechanisms by which the stress response provides cytoprotection, the capacity of HSP to subserve this function is of considerable interest from the perspective of elucidating the pathophysiology of organ damage and dysfunction in different diseases states.

HEAT STRESS RESPONSE REPLIES TO THE IMMUNE SYSTEM AND KEEPS QUIET THE SYSTEMIC INFLAMMATORY RESPONSE

The observations on HSP regulation suggest that there is a connection between in vivo stress proteins and disease states. Although the mechanism for HSP-mediated cytoprotection is not completely understood, one possible explanation is that this protective effect relates to the capacity of HSPs to block the synthesis and/or release of cytokines that play key roles in the febrile and inflammatory responses to stress [20]. Immunodominant antigens from a wide variety of pathogens have been found to be HSP. The major stress protein antigen recognized by antibodies in bacterial infections is HSP60 [21]. The sequence of the DNA clones has revealed that mycobacterial HSP70 and the HSP60 are the major targets of the murine antibody response to both *Mycobacterium tuberculosis* and *M. leprae*. The high degree of sequence conservation between host and pathogen stress proteins may provide a link between infection and autoimmunity. HSP65 is a molecule that is part self and part foreign to any organism with an immnune system. It is immunologically dominant and it elicits strong immune responses in individuals infected or exposed to various bacteria. Moreover, T-cell responses to HSP65 seem to be associated with autoimmune arthritis in both rats and humans. There is some evidence to suggest that a subset of human T cells specific for the 65 kDa antigen of *M. leprae* is able to recognize the corresponding HSP in human cells [22]. Murine macrophages stressed by viral infection or interferon (IFN)-γ become targets for anti-65 kDa cytotoxic T cells. This suggests that upregulation of HSP may indeed play a role in the pathology associated with autoimmune disease.

HSP have also been identified as immune targets in most major human parasitic infections. Antibodies to HSP70 have been identified in the sera of patients suffering from malaria, trypanosomiasis, leishmaniasis, schistosomiasis, and filariasis [23]. HSP90 is a target for antibodies in trypanosomiasis and a member of the small HSP family has been recognized in some patients with schistosomiasis. During viral infections there is increased synthesis of HSP that could, of course, be simply part of a non-specific induction of host genes. However, specific host-coded HSP may play a crucial role in viral replication. All types of mutual interactions are observed: viral induction of HSP synthesis, enhanced synthesis of viral proteins, and interference of heat shock and viral stress. Whether mammalian HSP70 is required for mammalian virus replication is not yet known. The sensitivity of virus multiplication to heat stress is well documented. Heat shock inhibits virus multiplication. Brief heat shock of host cells before viral infection inhibits the subsequent replication of herpes and pseudorabies virus [6]. The synthesis of the influenza B virus M protein in mammalian cells is specifically inhibited at 39°C. The inhibitory effects of fever on viral infections result i) from inhibition of the replicase, and ii) from liberation of lysosomal enzymes including RNAses which destroy viral RNA. Hence a reduced production of viral particles is observed. On the other hand, cytotoxic T lymphocytes that recognize HSP induced by the virus could limit the spread of the virus by killing infected cells, possibly before substantial amounts of mature virus are assembled, and by secreting IFN-γ [24].

In view of these observations, could immune responses to stress proteins have a role in protection against infection? One view is that they do not, since infection by any one pathogen does not generally protect an individual against infection by another. An alternative view is that immune responses to conserved stress protein determinants that developed early in life, probably during the establishment of natural microbial flora on the skin and in the gut, could provide a general level of protection against infection. This may help to explain the observation that, for many pathogens, only a fraction of infected individuals progress to clinical disease.

Irrespective of the mechanisms by which hyperthermia provides protection against subsequent noxious exposure, these observations are of interest from the perspective of the pathophysiology and clinical importance of fever. In most hospitalized patients, body temperature is recorded at least once daily. Fever has been recognized as a manifestation of disease since the dawn of civilization in the Fertile Crescent. Hippocrates said that fevers were the worst diseases. In the Antiquity, people died of fever, not microorganisms, which were then unknown. However, in the Modern Age fever was often regarded as favorable to the patient's survival. Fever is defined as an elevation of core body temperature above the normal level (>37.5°C in humans). Irreversible cell protein denaturation occurs at 42.5°C. Fever in the absence of detectable infection is a common finding in clinical practice. Trauma, drugs, inflammatory processes, malignant diseases, burns, dehydration, cell disruption, surgery, myocardial infarction or placental detachment are among the most common clinical conditions associated with a febrile response. The normal febrile response tends to be limited both in magnitude and in duration. Core temperatures in mammals can reach 40-41°C during fever, but it has been unclear whether such temperatures benefit or harm the host.

There is no evidence that fever is detrimental or that antipyretic therapy offers any significant benefit. Currently, fever is seen in the ICU environment as portending sinister outcomes. In many cases, it is treated as the origin of, rather than the response to, an illness. Many ICU physicians and nurses believe mistakenly that lowering the fever will improve the course of the illness. The observed correlation between hyperthermia and cytoprotection is consistent with data suggesting that the failure to mount an appropriate fever response is associated with increased mortality [25]. One of the first studies to examine the significance of hyperthermia in response to a bacterial infection was done by Kluger et al [26]. They used lizards inoculated with a bacterial suspension of live *Aeromonas hydrophila* to determine whether elevation in body temperature increases the resistance of the host to this infection. Infected animals were placed in a constant temperature chamber at different ambient temperatures, ranging from 34 to 42°C. An elevation in temperature following the experimental bacterial infection resulted in a significant increase in host survival throughout a 7-day period. Within 24 hours, 50% of the lizards maintained at 38°C were dead. However, lizards maintained at 40° and 42° had only 14 and 0 percent mortality, respectively (Figure 2).

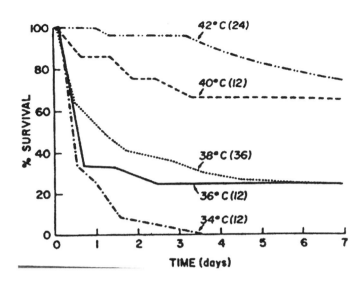

Figure 2. *Percentage survival of lizards injected with A. Hydrophila and maintained at temperatures of 34° to 42°C. The number of animals in each group is given in parentheses (From [26] with permission).*

In order to investigate whether the therapeutic benefits of fever might be engendered by HSP synthesis, Villar et al. [27] showed that thermal treatment of animals with intra-abdominal sepsis, produced by cecal ligation and perforation, induces the synthesis of HSP in the lung, heart and liver and is associated with the attenuation of organ damage and reduced mortality. This experimental model mimics many features of the human septic syndrome with the presence of enteric microorganisms and endotoxin in the blood. The authors studied two groups of animals (heated and unheated), and evaluated survival rate and pathological changes in the lung, heart and liver before and after cecal perforation, after cecum removal, and at 7 days. At 18 hours after perforation, 25% of the unheated animals died whereas none of the heated animals died. Seven days after cecal perforation, the protection was still evident, with 20% mortality compared to 70% in the non-stressed group. In addition, heated animals showed less histological evidence of lung and liver damage (Figure 3).

Since whole-body warming could be associated with a number of non-specific mechanisms unrelated to the induction of the heat shock response, Ribeiro et al [28] used sodium arsenite as a non-thermal means to induce the heat shock response and examined whether this could also provide protection in the same model of intra-abdominal sepsis. Following a single intravenous injection of sodium arsenite, HSP72 was detected in the lungs with a peak between 18 and 24 hours. Administration of 6 mg/kg of sodium arsenite 18 hours prior to performing cecal ligation and perforation was associated with a marked decrease in mortality at 18 and 24 hours after sepsis. The protection in the sodium arsenite treated animals appeared to follow the time course of HSP72 protein levels. Therefore, these studies support the hypothesis that HSPs are cytoprotective *in vivo*.

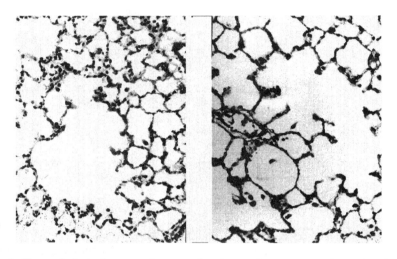

Figure 3. Histopathologic features of sepsis-induced acute lung injury. Left panel: unheated animal; representative example of the pathology of the lungs 18 hrs. after cecal ligation and perforation showing evidence of atelectasis, early hyaline membrane formation and acute inflammatory infiltrates. Right panel: heated animal; relatively normal architecture with occasional neutrophils present in the septa (HS stain x400) (from [27] with permission).

The mechanisms by which the heat shock response might provide cytoprotection are not known. However, Ribeiro et al [29] have demonstrated in endotoxin-stimulated alveolar macrophages that TNF-α levels were lower in the supernatant of LPS-treated cells, and that HSP72 coprecipitated with TNF-α from cells which had received stress treatment (heat stress and sodium arsenite) prior to endotoxin exposure. This finding suggests that HSP may participate in post-translational control of TNF-α release, binding with nascent TNF-α, and preventing its release from macrophages. Therefore, HSP determine whether TNF-α is released from the cell or is sent to the lysosomal machinery for degradation.

Several studies [30-32] have shown that the induction of the stress response by transient whole-body hyperthermia prior to the experimental sepsis can render animals resistant to the lethal effects of bacterial endotoxin. Ryan et al. [30] reported that administration of endotoxin from *E. coli* to nonheated rats resulted in 71% lethality; in contrast, all rats subjected to a single nonlethal heat stress 24 hr before endotoxin inoculation survived. This acquired resistance to endotoxin was not associated with the presence of endotoxemia immediately after the heat stress treatment. However, although they did not measure the expression of HSP, it is possible that in this model, the reduced lethality might be related to the reduced responsiveness of cells to endotoxin, resulting in reduced production of cytokines. Chu et al. [32] examined the effects of heat stress after the administration of *E. coli* endotoxin in rats. They found that survival rates in the heated animals were roughly double that of septic, unheated animals. This increase in survival could be related to the attenuation of plasma IL-1β concentrations, which were significantly lower at 2 hr after endotoxin administration in the heat stressed rats. In light of the broad cytoprotective role of heat shock response in animal models, Wong et al. [33] showed that the induction of HSP70 gene expression protected sheep pulmonary artery endothelial cells from cell death. In addition, they found inhibition of endotoxin-mediated superoxide anion generation, suggesting that an early step in endotoxin-induced apoptosis may be sensitive to HSP expression. On the other hand, the lack of HSP72 gene expression in the lungs of animals with fecal peritonitis might account for the high mortality rate of the septic insult [34]. Although the regulation of HSP expression in sepsis can be a multi-step process, Durand et al. [35] have recently reported that patients with the acute respiratory distress syndrome (ARDS) have an inability to mount a stress response, measured as HSP70 levels in blood monocytes, that correlates with disease severity and recovers over time while the patients are mechanically ventilated.

In patients with sepsis and septic shock, lactic acidosis develops as a result of organ hypoperfusion. Ischemia-reperfusion and hypoxia-reoxygenation can cause cellular damage and stress responses in several organs. Aoe et al. [36] analyzed HSP70 gene expression in the isolated rat liver exposed to various periods of ischemia/hypoxia-reperfusion. They found that HSP70 mRNA increased as the reperfusion period increased, suggesting that the accumulation of this messenger could be considered a marker of injury since it reflects the severity of reperfusion injuries. Deshpande et al. [37] have recently reported that the induction of heat shock response, prior to sepsis, markedly decreased lactate concentration in the plasma of septic rats. Several published clinical studies during the 70s and 80s showed a correlation between high levels of lactate and poor outcome in patients with sepsis and septic shock. By contrast, low levels of lactate and/or an ability to increase lactate clearance has been associated with good prognosis. Although the mechanisms by which the induction of the heat shock response might improved organ perfusion and attenuate organ damage are not fully understood, it has been demonstrated that the heat shock response inhibits cytokine-mediated expression of inducible nitric oxide synthetase (iNOS) [38]. As Deshpande et al. [37] have pointed out, organ protection may depend of the degree and duration of the heat stress. While a mild stress induces a protective response, a more potent stress stimulus induces apoptosis and an even stronger one leads to necrosis.

HEAT SHOCK PROTEINS: A NOVEL THERAPEUTIC AGENT FOR SEPSIS?

One cannot help wondering whether the genes and proteins involved in the complexities of the heat shock response might be important in human disease states and whether medically significant mutations that affect heat shock loci exist [39]. It is quite possible that this system of proteins is simply so important that such variations are incompatible with life. It has been shown that fibroblasts injected with monoclonal antibodies to HSP70 were unable to survive after a brief period of heat stress whereas cells injected with control antibodies survived a similar heat shock [40]. On the other hand, in transgenic animals engineered to express constitutively high levels of human inducible HSP70, the recovery of myocardial contractility after 30 min of ischemia is significantly better than in nontransgenic hearts. With the explosion of knowledge and technology in the fields of cellular and molecular biology, we will be able to study particular aspects of disease mechanisms in finer and finer detail. A further understanding of the role of the heat shock response may allow for the development of rational pharmacologic agents and to make them potential targets for therapeutic interventions. Future research could focus on novel strategies to turn on the HSP genes, as a potential therapy for sepsis, ALI and other critical care conditions.

ACKNOWLEDGEMENT

This work was supported in part by Fondo de Investigación Sanitaria (Spain) and the Canadian Institute of Health Research.

REFERENCES

1. Moldawer LL. Biology of proinflammatory cytokines and their antagonists. Crit Care Med 1994; 22:S3-S7
2. Thijs LG, Hack CE. Time course of cytokine levels in sepsis. Intensive Care Med 1995; 21:S258-S263
3. Christman JW, Holden EP, Blackwell TS. Strategies for blocking the systemic effects of cytokines in the sepsis syndrome. Crit Care Med 1995; 23:955-963
4. Greenman RL, Schein RMH, Martin MA, et al. A controlled clinical trial of E5 murine monoclonal IgM antibody to endotoxin in the treatment of Gram-negative sepsis. JAMA 1991; 266:1097-1102
5. Fisher CJ, Dhainaut JFA, Opal SM, et al. Recombinant human interleukin-1 receptor antagonist in the treatment of patients with sepsis syndrome. Results from a randomised, double-blind, placebo-controlled trial. JAMA 1994; 271:1836-1843
6. Nover L. Heat shock response. CRC Press, first edition, Boston, 1991
7. Burdon RH. Temperature and animal cell protein synthesis. In: Bowler K, Fuller BJ (eds) Temperature and Animal Cells. Company of Biologists Ltd, Cambridge, 1987.
8. Ritossa F. A new puffing pattern induced by temperature shock and DNP in Drosophila. Experientia 1962; 18:571-573
9. Tissiéres A, Mitchell HK, Tracy UM. Protein synthesis in salivary glands of D. melanogaster. Relation to chromosome puffs. J Mol Biol 1974; 84:389-398
10. Low-Friedrich I, Weisensee D, Mitrou P, et al. Cytokines induce stress protein formation in cultured cardiac myocytes. Basic Res Cardiol 1992; 87:12-18
11. Hunt C, Morimoto RI. Conserved features of eukaryotic HSP70 genes revealed by comparison with the nucleotide sequence of human HSP70. Proc Natl Acad Sci 1985; 82:6455-6459
12. Lindquist S, Craig EA. The heat shock proteins. Ann Rev Genet 1988; 22:631-677
13. Sanchez Y, Lindquist S. HSP104 required for induced thermotolerance. Science 1990; 248:1112-1115
14. Somero GN. Temperature and proteins: little things can mean a lot. News Physiol Sci 1996; 11:72-77
15. Barbe MF, Tytell M, Gower DJ, Welch WJ. Hyperthermia protects against light damage in the rat retina. Science 1988; 241:1817-1820
16. Villar J, Edelson JD, Post M, Mullen JBM, Slutsky AS. Induction of heat stress proteins is associated with decreased mortality in an animal model of acute lung injury. Am Rev Respir Dis 1993; 147:177-181
17. Winston BW, Villar J, Edelson JD, Piovesan J, Mullen JBM, Slutsky AS. Induction of heat stress proteins is associated with decreased mortality in an animal model of hyperoxic lung injury. Am Rev Respir Dis 1991; 143:A728 (abst)
18. Bowler K, Kashmeery AMS, Barker CJ. Heat sensitivity of tomour tissue. In: Bowler K, Fuller BJ (eds). Temperature and Animal Cells. Company of Biologists Ltd, Cambridge, 1987.
19. Burdon RH. Thermotolerance and the heat shock proteins. In: Bowler K, Fuller BJ (eds). Temperature and Animal Cells. Company of Biologists Ltd, Cambridge, 1987.
20. Villar J, Slutsky AS. Stress proteins and acute lung injury. In: Vincent JL (ed) Year Book of Intensive Care & Emergency Medicine. Springer-Verlag, Berlin, 1994, pp: 431-440
21. Shinnick TM, Vodkin MH, Williams JC. The Mycobacterium tuberculosis 65-kD antigen is a heat shock protein which corresponds to common antigen and to the Escherichia coli GroEL protein. Infect Immun 1988; 56:446-451
22. Polla BS, Young D. Heat shock proteins and immunity. Immunology Today 1989; 10(12):393-394

23. Young DB, Lathigra R, Mehlert A. Stress-induced proteins. In: Pardue ML, Feramisco JR, Lindquist S (eds), Alan R Liss Inc, New York, 1989

24. Koga T, Wand-Wurttenberg A, DeBruyn J, et al. T cells against a bacterial heat shock protein recognize stressed macrophages. Science 1989; 245:1112-1115

25. Styrt B, Sugerman B. Antipyresis and fever. Arch Intern Med 1990; 150:1589-1597

26. Kluger MJ, Ringler DH, Anver MR. Fever and survival. Science 1975; 188:166-168

27. Villar J, Ribeiro SP, Mullen JBM, Kuliszewski M, Post M, Slutsky AS. Induction of heat shock response reduces mortality rate and organ damage in a sepsis-induced acute lung injury model. Crit Care Med 1994; 22:914-921

28. Ribeiro SP, Villar J, Downey GP, Edelson JD, Slutsky AS. Sodium arsenite induces heat shock protein-72 kilodalton expression in the lungs and protects rats against sepsis. Crit Care Med 1994; 22:922-929

29. Ribeiro SP, Villar J, Downey GP, Edelson JD, Slutsky AS. Effects of the stress response in septic rats and LPS-stimulated alveolar macrophages: Evidence for TNF-α post-translational regulation. Am J Resp Crit Care Med 1996; 154:1843-1850

30. Ryan AJ, Flanagan SW, Moseley PL, Gisolfi CV. Acute heat stress protects rats against endotoxin shock. J Appl Physiol 1992; 73:1517-1522

31. Koh Y, Lim CM, Kim MJ, Shim TS, et al. Heat shock response decreases endotoxin-induced acute lung injury in rats. Respirology 1999; 4:325-330

32. Chu EK, Ribeiro SP, Slutsky AS. Heat stress increases survival rates in lipopolysaccharide-stimulated rats. Crit Care Med 1997; 25:1727-1732

33. Wong HR, Mannix RJ, Rusnak JM, et al. The heat-shock response attenuated lipopolysaccharide-mediated apoptosis in cultured sheep pulmonary artery endothelial cells. Am J Respir Cell Mol Biol 1996; 15:745-751

34. Villar J, Kuliszewski M, Ribeiro SP, Post M. Slutsky AS. Gene expression of HSP70 in the lung in an experimental model of sepsis-induced acute lung injury. Am J Respir Crit Care Med 1994; 149:A718 (Abst)

35. Durand P, Bachalet M, Brunet F, et al. Inducibility of the 70 kD heat shock protein in peripheral blood monocytes is decreased in human acute respiratory distress syndrome and recovers over time. Am J Respir Care Med 2000; 161:286-292

36. Aoe T, Inaba H, Kon S, et al. Heat shock protein 70 messenger RNA reflects the severity of ischemia/hypoxia-reperfusion injury in the perfused rat liver. Crit Care Med 1997; 25:324-329

37. Deshpande GG, Heidemann SM, Sarnaik AP. Heat stress is associated with decreased lactic acidemia in rat sepsis. Crit Care Forum 2000; 4:45-49

38. Wong HR, Ffinder JD, Wasserloos K, Pitt BR. Expression of iNOS in cultured rat pulmonary artery smooth muscle cells is inhibited by the heat shock response. Am J Physiol 1995; 269:L843-L848

39. Schroeder S, Reck M, Hoeft A, Stuber F. Analysis of two human leukocyte antigen-linked polymorphic heat shock protein 70 genes in patients with severe sepsis. Crit Care Med 1999; 27:1265-1270

40. Plumier JCL, Ross BM, Currie RW, et al. Transgenic mice expressing the human heat shock protein 70 have improved post-ischemic myocardial recovery. J Clin Invest 1995; 95:1854-1860

43

IMMUNODEPRESSION IN THE SURGICAL PATIENT AND INCREASED SUSCEPTIBILITY TO INFECTION

Martin K. Angele
Eugen Faist

Several studies indicate that organ failure is the leading cause of death in surgical patients [1]. Most cases of multiple organ dysfunction are precipitated by infection. Nonetheless, the outcome of organ dysfunction does not correlate well with the microbiology of multiple organ dysfunction syndrome (MODS) [2]. Several studies indicate that a causal relationship exists between surgical or traumatic injury and the predisposition of these patients to develop septic/infectious complications and/or multiple organ failure (MOF) [3-5]. The excessive inflammatory response together with a dramatic paralysis of cell-mediated immunity following major surgery [3,6] appears to be responsible for the increased susceptibility to subsequent sepsis.

In view of this, most of the scientific and medical research in this field has been directed towards measuring the progression and interrelationship of mediators which are activated or suppressed following major surgery. In most clinical studies, alterations in immune parameters of patients following surgery have been assessed due to evaluation of peripheral blood cell function and plasma levels of various mediators. Therefore, animal models have been utilized which simulate the clinical conditions. This has allowed us to better define the pathophysiology of the immunoinflammatory response following surgical trauma that reduces the patient's capability to resist subsequent life-threatening infectious complications.

This article will focus on the effect of blood loss and surgical injury on cell-mediated immune responses in experimental studies utilizing models of trauma and hemorrhagic shock which have defined effects on the immunoinflammatory response. Subsequently, each paragraph will discuss how the findings from these experimental studies correlate with data generated from surgical patients. Following this the effect of surgery on the susceptibility to polymicrobial sepsis and infection will be illustrated. These studies may generate new approaches for the treatment of immunodepression following major surgery which may be advantageous for decreasing the susceptibility to infection and for increasing the survival rate of the critical ill surgical patient.

MACROPHAGE FUNCTION FOLLOWING SURGERY

Macrophage Cytokine Release

Altered host defense mechanisms after major surgery or trauma are considered important for the development of infectious complications and sepsis.

Immune deterioration has also been reported in patients after trauma and surgery. In this respect, studies have shown areactivity of circulating monocytes towards stimulation with bacteria or endotoxin following surgical trauma [7]. This paralysis of monocyte cell function has been reported to persist for 3-5 days after trauma [8] and appears to be a potential risk factor for postoperative septic complications [7].

In contrast, other studies demonstrate an enhanced secretion of interleukin (IL)-1β and IL-10 by endotoxin-stimulated peripheral blood monocytes at different time points after surgery [9]. Differences in the severity of the surgical trauma might account for those divergent results.

In addition to cytokine release patterns, a high APACHE II score has been associated with an increased number of proinflammatory CD14+CD16+ monocytes [10]. Furthermore, high levels of CD14+CD16+ monocytes remained in patients with persistently high APACHE II scores [10].

Macrophage Antigen Presentation Following Major Surgery

Antigen presentation is defined as a process whereby a cell expresses antigen on its surface in a form capable of being recognized by a T-cell. The proteinacious antigen typically undergoes some form of processing in which it is degraded into small peptides which are capable of associating with major histocompatability complex (MHC) II for presentation to helper T-lymphocytes or in association with MHC I to become a target for cytotoxic T-lymphocytes [11]. However, for competent antigen presentation to take place the antigen presenting macrophage must provide a second co-stimulatory signal, in the form of a membrane and/or soluble factor. Impaired monocyte function and disruption of monocyte/T-cell interaction have been shown to be crucial for the development of septic complications in surgical patients [12]. In this respect, HLA-DR receptor expression is depressed in some surgical patients and correlates with sepsis severity and outcome [12]. Furthermore, a significant shift toward FcR+ monocyte subsets can be found. This subpopulation resembles activated macrophages characterized by high proinflammatory cytokine synthesis and suppressed antigen presentation. Similarly, Wakefield et al. demonstrated that an earlier recovery of the depressed HLA-DR expression was associated with a lower rate of septic complications [13].

It should be noted that a normal or enhanced capacity of peripheral blood monocytes to present bacterial superantigens and to stimulate T-cell proliferation after surgery has been found despite decreased HLA-DR antigen presentation [9]. Those changes were evident despite a significant loss of cell surface HLA-DR molecules. Thus, the level of MHC II protein expression does not necessarily predict the antigen-presenting capacity of monocytes obtained from surgical patients with uneventful postoperative recovery [9].

Moreover, MacLean et al. and Christou et al. have reported that the outcome of trauma patients is worsened when they exhibit a depressed delayed type hypersensitivity (DTH) reaction (which is antigen specific) [14,15]. Thus, depressed cell mediated immunity in patients following injury or major surgery, which is associated with an increased mortality from subsequent sepsis [16,17], is probably in part due to decreased antigen presenting capacity by macrophages.

These above findings collectively suggest the depression of macrophage antigen presentation capacity following injury or major surgery is an important factor contributing to the depression of cell mediated immunity, thereby, increasing subsequent susceptibility to infection. Interestingly, multiple factors which include decreased metabolic activity, anti-inflammatory cytokines, prostaglandins, and nitric oxide (NO) appear to be responsible for the depression of macrophage antigen presenting capacity.

These changes in macrophage function appear to be irreversible. Therefore, we treated patients undergoing major surgery with 15 μg granulocyte colony-stimulating factor (G-CSF) peri-operatively. The results indicate that G-CSF prevented the depressed lipopolysaccharide (LPS)-induced cytokine release by monocytes following major surgery. Moreover, administration of G-CSF normalized the depressed HLA-DR expression in surgical patients. It is our hypothesis, that G-CSF induces the release of new, unaltered monocytes postoperatively, thereby preventing immunosuppression. Whether these effects of G-CSF result in a decreased infection rate following major surgery remains to be determined in a larger clinical trial.

LYMPHOCYTE FUNCTION FOLLOWING HEMORRHAGIC SHOCK

Both experimental and clinical studies indicate that a wide range of traumatic injuries alter the ability of T-lymphocytes to respond to mitogenic activation, e.g., concanavalin A and phytohemagglutinin [18-23]. These studies demonstrate a decreased mitogenic response of lymphocytes in patients following general surgery, blunt trauma, and thermal injury [20-24]. Interestingly the degree of lymphocyte depression correlated with the complexity of the surgery. Similarly, following hemorrhagic shock, decreased splenocyte proliferative capacity in response to the T cell mitogen, concanavalin A, has been demonstrated extensively in our laboratory [18,19,25,26]. In addition, Hensler at al. showed a severe defect of T-lymphocyte proliferation and cytokine secretion *in vitro* following major surgery. In these studies, reduced cytokine secretion by T-lymphocytes was observed for IL-2, interferon (IFN)-γ, and tumor necrosis factor (TNF)-α during the early postoperative course [9]. Monocyte functions, however, were not altered, suggesting a predominant defect in the T-cell response rather than an impaired monocyte antigen-presenting capacity. Thus, suppression of T-cell effector functions during the early phase of the postoperative course may define a state of impaired defense against pathogens and increased susceptibility to infection and septic complications.

Similarly, the release of Th1 lymphokines, i.e., IL-2, IFN-γ, by splenocytes has been shown to be significantly depressed as early as 2 hr following experimental trauma and hemorrhagic shock [18,19,25,26] and this depression persists for up to 5 days following trauma-hemorrhage [26]. In contrast to Th1 lymphokines, the release of the anti-inflammatory Th2 lymphokine IL-10 has been shown to be increased after trauma-hemorrhage [18]. Neutralizing of IL-10 by addition of anti-IL-10 monoclonal antibodies to the culture media restored the depressed splenocyte proliferative capacity in splenocytes harvested from traumatized animals [18]. Thus, IL-10 following trauma-hemorrhage might contribute to the depressed splenocyte Th1 lymphokine release following trauma-hemorrhage. In addition to release patterns, T-lymphocyte subsets have been determined in patients with acute illness [27]. Those studies indicate that following major surgery both cell populations decrease [27]. Patients that develop septic complications, however, display a predominant decrease in CD 4 positive cells [28].

Moreover, changes in B-cell function have also been reported following surgical trauma. The capacity of splenic B-cells to produce antibodies is significantly decreased following trauma and blood loss [29,30]. In this regard, a decrease in overall serum levels of immunoglobulin was seen for up to 3 days after surgical trauma and blood loss [29,30]. The decreased IL-2 production by T-lymphocytes has been suggested to be responsible for the downregulation of antibody production by B-cells following severe injury, since T-cell lymphokines are a prerequisite for adequate B-cell proliferation and immunoglobulin secretion [3]. Whether restoration of T-cell function following severe injury and major surgery, however, restores the depressed B-cell function remains to be determined.

CIRCULATORY INFLAMMATORY MEDIATORS:

The observed immunodeficiency in trauma victims and patients following major surgery, however, has been found to be associated with enhanced concentrations of inflammatory cytokines reflecting activated immunocompetent cells in the same patient [31]. Thus, it appears that the depressed cell-mediated immune responses *in vitro* discussed in the above paragraphs reflects hyporesponsiveness to a second stimulus following massive activation *in vivo* [32].

In this respect, elevated levels of TNF-α, IL-1 and IL-6 in the plasma have been well described in both animal experiments [3,33,34] and patient studies [5,35-38] following trauma, severe blood loss, and sepsis. The sequence of cytokine release following trauma and hemorrhagic shock includes an increase in plasma TNF-α as early as 30 min after the onset of injury, peak TNF-α levels by 2 hr post-trauma and hemorrhage and a return towards baseline values at 24 hr [3,33] (Figure 1). In contrast to measurements using a bioassay [33], elevated plasma TNF-α levels were detectable at 24 hr post-trauma and blood loss with the ELISA technique [39]. This suggests that TNF-α detected 24 hr after injury might not be biologically active. In this regard, soluble TNF-α receptors have been isolated from the plasma which might neutralize the biological activity of circulating TNF-α [40]. Unlike TNF-α, plasma IL-6 levels are not

significantly elevated until 2 hr post-hemorrhage, and the levels remain
elevated up to 24 hr after the induction of hemorrhage [41].

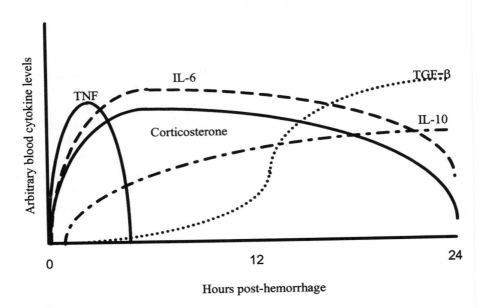

Figure 1. *Arbitrary blood cytokine levels during the first 24 hr following trauma and hemorrhagic shock. Levels of tumor necrosis factor (TNF)-α, interleukin (IL)-6, and transforming growth factor (TGF)-β were determined by specific bioassay. IL-10 was measured by ELISA and corticosterone by radioimmunoassay.*

Since *in vivo* administration of IL-1, IL-6, and TNF-α [42-45] induces a shock-like syndrome similar to that observed following severe blood loss and sepsis, it has been suggested that these cytokines may play a role in initiating the cascade of events that can lead to the development of multiple organ dysfunction following severe hemorrhagic shock.

Furthermore, the marked increase in the release of pro-inflammatory cytokines by Kupffer cells following trauma and blood loss in experimental studies has been reported to be associated with depressed immune functions [3]. This suggests that pro-inflammatory cytokines produced by Kupffer cells following hemorrhage act in an autocrine as well as a paracrine fashion to down regulate Kupffer cell and other macrophage populations. Furthermore, Kupffer cells, which represent the largest pool of macrophages in the body, were found to release increased amounts of IL-1, IL-6, and TNF-α following shock [42] and the selective reduction of this macrophage population by injection of gadolinium chloride significantly reduced plasma IL-6 levels following hemorrhage [46]. This leads to the conclusion that Kupffer cells are a significant source of the increased plasma levels of pro-inflammatory cytokines following trauma and hemorrhage and these cytokines can act to depress macrophage function. Whether or not Kupffer cells are the only contributor to the enhanced proinflammatory plasma levels following severe injury and major surgery remains to be determined.

In contrast to the early increase in pro-inflammatory cytokines in the plasma following trauma and shock, elevated plasma levels of the anti-inflammatory cytokine, transforming growth factor (TGF)-β, are not detectable until 24 hours after the insult [47]. Furthermore, this elevation in plasma TGF-β persisted until 72 hours after trauma and hemorrhage [47]. Neutralization of TGF-β antibodies restored the depressed antigen presentation to normal levels [47]. These results, along with the studies by Miller-Graziano et al. [48] indicate that the enhanced release of TGF-β is an additional factor responsible for the prolonged suppression of macrophage function following hemorrhagic shock.

In addition to pro- and anti-inflammatory cytokines numerous other mediators in the plasma have been reported to contribute to the depression of cell-mediated immune response following trauma and shock. In this respect, Eicosanoids have been extensively studied as agents involved in immunological responses[49-51]. Early following shock (2 hours) an increased release of prostaglandins and leukotrienes by macrophages occurs, leading to elevated plasma levels of eicosanoids [3,52]. Moreover, prostaglandin (PG)E$_2$ has been shown to inhibit cell-mediated immune function [53,54]. Conversely, administration of ibuprofen, an inhibitor of cyclooxygenase, to animals following severe blood loss prevented the depression of macrophage functions [55]. Ertel et al. [56] has also demonstrated that rodents which were pre-fed a fish oil diet high in omega-3-fatty acids that are known to inhibit the synthesis of PGE$_2$ *via* inhibition of arachidonic acid metabolism, had normal macrophage functions following hemorrhage.

Increased levels of circulating cytokines have also been reported following a variety of tissue insults in patients, including trauma, sepsis, thermal injury, and surgery [5,38,57,58]. In this regard, increased plasma IL-6 levels have been observed in patients during the first week following trauma [38]. Interestingly, levels of pro-inflammatory cytokines have been shown to be higher in trauma patients with severe blood loss compared to patients with trauma alone [5]. Moreover, in septic patients the increase of the pro-inflammatory cytokines IL-6 and TNF-α has been found to be much higher than in trauma victims without septic complications [38]. These findings suggest additive effects of trauma, blood loss, and septic complications on the immunoinflammatory response. Furthermore, proinflammatory cytokine levels as well as the duration of elevation appear to correlate with the severity of the insult. In this regard, elevated cytokine levels have been shown to persist for five days after gastrectomy compared to three days after mastectomy [58]. In addition, several clinical studies have shown an association between elevated plasma levels of proinflammatory cytokines and increased infectious complications and higher mortality rates [5,35,59-63]. In this respect, Calandra et al. reported a progressive decline in TNF-α levels in survivors of septic shock, whereas TNF-α levels remained persistently elevated after initial diagnosis and attempted treatment in non-survivors from septic shock [64].

The above studies suggest the important contribution of pro-inflammatory cytokines to the pathophysiological changes seen in surgical patients and trauma victims. Therefore determination of pro-inflammatory cytokine levels might become important for clinicians in the near future who encounter a trauma patients in the intensive care unit (ICU). Knowledge of the patient's cytokine levels may give some indication of the intracellular milieu and possibly insight into cellular changes taking place. This information might give the clinician a better understanding of how to treat such a critically ill trauma patient. More refinements towards the rapid and online measurements of cytokines are, however, needed before the full benefits of such information can be effectively translated to better management of trauma patients. Although various cytokine therapies in septic patients so far have not yielded satisfactory results, the lack of beneficial effects might be related to the timing and dose of anti-cytokine administration. It is our hypothesis that total blockade/neutralization of cytokines will not be helpful to the host. Instead, modulation of cytokine production/release by immune cells, i.e., macrophages, T-cells, leading to the restoration of cellular homeostasis might be a better approach for decreasing the susceptibility of trauma victims and patients following major surgery to subsequent sepsis and infection.

INCREASED SUSCEPTIBILITY TO INFECTION

Increased Susceptibility to Polymicrobial Sepsis

The studies mentioned above indicate depressed immunoresponsiveness after trauma and hemorrhage, which persists despite fluid resuscitation. To determine whether these observations translate into an actual reduction in the capacity of these traumatized animals to ward off infection of a clinically relevant nature, additional studies were conducted by Stephan et al. in which sepsis was induced three days after hemorrhagic shock. The results demonstrate an increased susceptibility of hemorrhaged animals to polymicrobial sepsis as evidenced by an increased mortality rate of hemorrhaged animals following subsequent sepsis (mortality of hemorrhaged animals following subsequent sepsis 100 % compared to 50 % in sham animals subjected to sepsis) [19,65]. Similarly, Zapata-Sirvent et al. have indicated that the mortality rate in response to a septic challenge was increased in mice [66]. Interestingly, restoration of the depressed immune responses following trauma and severe blood loss with immunomodulatory agents, i.e., flutamide (an androgen receptor blocker) was associated with increased survival rates following subsequent sepsis [65].

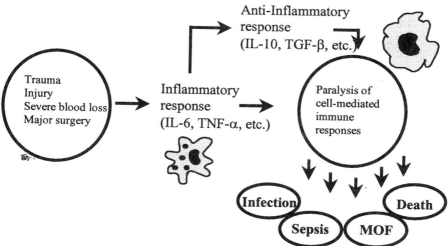

Figure 2. *Hypothesis of the cascade of events following major surgery that leads to the development of depressed immune responses and increased susceptibility to sepsis.*

Moreover, an association between the loss of immunocompetence in patients (paralysis of cell-mediated immunity) following traumatic injury and the development of sepsis and late death has been reported [16,17] (Figure 2). Furthermore, alterations in the levels of circulating E-selectin adhesion molecules after trauma and resuscitation have been found to be associated with an increased risk of infectious complications, organ failure and death [67]. In summary, these studies suggest that the immunodepression following injury and major surgery leads to an increased susceptibility to polymicrobial sepsis. Therefore, attempts to modulate the depressed immune responses in trauma victims might decrease the development of septic complications and multiple organ failure in those patients.

CONCLUSION

The above studies indicate that injury, trauma, and blood loss produce a marked suppression in cell mediated immunity and an increased susceptibility to subsequent sepsis and wound infection. Furthermore, global as well as differential effects can be observed on macrophages that are dependent on their anatomical location. Nonetheless, the use of a variety of immunomodulatory agents, e.g., dilitiazem, chloroquine, ibuprofen, IFN-γ, prolactin, metclopramide and flutamide have been shown to be helpful for the normalization of the altered immune responses following trauma and hemorrhage in experimental studies. The success in the use of immunomodulatory agents following hemorrhage in rodent models appears to be promising in the development of new therapeutic concepts for the treatment of immunosuppression and for decreasing the mortality from subsequent sepsis in humans. However, careful evaluation of both the benefits and potential adverse effects of therapy is needed before widespread clinical use can be envisioned. Recently, administration of G-CSF peri-operatively has been shown to prevent immunosuppression following major surgery. The enhanced release of new, unaltered monocytes appears to be responsible for the immunoenhancing effects of G-CSF. Larger clinical trials should be initiated to verify whether the immunoprotective effects of G-CSF are associated with a decreased susceptibility of surgical patients to infectious complications thereby decreasing the mortality rate.

In conclusion, the immunoinflammatory response and subsequent sepsis, is still one of the major causes of morbidity and mortality following major surgery. While significant advances have been made, it is important to further define the pathophysiology and identify the precise mechanisms responsible for the depression of the cell mediated immunity using experimental animal models. However, these animal models should take into consideration the various manipulations that the patient receives as well as the effect of gender, nutritional status, preexisting conditions etc. Only when models of injury begin to consider these factors, can effective treatment regimes for patients be developed.

REFERENCES

1. Carrico CJ, Meakins JL, Marshall, JC. Multiple organ failure syndrome. Arch Surg 1986; 121:196-208
2. Stahl GL, Bitterman H, Terashita Z, Lefer AM. Salutary consequences of blockade of platelet activating factor in hemorrhagic shock. Eur J Pharmacol 1988; 149:233-240
3. Chaudry IH, Ayala A. Immunological Aspects of Hemorrhage. (Medical Intelligence Unit). R.G. Landes Company, Austin, 1992
4. Stephan RN, Ayala A, Chaudry IH. Monocyte and lymphocyte responses following trauma. In: Schlag G, Redl H (eds) Pathophysiology of Shock, Sepsis and Organ Failure. Springer-Verlag, Berlin, 1993, pp:131-144
5. Roumen RM, Hendriks T, van der Ven-Jongekrijg J, et al. Cytokine patterns in patients after major surgery, hemorrhagic shock, and severe blunt trauma. Ann Surg 1993; 6:769-776
6. Faist E, Baue AE, Dittmer H. Multiple organ failure in polytrauma patients. J Trauma 1983; 23:775-787
7. Haupt W, Riese J, Mehler C, Weber K, Zowe M, Hohenberger W. Monocyte function before and after surgical trauma. Dig Surg 1998; 15:102-104
8. Faist E, Storck M, Hultner L, et al. Functional analysis of mnocyte activity through synthesis patterns of proinflammatory cytokines and neopterin in patients in surgical intensive care. Surgery 1992; 112:562-572
9. Hensler T, Ecker H, Eeg K, et al. Distinct mechanisms of immunosuppression as a consequence of major surgery. Infect Immun 1997; 65:2283-2291
10. Fingerle-Rowson G, Auers J, Kreuzer E, Fraunberger P, Blumenstein M, Ziegler-Heitbrock LH. Expansion of CD14+CD16+ monocytes in critically ill cardiac surgery patients. Inflammation 1998; 22:367-379
11. Ayala A, Ertel W, Chaudry IH. Trauma-induced suppression of antigen presentation and expression of major histocompatibility class II antigen complex in leukocytes. Shock 1996; 5:79-90
12. Schinkel C, Sendtner R, Zimmer S, Faist E. Functional analysis of monocyte subsets in surgical sepsis. J Trauma 1998; 44:743-748
13. Wakefield CH, Carey PD, Foulds S, Monson JR, Guillou PJ. Changes in major histocompatibility complex class II expression in monocytes and T cells of patients developing infection after surgery. Br J Surg 1993; 80:205-209
14. MacLean LD, Meakins JL, Taguchi K, Duignan J, Dhillon KS, Gordon J. Host resistance in sepsis and trauma. Ann Surg 1975; 182:207-211
15. Christou NV, Tellado JM. The impact of preexisting disease conditions for host defense integrity in traumatized and critically ill patients. In: Faist E, Meakins J, Schildberg FW (eds) Host Defense Dysfunction in Trauma, Shock and Sepsis. Springer-Verlag, Heidelberg, 1992, pp: 73-82

16. Levy EM, Alharbi SA, Grindlinger G, Black PH. Changes in mitogen responsiveness lymphocyte subsets after traumatic injury: relation to development of sepsis. Clin Immunol Immunopathol 1984; 32:224-233

17. Keane RM, Birmingham W, Shatney CM, Winchurch RA, Munster AM. Prediction of sepsis in the multitraumatic patient by assays of lymphocyte responsiveness. Surg Gynecol Obstet 1983; 156:163-167

18. Ayala A, Lehman DL, Herdon CD, Chaudry IH. Mechanism of enhanced susceptibility to sepsis following hemorrhage: Interleukin (IL)-10 suppression of T-cell response is mediated by eicosanoid induced IL-4 release. Arch Surg 1994; 129:1172-1178

19. Stephan RN, Kupper TS, Geha AS, Baue AE, Chaudry IH. Hemorrhage without tissue trauma produces immunosuppression and enhances susceptibility to sepsis. Arch Surg 1987; 122:62-68

20. Riddle PR, Berenbaum MC. Postoperative depression of the lymphocyte response to phytohaemagglutinin. Lancet 1969; i:746-748

21. O'Mahony JB, Palder SB, Wood JJ, et al. Depression of cellular immunity after multiple trauma in the absence of sepsis. J Trauma 1984; 24:869-875

22. Daniels JC, Sakai H, Cobb EK, Lewis SR, Larson DL, Ritzmann SE. Evaluation of lymphocyte reactivity studies in patients with thermal burns. J Trauma 1971; 11:595-607

23. Sakai H, Daniels JC, Lewis SR, Lynch JB, Watson DL, Ritzmann SE. Reversible alterations of nucleic acid synthesis in lymphocytes after thermal burns. J Reticuloendothelial Soc 1972; 11:19-28

24. Abraham E, Chang YH. The effects of hemorrhage on mitogen-induced lymphocyte proliferation. Circ Shock 1985; 15:141-149

25. Angele MK, Ayala A, Cioffi WG, Bland KI, Chaudry IH. Testosterone: The culprit for producing splenocyte depression following trauma-hemorrhage. Am J Physiol 1998; 274:C1530-C1536

26. Zellweger R, Ayala A, DeMaso CM, Chaudry IH. Trauma-hemorrhage causes prolonged depression in cellular immunity. Shock 1995; 4:149-153

27. Feeney C, Bryzman S, Kong L, Brazil H, Deutsch R, Fritz LC. T-lymphocyte subsets in acute illness. Crit Care Med 1995; 23:1680-1685

28. O'Mahony JB, Wood JJ, Rodrick ML, Mannick JA. Changes in T lymphocyte subsets following injury. Assessment by flow cytometry and relationship to sepsis. Ann Surg 1985; 202:580-586

29. Abraham E, Freitas AA. Hemorrhage in mice induces alterations in immunoglobulin secreting B-cells. Crit Care Med 1989; 17:1015-1019

30. Abraham E, Freitas AA. Hemorrhage produces abnormalities in lymphocyte function and lymphokine generation. J Immunol 1989; 142:899-906

31. Fuchs D, Gruber A, Wachter H, Faist E. Activated cell-mediated immunity and immunodeficiency in trauma and sepsis. In: Faist E, Baue AE, Schildberg FW (eds). The Immune Consequences of Trauma, Shock and Sepsis: Mechanisms and Therapeutic Approaches. Pabst Science Publishers, Lengerich, 1996, pp:235-239

32. Fuchs D, Malkovsky M, Reibnegger G, Werner ER, Forni G, Wachter H. Endogenous release of interferon-gamma and diminished response of peripheral blood mononuclear cells to antigenic stimulation. Immunol Lett 1989; 23:103-108

33. Ayala A, Perrin MM, Meldrum DR, Ertel W, Chaudry IH. Hemorrhage induces an increase in serum TNF which is not associated with elevated levels of endotoxin. Cytokine 1990; 2:170-174

34. Ayala A, Wang P, Ba ZF, Perrin MM, Ertel W, Chaudry IH. Differential alterations in plasma IL-6 and TNF levels following trauma and hemorrhage. Am J Physiol 1991; 260:R167-R171

35. Damas P, Reuter A, Gysen P, Demonty J, Lamy M, Franchimont P. Tumor necrosis factor and interleukin-1 serum levels during severe sepsis in humans. Crit Care Med 1989; 17:975-978
36. Damas P, Ledoux D, Nys M, et al. Cytokine serum level during severe sepsis in human IL-6 as a marker of severity. Ann Surg 1992; 215:356-362
37. Romagnani S. Th1 and Th2 in human diseases. Clin Immunol Immunopathol 1996; 80:225-235
38. Martin C, Boisson C, Haccoun M, Thomachot L, Mege JL. Patterns of cytokine evolution (tumor necrosis factor-α and interleukin-6) after septic shock, hemorrhagic shock, and severe trauma. Crit Care Med 1997; 25:1813-1819
39. Ertel W, Morrison MH, Ayala A, Perrin MM, Chaudry IH. Anti-TNF monoclonal antibodies prevent haemorrhage-induced suppression of Kupffer cell antigen presentation and MHC class II antigen expression. Immunology 1991; 74:290-297
40. Porteu F, Nathan C. Shedding of tumor necrosis factor receptors by activated human neutrophils. J Exp Med 1990; 172:599-607
41. Ertel W, Morrison MH, Ayala A, Chaudry IH. Chloroquine attenuates hemorrhagic shock induced suppression of Kupffer cell antigen presentation and MHC class II antigen expression through blockade of tumor necrosis factor and prostaglandin release. Blood 1991; 78:1781-1788
42. Wong GC, Clark SC. Multiple actions of interleukin 6 within a cytokine network. Immunol Today 1988; 9:137-139
43. Okusawa S, Gelfand JA, Ikejima T, Connolly RJ, Dinarello CA. Interleukin-1 induces a shock like state in rabbits. Synergism with tumor necrosis factor and the effects of cyclooxygenase inhibition. J Clin Invest 1988; 81:1162-1172
44. Tracey KJ, Lowry SF, Fahey TJI, et al. Cachectin/tumor necrosis factor induces lethal shock and stress hormone responses in the dog. Surg Gynecol Obstet 1987; 164:415-422
45. Lejeune P, Lagadec P, Onier N, Pinnard D, Ohshima H, Jeannin JF. Nitric oxide involvement in tumor-induced immunosuppression. J Immunol 1994; 152:5077-5083
46. O'Neill PJ, Ayala A, Wang P, et al. Role of Kupffer cells in interleukin-6 release following trauma- hemorrhage and resuscitation. Shock 1994; 1:43-47
47. Ayala A, Meldrum DR, Perrin MM, Chaudry IH. The release of transforming growth factor-□ following hemorrhage: Its role as a mediator of host immunosuppression. FASEB J 1992; 6:A1604 (Abst)
48. Miller-Graziano CL, Szabo G, Griffey K, Metha B, Kodys K, Catalano D. Role of elevated monocyte transforming growth factor beta (TGF- beta) production in posttrauma immunosuppression. J Clin Immunol 1991; 11:95-102
49. Waal Malefyt R, Abrams J, Bennett B, Figdor CG, Vries JE. Interleukin 10 (IL-10) inhibits cytokine synthesis by human monocytes: An autoregulatory role of IL-10 produced by monocytes. J Exp Med 1991; 174:1209-1220
50. Faist E, Mewes A, Baker CC, et al. Prostaglandin E$_2$ dependent suppression of interleukin-2 production in patients with major trauma. J.Trauma 1987; 27:837-848
51. Knapp W, Baumgartner G. Monocyte-mediated suppression of human B lymphocyte differentiation in vitro. J Immunol 1978; 121:1177-1183
52. Johnston PA, Selkurt EE. Effect of hemorrhagic shock on renal release of prostaglandin E. Am J Physiol 1976; 230:831-838
53. Bonta IL, Parnham MJ. Immunomodulatory-antiinflammatory functions of E-type prostaglandins. Minireview with emphasis on macrophage mediated effects. Int J Immunopharmacol 1982; 4:103-109
54. Plaut M. The role of cyclic AMP in modulating cytotoxic T lymphocytes. I. In vivo-generated cytotoxic lymphocytes, but not in vitro- generated cytotoxic lymphocytes, are inhibited by cyclic AMP- active agents. J Immunol 1979; 123:692-701

55. Chaudry IH, Ayala A. Immune consequences of hypovolemic shock and resuscitation. Curr Opin Anaesthesiology 1993; 6:385-392
56. Ayala A, Chaudry IH. Dietary n-3 polyunsaturated fatty acid modulation of immune cell function pre- or post-trauma. Nutrition 1995; 11:1-11
57. Beutler B. Tumor necrosis factor and other cytokines in septic syndrome. In: Vincent JL (ed) Sepsis. Springer-Verlag, Berlin, 1994 pp: 107-121
58. Shirakawa T, Tokunaga A, Onda M. Release of immunosuppressive substances after gastric resection is more prolonged than after mastectomy in humans. Int Surg 1998; 83:210-214
59. Feldbush TL, Hobbs MV, Severson CD, Ballas ZF, Weiler JM. Role of complement in the immune response. Fed Proc 1984; 43:2548-2552
60. Marks JD, Marks CB, Luce JM, et al. Plasma tumor necrosis factor in patients with septic shock. Am Rev Respir Dis 1990; 141:94-97
61. Marano MA, Fong Y, Moldawer LL, et al. Serum cachectin/tumor necrosis factor in critically ill patients with burns correlates with infection and mortality. Surg Gynecol Obstet 1990; 170:32-38
62. Waage A, Halstensen A, Espevik T. Association between tumor necrosis factor in serum and fatal outcome in patients with meningococcal disease. Lancet 1987; i:355-357
63. Waage A, Brandtzaeg P, Halstensen A, Kierulf P, Espevik T. The complex pattern of cytokines in serum from patients with meningococcal septic shock. Association between interleukin 6, interleukin 1, and fatal outcome. J Exp Med 1989; 169:333-338
64. Molloy RG, Mannick JA, Rodrick ML. Cytokines, sepsis and immunomodulation. Br J Surg 1993 80:289-297
65. Angele MK, Wichmann MW, Ayala A, Cioffi WG, Chaudry IH. Testosterone receptor blockade after hemorrhage in males: Restoration of the depressed immune functions and improved survival following subsequent sepsis. Arch Surg 1997; 132:1207-1214
66. Zapata-Sirvent RL, Hansbrough JF, Cox MC, Carter WH. Immunologic alterations in a murine model of hemorrhagic shock. Crit Care Med 1992; 20:508-517
67. Simons RK, Hoyt DB, Winchell RJ, Rose RM, Holbrook T. Elevated selectin levels after severe trauma: A marker for sepsis and organ failure and a potential target for immounomodulatory therapy. J Trauma 1996; 41:653-662

44

THE PLACE OF CORTICOSTEROIDS

Djillali Annane
Eric Bellissant

Since the discovery of cortisone by Reichstein and Kendall in 1937, corticosteroids have been recognized as invaluable drugs in numerous inflammatory conditions. Indeed, corticosteroids were proposed to treat patients with severe infection as early as 1940 [1]. There are now more than 2,000 publications reporting the effects of corticosteroids in human sepsis and septic shock, including almost fifty controlled clinical trials and a dozen reviews. The first systematic review of the literature was published in 1974 and exhorted physicians to conduct well designed, randomized, controlled trials to resolve the controversy surrounding the use of corticosteroids as adjunctive therapy to severe infection [2]. The last systematic reviews were published 20 years later and reported two meta-analyses of all available randomized controlled trials performed between 1966 and 1993 [3,4]. These meta-analyses reached the conclusion that there was no evidence for a beneficial effect of corticosteroids in patients with sepsis and septic shock. However, given the recent advances in the understanding of the mechanisms of host defense against inflammation and of action of corticosteroids, several physicians still believe to be on the right track in studying corticosteroids to reduce the unacceptable high mortality rate from septic shock. In this chapter, the reader will find an overview of the current knowledge on the role of endogenous corticosteroids in host defense against sepsis and on the effects of the administration of exogenous corticosteroids in sepsis and septic shock.

ROLE OF ENDOGENOUS CORTICOSTEROIDS IN HOST RESPONSE TO SEPSIS

It is well established that a stress like sepsis causes the activation of the hypothalamic-pituitary adrenal (HPA) axis. This activation releases cortisol which exerts a key role in host defenses through anti-inflammatory and vascular effects (Table 1).

	Cortisol effects	
	Potentially favorable	**Potentially deleterious**
Immune cascade	Prevents inflammatory cells migration by: • Blocking chemokines like MCP-1, IL-8 and MIP-1α • Stimulating the synthesis of lipocortin-1 Blocks the synthesis of: • IL-2, IL-3, IL-4, IL-5, IFN-γ and GM-CSF by T-cells • IL-1, IL-6, IL-8, IL-12, TNF-α and MIP-1α by monocytes • IL-8 by neutrophils Blocks the expression of: • Endothelial cells adhesion molecules Inhibits the synthesis of: • Soluble PLA$_2$ • Inducible COX-2 • Inducible NOS Acts synergistically with: • IL-6 to induce production of acute phase proteins in the liver • Anti-inflammatory mediators like IL-1ra and IL-10.	Induces the synthesis of macrophage MIF
Vascular beds	Increases vasoconstrictor response to: epinephrine, norepinephrine, phenylephrine and angiotensin II Improves renal blood flow Increases vessels wall content in salt and water	Not known

COX-2 : cyclooxygenase-2, GM-CSF : granulocyte macrophage colony stimulating factor, IFN-γ : interferon-γ, IL : interleukin, MCP-1 : monocyte chemo-attractant protein-1, MIF : migration inhibitory factor, MIP-1α : macrophage inflammatory peptide-1α, NOS : nitric oxide synthase, PLA$_2$: phospholipase A$_2$, TNF-α : tumor necrosis factor-α.

Table 1. Effects of cortisol in sepsis

Anti-inflammatory Effects of Endogenous Corticosteroids

The activation of the HPA axis results in a dramatic reduction of the intensity of the immune response to sepsis, as almost all the components of this response are virtually inhibited by cortisol. Indeed, cortisol prevents the migration of inflammatory cells from circulation to tissues and blocks the synthesis or the action of most pro-inflammatory mediators, including several interleukins (IL-1, IL-2, IL-3, IL-6), interferon-γ (IFN-γ), granulocyte macrophage colony stimulating factor (GM-CSF), tumor necrosis factor-α (TNF-α), cell adhesion molecules, phospholipase A_2 (PLA$_2$), cyclooxygenase-2 (COX-2), and inducible nitric oxide synthase (iNOS) [5]. Corticosteroids repress the gene expression of various inflammatory molecules through transcriptional interference between the activated glucocorticoid receptor and both activator protein-1 (AP-1) [6,7] and nuclear factor-κB (NF-κB) [8,9]. In addition, corticosteroids also inhibit NF-κB activation by induction of IκBα expression resulting in sequestration of NF-κB dimers in the cytoplasm [10,11]. These anti-inflammatory effects of corticosteroids may be counteracted by the overexpression of AP-1 and NF-κB, which is induced, for instance, by IL-2 and IL-4 [12], and by the macrophage migration inhibitory factor (MIF) [13]. Cortisol potentiates IL-6 induced production of acute phase proteins in the liver [14] and acts synergistically with anti-inflammatory mediators like IL-1ra and IL-10 [15]. Finally, cortisol, through the control of the synthesis of the regulatory cytokines IL-4, IL-10, IL-12 and IFN-γ favors T helper 2 type immune response and enhances humoral more than cellular immunity [16].

Vascular Effects of Endogenous Corticosteroids

Hypertension is a well known complication of chronic corticosteroid excess as observed in Cushing's syndrome. This hypertension occurs rapidly and is independent of salt intake. Conversely, the decrease in vascular resistance is a common feature of adrenal insufficiency [17]. In rats, RU 486, a corticosteroid antagonist, decreases vascular resistance, and blunts systemic and renal vascular responses to norepinephrine and angiotensin II, demonstrating the role of endogenous corticosteroids in blood pressure regulation [18]. In experimental sepsis, endogenous corticosteroids have been shown to inhibit iNOS, and hence to account for the cardiovascular tolerance to endotoxin [19]. *In vitro* studies on rat aorta smooth muscle cells have also suggested that stimulation of the phosphoinositide system is involved in vascular effects of corticosteroids since it influences intracellular free calcium and thus vascular tone and blood pressure [20]. In fact, the mechanisms by which endogenous corticosteroids maintain cardiovascular homeostasis remain incompletely understood.

Activation of the HPA Axis in Sepsis

A little bit more than one century ago, it was observed that glucosuria occurs during infection. In 1936, Hans Selye described that stress induces enlargement of adrenal glands as a part of the general body adaptation to various challenges [21]. The entire HPA axis is now well recognized as being a key component of the stress system [5]. There is a body of evidence that the HPA axis is activated in sepsis. In dogs challenged by lethal injections of endotoxin, blood cortisol levels are elevated along with maximal concentrations of cortisol in the adrenal venous effluent [22]. In human septic shock, investigations using sodium succinate ester of cortisol demonstrated that adrenal secretory activity is increased and that a decrease in plasma cortisol clearance only occurs in moribund patients [23]. In sepsis, the HPA axis is activated through two main pathways [5]. The first pathway is a systemic pathway: TNF-α, IL-1 and IL-6 activate the HPA axis independently and when combined their effects are synergistic [5]. In plasma, IL-6, rather than IL-1β, may be the major determinant of the individual variation of HPA axis responses to lipopolysaccharides (LPS), activating vagal afferents at the level of the brain stem [24]. The second pathway uses the neural routes of communication between the site of inflammation and the brain. Indeed, sub-diaphragmatic vagotomy has been shown to reduce HPA axis activation and fever response to intravenous challenge with LPS, TNF-α or IL-1β, albeit elevated circulating cytokines levels [25,26].

Disruption of the HPA Axis in Severe Sepsis

The observations by Waterhouse [27] and Friderichsen [28] of bilateral hemorrhage of the adrenal glands were the first evidence of a disruption of the HPA axis during severe sepsis. In fact, besides obvious anatomical damage of the HPA axis, numerous experimental and clinical investigations have suggested that a reversible dysfunction of the HPA axis may occur during sepsis [29]. Occult adrenal insufficiency and peripheral resistance to corticosteroids are the two main features of this dysfunction.

Occult Adrenal Insufficiency

More than 50 % of patients with septic shock have an occult adrenal insufficiency defined by a blunted cortisol response to a short corticotrophin test (i.e., less than 9 µg/dl of cortisol increase after 250 µg of tetracosactrin) [30]. Septic shock patients with relative adrenal insufficiency are more likely to have impaired pressor responsiveness to norepinephrine [31]. The probability of survival in these patients is lower than that of patients with normal adrenal function [30,31]. Cortisol response to corticotrophin is not related to baseline cortisol levels in septic shock. Nevertheless, the higher baseline cortisol levels the higher the mortality rate among patients with relative adrenal insufficiency [30]. High IL-6 plasma levels may be the main determinant of the disruption of the HPA axis in sepsis [24, 32].

Corticosteroid Resistance Syndrome

The corticosteroid resistance syndrome may be responsible for excessive immune-mediated inflammation in several disorders, including rheumatoid arthritis, corticosteroid-resistant asthma, acquired immunodeficiency syndrome (AIDS) and chronic degenerative osteoarthritis [5]. In patients with sepsis and septic shock, the sensitivity of peripheral blood mononuclear cells to corticosteroids is generally up-regulated, except at the site of infection given the high concentrations of cytokines [33]. Indeed, several cytokines, like IL-2 and IL-4, may induce an overexpression of NF-κB that interferes with the glucocorticoid receptor function [10,11]. The decreased affinity and decreased binding capacity of the glucocorticoid receptor have been shown in T cells incubated with various cytokines [34,35] and in peripheral blood mononuclear leukocytes from patients with sepsis or septic shock [36]. Moreover, a negative correlation has been established between body temperature and the number of glucocorticoid receptors in patients with sepsis or septic shock [36].

Thus, endogenous corticosteroids have an important role in the regulation of immune response and possess favorable cardiovascular effects in sepsis. The high probability that sepsis is associated with an inappropriate activation of the HPA axis provides a clear therapeutic rationale for the study of corticosteroids in patients with septic shock.

EFFECTS OF EXOGENOUS CORTICOSTEROIDS IN SEPSIS

In severe sepsis, among the various effects of corticosteroids, the effects on hemodynamics and inflammatory process are potentially beneficial.

Exogenous Corticosteroids and Cardiovascular Failure in Sepsis

Physicians have known for a long time that corticosteroids induce vasoconstriction [37]. Experimental studies have suggested that this effect might result from iNOS and COX-2 inhibition [38,39]. Moreover, studies in dogs and cats have also demonstrated that cortisol and aldosterone increase the vasoconstrictor response to epinephrine [40]. In human volunteers, hydrocortisone has been shown to prevent endotoxin-induced hyporesponsiveness to norepinephrine in the venous vascular bed. This effect was not mediated through nitric oxide (NO) or prostanoid synthesis inhibition [41]. Similarly, in patients with septic shock, hydrocortisone was shown to restore pressure response to norepinephrine and phenylephrine [31,42]. This effect was more pronounced in patients with impaired adrenal function reserve [31] and was probably mediated neither by sympathetic or renin-angiotensin systems nor by NO [42]. Finally, two small placebo-controlled randomized trials have demonstrated that prolonged treatment (5 days or more) with low doses (about 300 mg daily) of hydrocortisone increases mean arterial pressure and systemic vascular resistance and shortens the need for vasopressor therapy in patients with catecholamine-dependent septic shock [43,44].

Exogenous Corticosteroids and the Systemic Inflammatory Response to Sepsis

The anti-inflammatory effects of high doses of corticosteroids are well known and will not be reviewed here [5]. However, the effects of low doses of hydrocortisone on the systemic inflammatory response to sepsis deserve to be discussed. In healthy volunteers challenged with LPS, hydrocortisone (3 μg/kg/min for 6 hours) was shown to prevent the expected rises in temperature and pulse rate and to decrease the peak plasma levels of epinephrine, C-reactive protein (CRP) and TNF-α, but not of IL-6 [45]. Interestingly, these effects of hydrocortisone were only observed when it was administered immediately before, or concomitant to, LPS exposure. When hydrocortisone was infused 12 or 144 hours before LPS exposure, circulating levels of TNF-α and IL-6 were higher than those observed with LPS alone suggesting that corticosteroid withdrawal induced rebound phenomenon. In subsequent experiments in healthy volunteers challenged with LPS, hydrocortisone was shown to enhance the release of anti-inflammatory cytokines, like IL-1 receptor antagonist (IL-1ra), soluble TNF receptor (sTNF-R) [46], and IL-10 [47]. In patients with septic shock, prolonged treatment with low doses of hydrocortisone (about 300 mg for 5 days) was associated with a significant reduction of the systemic inflammatory response syndrome, as shown by decreases in core temperature, heart rate and inflammatory markers such as phospholipase A_2 (PLA_2) and CRP [48]. This study also showed that the withdrawal of exogenous hydrocortisone may amplify the systemic inflammatory response syndrome and was associated with a relapse of shock. The effect of prolonged treatment with low doses of hydrocortisone (about 300 mg for 3 days) on the markers of inflammation in septic shock patients has been scrutinized in another study [49]. Hydrocortisone was shown to dramatically decrease plasma levels of proinflammatory cytokines and of nitrites/nitrates, and tended to decrease the concentrations of soluble adhesion molecules.

Exogenous Corticosteroids and Survival from Sepsis

Effect of High Dose Corticosteroids

Corticosteroids have been shown to improve survival in various experimental models of septic shock [13,50,51]. In humans, initial research used high doses of corticosteroids in sepsis treatment. These high doses proved to be effective in severe sepsis due to typhoid fever [52], *Pneumocystis carinii* pneumonia in AIDS patients [53], and bacterial meningitis in children [54]. However, a systematic review with a meta-analysis of the studies with corticosteroids, including 10 placebo-controlled randomized trials with a total of 1329 patients in sepsis or septic shock, did not find similar results in other cases of sepsis [3]. This review did not find any significant difference between groups in absolute mortality rates, but showed significant heterogeneity across studies. Another systematic review with a meta-analysis of the studies with corticosteroids included nine placebo-controlled randomized trials with a total of 1232 patients in sepsis or septic shock [4]. The authors did not include one study [55] since they had not been able to clarify whether the treatment had been allocated in a random order or not. This meta-analysis did not find any significant difference between groups in relative risk of death, but showed significant heterogeneity across studies. Further, both reviews did not show any significant increase in gastrointestinal bleeding or superinfection associated with corticosteroids. Finally, it must be emphasized that: 1) the reviews covered the clinical trials published between 1966 and 1993; and 2) they did not exclude a possible benefit of stress doses (i.e., less than 500 mg of hydrocortisone per day) administered for longer duration (i.e., more than two days).

Effect of Low Dose Corticosteroids

Almost 40 years ago, a placebo-controlled randomized trial evaluated the effectiveness of hydrocortisone given at decreasing doses (from 300 mg to 50 mg by 50 mg steps per day) for six days [56]. This study failed to demonstrate any beneficial effect of this strategy on survival in septic patients. However, it must be underlined that the study population included both children and adults, that meningitis accounted for almost half of the population included, and that there were significantly more patients with fulminant staphylococcal infections in the hydrocortisone group. In addition, the distribution of prognostic factors other than age, the appropriateness of antibiotherapy and supportive care, i.e. fluid replacement and vasopressor therapy, were not discussed. These important points probably explain the fairly large variability observed in mortality rates (from 20 to 70 %) within the five participating centers. Thus, the results of this study seem difficult to apply to septic patients treated in modern intensive care units (ICUs).

Almost 20 years ago, a small quasi-randomized trial investigated the effectiveness of stress doses of hydrocortisone in 18 critically ill patients with presumed adrenocortical insufficiency [57]. This study showed a significant dramatic improvement in survival rates in patients treated with 100 mg of hydrocortisone twice daily as compared to those of the control group (90 vs. 12.5%). In a more recent study, prolonged treatment with low doses of hydrocortisone was associated with an interesting, although non significant, trend toward reduced 28-day mortality (32 vs. 63%) [43]. A non significant improvement in survival with prolonged low doses of hydrocortisone in catecholamine-dependent septic shock was also shown in another small study [58]. Finally, we have recently completed a multicenter, placebo-controlled, randomized, double-blind study to determine if a combination of hydrocortisone (50 mg intravenous bolus four times per day) and fludrocortisone (50 µg orally once a day) given for seven days improves survival from septic shock, particularly in patients with occult adrenal insufficiency. This study, which included 300 patients, should allow a definitive conclusion on the therapeutic value of corticosteroids for septic shock.

CONCLUSION

Apart from in severe sepsis related to specific diseases like chloramphenicol-treated typhoid fever, *Pneumocystis carinii* pneumonia in AIDS patients and bacterial meningitis in children, short courses of high doses of corticosteroids should not be given to patients with sepsis and septic shock. Conversely, prolonged treatment with stress doses of hydrocortisone reduces the need for vasopressors, increases the probability of shock reversal in patients with catecholamine-dependent septic shock, and may impact favorably on survival.

REFERENCES

1. Perla D, Marmorston J. Suprarenal cortical hormone and salt in the treatment of pneumonia and other severe infections. Endocrinology 1940; 27:367-374
2. Weitzman S, Berger S. Clinical trial design in studies of corticosteroids for bacterial infections. Ann Intern Med 1974; 81:36-42
3. Lefering R, Neugebauer EA. Steroid controversy in sepsis and septic shock: a meta-analysis. Crit Care Med 1995; 23:1294-1303
4. Cronin L, Cook DJ, Carlet J, et al. Corticosteroid treatment for sepsis: a critical appraisal and meta-analysis of the literature. Crit Care Med 1995; 23:1430-1439
5. Chrousos GP. The hypothalamic-pituitary-adrenal axis and immune-mediated inflammation. N Engl J Med 1995; 332:1351-1362
6. Akerblom IE, Slater EP, Beato M, Baxter JD, Mellon PL. Negative regulation by glucocorticoids through interference with a cAMP responsive enhancer. Science 1988; 241:350-353
7. Diamond MI, Miner JN, Yoshinaga SK, Yamamoto KR. Transcription factor interactions: selectors of positive or negative regulation from a single DNA element. Science 1990; 249:1266-1272
8. Ray A, Prefontaine KE. Physical association and functional antagonism between the p65 subunit of transcription factor NF-kappa B and the glucocorticoid receptor. Proc Natl Acad Sci USA 1994; 91:752-756
9. Mukaida N, Morita M, Ishikawa Y, et al. Novel mechanism of glucocorticoid-mediated gene repression. Nuclear factor-kappa B is target for glucocorticoid-mediated interleukin 8 gene repression. J Biol Chem 1994; 269:13289-13295
10. Scheinman RI, Cogswell PC, Lofquist AK, Baldwin AS Jr. Role of transcriptional activation of I kappa B alpha in mediation of immunosuppression by glucocorticoids. Science 1995; 270:283-286
11. Auphan N, DiDonato JA, Rosette C, Helmberg A, Karin M. Immunosuppression by glucocorticoids: inhibition of NF-kappa B activity through induction of I kappa B synthesis. Science 1995; 270:286-290

12. Yang-Yen HF, Chambard JC, Sun YL, et al. Transcriptional interference between c-jun and the glucocorticoid receptor: mutual inhibition of DNA binding due to direct protein-protein interaction. Cell 1990; 62:1205-1215

13. Calandra T, Bernhagen J, Metz CN, et al. MIF as a glucocorticoid-induced modulator of cytokine production. Nature 1995; 377:68-71

14. Hirano T, Akira S, Taga T, Kishimoto T. Biological and clinical aspects of interleukin 6. Immunol Today 1990; 11:443-449

15. Webster EL, Torpy DJ, Elenkov IJ, Chrousos GP. Corticotropin-releasing hormone and inflammation. Ann NY Acad Sci 1998; 840:21-32

16. Ramirez F, Fowell DJ, Puklavec M, Simmonds S, Mason D. Glucocorticoids promote a TH2 cytokine response by CD4+ T cells in vitro. J Immunol 1996; 156:2406-2412

17. Swingle WW, Pfiffner JJ, Vars HM, et al. The function of the adrenal cortical hormone and the cause of death from adrenal insufficiency. Science 1933; 77:58-64

18. Grunfeld JP, Eloy L. Glucocorticoids modulate vascular reactivity in the rat. Hypertension 1987; 10:608-618

19. Szabo C, Thiemermann C, Wu CC, Perretti M, Vane JR. Attenuation of the induction of nitric oxide synthase by endogenous glucocorticoids accounts for endotoxin tolerance in vivo. Proc Natl Acad Sci USA 1994; 91:271-275

20. Steiner A, Vogt E, Locher R, Vetter W. Stimulation of the phosphoinositide signalling system as a possible mechanism for glucocorticoid action in blood pressure control. J Hypertens Suppl 1988; 6:S366-S368

21. Selye HA. A syndrome produced by diverse nocuous agents. Nature 1936; 138:32

22. Melby JC, Egdahl RH, Spink WW. Effect of brucella endotoxin on adrenocortical function in the dog. Fed Proc 1957; 16:425-429

23. Melby JC, Spink WW. Comparative studies on adrenal cortical function and cortisol metabolism in healthy adults and in patients with shock due to infection. J Clin Invest 1958; 37: 1791-1798

24. Lenczowski MJ, Schmidt ED, Van Dam AM, Gaykema RP, Tilders FJ. Individual variation in hypothalamus-pituitary-adrenal responsiveness of rats to endotoxin and interleukin-1 beta. Ann N Y Acad Sci 1998; 856:139-147

25. Bluthe RM, Walter V, Parnet P, et al. Lipopolysaccharide induces sickness behaviour in rats by a vagal mediated mechanism. C R Acad Sci III 1994; 317:499-503

26. Gaykema RP, Dijkstra I, Tilders FJ. Subdiaphragmatic vagotomy suppresses endotoxin-induced activation of hypothalamic corticotropin-releasing hormone neurons and ACTH secretion. Endocrinology 1995; 136:4717-4720

27. Waterhouse R. Case of suprarenal apoplexy. Lancet 1911; 1:577

28. Friderichsen C. Nebennierenapoplexie bei kleinen Kindern. Jb Kinderheilk 1918; 87:109

29. Annane D, Bellissant E, Bollaert PE, et al. The hypothalamo-pituitary axis in septic shock. Br J Intensive Care 1996; 6:260-268

30. Annane D, Sébille V, Troché G, Raphaël JC, Gajdos P, Bellissant E. A 3-level prognostic classification in septic shock based on cortisol levels and cortisol response to corticotropin. JAMA 2000; 283:1038-1045

31. Annane D, Bellissant E, Sébille V, et al. Impaired pressor sensitivity to noradrenaline in septic shock patients with and without impaired adrenal function reserve. Br J Clin Pharmacol 1998; 46:589-597

32. Soni A, Pepper GM, Wyrwinski PM, et al. Adrenal insufficiency occurring during septic shock: incidence, outcome, and relationship to peripheral cytokine levels. Am J Med 1995; 98:266-271

33. Molijn GJ, Spek JJ, van Uffelen JC, et al. Differential adaptation of glucocorticoid sensitivity of peripheral blood mononuclear leukocytes in patients with sepsis or septic shock. J Clin Endocrinol Metab 1995; 80:1799-1803

34. Almawi WY, Lipman ML, Stevens AC, Zanker B, Hadro ET, Strom TB. Abrogation of glucocorticoid-mediated inhibition of T cell proliferation by the synergistic action of IL-1, IL-6, and IFN-gamma. J Immunol 1991; 146:3523-3527

35. Kam JC, Szefler SJ, Surs W, Sher ER, Leung DY. Combination of IL-2 and IL-4 reduces glucocorticoid receptor-binding affinity and T cell response to glucocorticoids. J Immunol 1993; 151:3460-3466

36. Molijn GJ, Koper JW, van Uffelen CJ, et al. Temperature-induced down-regulation of the glucocorticoid receptor in peripheral blood mononuclear leucocyte in patients with sepsis or septic shock. Clin Endocrinol 1995; 43:197-203

37. McKenzie AW, Stoughton RB. Methods for comparing percutaneous absorption of steroids. Archs Derm 1962; 86:608-610

38. Thiemermann C, Vane JR. Inhibition of nitric oxide synthesis reduces the hypotension induced by bacterial lipopolysaccharides in the rat in vivo. Eur J Pharmacol 1990; 182:591-595

39. Paya D, Gray GA, Fleming I, Stoclet JC. Effect of dexamethasone on the onset and persistence of vascular hyporeactivity induced by E. coli lipopolysaccharide in rats. Circ Shock 1993; 41:103-112

40. Yard AC, Kadowitz PJ. Studies on the mechanism of hydrocortisone potentiation of vasoconstrictor responses to epinephrine in the anesthetized animal. Eur J Pharmacol 1972; 20:1-9

41. Bhagat K, Collier J, Vallance P. Local venous responses to endotoxin in humans. Circulation 1996; 94:490-497

42. Bellissant E, Annane D. Effect of hydrocortisone on phenylephrine - mean arterial pressure dose-response relationship in septic shock. Clin Pharmacol Ther 2000; 68:293-303

43. Bollaert PE, Charpentier C, Levy B, Debouverie M, Audibert G, Larcan A. Reversal of late septic shock with supraphysiologic doses of hydrocortisone. Crit Care Med 1998; 26:45-650

44. Briegel J, Forst H, Haller M, et al. Stress doses of hydrocortisone reverse hyperdynamic septic shock: a prospective, randomized, double-blind, single-center study. Crit Care Med 1999; 27:723-732

45. Barber AE, Coyle SM, Marano MA, et al. Glucocorticoid therapy alters hormonal and cytokine responses to endotoxin in man. J Immunol 1993; 150:1999-2006.

46. Barber AE, Coyle SM, Fischer E, et al. Influence of hypercortisolemia on soluble tumor necrosis factor receptor II and interleukin-1 receptor antagonist responses to endotoxin in human beings. Surgery 1995; 118:406-410

47. van der Poll T, Barber AE, Coyle SM, Lowry SF. Hypercortisolemia increases plasma interleukin-10 concentrations during human endotoxemia – a clinical research center study. J Clin Endocrinol Metab 1996; 81:3604-3606

48. Briegel J, Kellermann W, Forst H, et al. Low-dose hydrocortisone infusion attenuates the systemic inflammatory response syndrome. The phospholipase A2 study group. Clin Investig 1994; 72:782-787

49. Key D. Effects of hydrocortisone on the immune response in patients with septic shock – results from a double-blind cross-over study. J Anaesth Intensive 1999; 1:S195-S196

50. Hinshaw LB, Beller BK, Chang AC, et al. Corticosteroid/antibiotic treatment of adrenalectomized dogs challenged with lethal E. Coli. Circ Shock 1985; 16: 265-277.

51. Fabian TC, Patterson R. Steroid therapy in septic shock. Survival studies in a laboratory model. Am Surg 1982; 48:614-617

52. Hoffman SL, Punjabi NH, Kumala S, et al. Reduction of mortality in chloramphenicol-treated severe typhoid fever by high-dose dexamethasone. N Engl J Med 1984; 310:82-88

53. Gagnon S, Boota AM, Fischl MA, Baier H, Kirksey OW, La Voie L. Corticosteroids as adjunctive therapy for severe Pneumocystis carinii pneumonia in the acquired

immunodeficiency syndrome. A double-blind, placebo-controlled trial. N Engl J Med 1990; 323:1440-1450

54. Odio CM, Faingezicht I, Paris M, et al. The beneficial effects of early dexamethasone administration in infants and children with bacterial meningitis. N Engl J Med 1991; 324:1525-1531

55. Rogers J. Large doses of steroids in septicaemic shock. Br J Urol 1970; 42: 742.

56. Cooperative Study Group. The effectiveness of hydrocortisone in the management of severe infections. JAMA 1963; 183:462-465

57. McKee JI, Finlay WE. Cortisol replacement in severely stressed patients. Lancet 1983; 1:484

58. Chawla K, Kupfer Y, Tessler S. Hydrocortisone reverses refractory septic shock. Crit Care Med 1999; 27:A33 (Abst)

45

THE PLACE OF IMMUNONUTRITION

Ben L. Zarzaur
Kenneth A. Kudsk

Following severe trauma or major surgical procedures, patients often have delayed ability to resume oral intake. While this is well tolerated in well-nourished patients for a short period of time, a delay in oral resumption of nutrients often leads to progressive protein depletion, altered host defenses, and high rates of pneumonia, intra-abdominal abscess formation, anastomotic leaks, and wound dehiscences [1-3]. To counteract these deleterious effects, specialized nutritional support with either parenteral or enteral feeding has been utilized over the past thirty years.

Over the last two decades, it has become clear that there are benefits gained when nutrients are delivered via the gastrointestinal tract that are not gained when these nutrients are delivered parenterally. In particular, patients appear to be at less risk of pneumonia and intra-abdominal abscess formation, suggesting alterations in respiratory immunity and peritoneal protection [1-3]. Recently, studies suggest that the addition of specific immunonutrients to enteral feeding provides additional benefits. Several immune-enhancing diets have been formulated and tested in different patient populations. While there is less debate regarding the benefits of enteral delivery, the use of immune-enhancing diets as a general diet remains controversial. There are, however, significant clinical data suggesting that certain subpopulations of patients may benefit from these formulas. On the other hand, there may be some increased risk with these diets in a small subpopulation of patients with preexisting upregulation of the immune system.

Author [ref]	Study Design	Patient Population	Formula	Conclusions and Problems
Daly et al [11]	Randomized, prospective, double blind trial	85 patients undergoing major abdominal surgery for upper gastrointestinal cancer (UGI CA)	41 patients (pt) received an IED with arginine, ω-3 Fatty acids and nucleotides 44 pt received a standard enteral diet (SED)	77 pt were eligible for analysis. Diets were not isonitrogenous. The mean albumin level was 3.3 ± 0.8g/dL for the IED group and 3.0 ± 1.2g/dL for the control group. There were 70% fewer infectious and wound complications in the IED group ($p=.02$ vs the SED group). Hospital stay was reduced 22% among those in the IED group when compared to the SED group.
Daly et al [12]	Randomized, prospective, double blind trial	60 pt undergoing major abdominal surgery for UGI CA	18 pt received an IED with arginine, ω-3 Fatty acids and nucleotides postoperatively and as an outpatient during chemotherapy and radiation 12 pt received the IED while an inpatient only 19 pt received a SED postoperatively and as an outpatient during chemotherapy and radiation 11 pt received a SED while an inpatient only	Diets were nearly isonitrogenous and isocaloric. Pt were moderately malnourished with mean albumin levels of 3.3 ± 0.6g/dL for the IED group and 3.2 ± 0.5g/dL for the control group. The IED pt group displayed 33% fewer infectious complications when compared to the SED group ($p<.005$). The IED pt group had a 6 day reduction in hospital stay when compared to the SED group ($p<.03$). There was no difference in mortality. Pt who received enteral feeding during outpatient treatment were significantly less intolerant to the treatments than the non-fed group.
Braga et al [18]	Randomized, prospective trial	77 pt undergoing curative surgery for gastric or pancreatic CA	26 pt received an IED with arginine, ω-3 Fatty acids and nucleotides 24 pt received a SED 27 pt received total parenteral nutrition (TPN)	All diets were isonitrogenous and isocaloric. The mean albumin levels for the 3 groups were 3.98 ± 5.4g/dL for the IED group, 3.78 ± 5.2g/dL for the SED group and 3.79 ± 3.2g/dL for the TPN group. The IED group showed a significant drop in sepsis scores for pt fed the IED ($p<.05$ vs the parenteral group). There was a trend towards a reduction in infectious complications among the IED group pt when compared to the SED group. There was also a trend towards a decrease in the sepsis scores for the IED group when compared to the SED group.
Schilling et al [15]	Randomized, prospective trial	45 pt undergoing elective abdominal surgery for UGI CA	14 pt received an IED with arginine, ω-3 Fatty acids and nucleotides 14 pt received a SED 13 pt received a low calorie TPN with fat and carbohydrates only	The diets were neither isonitrogenous nor isocaloric. No data regarding preoperative nutritional status was recorded. There was a trend towards a decrease in infectious complications and hospital length of stay among the IED group compared to the other two groups. This study had low statistical power secondary to small sample size.
Heslin et al [34]	Randomized, prospective trial	195 pt undergoing abdominal surgery for UGI CA	97 pt received an IED with arginine, ω-3 Fatty acids and nucleotides 98 pt received standard postoperative care with crystalloids and dextrose	Control group pt received only IV fluids. Pt in both groups, similar to the Braga study in 1995, were well nourished (Albumin ≥ 4.0 g/dL). No difference was found between the two groups with regard to infectious complications, mortality, or hospital length of stay.

Study	Design	Population / Intervention	Results
Gianotti et al [16]	Randomized, prospective double blind trial	260 pt undergoing elective abdominal surgery for UGI CA. 87 pt received an IED with arginine, ω-3 fatty acids and nucleotides. 87 pt received a SED. 86 received TPN	The diets were isonitrogenous and isocaloric. The mean albumin levels were $3.79 \pm .35$g/dL and 3.82 ± 39g/dL for the IED and SED groups respectively. There was a trend towards fewer infectious complications in the IED group compared to the SED group. There was a significant difference in infectious complications between the IED group and the TPN group ($p=.06$).
Senkal et al [21]	Randomized, prospective double blind, multicenter trial	164 pt undergoing elective abdominal surgery for UGI CA. 10 pt dropped out for various reasons. 77 pt received an IED with arginine, ω-3 fatty acids and nucleotides. 77 patients received a SED	The diets were isonitrogenous and isocaloric. There was a significant reduction in infections after postoperative day 5 in the IED group when compared to the SED group ($p<.05$).
Braga et al [19]	Randomized, prospective trial	166 pt undergoing elective abdominal surgery for UGI CA. 55 pt received an IED with arginine, ω-3 fatty acids and nucleotides. 55 pt received a SED. 55 received TPN	All diets were isonitrogenous and isocaloric. The mean albumin levels were 3.81 ± 23g/dL, $3.73 \pm .39$g/dL and $3.76 \pm .35$ for the IED, SED and TPN groups respectively. Those pt with weight loss >10% body weight in the previous 6 months were stratified as malnourished. The infectious complication rate was 7.3% higher in the malnourished group than in the well nourished group. Among malnourished patients, the infectious complications rate was significantly lower in the IED group than in the TPN group ($p<.05$). Among all pt, sepsis scores of pt fed the IED were significantly lower than those fed the SED or TPN ($p<.05$ vs both groups).
Braga et al [20]	Randomized, prospective, double blind trial	206 pt with CA of stomach, colorectum or pancreas. 111 pt were eligible for analysis. 102 pt received 1 L/day of an IED with arginine, ω-3 fatty acids and nucleotides for 7 days preoperatively with continuation of the diet 6 hrs postoperatively. 104 pt received a 1 L/day of a SED for 7 days preoperatively with continuation 6 hrs postoperatively	The diets were isonitrogenous and isocaloric. The mean albumin levels were $3.93 \pm .42$g/dL and $3.91 \pm .46$g/dL for the IED and SED groups respectively. The IED group had significantly fewer infectious complications than the SED group ($p=.02$). There was also a decrease in length of hospital stay postoperatively for the IED fed pt ($p=.01$).
Senkal et al [35]	Randomized, prospective, double blind trial	154 pt with UGI CA scheduled for elective surgery. 89 pt received 1 L/day of an IED with arginine, ω-3 fatty acids and nucleotides for at least 5 days preoperatively with the same diet continued postoperatively. 89 pt received 1 L/day of a SED for at least 5 days preoperatively with the same diet continued postoperatively	All diets were isocaloric and isonitrogenous. Pt fed the IED had significantly fewer infectious complications than the control group ($p<.05$). After postoperative day 3, pt fed the IED had fewer infectious complications than the SED group ($p<.04$).

Table 1. Immune-enhancing diets (IED) in the general surgery population.

COMPONENTS OF IMMUNE-ENANCING DIETS

Several specific nutrients or substances have been shown to have beneficial effects upon immunity and healing in animal models. Commercially available diets usually contain a mixture of these specific nutrients.

Omega-3 Fatty Acids

Fatty acids make up the phospholipid lipid bilayer of all human cells. The human body is incapable of synthesizing polyunsaturated fatty acids (PUFAs), such as omega-3 or omega-6 fatty acids, but can incorporate them into the phospholipid bilayer structure if these fatty acids are provided in the diet. This membrane phospholipid serves as a source of fatty acids for the arachidonic acid cascade during stress or sepsis. When omega-6 fatty acids are metabolized, immunosuppressive prostaglandins of the two and four series are produced. Omega-3 fatty acid metabolism, however, results in production of prostaglandins or leukotrienes of the 3- and 5-series which are neither proinflammatory nor immunosuppressive. Therefore, a diet enriched in omega-3 fatty acids has been shown in experimental models to have beneficial immunologic effects [4]. Vegetable oils are primarily composed of omega-6 fatty acids; fish oil and canola oil provide omega-3 fatty acids.

Glutamine

Glutamine is a key amino acid involved in the stress response. It is the most abundant amino acid in the body and, following stress and injury, its production is upregulated in the muscle cell for release into the blood where it provides an important fuel for rapidly proliferating cells such as enterocytes, and immunocytes. Its effects upon these cells have been extensively studied in animal models. For example, supplementation of parenteral nutrition with glutamine prevents atrophy of the mucosa and reduction in cells of the gut-associated lymphoid tissue (GALT) [5]. Functionally, glutamine supplementation reduces bacterial translocation, bacteremia, and mortality following sepsis in animal experiments [6].

Arginine

Normally, arginine is a nonessential amino acid synthesized by the human body. Following injury and during stress, it becomes a conditionally essential amino acid necessary for tissue growth and healing. Arginine increases thymic cellularity, augments natural killer cell activity and enhances macrophage tumor cytotoxicity in animal models [7,8]. In human volunteers, arginine improved T cell responses compared to non-supplemented patients [9].

Nucleotides

Nucleotides are important in purine and pyrimidine synthesis for rapidly dividing cells of the immune system. Mice fed diets containing nucleotides have increased natural killer cell activity and improved survival to sepsis induced by *Candida* or *Staphylococcus* species [10].

CLINICAL USE OF IMMUNE-ENHANCING DIETS

A number of clinical studies have been performed in general surgical patients undergoing major gastrointestinal procedures and in critically injured trauma patients. Compelling data suggest that certain patient populations benefit from immune-enhancing diets while other populations demonstrate no clear effect. There is a small, but significant, subset of critically ill septic patients in whom immune-enhancing diets may be detrimental but this evidence is preliminary, incomplete, and contradictory. The published clinical trials to date are tabulated in Tables 1-5.

Several issues must be kept in mind when reviewing these data. First, there is no single standard formula which is considered 'immune-enhancing', and the various formulas contain one or more of the nutrients previously discussed. Second, many of the studies have been criticized for providing control diets that are not isocaloric or isonitrogenous to the immune-enhancing diet. Finally, outcome measures vary between trials and have included markers of infection, wound problems, length of stay, cost, and mortality. Many outcome measurements, e.g., intensive care unit (ICU) stay, can be influenced by uncontrolled non-dietary factors such as physician preference, early mortality, and hospital policy. Therefore, blinded studies with appropriate control diets provide the most valuable information.

Author [ref]	Study Design	Patient Population	Formula	Conclusions and Problems
Brown et al [24]	Randomized, prospective trial	41 consecutive pt with major trauma who required enteral nutritional support	19 pt received an IED with arginine, ω-3 Fatty acids β-carotene 18 pt received a standard enteral diet (SED) 37 pt completed the study	Diets were neither isonitrogenous nor isocaloric. Pt in the IED group received feeds earlier than the SED group, and they received more nutritional support as a whole than the SED group. Pt fed the IED had significantly less infectious complications than those fed the SED.
Moore et al [21]	Randomized, prospective, multicenter trial	114 severely injured trauma pt. 98 pt eligible for analysis	51 pt received an IED with arginine, ω-3 Fatty acids and nucleotides 47 pt received a SED	Diets were not isonitrogenous. The study had a small sample size. The mean ISS for the IED group was 20.6 ± 1.2 and 21.8 ± 1.2 for the control group. Pt receiving the IED had significantly fewer intrabdominal abscesses and multisystem organ failure (p= .023 for both vs the SED group).
Kudsk et al [22]	Randomized, prospective, blinded trial	35 severely injured trauma pt	17 pt received an IED with arginine, ω-3 Fatty acids and nucleotides 18 pt received a SED Contemporaneous controls were severely injured pt without enteral access and unable to be fed	The diets were isonitrogenous and isocaloric. Pt in the IED group had a mean ISS of 25.1 ± 3.3; pt in the control group had a mean ISS of 28.4 ± 2.9. Pt fed the IED had significantly fewer infections than the SED group (p= .02) or the unfed control group (p= .002). The unfed control group had the most infectious complications and use of antibiotics. The IED group had significantly fewer intra-abdominal abscess formation than the other two groups (p= .05). Pt in the IED group had significantly shorter hospital stays when compared to the other two groups (p= .03 for both groups). Pt in the IED group had shorter ICU stays and number of ventilator days compared to the other two groups, although this did not reach statistical significance.
Mendez et al [26]	Randomized, prospective, blinded trial	59 severely injured trauma pt	22 pt received an IED with arginine, ω-3 Fatty acids and nucleotides 21 pt received a SED	The diets were isonitrogenous but not isocaloric. The mean ISS was 28.2 ± 2.1 for the IED group and 32.2 ± 2.3 for the control group. There was a trend towards increased hospital stay, infectious complications and ventilator days among the IED group although this did not reach statistical significance. However, the IED group had more pt with ARDS prior to entry into the study (45% vs 19% for the SED group).
Weimann et al [25]	Randomized, prospective, double blind, controlled trial	32 severely injured trauma pt	16 pt received an IED with arginine, ω-3 Fatty acids and nucleotides 13 pt received a SED	The diets were isonitrogenous and isocaloric. The mean ISS were 39.6 ± 11.4 and 40.5 ± 9.2 for the IED and SED groups respectively. While the pt fed the IED had significantly less SIRS between hospital days 8-14 than the SED group (p<.001), there was no difference in mortality and infectious complications.

Table 2. Immune-enhancing diets (IED) in the trauma population

An important issue in interpreting these studies is patient selection. Recruitment of patients at low risk of nutrition-related complications into studies dilutes any potential beneficial effect of an immune-enhancing diet compared to any control. For example, when well-nourished patients at low risk of significant complications are entered into randomized, controlled studies, low rates of infectious complications or wound problems do not necessarily reflect ineffectiveness of an immune-enhancing diet but rather reflect the low-risk patient population. Similar observations have been made in trauma studies where low-risk patients stratified by the abdominal trauma index (ATI) or injury severity score (ISS) have few complications with little nutritional effect. One would not expect to see improved outcome in this low-risk population even if there were improved immunological defenses with an immune-enhancing diet. Therefore, the patient population selected for entry into a study influences outcome.

Clear Evidence of Benefit from an Immune-Enhancing Diet

Major Elective Upper Gastrointestinal Surgery

There is ample evidence that an immune-enhancing diet improves the postoperative outcome of patients undergoing major upper gastrointestinal surgery. This benefit is most clearly realized in patients who are nutritionally deficient prior to surgery.

In 1992, Daly et al. randomized 85 patients undergoing upper GI surgery for malignancy to jejunal feedings with advancement to goal by postoperative day 4. A special diet containing arginine, omega-3 fatty acids, and nucleotides was compared with a nonisonitrogenous, isocaloric control. The immune-enhancing diet group sustained significantly fewer infectious and wound-related problems and had a shorter length of stay. There was no difference in mortality, a trend found in all studies performed in elective general surgical patients [11]. Subsequently, Daly's group tested an immune-enhancing diet against an isocaloric, isonitrogenous diet and again demonstrated a significant reduction in infectious complications with a reduced length of stay [12].

The importance of patient selection is shown in a study by Heslin et al. [13] who noted no benefits with the same immune-enhancing diet used by Daly et al., compared to IV fluids alone in patients undergoing curative resection of upper GI tumors. Tube feedings were started within 24 hours of surgery in the immune-enhancing diet group and advanced to goal. The control group received IV fluids alone until return of normal bowel function or postoperative day 10 at which time either enteral or parenteral nutrition was instituted. There were no differences in any outcome variable between the immune-enhancing diet and control group including postoperative infectious complications. However, the patients entered into the study differed from the Daly studies in a very important criteria. Patients in the Heslin study were better nourished with an average preoperative albumin of 4.0-4.1 g/dl and had minimal preoperative weight loss while patients entered into Daly's study had average preoperative albumins of 3.1-3.3 g/dl. In addition, 30-40% of patients sustained at least 10% of weight loss preoperatively. These results reinforce the need for appropriate patient selection in randomized, prospective studies and demonstrate that an immune-enhancing diet (and probably nutrition support in general) is unnecessary in patients at a low risk of malnutrition-related complications.

Studies by Senkal et al. [14], Schilling et al. [15], and several studies by Gianotti et al. [16] and Braga et al. [17-20] confirm the benefits of an immune-enhancing diet in at-risk general surgery patients undergoing major upper gastrointestinal surgery. A notable observation is that as the average albumin of patient populations decreased, the effectiveness of therapy with an immune-enhancing diet appeared to improve. For example, Braga et al. entered patients with an average albumin of approximately 3.9 g/dl and noted significant reduction in sepsis scores and only a trend to reduced infectious complications in the immune-enhancing diet group. In studies with more malnourished patients, however, clearer outcomes with reduction in infectious complications were evident.

Two other issues of feeding in general surgical patient populations are worth mentioning. In a study by Daly et al. [12], jejunal feeding with an immune-enhancing diet was continued in the postoperative period while the patients were receiving outpatient chemotherapy and radiation. In this group, there was a significantly lower rehospitalization rate for both infectious and noninfectious reasons when compared with unfed patients, indicating a benefit from postoperative feeding in patients undergoing immunosuppressive treatments with radiation and chemotherapy. Second, at-risk patients may benefit from preoperative 'loading' with an immune-enhancing diet. Patients undergoing curative resection for upper gastrointestinal tumors were instructed to drink either an isonitrogenous, isocaloric enteral formula or an immune-enhancing diet containing arginine, nucleotides, and omega-3 fatty acids for seven days prior to operations. Diets were continued postoperatively. Infectious complications decreased significantly in the immune-enhancing diet group compared with the control group, indicating that preoperative supplementation with these specialty nutrients may be beneficial [14,20]. This concept of loading is evident in the study by Senkal et al. [21] in which the immune-enhancing diet was compared to an isonitrogenous, isocaloric diet administered following elective abdominal surgery for upper GI carcinoma. While there was no difference in early postoperative infections, infectious complications after postoperative day 5 dropped significantly in the immune-enhancing diet group. These observations are consistent with a delay between incorporation of nutrients into cell membranes and their effect on metabolism and cellular defenses.

Moderate to Severely Injured Trauma Patients

The ISS and ATI are commonly used to quantitate severity of injury following blunt and penetrating trauma. The ISS reflects global body injury to the head, chest, abdomen, pelvis, lower extremities, and soft tissues while the ATI quantifies the magnitude and severity of intra-abdominal injuries. These scoring systems allow patients to be stratified by ISS (> 17) or ATI (> 18) into patient populations at high risk of infectious complications.

The trauma studies investigating immune-enhancing diets are heterogenous both in patient populations and in type of diet used. Five studies used three different immune-enhancing diets and five different control diets. Several of the studies had low patient numbers. Despite these restrictions, several observations can be made from the available data. Moore et al. [22] randomized 98 trauma victims with moderate degrees of injury to an immune-enhancing diet enriched with arginine, omega-3 fatty acids, glutamine, and nucleotides or a standard nonisonitrogenous, isocaloric diet. Patients receiving the immune-enhancing diet sustained significantly fewer intra-abdominal abscesses and a reduction in multiple organ dysfunction syndrome compared to patients receiving a standard diet. The average ATI for the control and immune-enhancing diet groups were similar (21.8 ± 1.4 and 19.0 ± 1.3, respectively) and there were no differences in the average ISS between the two groups (21.8 ± 1.2 and 20.6 ± 1.2, respectively).

In a subsequent study, Kudsk et al. [23] limited entry to patients with more severe degrees of trauma (an ATI ≥ 25 or an ISS ≥ 20) who had jejunostomy tubes placed at the time of their laparotomy for intra-abdominal injuries. Patients were randomized to either an immune-enhancing diet containing arginine, omega-3 fatty acids, glutamine, and nucleotides or an isonitrogenous, isocaloric control. Patients receiving the immune-enhancing diet sustained significantly fewer septic complications, especially intra-abdominal abscess formation. Hospital stay was significantly shorter and there were few pulmonary infections. A third group of patients eligible by severity of injury but without jejunostomy tube placement received little or no nutrition support. This unfed group had the highest incidence of major sepsis, intra-abdominal abscess formation, pneumonia, length of stay, and hospital charges.

Brown et al. [24] randomized 41 consecutive trauma patients who required enteral nutrition support to either an immune-enhancing diet with arginine, omega-3 fatty acids, and beta-carotene or a nonisonitrogenous, nonisocaloric control diet. While there was a significant reduction in pneumonia with the immune-enhancing diet as well as an overall reduction in septic complications, an important variable confounded the interpretation of this study. Patients randomized to the immune-enhancing diet had significantly more jejunostomies, were successfully fed earlier, and received more nutrition support than the control group who were fed intragastrically. Thus, the reduction in pneumonia in the immune-enhancing diet group could be due to the diet, intrajejunal feeding, or to earlier, more successful enteral nutrition.

Weimann et al. [25] studied 32 patients receiving either an immune-enhancing diet with arginine, omega-3 fatty acids, and nucleotides or an isonitrogenous, isocaloric control diet and noted no differences between the groups. A comparable incidence of pneumonia, sepsis, bacteremia, urinary tract infection, and central venous line infections occurred in the two groups. These patients, however, were extremely injured with an average ISS of 39.6 $\pm$ 11.4 for the immune-enhancing diet and 40.5 $\pm$ 9.2 for the control groups; mortality was almost 50%. Complications in such a severely injured group may not be affected by nutrition support with or without an immune-enhancing diet.

A final trauma study indicates a *potential* risk of immune-enhancing diet administration due to an augmented inflammatory response. Mendez et al. [26] randomized critically injured patients with an ISS > 13 to either a standard enteral diet or an immune-enhancing diet enriched with arginine, omega-3 fatty acids, and the trace elements, selenium, chromium, molybdenum, and taurine. Patients receiving the immune-enhancing diet had prolonged hospital stays, prolonged ventilator days, and more pneumonia than the control patients. However, the acute respiratory distress syndrome (ARDS) was present in 45% of patients receiving the immune-enhancing diet *prior to enrollment* compared to 19% of patients in the control group. Therefore, the outcomes could reflect either an upregulation in the inflammatory response by the immune-enhancing diet or a breakdown in the randomization process with more severely injured patients randomized to the immune-enhancing diet group. The rate of pneumonia could, of course, be influenced by the pre-existing ARDS.

Author [ref]	Study Design	Patient Population	Formula	Conclusions and Problems
Saffle et al [28]	Randomized, prospective, double-blind trial	49 severely burned patients (pt).	25 pt received an IED with arginine, ω-3 Fatty acids, & nucleotides 24 patients received a standard enteral diet (SED)	The diets were neither isonitrogenous nor isocaloric. There was no difference in infectious complications, mortality, length of stay or hospital cost between the two groups. This study had a small sample size. There were a large number of patients in each group that had inhalation injuries (71% for the control group and 56% for the IED group) which might have influenced the results when compared to the other burn study.
Gottschlich et al [27]	Randomized, prospective, double-blind trial	50 severely burned Pt	17 pt received an IED with arginine & fish oil 17 pt received a stress formula 14 pt received a SED	The pt who received the IED had a lower infection rate (p<.03) and length of stay per percent body surface area burn (p<.02) than those fed the SED and stress formula.

Table 3. Immune-enhancing diets (IED) in the burn population

Author [ref]	Study Design	Patient Population	Formula	Conclusions and Problems
Chendrasekhar et al [29]	Randomized prospective trial	20 patients (pt) with severe closed head injury (CHI)	11 pt received an IED with arginine, ω-3 Fatty acids, & nucleotides 9 pt received a standard enteral diet (SED)	A small number of pt were involved in this study. The diets were neither isonitrogenous nor isocaloric. Infectious complications were significantly lower in the IED group when compared to the SED group (p<.0001). All pt in the IED group had infections as opposed to 9.1% in the SED group.
Minard et al (JPEN 1998; 22:59 (abst)	Randomized, prospective trial	30 pt. with severe CHI were enrolled and 27 pt were eligible for analysis	All patients received an IED with arginine, ω-3 Fatty acids, & nucleotides 12 pt were randomized to receive endoscopically placed jejunostomies and early feeding 15 pt were randomized to receive feedings after the gastric ileus had resolved	A small number of pt were involved in this study. There were a large number of deaths in the late feeding group. There was no difference between those fed early and those fed late with regard to infectious complications, ICU stay, and length of hospital stay. There is no advantage to endoscopic placement of a feeding naso-jejunal tube in this patient population for very early feeding.

Table 4. Immune-enhancing diets (IED) in the head injury population

Author [ref]	Study Design	Patient Population	Formula	Conclusions and Problems
Bower et al [31]	Randomized, prospective, double-blind, multicenter trial	326 critically ill patients (pt) following trauma, major surgery or sepsis 296 pt were eligible for analysis after randomization	167 pt received an IED with arginine, ω-3 FA, & nucleotides 159 pt received a standard enteral diet (SED)	Diets were neither isonitrogenous nor isocaloric. Many of the patients were trauma patients (235/826). Pt who reached the minimal feeding criteria had significantly decreased length of stay but with an increase in mortality among the septic pt (approached statistical significance). These results support the idea of a minimal effective dose per day of an IED that must be delivered in order to obtain maximal benefit.
Galban et al [33]	Randomized, prospective, multicenter trial	181 critically ill ICU patients 176 pt were eligible for analysis	89 pt received an IED with arginine, ω-3 Fatty acids, & nucleotides 87 pt received a high protein SED	There was a significant decrease in mortality among the IED fed patients when compared to the SED group (p < 05). The number of infectious complications was significantly lower in the IED group than in the SED group.
Atkinson et al [32]	Randomized, prospective, double blind trial	390 critically ill ICU patients	197 pt received an IED with arginine, ω-3 Fatty acids, & nucleotides 193 pt received a SED	The diets were isonitrogenous and isocaloric. Those who were successfully fed the IED were able to be removed from the ventilator sooner than the SED group and had a shorter length of ICU and hospital stay. While the patients in the IED group had higher mortality than the SED group, the pt in the IED group had higher APACHE II scores upon entering the study. These results support the idea of the early institution of an IED in order to get the maximal benefit.
Snyder-man et al [36]	Randomized, prospective, dual center trial	136 Pt. With head and neck CA requiring surgery	82 pt received an IED with arginine, ω-3 Fatty acids, & nucleotides 47 pt received an SED (6 different diets)	The diets were neither isonitrogenous nor isocaloric. Six different control diets were used. Infectious complications were not clearly defined. The authors found a significant reduction in infectious complications in the IED group when compared to the SED group (p <04). There was a trend towards shorter ICU stays for the IED group (p<08).

Table 5. Immune-enhancing diets (IED) in the intensive care unit and head and neck cancer populations

In summary, the perceived effects of an immune-enhancing diet in the trauma population are on reduced septic complications and, in particular, a reduction in intra-abdominal abscess formation following celiotomy. Caution should be used when considering an immune-enhancing diet in patients with preexisting evidence of multiple organ dysfunction and ARDS.

Patients Who Might Benefit from Immune-Enhancing Diets

Burns

Two studies have been performed in the burn population. Gottschlich et al. [27] studied 50 severely burned patients receiving an immune-enhancing diet enriched with arginine and fish oil versus a standard diet or a specialty stress formula (Trauma-Cal). Patients who received the immune-enhancing diet showed a reduction in the wound infection rate, a shorter length of stay for percent body surface area burn, a reduced incidence of diarrhea, and increased glucose tolerance.

Saffle et al. [28], however, noted no differences between patients receiving an immune-enhancing diet enriched with arginine, omega-3 fatty acids, and nucleotides and a nonisonitrogenous, nonisocaloric control diet. The sample size was small which decreases its statistical power, but there was no difference in regard to infectious complications, mortality, length of stay, or hospital costs.

Head-injured Patients

In one small study of 20 patients with severe closed-head injury who were randomized to a nonisonitrogenous, nonisocaloric control diet or an immune-enhancing diet enriched with arginine, omega-3 fatty acids, and nucleotides. One hundred percent of patients receiving the control diet sustained infectious complications. Of the patients receiving the immune-enhancing diet, only 9% had infectious complications [29].

In a larger study by Minard et al. [30], head-injured patients were randomized to either endoscopic placement of a nasojejunal tube with early institution of an immune-enhancing diet enriched with omega-3 fatty acids, nucleotides, and arginine or to intragastric feeding with a small-bore nasogastric tube. Feedings were instituted within 36 hours of admission following endoscopic placement and within approximately 72 hours in the patients receiving intragastric feeding. There was no difference in infectious complications, ICU stay, or length of stay with either group. The authors concluded that there was no additional benefit by attempting to institute an immune-enhancing diet prior to normal recovery from gastroparesis in severely head-injured patients.

Intensive Care Unit Patients

Three studies have examined ICU populations. Bower et al. [31], noted that patients receiving an immune-enhancing diet enriched with omega-3 fatty acids, arginine, and nucleotides had shorter hospital stays compared to a nonisonitrogenous, nonisocaloric control diet. A majority of these patients were trauma patients. The study has been criticized for excessive post hoc analysis of outcome which demonstrated that successfully fed patients (receiving > 821 ml/day) had significantly shorter hospital stays than other groups. Patients admitted for sepsis appeared to have a reduction in length of stay and nosocomial infections; however, the mortality rate in this group appeared to be excessively high and approached statistical significance, leading to a concern that in some subpopulations, an immune-enhancing diet can aggravate the clinical condition.

Atkinson et al. [32] randomized 390 critically ill ICU patients to either an immune-enhancing diet enriched with arginine, omega-3 fatty acids, nucleotides, or a standard isonitrogenous, isocaloric control diet. Patients successfully fed with the immune-enhancing diet were weaned from the ventilator sooner and had a shorter length of stay. A clear benefit was noted in patients who received more than 3 liters of the immune-enhancing diet over the first 72 hours following admission. An unblinded study by Galban et al. [33] recruited medical and surgical ICU patients showing a significant reduction in infectious complications in patients fed an immune-enhancing diet containing omega-3 fatty acids, arginine, and nucleotides. Most of the benefit was noted in the patients who were moderately ill based on APACHE II scores.

Potential Risks with Immune-Enhancing Diets

As pointed out in a few studies, authors have suspected an increase in the proinflammatory responses following trauma and an increase in mortality of patients with preexisting infectious complications and sepsis. A recent unpublished study of an experimental formula also noted an increase in mortality in a blinded prospective study if there was preexisting sepsis. Unfortunately, these data have not been available for analysis of patient populations, selection bias, comorbidities, and other explanations for increased mortality. The potential for adverse effects in this small segment of septic patients must be addressed in further studies.

Institution of Immune-Enhancing Diets

There are no clear guidelines for the use of these formulas, but certain recommendations can be made using the available studies. The diet should be administered as soon as safely possible after trauma or ICU admission. In patients undergoing elective resection of upper gastrointestinal malignancies, who are at risk of starvation-induced malnutrition, consideration should be given to preoperative administration of an immune-enhancing diet for 7 to 10 days prior to surgery. Postoperatively, approximately 3,000 to 3,500 cc *total* must be administered over the first 3 days following surgery to achieve effects. Diet progression, however, must be limited by tolerance which requires close patient observation, particularly when feedings are delivered beyond the ligament of Treitz. Because of the potential for bowel necrosis, under no circumstances should these or any enteral feeding formula be administered to patients who are hemodynamically unstable, are receiving high doses of pressors, or have suspected reduced splanchnic blood flow. The diet should be continued for 5 to 7 days or longer until the patient is at reduced risk of subsequent septic complications.

CONCLUSION

While there has been much progress toward understanding the relationship between route and type of nutrition and its effects upon the immune system, the field is still relatively young. Several clinical studies have shown that enteral supplementation with immune-enhancing nutrients can be beneficial in certain subpopulations. In particular, moderate to severely injured trauma patients who are expected to survive their injuries and patients undergoing elective upper GI surgery who are at risk of malnutrition-related complications appear to benefit from these supplemented diets. More study is necessary in patient populations with head injuries, burns, or medical ICU patients in order to determine the usefulness of immune-enhancing diets in these settings. In particular, more study must be directed to determining the correct dose and length of therapy required for these diets to be effective. Further study is necessary to define any increased inflammatory response or mortality rates in a small group of patients with preexisting inflammatory responses or sepsis.

REFERENCES

1.   Kudsk KA, Croce MA, Fabian TC, et al. Enteral versus parenteral feeding. Effects on septic morbidity after blunt and penetrating abdominal trauma. Ann Surg 1992; 215:503-513
2.   Moore FA, Feliciano DV, Andrassy RJ, et al. Early enteral feeding, compared with parenteral, reduces postoperative septic complications: the results of a meta-analysis. Ann Surg 1992; 216:172-183
3.   Moore EE, Jones TN. Benefits of immediate jejunostomy feeding after major abdominal trauma—a prospective, randomized study. J Trauma 1986; 26:874-879
4.   Pomposelli JJ, Flores E, Hirschberg Y, et al. Short-term TPN containing ω-3 fatty acids ameliorate lactic acidosis induced by endotoxin in guinea pigs. Am J Clini Nutr 1990; 52:548-552
5.   Kudsk K, Janu P, Renegar K. Effect of glutamine-enriched TPN on small intestine gut-associated lymphoid tissue and upper respiratory tract immunity. Surgery 1997; 121:542-549
6.   O'Dwyer ST, Smith RJ, Hwang TL, et al. Maintenance of small bowel mucosa with glutamine-enriched parenteral nutrition. J Parenter Enteral Nutr 1989; 13:579-585
7.   Barbul A. Arginine and immune function. Nutr Suppl 1990; 6:53-58
8.   Reynolds JV, Daly JM, Zhang S, et al. Immunomodulatory mechanisms of arginine, Surgery 1988; 104:142-151
9.   Barbul A, Sisto DA. Wasserkrug HL, et al. Arginine stimulates lymphocyte immune response in healthy human beings. Surgery 1981; 90:244-251
10. Fanslow WC, Kulkarni AD, Van Buren CT, et al. Effect of nucleotide restriction and supplementation on resistance to supplemental murine candidiasis. J Parenter Enteral Nutr 1988; 12:49-52
11. Daly JM, Lieberman MD, Goldfine J, et al. Enteral nutrition with supplemental arginine, RNA, and omega-3 fatty acids in patients after operation: immunologic, metabolic, and clinical outcome. Surgery 1992; 112:56-67
12. Daly JM, Weintraub FN, Shou J, et al. Enteral nutrition during multimodality therapy in upper gastrointestinal cancer patients. Ann Surg 1995; 221:327-338
13. Heslin MJ, Latkany L, Leung D, et al. A prospective, randomized trial of early enteral feeding after resection of upper gastrointestinal malignancy. Ann Surg 1997; 226:567-577
14. Senkal M, Mumme A, Eickhoff V, et al. Early postoperative enteral immunonutrition: clinical outcome and cost-comparison analysis in surgical patients. Crit Care Med 1997; 25:1489-1496
15. Schilling J, Vranjes N, Firez W, et al. Clinical outcome and immunology of postoperative arginine, ω-3 fatty acids, and nucleotide-enriched enteral feeding; a randomized prospective comparison with standard enteral and low calorie/low fat IV solutions. Nutrition 1996; 12:423-429
16. Gianotti L, Braga M, Vignali A, et al. Effect of route of delivery and formulation of postoperative nutritional support in patients undergoing major operations for malignant neoplasms. Arch Surg 1997; 132:1222-1230
17. Braga M, Vignali A, Gianotti L, et al. Immune and nutritional effects of early enteral nutrition after major abdominal operations. Eur J Surg 1996; 162:105-112
18. Braga M, Vignali A, Gianotti L, et al. Benefits of early postoperative enteral feeding in cancer patients. Infusionsther Transfusionsmed 1995; 22:280-284
19. Braga M, Gianotti L, Vignali A, et al. Artificial nutrition after major abdominal surgery: Impact of route of administration and composition of the diet. Crit Car Med 1998;26:24-30.

20. Braga M, Gianotti L, Radaelli G, et al. Perioperative immunonutrition in patients undergoing cancer surgery. Arch Surg 1999; 134:428-433
21. Senkal M, Mumme A, Eickhoff U, et al. Early postoperative enteral immunonutrition: clinical outcome and cost-comparison analysis in surgical patients. Crit Care Med 1997; 25:1489-1496
22. Moore FA, Moore EE, Kudsk KA, et al. Clinical benefits of an immune-enhancing diet for early postinjury enteral feeding. J Trauma 1994; 37:607-615
23. Kudsk KA, Minard G, Croce MA, et al. A randomized trial of isonitrogenous enteral diets after severe trauma. An immune-enhancing diet reduces septic complications. Ann Surg 1996; 224:531-540
24. Brown RO, Hunt H, Mowatt-Larssen CA, et al. Comparison of specialized and standard enteral formulas in trauma patients. Pharmacotherapy 1994; 14:314-320
25. Weimann A, Bastian L, Bischoff WE, et al. Influence of arginine, omega-3 fatty acids and nucleotide-supplemented enteral support on systemic inflammatory response syndrome and multiple organ failure in patients after severe trauma. Nutrition 1998; 14:165-172
26. Mendez C, Jurkovich GJ, Garcia I, et al. Effects of an immune-enhancing diet in critically injured patients. J Trauma 1997; 42:933-940
27. Gottschlich MM, Jenkins M, Warden GD, et al. Differential effects of three enteral dietary regimens on selected outcome variables in burn patients. J Parenter Enteral Nutr 1990; 14:225-236
28. Saffle JR, Wiebke G, Jennings K, et al. Randomized trial of immune-enhancing enteral nutrition in burn patients. J Trauma 1997; 42:793-802
29. Chendrasekhar A, Fagerli JC, Prabhakar B, et al. Evaluation of an enhanced diet in patients with severe closed head injury. Crit Care Med 1997; 25:SA80 (Abst)
30. Minard G, Kudsk KA, Melton S, et al. Early versus delayed feeding with an immune-enhancing diet in patients with severe head injuries. J Parenter Enteral Nutr 2000; 24:145-149
31. Bower RH, Cerra FB, Bershadsky B, et al. Early enteral administration of a formula (Impact) supplemented with arginine, nucleotides, and fish oil in intensive care unit patients: results of a multicenter, prospective, randomized, clinical trial. Crit Cre Med 1995; 23:436-49
32. Atkinson S, Sieffert E, Bihari D. A prospective, randomized, double-blind, controlled clinical trial of enteral immunonutrition in the critically ill. Crit Care Med 1998; 26:1164-1172
33. Galbán C, Celaya S, Marco P, et al. An immune enhancing enteral diet reduces mortality and episodes of bacteriemia in septic ICU patients. J Parenter Enteral Nutr 1998; 22:S13 (Abst)
34. Heslin MJ, Latkany L, Leung D, et al. A prospective, randomized trial of early enteral feeding after resection of upper gastrointestinal malignancy. Ann Surg 1997; 226:567-577
35. Senkal M, Zumtobel V, Bauer KH, et al. Outcome and cost-effectiveness of perioperative enteral immunonutrition in patients undergoing elective upper gastrointestinal tract surgery: a prospective randomized study. Arch Surg 1999; 134:1309-1316
36. Snyderman CH, Kachman K, Molseed L, et al. Reduced postoperative infections with an immune-enhancing nutritional supplement. Laryngoscope 1999; 109:915-921

46

INTERFERENCE WITH THE COAGULATION SYSTEM

Lambert G. Thijs

In patients with severe sepsis or septic shock, systemic activation of the coagulation system as well as early activation with subsequent inhibition of the fibrinolytic system are common features [1-5]. Using newly developed highly sensitive assays to measure activation products of coagulation, activation of coagulation can be detected even in most patients with uncomplicated sepsis [6]. The most pronounced clinical manifestation of these alterations is disseminated intravascular coagulation (DIC), which is characterized by generation and deposition of fibrin in the microvasculature with widespread microvascular thrombosis in various organs. The progressive inhibition of the fibrinolytic system may ultimately result in impaired fibrin dissolution and aggravate the formation of microthrombi. In addition, depletion of coagulation proteins and platelets, mainly due to the extensive and ongoing activation of the coagulation system may induce severe bleeding complications [7].

Sepsis is the most common cause of acute DIC and DIC is a frequent complication of sepsis with major implications for morbidity and mortality. There is evidence that activation of the coagulation system contributes to the development of organ failure and death [3,5]. The reported incidence and prevalence of DIC in sepsis varies widely depending on type of patients and definitions used to characterize DIC. The prevalence of DIC in patients included in recent large-scale clinical trials in sepsis ranged from 7.5 to 49 % and is generally higher in patients with than in patients without shock [8-11]. In a large prospective study the incidence of DIC in sepsis was 16 %, in severe sepsis 18 % and in septic shock 38 % [12].

IMBALANCE BETWEEN COAGULATION AND FIBRINOLYSIS

In sepsis, coagulation is primarily driven by the tissue factor (TF)-dependent pathway and amplified by activation of various factors of the contact activation-dependent pathway [13]. Several mediators of sepsis (e.g., tumor necrosis factor [TNF], interleukin [IL]-1, endotoxin) can induce TF on endothelial cells and monocytes, which binds to and activates factor VII. Subsequently, the factor VII/TF complex activates a number of proteolytic processes, ultimately resulting in fibrin clot formation. In this process thrombin is generated which binds to antithrombin (AT) to form thrombin-antithrombin (TAT) complexes which are sensitive markers of *in vivo* thrombin generation. Elevated levels of circulating TAT complexes are generally found in septic patients even in the absence of clinically overt DIC [4,5,6,14,15]. These levels are related to the severity of sepsis i.e. highest levels are found in the most severe forms of sepsis [6].

The fibrinolytic system is also activated in sepsis [13]. The importance of this system is its capacity to remove (micro) thrombi and maintain blood fluidity and thereby preserve the microcirculation from irreversible damage. Fibrinolysis is initiated mainly by the release of tissue-type plasminogen activator (t-PA) released from endothelial cells. t-PA converts plasminogen into plasmin which among other proteolytic functions enzymatically degrades fibrin into fibrin degradation products. Fibrinolysis is regulated at two levels. First, t-PA can bind to plasminogen activator inhibitor type I (PAI-1) to form complexes which loose the ability to activate plasminogen. High circulating levels of t-PA antigen can usually be found in septic patients [2,4,16]. In contrast, t-PA activity can often not be detected or is only moderately elevated [2,17], suggesting that t-PA activity is inhibited by PAI-1. Indeed, plasma levels of PAI-1 antigen [1,4,17,18] and PAI-1 activity [2,16,19] are markedly increased in patients with severe sepsis. Second, free plasmin is rapidly bound to circulating α2-antiplasmin, thereby forming plasmin-antiplasmin (PAP) complexes which are direct markers of *in vivo* plasmin generation. In many patients with sepsis elevated levels of circulating PAP complexes can be found, indeed indicating activation of the fibrinolytic system [5,15].

Dynamic studies in human volunteers subjected to low dose endotoxin, and in animal models of sepsis, have demonstrated early activation of fibrinolysis before significant thrombin generation can be detected in plasma whereas fibrinolysis is already offset by the release of PAI-1 when thrombin generation becomes maximal [20,21]. So, there is a remarkable imbalance between coagulation and fibrinolysis resulting in a procoagulant state several hours after the challenge. This imbalance can be assessed by the ratio of the levels of TAT and PAP complexes. An elevated TAT/PAP ratio which may reflect a procoagulant state has been demonstrated in many patients with sepsis [5,15]. The TAT/PAP ratio is higher in patients who develop organ dysfunction than those who do not and higher in non-survivors than in survivors [5,15]. Apparently, in sepsis, a dynamic process of coagulation and fibrinolysis is ongoing, whereas the latter is counteracted with resulting impaired fibrinolysis and an imbalance between coagulation and fibrinolysis. These abnormalities have major pathophysiological, and therefore, clinical implications as the fibrinolytic capacity to counteract widespread vital organ microvascular thrombosis becomes insufficient which seems to contribute to the development of (multiple) organ dysfunction and mortality.

THERAPEUTIC STRATEGIES

The proper management of septic patients with DIC remains controversial. Adequate clinical trials on DIC treatment in general are scarce, probably related to the complexity of the syndrome, lack of generally accepted definitions and its variable and unpredictable course. The clinical picture of simultaneously occurring risk of bleeding due to coagulation factor consumption (and trombocytopenia) and widespread systemic microvascular thrombosis does not directly indicate which treatment should be instituted. There is general agreement that adequate treatment of the septic process is the cornerstone of management. Plasma and platelet substitution are advocated in bleeding patients and in those requiring invasive procedures or who are otherwise at risk for bleeding complications [22]. The efficacy of this treatment has, however, not been proven in randomized controlled trials. This therapeutic approach is symptomatic as it substitutes deficiencies acquired during the clotting process. Since coagulation activation with impaired fibrinolytic capacity seems to have a pathogenetic role in sepsis, interference with these processes becomes a potential therapeutic option even in patients without clinically overt DIC.

Interference with the Fibrinolytic System

Since the fibrinolytic impairment in sepsis appears to be related to high circulating levels of PAI-1, strategies directed against this fibrinolysis inhibitor might be of benefit. Anti-PAI-1 strategies have been shown to have beneficial effects in initial experimental studies [23], but clinical studies remain to be done. Alternatively, administration of t-PA can enhance fibrinolysis and some case reports suggest improvement of the clinical condition of patients with meningococcemia and DIC after t-PA treatment [24,25]. Controlled clinical trials are, however, as yet not available.

Anticoagulants

Experimental studies have shown that heparin can at least partly inhibit the activation of coagulation in sepsis [26]. A beneficial effect of heparin on clinically important outcome events in patients with DIC has never been demonstrated in a controlled clinical trial. Although in an experimental sepsis model heparin could ameliorate organ damage [27], there is no evidence that this also occurs in human sepsis. There is at present no sound evidence in favor of the use of heparin as routine treatment, except possibly in patients with clinical signs of extensive fibrin deposition like purpura fulminans or severe acral ischemia [28]. The risk of bleeding in patients with DIC who are prone to bleeding is, however, a major concern.

Antithrombin Concentrates

AT is an important physiologic regulator of blood coagulation as it inhibits the clotting process at several levels. In addition to its function as a specific thrombin inhibitor with which it forms the TAT complex, AT has the capacity to inhibit the contact factors XIIa (FXIIa) and XIa (FXIa) and kallikrein. Its inhibitory profile also includes FIXa and FXa and AT may function with heparin or in concert with TFPI to inactivate tissue factor/FVIIa complexes [29,30].

AT circulates as a monomer in the plasma and is also found on the cell surface of endothelial cells. It contains a heparin-binding domain and a serine-binding domain at the active site of the molecule. Glycosaminoglycans such as heparan-sulfate present on endothelial cell surfaces activate AT, and heparin competitively inhibits the binding of AT to heparan sulfate, but by itself activates AT. In the absence of heparin, AT binds to endothelial surfaces and functions as an anticoagulant, thereby blocking the intrinsic thrombogenic activity of (sub)endothelial surfaces. In sepsis, AT activity is rapidly depleted, primarily as a result of complex formation with multiple activated clotting factors, particularly in patients who progress to septic shock [31]. In addition, proteolytic inactivation of AT by activated neutrophil products (e.g., elastase) further reduces AT activity, whereas decreased synthesis by the liver (AT is a negative acute phase protein), leakage from the intravascular compartment and dilution by volume therapy may contribute to low plasma AT activity. Severely depressed AT levels are predictive of a fatal outcome in many studies in septic patients [3,31]. Serial studies demonstrate a slow spontaneous recovery toward normal levels in survivors, whereas AT concentrations typically remain low in nonsurvivors [3,4]. Loss of AT activity (and also of protein C activity, *vide infra*) impairs an endogenous control mechanism for thrombin generation, resulting in a potentially lethal state of systemic activation of coagulation and inflammatory processes. Thrombin promotes platelet aggregation in the microvasculture and promotes expression or upregulation of, e.g., P- and E-selectins, intercellular adhesion molecule (ICAM)-1 and induces release of several proinflammatory mediators.

These processes promote neutrophil activation and neutrophil-platelet-endothelium interactions as part of a generalized inflammatory response. Also, microvascular thrombosis may cause tissue ischemia which in turn is a strong stimulus for proinflammatory cytokine generation. Therefore, AT supplementation to restore sufficient plasma anticoagulant activity to prevent or reduce systemic coagulation activation seems a rational approach. Moreover, experimental studies have shown that AT, in addition to its anticoagulant effects, also has anti-inflammatory properties. AT bound to endothelial surfaces stimulates endothelial cells to release prostacyclin *in vitro* [32,33]. *In vivo*, administration of AT increases plasma levels of prostacyclin [34,35]. Prostacyclin is a potent inhibitor of platelet aggregation and inhibits synthesis of pro-inflammatory cytokines and attenuates neutrophil activation, thereby reducing neutrophil degranulation and release of elastase and oxygen radicals [35,36]. AT is able to prevent the endotoxin-induced accumulation of leukocytes in the lungs and to inhibit the increase in pulmonary microvascular permeability in the animal model [35,36]. Also, ischemia/reperfusion-induced injury in the liver can be prevented by AT infusion [37]. This compound increases the hepatic levels of prostacyclin, which promotes the increase in hepatic tissue flow and reduces leukocyte activation. Moreover, intravital microscopy has demonstrated that AT can reduce neutrophil rolling and adhesion during reperfusion in another ischemia/reperfusion model [38]. There is evidence that prevention of endotoxin or ischemia/reperfusion-induced tissue injury by AT is largely independent of its anticoagulant activity. These anti-inflammatory activities of AT are only seen in the absence of therapeutic doses of heparin, which interferes with the interaction of AT with heparan sulfate on endothelial surfaces. Additionally, these effects are observed primarily at supraphysiological levels of AT [36].

Many studies on the use of AT in experimental models of sepsis have shown that this compound is protective, reducing morbidity and mortality in septic animals [39,40]. This has been demonstrated in endotoxin models, in models using a live bacterial challenge with Gram-negative or Gram-positive bacteria and with a polymicrobial challenge in a variety of animal species ranging from mice to subhuman primates [39]. AT has been effective alone, or in combination with other agents [40], with or without antibiotic treatment, as a pretreatment or as a salvage therapy after established sepsis [39]. These studies suggest that plasma levels of AT must be maintained at levels markedly higher than normal to be efficacious in animal models of sepsis.

There also has been considerable experience with the use of AT in septic patients over the past decades [41,42]. Numerous uncontrolled studies on AT in sepsis have shown that AT may have beneficial effects. The first larger and randomized study in patients in shock (about one third with septic shock) compared heparin, AT, and their combination, and showed that the duration of symptoms of DIC was significantly reduced in both groups receiving AT, whereas addition of heparin resulted in more blood loss [43]. A follow-up study in a similar group of patients comparing heparin versus AT showed that patients receiving AT had a significant lower mortality rate [44]. In both studies, however, there was no control group. The first prospective, randomized, double-blind placebo-controlled phase II clinical trial included patients with septic shock and DIC and showed a significant improvement in DIC symptoms with a positive trend to improved outcome in the AT group [45]. A second phase II placebo-controlled trial in severely ill septic patients also showed a positive trend towards improved outcome in favor of the treated group [46]. Similarly, a third phase II study in severe sepsis resulted in reduction in ICU stay and also a positive trend towards a better outcome for the treated group [46]. A meta-analysis of the collected clinical experience with these three phase II clinical trials comprising 122 patients shows that the therapeutic use of AT in patients with severe sepsis was associated with an overall reduction in the relative risk of mortality over a 30 day follow-up period of 22.9 % (45 % placebo vs 35 % AT; p=NS) [46].

In contrast, another prospective double-blind, placebo-controlled clinical trial in 34 patients with an inflammatory process and clinical signs of infection, showed a statistically non-significant higher mortality rate in patients receiving AT than in controls (22.2 versus 12.5 %) [47]. There was, however, a low incidence of DIC and a low overall mortality rate in this study group. This may indicate that AT could be of benefit in the most sick patients rather than in patients with mild disease. This concept is further supported by the results of another double-blind, placebo-controlled trial including 120 patients with sepsis and/or post-surgical complications including 56 patients with septic shock [48]. The difference in overall mortality was small with a relative reduction of 7% in the treated group. In patients with septic shock, however, administration of AT concentrate resulted in a statistically significant reduction in 30-day all-cause mortality of 20%. Due to the fact that the subgroup analysis of the septic shock patients was not *a priori* defined in the study protocol, the results are statistically unconfirmed. Interestingly, long-term AT supplementation in patients with severe sepsis resulted in disappearance of DIC, a progressive rise in PaO_2/FiO_2, a decrease in the pulmonary artery pressure/mean arterial pressure (PAP/MAP) ratio, prevention of the rise in serum bilirubin concentrations and less need for renal support therapy when compared to control patients [49]. Also, this therapeutic approach was associated with attenuation of the systemic inflammatory response as assessed by downregulation of IL-6 and soluble endothelial adhesion molecules (sE-selectin, sICAM) [50]. On the other hand, there was no statistically significant effect on IL-8 and elastase levels or total leukocyte count. In septic patients, therefore, AT seems to be more effective in the modulation of the monocytic and endothelial response than in the modulation of leukocyte degranulation [50].

These clinical data support a potential therapeutic role for AT in severely septic patients. However, while phase II clinical trial results are suggestive of a clinically meaningful reduction in mortality in sepsis, the first results of a large scale phase III clinical trial show no effect on outcome.

PROTEIN C CONCENTRATES

The protein C-protein S pathway also is an important endogenous anticoagulant system. The circulating inactive protein C is activated and rapidly converted to the serine protease, activated PC (APC), by a complex between thrombin and thrombomodulin, which is primarily present on endothelial cells. The unique feature of the protein C-protein S pathway, therefore, is its ability to generate an anticoagulant response proportional to the thrombotic stimulus. APC binds to free protein S and this complex inactivates FVa and FVIIIa. In addition, APC binds to and inhibits PAI-1 activity, thereby promoting fibrinolysis.

Protein serves as a cofactor for APC and exists in two forms: as free protein which is active and as an inactive form complexed to C4b-binding protein (C4b-BP), which therefore is an inhibitor of protein S activity. Inactivation of protein C is mediated by protein C-inhibitor, α_1-antitrypsin and α_2-macroglobulin.

The protein C-protein S anticoagulant pathway function is reduced in sepsis. *In vitro*, endotoxin and proinflammatory cytokines (TNF, IL-1) can downregulate thrombomodulin expression on endothelial cells and TNF has been shown to reduce protein S synthesis in these cells [13]. In sepsis, recruitment of neutrophils with release of oxidants and proteases which can cleave thrombomodulin, in addition impairs protein C activity. Large increases in circulating thrombomodulin as observed in septic shock, probably result from this neutrophil elastase mediated proteolytic cleavage of endothelial cell-associated thrombomodulin [51].The acute phase proteins C4bBP and α_1-

antitrypsin increase during sepsis and bind protein S and APC respectively, thereby reducing their anticoagulant activity

In patients with severe sepsis, plasma levels of protein C are almost uniformly decreased, lowest levels occurring in patients with septic shock and nonsurvivors [1,3,52,53]. An acute, severe and prolonged decrease in protein C activity has been found in nonsurvivors, whereas in survivors serial measurements demonstrate a gradual return toward normal levels [1,3,4]. A major mechanism inducing a decline in protein C activity is most likely consumption during the coagulation process, whereas above mentioned mechanisms also interfere with protein C activation or activity. Changes in protein S levels in sepsis are not uniform. Levels of free and total protein S may be lowered or normal [1,3,52,54].

Protein C administration in animal models of sepsis has protective effects. Infusion of APC in the baboon model prevented the coagulopathic, hepatotoxic and lethal effects of infusion with a lethal dose of live *E coli* microorganisms [55]. Conversely, blocking protein C activation with an anti-protein C monoclonal antibody caused an enhanced pathologic response to infusion of sublethal concentrations of live *E. coli*, ultimately resulting in death, which could be prevented by APC infusion [55]. Infusion of C4b-BP in baboons challenged with a sublethal dose of live *E. coli* resulted in rapid consumption of fibrinogen, a rise in circulating TNF levels, organ damage and ultimately death [56]. Also, restoration of the protein C system with supplementation of a slight excess of protein S in addition to C4b-BP prevented DIC, organ damage and elaboration of elevated TNF levels [56]. These results indicate that the protein C system is a major regulator of microvascular thrombosis in sepsis and also modulates the inflammatory response. *In vitro* studies have shown that APC inhibits TNF production by endotoxin-stimulated human blood monocytes [57]. It also prevents interferon (IFN)-γ-mediated Ca^{2+} transients and cellular proliferation [58] and inhibits leukocyte adhesion to selectins [59]. Activated protein C infused in an animal model prevented the endotoxin-induced increase in pulmonary microvascular permeability and pulmonary accumulation of leukocytes [60]. Similarly, recombinant human soluble thrombomodulin reduces endotoxin-induced pulmonary vascular injury via protein C activation [61]. These effects are independent of the anticoagulant effects of these compounds and seem to be dependent on their ability to inhibit leukocyte activation [60,61].

There are limited published data on the use of protein C concentrates in patients with sepsis. Anecdotal reports in patients with severe (meningococcal) sepsis have shown that protein C infusion is associated with reversal of organ dysfunction and clinical improvement [62,63]. A recent observational study in 12 patients with severe meningococcal sepsis showed that no mortality occurred when protein C was infused to obtain normal plasma levels [64]. A prospective, randomized, double-blind, placebo-controlled phase II clinical trial in patients with severe sepsis showed a reduction in mortality (40% relative risk reduction, p=0.21) in the high dose treatment group [65,66]. This was associated with a trend towards decreased time on the ventilator, in the ICU and in the hospital. It was also associated with lower levels of D-dimers and a larger decrease in IL-6 plasma levels. Finally, the preliminary results of a large multicenter phase III trial show a statistically significant reduction in mortality in patients treated with recombinant APC [67].

TISSUE FACTOR PATHWAY INHIBITOR (TFPI)

TFPI, a multivalent inhibitor with three tandemly arranged Kunitz-type protease inhibitor domains, is a serine protease inhibitor that inhibits FXa directly and the FVIIa/TF catalytic complex in a FXa dependent fashion [68]. The endothelium is the primary site of TFPI synthesis and endothelial cell bound TFPI is thought to be the major pool of TFPI and is heparin releasable. In plasma, TFPI is primarily complexed with lipoproteins and also platelets can store TFPI. Several proteases including leukocyte elastase have been shown to specifically cleave TFPI [69].

In contrast to AT and protein C, plasma levels of TFPI are increased rather than decreased in sepsis [31]. *In vitro* studies have shown that exposure of endothelial cells to endotoxin, TNF or thrombin causes enhanced export of TFPI to the cell surface, suggesting that this inhibitor provides a protective mechanism for the microvasculature [70,71]. The mechanisms of increased TFPI levels have not been fully elucidated but they could reflect endothelial cell damage and indicate a depletion of the endothelial cell bound TFPI pool with loss of its protective function. The rationale for use of TFPI for the treatment of sepsis stems from these considerations.

Several studies have shown that TFPI improves survival in various lethal animal models of sepsis: a rabbit peritonitis model [72], a porcine peritonitis-induced septic shock model [73] and a baboon bacteremia model [74,75]. TFPI has been shown to be effective when administered early after the challenge or as late as four hours. In these models rTFPI had highly pronounced effects on laboratory variables, including coagulation and inflammatory markers [74-76]. Interestingly, TFPI treatment significantly attenuated the IL-6 and IL-8 responses to sepsis [73-76], whereas TNF levels were either not affected [74] or lowered [73]. TFPI-treated survivors had lower levels of soluble Fas, a marker of apoptosis [76], suggesting maintenance of cell membrane integrity as direct effects of rTFPI. Moreover, attenuation of the sepsis-related drop in blood pressure by TFPI has been reported [75] as well as an increase in cardiac output [73].

In normal volunteers rTFPI was found to be well tolerated with no clinically significant bleeding (Braeckman et al., unpublished data).In a phase II clinical trial in patients with severe sepsis this compound proved to be safe with a trend towards reduced mortality in the TFPI-treated group. Recently a large multicenter placebo controlled phase III clinical trial has been completed to test whether TFPI can improve survival in patients with sever sepsis.

In summary, recent studies have shown that interference with the coagulation system using infusions of recombinant APC indeed improves patient outcome in sepsis. Although both AT, which did not show an effect on mortality in a large phase III study, and APC have anticoagulant and anti-inflammatory effects, their mechanism of action is different. Moreover, APC also has fibrinolytic activities, which AT does not have. This may possibly explain the varying outcome of the respective phase III trials.

REFERENCES

1.   Hesselvik JF, Blombäck M, Brodin B, et al. Coagulation, fibrinolysis, and kallikrein systems in sepsis: relation to outcome. Crit Care Med 1989; 17:724-733
2.   Voss R, Matthias FR, Borkowski G, et al. Activation and inhibition of fibrinolysis in septic patients in an internal intensive care unit. Br J Haematol 1990; 75: 99-105
3.   Fourrier F, Chopin C, Goudemand J, et al. Septic shock, multiple organ failure, and disseminated intravascular coagulation. Compared patterns of antithrombin III, protein C, and protein S deficiencies. Chest 1992; 101:816-823
4.   Lorente JA, García-Frade LJ, Landín L, et al. Time course of hemostatic abnormalities in sepsis and its relation to outcome. Chest 1993; 103:1536-1542
5.   Kidokoro A, Iba T, Fukunaga M, et al. Alterations in coagulation and fibrinolysis during sepsis. Shock 1996; 5:223-228
6.   Mavrommatis AC, Theodoridis Th, Orfanidou A, et al. Coagulation system and platelets are fully activated in uncomplicated sepsis. Crit Care Med 2000; 28:451-457
7.   Levi M, Ten Cate H, Van der Poll T, et al. Pathogenesis of disseminated intravascular coagulation in sepsis. JAMA 1993; 270:975-979
8.   Abraham E, Wunderink R, Silverman H, et al. Efficacy and safety of monoclonal antibody to human tumor necrosis factor ' in patients with sepsis syndrome. JAMA 1995; 273:934-941
9.   Bone RC, Balk RA, Fein AM, et al. A second large controlled clinical study of E5, a monoclonal antibody to endotoxin: Results of a prospective, multicenter, randomized, controlled trial. Crit Care Med 1995; 23:994-1005
10.   Cohen J, Carlet J, Intersept study group: INTERSEPT: an international, multicenter, placebo-controlled trial of monoclonal antibody to human tumor necrosis factor-' in patients with sepsis. Crit Care Med 1996; 24:1431-1440
11.   Abraham E, Anzueto A, Gutierrez G, et al. Double-blind randomised controlled trial of monoclonal antibody to human tumour necrosis factor in treatment of septic shock. Lancet 1998; 351:929-933

12. Rangel-Frausto MS, Pittet D, Costigan M, et al. The natural history of the systemic inflammatory response syndrome (SIRS). A prospective study. JAMA 1995; 273:117-123

13. Vervloet MG, Thijs LG, Hack CE. Derangements of coagulation and fibrinolysis in critically III patients with sepsis and septic shock. Thromb Haemostas 1998; 24:33-44

14. Wuillemin WA, Fijnvandraat K, Derkx BHF, et al. Activation of the intrinsic pathway of coagulation in children with meningococcal septic shock. Tromb Heamostas 1995; 74:1436-1441

15. Thijs LG, De Boer JP, De Groot MCM, et al. Coagulation disorders in septic shock. Intensive Care Med 1993; 9:S8-S15

16. Mesters RM, Florke N, Ostermann H, et al. Increase of plasminogen activator inhibitor levels predicts outcome of leukocytopenic patients with sepsis. Thromb Haemostas 1996; 75: 902-907

17. Haj MA, Neilly IJ, Robbie LA, et al. Influence of white blood cells on the fibrinolytic response to sepsis: studies of septic patients with or without severe leukopenia. Br J Haematol 1995; 90: 541-547

18. Kruithof EKO, Calandra T, Pralong G, et al, Evolution of plasminogen activator inhibitor type I in patients with septic shock-Correlation with cytokine concentrations. Fibrinolysis 1993; 7: 117-121

19. Gando S, Kameue T, Nanzaki S, et al. Disseminated intravascular coagulation is a frequent complication of systemic inflammatory response syndrome. Thromb Haemostas 1996; 75: 224-228

20. Van Deventer SJH, Büller HR, Ten Cate JW, et al. Experimental endotoxemia in humans: analysis of cytokine release and coagulation, fibrinolytic and complement pathways. Blood 1990; 76:2520-2526

21. De Boer JP, Creasy AA, Chang A, et al. Activation patterns of coagulation and fibrinolysis in baboons following infusion with lethal or sublethal dose of escherichia coli. Circ Shock 1993; 39: 59-67

22. Levi M, De Jonge E, Van der Poll T, et al. Disseminated intravascular coagulation. Thromb Haemostas 1999; 82: 695-705

23. Levi M, Biemond BJ, Van Zonneveld AJ, et al. Inhibition of plasminogen activator inhibitor-1 (PAI-1) activity results in promotion of endogenous fibrinolysis and inhibition of thrombosis in experimental models. Circulation 1992; 83: 305-312

24. Zenz W, Muntean W, Zobel G, et al. Treatment of fulminant meningococcenia with recombinant tissue plasminogen activator. Thromb Haemostas 1995; 74: 802-803

25. Aiuto LT, Barone SR, Cohen PS, et al. Recombinant tissue plasminogen activator restores perfusion in meningococcal purpura fulminans. Crit Care Med 1997; 25: 1079-1082

26. Du Toit HJ, Coetzee AR, Chalton DO. Heparin treatment in thrombin-induced disseminated intravascular coagulation in the baboon. Crit Care Med 1991; 19:1195-1200

27. Tanaka T, Tsujinaka T, Kambayashi J-I, et al. The effect of heparin on multiple organ failure and disseminated intravascular coagulation in a sepsis model. Thromb Res 1990; 60: 321-330

28. De Jonge E, Levi M, Stoutenbeek CP, et al. Current drug treatment strategies for disseminated intravascular coagulation. Drugs 1998; 55: 767-777

29. Jesty J, Lorenz A, Rodriguez J, et al. Initiation of tissue factor pathway of coagulation in the presence of heparin:control by antithrombin III and tissue factor pathway inhibitor. Blood 1996; 15:2301-2307

30. Hamamoto T, Kisiel W. The effect of heparin on the regulation of factor VIIa-tissue factor activity by tissue factor pathway inhibitor. Blood Coagul Fibrinolysis 1996; 7:470-476

31. Mesters RM, Mannucci PM, Coppola R, et al. Factor VIIa and antithrombin III activity during severe sepsis and septic shock in neutropenic patients. Blood 1996; 88:881-886

.

32. Yamauchi T, Umeda F, Inoguchi T, et al. Antithrombin III stimulates prostacyclin production by cultured aortic endothelial cells. Biochem Biophys Res Commun 1989; 163:1404-1411

33. Horie S, Ichii H, Kazama M. Heparin-like glycosaminoglycan is a receptor for antithrombin III-dependent but not thrombin-dependent prostacyclin production in human endothelial cells. Thromb Res 1990; 59:899-904

34. Uchiba M, Okajima K, Murakami K, et al. Effects of antithrombin III (AT III) and TRP49-modified AT III on plasma level of 6-Keto-PGF1α in rats. Thromb Res 1995; 80:201-208

35. Uchiba M, Okajima K, Murakami K. Et al. Attenuation of endotoxin-induced pulmonary vascular injury bu Antithrombin III. Am J Physiol 1996; 270:L921-L930

36. Uchiba M, Okajima K, Murakami K. Effects of various doses of Antithrombin III on endotoxin-induced endothelial cell injury and coagulation abnormalities in rats. Thromb Res 1998; 89:233-241

37. Harada N, Okajima K, Kushimoto S, et al. Antithrombin reduces ischemia/reperfusion injury of rat liver by increasing the hepatic level of prostacyclin. Blood 1999; 93:157-164

38. Ostrovsky L, Woodman RC, Payne D, et al. Antithrombin III prevents and rapidly reverses leukocyte recruitment in ischemia/reperfusion. Circulation 1997; 96:2302-2310

39. Dickneite G. Antithrombin III in animal models of sepsis and organ failure. Semin Thromb Haemostas 1998; 24:61-69

40. Giebler R, Schmidt U, Koch S, et al. Combined antithrombin III and C1-esterase inhibitor treatment decreases intravascular fibrin deposition and attenuates cardiorespiratory impairment in rabbits exposed to Escherichia coli endotoxin. Crit Care Med 1999; 27:597-604

41. Eisele B, Lamy M. Clinical experience with antithrombin III concentrates in critically ill patients with sepsis and multiple organ failure. Semin Thromb Haemostas 1998; 24:71-80

42. Balk R, Emerson T, Fourrier F, et al. Therapeutic use of antithrombin concentrate in sepsis. Semin Thromb Haemostas 1998; 24:183-194

43. Blauhut B, Kramar H, Vinazzer H, et al. Substitution of antithrombin III in shock and DIC: A randomized study. Thromb Res 1985; 39:81-89

44. Vinazzer H. Therapeutic use of antithrombin III in shock and disseminated intravascular coagulation. Semin Thromb Hemostas 1989; 15:347-352

45. Fourrier F, Chopin C, Huart J-J, et al. Double-blind, placebo-controlled trial of antithrombin III concentrates in septic shock with disseminated intravascular coagulation. Chest 1993; 104:882-888

46. Eisele B, Lamy M, Thijs LG,et al. Anti-thrombin III in patients with severe sepsis: a randomized, placebo-controlled, double-blind, multicenter trial plus a meta-analysis on all randomized-placebo-controlled, double-blind trials with antithrombin III in severe sepsis. Intensive Care Med 1998; 24:663-672

47. Balk R, Bedrosian C, McCormick L, et al. Prospective double-blind, placebo-controlled trial of AT III substitution in sepsis. In: Roussos C, edn. 8th European Congress of Intensive Care Medicine. Bologna: Monduzzi Editore: 1995; 7-11

48. Baudo F, Caimi TM, deCataldo F, et al. Antithrombin III (AT III) replacement therapy in patients with sepsis and/or post surgical complications: a double-blind, randomized, multicenter trial. Intensive Care Med 1998; 24:336-342

49. Inthorn D, Hoffmann JM, Hartl WH, et al. Antithrombin III supplementation in severe sepsis: beneficial effects on organ dysfunction. Shock 1997; 8:328-334.

50. Inthorn D, Hoffmann JN, Harti WH, et al. Effect of Antithrombin III supplementation on inflammatory response in patients with severe sepsis. Shock 1998; 10:90-96

51. Boehme MWJ, Deng Y, Raeth U, et al. Release of thrombomodulin from endothelial cells by concerted action of TNF-α and neutrophils: in vivo and in vitro studies. Immunol 1996; 87:134-140

52. Leclerc F, Hazelzet J, Jude B, et al. Protein C and S deficiency in severe infectious purpura of children: a collaborative study of 40 cases. Intensive Care Med 1992; 18:202-205

53. Hesselvik JF, Malm J, Dahlbäck B, et al. Protein C, protein S and C4b-binding protein in severe infection and septic shock. Tromb Haemostas 1991; 65:126-129

54. Alcaraz A, Espana F, Sánchez-Cuenca J, et al. Activation of the protein C pathway in acute sepsis. Thromb Res 1995; 79:83-93

55. Taylor FB, Chang A Jr, Esmon CT, et al. Protein C prevents the coagulation and lethal effects of escherichia coli infusion in the baboon. J Clin Invest 1987; 79:918-925

56. Taylor F, Chang A, Ferrell G, et al. C4b-binding protein exacerbates the host response to Escherichia coli. Blood 1991; 78:357-363

57. Grey ST, Tsuchida A, Hau H, et al. Selective inhibitory effects of the anticoagulant activated protein C on the responses of human mononuclear phagocytes to LPS, IFN-gamma, or phorbol ester. J Immunol 1994; 153:3664-3672

58. Hancock WW, Grey ST, Hau L, et al. Binding of activated protein C to a specific receptor on human mononuclear phagocytes inhibits intracellular calcium signaling and monocyte-dependent proliferative responses. Transplantation 1995; 60:1525-1532

59. Grinnell BW, Hermann RB, Yan SB. Human protein C inhibits selectin-mediated cell adhesion: Role of unique fucosylated oligosaccharide. Glycobiology 1994; 4:221-226

60. Murakami K, Okajima K, Uchiba M, et al. Activated protein C attenuates endotoxin-induced pulmonary vascular injury by inhibiting activated leukocytes in rats. Blood 1996; 87:642-647

61. Uchiba M, Okajima K, Murakami K, et al. Recombinant human soluble thrombomodulin reduces endotoxin-induced pulomonary vascular injury via protein C activation in rats. Thromb Haemostas 1995; 74:1265-1270

62. Rivard GE, David M, Farrell C, et al. Treatment of purpura fulminans in meningococcemia with protein C concentrate. J Pediatr 1995; 126:646-652

63. Gerson WT, Dickerman JD, Bovill EG, et al. Severe acquired protein C deficiency in purpura fulmimans associated with disseminated intravascular coagulation: treatment with protein C concentrate. Pediatrics 1993; 91:418-422

64. Smith OP, White B, Vaughan D, et al. Use of protein-C concentrate, heparin, and haemodiafiltration in meningocuccus-induced purpura fulminans. Lancet 1997; 350:1590-1593

65. Hartman DL, Bernard GR, Helterbrand JD, et al. Recombinant human activated protein C (rhAPC) improves coagulation abnormalities associated with severe sepsis. Intensive Care Med 1998; 24:S77(Abstr.)

66. Bernard GR, Hartman DL, Helterbrand JD, et al. Recombinant human activated protein C (rhAPC) produces a trend toward improvement in morbidity and 28 day survival in patients with severe sepsis. Crit Care Med 1998; 27:S4 (Abst)

67. Bernard GR, Vincent JL, Laterre PF, et al. Efficacy and safety of recombinant human activated protein C for severe sepsis. N Engl J Med 2001; 344:699-709

68. Broze GJ, Miletich JP. Characterization of the inhibition of tissue factor in serum. Blood 1987; 69:150-155

69. Higuchi DA, Wun T-C, Likert KM, et al. The effect of leukocyte elastase on tissue factor pathway inhibitor. Blood 1992; 79:1712-1719

70. Lupu C, Goodwin CA, Westmuckett AD, et al. Tissue factor pathway inhibitor in endothelial cells colocalizes with glycolipid microdomain caveolae. Regulatory

mechanism(s) of the anticoagulant properties of the endothelium. Arterioscler Thromb Vasc Biol 1997; 17:2964-74

71.   Sevinsky JR, Rao LVM, Ruf W. Ligand-induced protease receptor translocation into caveolae: A mechanism for regulating cell surface proteolysis of the tissue factor dependent coagulation pathway. J Cell Biol 1996; 133:293-304

72.   Camerota AJ, Creasey AA, Patla V, et al. Delayed treatment with recombinant human tissue factor pathway inhibitor improves survival in rabbits with gram-negative peritonitis. J Infect Dis 1998; 177:668-76

73.   Goldfarb RD, Glock D, Johnson K, et al. Randomized, blinded, placebo-controlled trial of tissue factor pathway inhibitor in porcine septic shock. Shock 1998; 10:258-64

74.   Creasey AA, Chang ACK, Fiegen L, et al. Tissue factor pathway inhibitor reduces mortality from Escherichia coli septic shock. J Clin Invest 1993; 91:2850-60

75.   Carr C, Bild GS, Chang ACK, et al. Recombinant E. coli-derived tissue fator pathway inhibitor reduces coagulopathic and lethal effects in the baboon gram-negative model of septic shock. Circ Shock 1995; 44:126-37

76.   Jansen P, Van Lopik T, Lubbers Y. The coagulant-inflammatory axis in the baboon response to E.coli: Effects of tissue factor pathway inhibitor on hemostatic balance, the cytokine network and the release of apoptosis marker sFas. In: Jansen P: Thesis 1997; p 95-107, University of Amsterdam

47

HEMOFILTRATION AND PLASMAPHERESIS

Peter Rogiers

In this chapter we will discuss the strategy of blood purification using extracorporeal therapies such as hemofiltration, plasmapheresis and hemoperfusion. In the first two techniques modified 'hemodialysis' machines are used to pump the blood through a filter and replace the ultrafiltrate by a substitution fluid. In the hemofiltration techniques high-flux hemofiltration membranes are commonly used allowing passage of molecules up to 20 kDa, and replacing the ultrafiltrate by an isotonic crystalloid solution containing physiologic concentrations of ions and using lactate or bicarbonate as a buffer. In plasmapheresis, plasmafiltration membranes are used to separate plasma from cellular elements in the blood. Plasma is replaced by the same crystalloid solutions in combination with human albumin and sometimes fresh frozen plasma. Hemoperfusion techniques involve no, or only minimal, convective transport of fluid and solutes across the membrane, but instead, adsorption of proteins to the membrane surface occurs.

HEMOFILTRATION

In Vivo Experimental Studies in Sepsis and Septic Shock

Animal studies on hemofiltration have yielded various results, in part due to differences in design, differences in model of sepsis and endpoints of the studies, differences in volume of ultrafiltration, and differences in membrane.

Role of the Experimental Model and Endpoints

In most of the studies, endotoxin was administered either by intravenous bolus or by short infusion. Also in most of these studies fluid resuscitation was minor or sometimes even absent, resulting in a hypodynamic state with low blood pressure and low cardiac output within a few hours. The onset of hemofiltration was within 30-60 min after the administration of endotoxin. The duration of hemofiltration was limited to a few hours and the experimental observation was also kept short, ranging from 180 to 360 minutes and focusing on hemodynamic parameters. In most of these studies hemofiltration improved cardiac function. One should however question the relevance of these models. Indeed, human sepsis and septic shock is rather characterized by a hyperdynamic state with high cardiac output and low arterial blood pressure due to low systemic vascular resistance needing vasopressor therapy. Therefore, some authors tried to mimick this situation by inducing peritonitis or pancreatitis or gut ischemia and reperfusion. In these studies hemodynamics and survival after 24 h or several days were the endpoints.

During septic shock in dogs due to peritoneal fecal clot implantation, Freeman et al. [1] demonstrated that moderate-volume continuous arteriovenous hemofiltration (CAVH, 60 ml/kg/h) failed to improve hemodynamics or survival rate at 18 hours. In a cecal ligation and rupture model in awake pigs [2], the animals were in a septic state, but no shock during 72 hours. Hemofiltration (8 ml/kg/h) modulated the immune response expressed by a decrease of polymorphonuclear phagocytosis of Candida. In another model of gut ischemia and reperfusion in pigs, Grootendorst et al. [3] reported that continuous veno-venous hemofiltration (CVVH, 172 ml/kg/h), started before clamping of the superior mesenteric artery, significantly increased arterial blood pressure, improved cardiac function, reduced macroscopic gut damage, and improved 24-hour survival. In a model of severe pancreatitis in pigs Yekebas et al. [4] showed that survival time was doubled with hemofiltration. In pigs with *Staphylococcus aureus* sepsis but no shock, Lee et al. [5] showed that CAVH (133 ml/kg/h) did not influence arterial blood pressure, but increased survival from 33 hours in the control group to 70 hours in the hemofiltered group. In another study using the same model, survival increased from 56 hours in the control group to 103 hours in the hemofiltration group [6]. We [7] recently investigated the potential role of hemofiltration (100 ml/kg /h) in acute ovine septic shock due to peritonitis and found no positive effects on hemodynamics or outcome compared to control animals.

Role of Ultrafiltration Volume

Some authors found only minor or even no effects of hemofiltration on hemodynamics while others demonstrated impressive hemodynamic improvement. These discrepancies may be explained by differences in ultrafiltration rate. Only minor or even no effects may occur with low-volume hemofiltration, whereas high-volume hemofiltration can markedly improve hemodynamics in experimental endotoxic shock. In a pig model of endotoxin infusion Staubach et al. [8] observed some hemodynamic improvement with hemofiltration, but survival time was not influenced. During endotoxic shock in pigs, Stein et al. [9] showed that low-volume CAVH (20 ml/kg/h) did not significantly influence hemodynamics. In a dog model of live *E. coli* sepsis, Gomez et al. [10] showed that low-volume (27 ml/kg/h) CAVH increased cardiac contractility, but the hemodynamic variables were not significantly compromised during their study. In a canine model of live *E. coli* sepsis, the same group of investigators [11] reported that the combination of low-volume CAVH (16 ml/kg/h) and phenylephrine could restore stroke volume and blood pressure, suggesting that low-volume CAVH alone may not be sufficient to improve hemodynamics in these conditions. In another study from the same group in a canine model of *Pseudomonas* pneumonia early hemofiltration improved cardiac function, whereas late hemofiltration had no effects [12]. In a study also using low-volume hemofiltration (33 ml/kg/h), Murphey and coworkers were not able to demonstrate any cardiopulmonary improvement in a porcine model of acute endotoxin shock [13]. In an endotoxin infusion model in piglets, Reeves et al. [14] observed no positive hemodynamic effects during hemofitration (40 ml/kg/h). However in endotoxic rats, Heidemann et al. [15] reported an to improved short term survival with CAVH (22-48 ml/kg/h) and this was associated with the removal of thromboxane.

Bearing in mind that the removal of the so-called 'middle-molecules' is a convective process, Grootendorst et al. [16,17] decided to apply much higher volumes of ultrafiltration. In pigs with endotoxic shock high-volume CVVH (162 ml/kg/h or 6 l/h) was associated with greater arterial blood pressure and cardiac output, as well as right ventricular ejection fraction. We [18] studied the effects of CVVH with two different ultrafiltrate rates (107 and 214 ml/kg/h or 3 and 6l/h respectively) in a canine model of acute endotoxic shock and demonstrated positive hemodynamic effects in the high-flow but not in the low-flow group.

Role of the Membrane

Hemofilters were originally designed for treatment of chronic renal failure. Until recently, cuprophane, a cellulose-based material, was the most commonly used membrane material. Triacetate and hemophane are examples of modified cellulose structure, which enhances biocompatibility. Most of these cellulosic membranes are low-flux, i.e. permeable to smaller, lower-molecular weight molecules. Synthetic polymers used for hemofilters are polycarbonate, polysulphone, polyacrylonitrile (PAN and AN69) and polymethylmethacrylate (PMMA). Most of these synthetic membranes are high-flux, i.e. permeable to larger, higher-molecular-weight molecules. Synthetic membranes are generally more biocompatible than cellulose membranes. For their biocompatibility and high permeability, synthetic membranes are widely used for hemofiltration, allowing convective removal of small molecules such as urea and creatinine and also ions. These membranes have a sieving coefficient of 0.55 for myoglobin, whose molecular weight is 17000 Da, i.e., very close to that of tumor necrosis factor (TNF)-α (16500 Da) (Table 1). By using these membranes, the TNF-α monomer and various cytokines responsible for myocardial dysfunction can theoretically be removed by convection. Polysulphone or polyamide membranes were used in most studies.

Since the biological form of TNF is a trimer that has a molecular weight that is too big to pass hemofiltration membranes, substantial removal can only take place by using adsorptive devices or membranes with high permeability. The physicochemical stucture of the membrane is also very important in terms of protein interaction. The asymmetrical microporous membranes like polysulphone and polyamide can only adsorb at the surface area, whereas the AN69 membrane has a symmetrical hydrogel structure with a high hydrophylicity and negative charges, resulting in protein binding capacities over the entire breadt of the membrane and therefore a much larger adsorbing capacity. We recently compared two membranes in an acute canine endotoxic shock model and found that CVVH with PAN (AN69) membrane but not with polysulphone membrane, improved cardiac performance (Rogiers et al. unpublished data). These effects were immediately seen and lasted for 4 hours, suggesting an adsorptive mechanism.

Hemofiltration with high-pore membranes has also recently been shown to be beneficial in sepsis. By enlarging filter pore size the cut-off point of the membrane increases from 40 kDa to about 80 kDa, resulting in convective removal of larger molecules responsible for the sepsis syndrome. Two experimental studies showed hemodynamic improvement [19] and increased survival rates with this technique [5].

Removal of Mediators of Sepsis

Is there experimental or clinical evidence that hemofiltration can remove mediators, like eicosanoids, cytokines (TNF-α, interleukin [IL]-1, IL-6, IL-8, endothelin and platelet activating factor [PAF])?

Membrane	Surface (m²)	Convect	Adsor	Cut-off point	Sieving coeff	Fiber diameter (µm)	Fiber wall thickness (µm)
Polysulphone (PSHF, Baxter, Irvine, USA)	0.3-1.25	Yes	no	20-40 kDa	0.51 myoglobin 0.02 albumin	200	40
AN69 (Multiflow, Hospal-Cobe, Lyon, France)	1.0	Yes	yes	20-40 kDa	0.55 myoglobin 0.01 albumin	215	50
PAES (Hospal-Cobe, Lyon, France)	1.15	Yes	no	10-30 kDa	0.12 myoglobin 0.01 albumin	240	50
Polyamide (P1SH, P2SH, P5SH, Gambro, Hechingen)	0.6-1.4	Yes	no	50-100 kDa	0.97 myoglobin 0.70 albumin	215	50
Cellulose triacetate (FB-190U, Nissho-Nipro, Osaka, Japan)	1.9	Yes	no	20-40 kDa	0.22 myoglobin	200	15

Convect: convection; adsor: adsorption; coeff: coefficient

Table 1. Hemofiltration membrane characteristics

Experimental Studies *in Vitro*

Many *in vitro* studies have shown that especially the synthetic membranes can remove inflammatory proteins from the solution to which they were added. This *in vitro* removal is mainly caused by adsorption and much less by convection, and not at all by diffusion. Lonneman et al.[20] showed significant removal of TNF and IL-1, using AN69 and polysulphone membranes in an *in vitro* dialysis system. These observations were confirmed by others [21-23]. *In vitro*, hemofiltration of a 1% albumin solution containing TNF and IL-1 through a variety of filters, resulted in higher sieving coefficients of the two cytokines than expected. This was due to a 32 % binding effect by the membranes [22]. Because of its high molecular weight, endotoxin cannot be readily removed from the circulation, but endotoxin fragments can be eliminated. Also PAF can be removed by convection and adsorption [24].

Clinical Studies

Studies describing the potential role of hemofiltration in the removal of inflammatory proteins are presented in Table 2. Despite removal of mediators with hemofiltration, plasma levels seldom decrease, largely because these substances have an endogenous clearance that largely exceeds the clearance by extracorporeal techniques. Moreover the plasma half-life is very short, from 6 to 17 min [49], so that hemofiltration can only remove a small fraction of inflammatory mediators. Therefore, some authors consider hemofiltration in sepsis as futile [50,51]. Nevertheless, recently the clinical application of high-volume hemofiltration gained importance again. In a prospective cohort analysis Oudemans-van Straaten et al. showed that the observed mortality was lower than predicted in 306 patients treated with high-volume hemofiltration [52]. In another prospective randomized study, 425 patients with acute renal failure were treated with hemofiltration using three different ultrafiltration rates (20, 35 and 45 ml/kg/h). Survival was significantly greater in the groups with the higher ultrafiltration rates than in the lower rate group [53].

PLASMAPHERESIS

Plasmapheresis represents a more complete way to remove inflammatory mediators. During plasma exchange, plasma from healthy donors is used to replace the plasma from the patient. In animal models this technique has yielded various results. In a canine model of septic shock due to peritonitis, Natanson and colleagues observed worsened hemodynamics and decreased survival time with plasmapheresis [54]. On the other hand, Stegmayr [55] found a surprisingly high survival rate of 80% in patients with multiple organ failure (MOF) submitted to plasmapheresis. Similar results were previously reported in uncontrolled clinical studies including very small patient numbers [56,57].

In a recent randomized, controlled clinical trial, Reeves et al. [58] found that plasmapheresis had no effect on survival in septic patients, despite a reduction in plasma levels of C-reactive protein, C3, haptoglobin and alpha-1 antitrypsin. In another clinical trial in patients with surgical sepsis, Schmidt et al. found a significant reduction in mortality in the group treated with combined hemofiltration and plasmapheresis [59].

Ref	Author	Year	Patients	Membrane	Mediator
25	Gotloib	1986	24, septic ARDS	CU	TXB2
26	Coraim	1986	36, resp failure after CABG	PS	myocardial depressing factor
27	Mc Donald	1990	12, septic ARF	AN69	TNF-α, IL-1β
28	Kierdorf	1992	10, MOF	AN69	TNF-α
29	Tonnessen	1993	9, septic shock and ARF	PS	TNF-α, IL-1β, IL-6
30	Bellomo	1993	18, septic ARF	AN69	TNF-α, IL-1β
31	Andreasson	1993	9, CABG	PA	complement
32	Millar	1993	18, CABG	PA	TNF-α, IL-6, IL-8
33	Journois	1994	32, CABG in children	PS	TNF-α, IL-6, IL-8, complement
34	Elliott	1994	77		TNF-α, IL-1β
35	Bellomo	1995	10, septic ARF	AN69	IL-6, IL-8
36	Hoffmann	1995	16, MOF	PA	TNF-α, IL-1, IL-6, IL-8, complement
37	Sander	1995	16, septic shock	AN69	TNF-α, IL-6
38	Braun	1995	30, SIRS	PA/AN69	TNF-α, IL-6, complement
39	Hoffmann	1996	16, severe sepsis	PA	complement
40	Boldt	1996	14, SIRS and ARF	PS	sELAM-1, sICAM-1, sVCAM-1, sGMP-140
41	Wakabayashi	1996	6, SIRS		IL-6, IL-8
42	Gashe	1996	7, ARF	AN69, PA	factor D
43	Journois	1996	20, CABG in children	AN69	TNF-α, IL-1, IL-6, IL-8, IL-10, complement
44	Heering	1997	33, ARF, septic and cardovascular	PS	TNF-α, IL-1, IL-6, IL-8, IL-10, IL-2, IL-1ra, IL-2R, IL-6R, TNF-R
45	Sander	1997	26, SIRS	AN69	TNF-α, IL-6
46	van Bommel	1997	9, SIRS and ARF	AN69	TNF-α, sTNF R, IL-1ra
47	Kellum	1998	13, ARF	AN69	TNF-α, IL-6, IL-10, sL-selectin, endotoxin
48	De Vriese	1999	15, septic ARF	AN69	TNF-α, IL-1, IL-6, IL-10, IL-1ra, sTNFR, IL-10, IL-1ra,

CU = cuprophane ; TX = thromboxane ; TNF = tumor necrosis factor ; PS = polysulphone ; PA = polyamide; IL = interleukin; SIRS = systemic inflammatory response syndrome; ARF = acute respiratory failure

Table 2. *Clinical studies on mediator removal with hemofiltration*

Extracorporeal devices could be coupled plasma filtration and adsorption (CPFA). With this innovative technique, plasma is first separated by a conventional plasmafiltration system before running over an adsorptive column and being returned to the patient. The potential advantage is that activation of neutrophils and cytokine release is minimal or even absent, since all cells are first separated from the plasma before reaching the adsorptive column. *In vitro*, Tetta et al. [60] showed efficient removal of cytokines from the plasma. *In vivo* the same authors demonstrated an improved survival in rabbits treated with this technique in a model of endotoxin shock [61]. In a prospective, controlled, randomized trial in patients with septic shock, the CPFA system showed a reduction in norepinephrine requirements and improved hemodynamic stability [62].

HEMOPERFUSION WITH ADSORPTIVE DEVICES

Adsorption is defined as the removal of molecules by binding on the surface of a material. This binding can occur by different processes such as hydrophobic interaction, hydrogen binding, electrostatic interaction, covalent binding and chemical conversion [63]. In case of hemoperfusion these adsorptive materials are used to remove various 'toxic' substances from the blood, in a selective or a non-selective way [64].

Activated charcoal has been widely used to remove toxins and pyrogens from industrial and pharmaceutical preparations. Hemoperfusion with activated charcoal has been described more than 35 years ago. With the development of new technology more bio-compatible, polymer-coated cartridges are available. *In vitro* experiments have shown that activated charcaol can effectively remove endotoxin from plama [65]. Few experimental *in vivo* data are available. In one study in canine endotoxic shock activated charcoal hemoperfusion effectively removed endotoxin from the plasma, but no data on survival were available [66]. In another study [67] comparing different extracorporeal therapies in canine *E coli* sepsis, only plasma exchange improved survival.

Another more specific adsorption of endotoxin can be performed with the use of polymyxin (PMX-F) [68]. The endotoxin-neutralizing capacity of PMX-F has been tested *ex vivo* by incubating PMX-F with *E. coli* endotoxin, and subsequently injecting the solution intravenously in mice or rabbits. All *ex vivo* experiments showed marked improved survival in animals treated with the mixed PMX-F/endotoxin solution compared with pure endotoxin [69,70]. *In vivo*, Sato et al.[71] showed that hemoperfusion using a polymyxin B fiber column can decrease circulating endotoxin and TNF levels in live *E. coli* shock in dogs. They also showed the technique can dramatically improve survival from murine endotoxic shock [72]. Several uncontrolled trials were published, showing decrease of endotoxin levels and reversal of the hyperdynamic syndrome [73,74]. No conclusions can be drawn from the mortality data since these studies were uncontrolled. A second problem is that hemoperfusion was initiated rather late in the phase of sepsis, whereas earlier application could possibly be more beneficial and maybe prevent organ failure and death. Recently however, a prospective clinical study in 70 septic patients, showed polymyxin-B hemoperfusion resulted in improved cardiac function and increased survival rate [75].

Other more specific extracorporeal devices are being designed and studied. A multicenter study is being performed with a hemoperfusion system using albumin to scavenge endotoxin. With modern technologies, polyclonal TNF and IL-1 antibodies can be coupled on microspheric adsorbents. With these systems a much higher clearance of pro-inflammatory cytokines can be obtained than with conventional hemofiltration [76].

One of the latest developments and results of modern bio-engineering is the bio-artificial kidney. Recent reports with this bioartificial renal tubule assist device showed improved metabolic and endocrinological functions [77]. Whether this has a role to play in sepsis remains to be investigated.

CONCLUSION

Sepsis and septic shock remain a very complex matter. It is only by a better knowledge of the pathophysiology of this syndrome and a better insight into the role of the various pro-and anti-inflammatory mediators that new treatments can be tested. Hemofiltration or hemoperfusion remain invasive, with potential side effects for the patient. Hence, experimental research remains very important and should be performed before the onset of clinical trials in patients.

REFERENCES

1. Freeman BD, Yatsiv I, Natanson C, et al. Continuous arteriovenous hemofiltration does not improve survival in a canine model of septic shock. J Am Coll Surg 1995; 180:286-292
2. DiScipio AW, Burchard KW. Continuous arteriovenous hemofiltration attenuates polymorphonuclear leukocyte phagocytosis in porcine intra-abdominal sepsis. Am J Surg 1997; 173:174-180
3. Grootendorst AF, van Bommel EF, van Leengoed LA, et al. High volume hemofiltration improves hemodynamics and survival of pigs exposed to gut ischemia and reperfusion. Shock 1994; 2:72-78
4. Yekebas EF, Treede H, Knoefel WT, et al. Influence of zero-balanced hemofiltration on the course of severe experimental pancreatitis in pigs. Ann Surg 1999; 229:514-522

5.   Lee PA, Matson JR, Pryor RW et al. Continuous arteriovenous hemofiltration therapy for Staphylococcus aureus induced septicemia in immature swine. Crit Care Med 1993; 21:914-924
6.   Lee PA, Weger GW, Pryor RW et al. Effects of filter pore size on efficacy of continuous arteriovenous hemofiltration therapy for Staphylococcus aureus- induced septicemia in immature swine. Crit Care Med 1998; 26:730-737
7.   Rogiers P, Sun Q, Pauwels D, et al . Hemofiltration does not reverse hemodynamic changes in acute ovine septic shock. Am J Resp Crit Care Med 2000; 161:A 885 (Abst)
8.   Staubach KH, Rau HG, Kooistra A, et al. Can hemofiltration increase survival time in acute endotoxemia - a porcine shock model. Progr Clin Biol Res 1989; 308:821-826
9.   Stein B, Pfenninger E, Grunert A et al. Influence of continuous hemofiltration on hemodynamics and central blood volume in experimental endotoxic shock. Intensive Care Med 1990; 16:494-499
10. Gomez A, Wang R, Unruh H, et al. Hemofiltration reverses left ventricular dysfunction during sepsis in dogs. Anesthesiology 1990; 73:671-685
11. Mink SN, Jha P, Wang R, et al. Effects of continuous arteriovenous hemofiltration with systemic vasopressor therapy on depressed left ventricular contractility and tissue oxygen delivery in canine Escherichia coli sepsis. Anesthesiology 1995; 83:178-190
12. Mink SN, Li X, Bose D, et al. Early but not delayed continuous arteriovenous hemofiltration improves cardiovascular function in sepsis in dogs. Intensive Care Med 1999; 25:733-743
13. Murphey ED, Fessler JF, Bottoms GD, et al. Effects of continuous venovenous hemofiltration on cardiopulmonary function in a porcine model of endotoxin-induced shock. J Vet Res 1997; 58:408-413
14. Reeves JH, Butt WW. Hemodynamic effects of arteriovenous and venovenous hemofiltration in piglets. Pediatr Nephrol 1996; 10:58-63
15. Heidemann SM, Ofenstein JP, Sarnaik AP. Efficacy of continuous arteriovenous hemofiltration in endotoxic shock. Circ Shock 1994; 44:183-187
16. Grootendorst AF, van Bommel EFH, van der Hoven B, et al. High-volume hemofiltration improves hemodynamics of endotoxin-induced shock in the pig. J Crit Care 1992; 7:67-75
17. Grootendorst AF, van Bommel EFH, van der Hoven B, et al. High volume hemofiltration improves right ventricular function of endotoxin induced shock in the pig. Intensive Care Med 1992; 18:235-240
18. Rogiers P, Zhang H, Smail N, et al. CVVH improves cardiac performance by mechanisms other than TNF attenuation during endotoxic shock. Crit Care Med 1999; 27:1848-1855
19. Kline JA, Gordon BE, Williams et al. Large-pore hemodialysis in acute endotoxin shock. Crit Care Med 1999; 27:588-96
20. Lonneman G, Schindler R, Dinarello CA, et al. Removal of cytokines by hemodialysis membrane in vitro. In: Faist E, Meakins J, Schildberg FW [eds] Host defense dysfunction in trauma, shock and sepsis. Springer, Berlin, Heidelber, New York 1993, 613-623
21. Barrera P, Janssen EM, Demacker PN, et al. Removal of interleukin-1 beta and TNF from human plasma by in vitro dialysis with polyacrylonitrile membranes. Lymphokine Cytokine Res 1992; 11:99-104
22. Goldfarb S, Golper TA. Pro-inflammatory cytokines and hemofiltration membranes. J Am Soc Nephrol 1994; 5:228-232
23. Nagaki M, Hughes RD, Lau JYN, et al. Removal of endotoxin and cytokines by adsorbents and the effects of plasma protein binding. Int J Artif Organs 1991; 14:43-50
24. Ronco C, Tetta C, Lupi A, et al. Removal of platelet-activating factor in experimental continuous arteriovenous hemofiltration. Crit Care Med 1995; 23:99-107
25. Gotloib L, Barzilay E, Shustak A, et al. Hemofiltration in septic ARDS. The artificial kidney as an artificial endocrine lung. Resuscitation 1986; 13:123-132

26. Coraim FJ, Coraim HP, Ebermann R, et al. Acute respiratory failure after cardiac surgery: clinical experience with the application of continuous arteriovenous hemofiltration. Crit Care Med 1986; 14:714-718

27. Mc Donald BR, Mehta RL. Transmembrane flux of IL-1B and TNF-a in patients undergoing continuous arteriovenous hemodialysis. J Am Soc Nephrol 1990; 1:368A

28. Kierdorf H, Melzer H, Weissen D, et al. Elimination of tumor necrosis factor by continuous venovenous hemofiltration. Ren Fail 1992; 14:98 (Abst)

29. Tonnesen E, Hansen MB, Höhndorf K, et al. Cytokines in plasma and ultrafiltrate during continuous arteriovenous hemofiltration. Anaesth Intens Care 1993; 21:752-758

30. Bellomo R, Tipping P, Boyce N. Continuous veno-venous hemofiltration with dialysis removes cytokines from the circulation of septic patients. Crit Care Med 1993; 21:522-526

31. Andreasson S, Göthberg S, Berggren H, et al. Hemofiltration modifies complement activation after extracorporeal circulation in infants. Ann Thorac Surg 1993; 56:1515-1517

32. Millar AB, Armstrong L, van der Linden. Cytokine production and hemofiltration in children undergoing cardiopulmonary bypass. Ann Thorac Surg 1993; 56:1499-1502

33. Journois D, Pouard P, Greeley WJ, et al. Hemofiltration during cardiopulmonary bypass in pediatric cardiac surgery. Anesthesiology 1994; 81:1181-1189

34. Elliott D, Wiles C, Reynolds H, et al. Removal of cytokines in septic patients using continuous venovenous hemodiafiltration. Crit Care Med 1994; 22:718-719

35. Bellomo R, Tipping P, Boyce N. Interleukin-6 and interleukin-8 extraction during continuous venovenous hemodiafiltration in septic acute renal failure. Renal Failure 1995; 17:457-466

36. Hoffmann J, Hartl W, Deppisch, et al. Hemofiltration in human sepsis: evidence for elimination of immunomodulary substances. Kidney Int 1995; 48:1563-1570

37. Sander A, Armbruster W, Sander B, et al. The influence of continuous hemofiltration on cytokine elimination and cardiovascular stability in the early phase of sepsis. Contrib Nephrol 1995; 116:99-103

38. Braun N, Rosenfeld S, Giolai M, et al. Effect of continuous hemodiafiltration on IL-6, TNF-alpha, C3a and TCC in patients with SIRS/septic shock using two different membranes. Contrib Nephrol 1995; 116:89-98

39. Hoffmann J, Hartl W, Deppisch R, et al. Effect of hemofiltration on hemodynamics and systemic concentrations of anaphylatoxins and cytokines in human sepsis. Intensive Care Med 1996; 22:1360-1367

40. Boldt J, Müller M, Heesen M, et al. The effects of pentoxifylline on circulating adhesion molecules in critically ill patients with acute renal failure treated by continuous haemofiltration. Intensive Care Med 1996; 22:305-311

41. Wakabayashi Y, Kamijou Y, Soma K, et al. Removal of circulating cytokines by continuous haemofiltration in patients with systemic inflammatory response syndrome or multiple organ dysfunction syndrome. Br J Surg 1996; 83:393-394

42. Gasche Y, Pascual M, Suter PM, et al. Complement depletion during haemofiltration with polyacrilonitrile membranes. Nephrol Dial Transplant 1996; 11:117-119

43. Journois D, Israel-Biet D, Pouard P, et al. High-volume, zero-balanced hemofiltration to reduce delayed inflammatory response to cardiopulmonary bypass in children. Anesthesiology 1996; 85:965-976

44. Heering P, Morgera S, Schmitz FJ, et al. Cytokine removal and cardiovascular hemodynamics in septic patients with continuous veno-venous hemofiltration. Intensive Care Med 1997; 23:288-296

45. Sander A, Armbruster W, Sander B, et al. Hemofiltration increases IL-6 clearance in early systemic inflammatory response syndrome, but does not alter IL-6 and TNF-alpha plasma concentrations. Intensive Care Med 1997; 23:878-884

46. van Bommel EF, Hesse CJ, Jutte NH, et al. Impact of continuous hemofiltration on cytokines and cytokine inhibitors in oliguric patients suffering from systemic inflammatory response syndrome. Ren Fail 1997; 19:443-454

47. Kellum JA, Johnson JP, Kramer D, et al. Diffusive vs convective therapy: effects on mediators of inflammation in patients with severe systemic inflammatory response syndrome. Crit Care Med 1998; 26:1995-2000

48. De Vriese AS, Colardyn FA, Philippé JJ, et al. Cytokine removal during continuous hemofiltration in septic patients. J Am Soc Nephrol 1999; 10:846-853

49. Grooteman MPC, Groeneveld ABJ. A role for plasma removal during sepsis? Intensive Care Med 2000; 26:493-495

50. Schetz M, Ferdinande P, Van den Berghe G, et al. Removal of pro-inflammatory cytokines with renal replacement therapy: sense or nonsense? Intensive Care Med 1995; 21:169-176

51. Rodby RA. Hemofiltration for SIRS: Bloodletting, twentieth century style? Crit Care Med 1998; 26:1940-1942

52. Oudemans-van Straaten, HM, Bosman RJ, van der Spoel JI, et al. Outcome of critically ill patients treated with intermittent high-volume hemofiltration: a prospective cohort analysis. Intensive Care Med 1999; 25:814-21

53. Ronco C, Bellomo R, Homel P, et al. Effects of different doses in continuous veno-venous hemofiltration on outcomes of acute renal failure: a prospective randomized trial. Lancet 2000; 355:26-30

54. Natanson C, Hoffman WD, Koev LA, et al. Plasma exchange does not improve survival in a canine model of human septic shock. Transfusion 1993; 33:243-248

55. Stegmayr BG. Plasmapheresis in severe sepsis or septic shock. Blood Purification 1996; 14:94-101

56. van Deuren M, Santman FW, van Dalen R, et al. Plasma and whole blood exchange in meningococcal sepsis. Clin Infect Dis 1992; 15:424-430

57. Mc Clelland P, Williams PS, Yaqoob M, et al. Multiple organ failure: a role for plasma exchange. Intensive Care Med 1990; 16:100-103

58. Reeves JH, Butt WW, Shann F, et al. Continuous plasmafiltration in sepsis syndrome. Crit Care Med 1999; 27:2096-2104

59. Schmidt J, Mann S, Mohr VD, et al. Plasmapheresis combined with continuous hemofiltration in surgical patients with sepsis. Intensive Care Med 2000; 26:532-537

60. Tetta C, Cavaillon JM, Schulze M, et al. Removal of cytokines and activated complement components in an experimental model of continuous plasma filtration coupled with sorbent adsorption. Nephrol Dial Transplant 1998; 13:1458-1464

61. Tetta C, Gianotti L, Cavaillon JM, et al. Continuous plasmafiltration coupled with sorbent adsorption in a rabbit model of gram-negative sepsis. J Am Soc Nephrol. 1998; 9:588A

62. Brendolan A, Irone M, Digno A, et al. Coupled plasma filtration-adsorption technique [CPAT] in sepsis-associated acute renal failure: hemodynamic effects. J Am Soc Nephrol. 1998; 9:127A

63. Winchester JF. Hemoperfusion. In: Maher JF (ed) Replacement of Renal Function by Dialysis. Kluwer Academic Publishers, Dordrecht, The Netherlands, 1989, pp 439-459

64. Jaber BL, Pereira BJG. Extracorporeal adsorbent-based strategies in sepsis. Am J Kidney Dis 1997; 30:44-56

65. Bysani GK, Shenep JL, Hildner WK, et al. Detoxification of plasma containing lipopolysaccharide by adsorption. Crit Care Med 1990; 18:67-71

66. Bende S, Bertok L. Elimination of endotoxin from the blood by extracorporeal activated charcaol hemoperfusion in experimental canine endotoxic shock. Circ Shock 1986; 19:239-244

67. Asanuma Y, Takahashi T, Kato T, et al. Treatment of endotoxin shock due to gram-negative bacteremia using extracorporeal circulation. Jpn J Gastroenterol 1989; 86:246-252

68. Jaber BL, Barrett TW, Cendoroglo Neto M, et al. Endotoxin removal by polymyxin-B immobilized derivative fibers during in vitro hemoperfusion of 10% human plasma. ASAIO J 1998; 44:54-61

69. Hanasawa K, Tani T, Kodama M. New approach to endotoxic and septic shock by means of polymyxin B immobilized fiber. Surg Gynecol Obstet 1989; 168:323-331

70. Kodama M, Hanasawa K, Tani T. New therapeutic method against septic shock-Removal of endotoxin using extracorporeal circulation. Adv Exp Med Biol 1990; 256:653-664

71. Sato T, Orlowski JP, Zborowski M. Experimental study of extracorporeal perfusion for septic shock. ASAIO J 1993; 39:M790-M793

72. Cheadle WG, Hanasawa K, Gallinaro RN, et al. Endotoxin filtration and immune stimulation improve survival from gram-negative sepsis. Surgery 1991; 110:785-792

73. Kodama M, Aoki H, Tani T, et al. Hemoperfusion using a polymyxin B immobilized fiber columnfor the removal of endotoxin. In: Levin J, Alving CR, Munford RS, Stutz PL (eds) Bacterial Endotoxin: Recognition and Effector Mechanisms. Elsevier Science, Amsterdam, The Netherlands, 1993, pp 389-398

74. Aoki H, Kodama M, Tani T, et al. Treatment of sepsis by extracorporeal elimination of endotoxin using polymyxin B-immobilized fiber. Am J Surg 1994; 167:412-417

75. Tani T, Hanasawa K, Endo Y, et al. Therapeutic apheresis for septic patients with organ dysfunction: hemoperfusion using a polymyxin B immobilized column. Artif Organs 1998; 22:1038-1044

76. Weber C, Falkenhagen D. Extracorporeal removal of proinflammatory cytokines by specific adsorption onto microspheres. ASAIO J 1996; 42:M908-M911

77. Humes HD, Mac Kay SM, Funke AJ, et al. Tissue engineering of a bioartificial renal tubule assist device: in vitro transport and metabolic characteristics. Kidney Int 1999; 55:2502-2514

48

ENDOTOXIN ANALOGS IN THE TREATMENT OF SEPTIC SHOCK

Mark E. Astiz

Endotoxin (lipopolysaccharide, LPS), an essential component of the outer membrane of Gram-negative bacteria, plays a central role in the pathogenesis of septic shock related to gram-negative bacterial infections. Endotoxin levels have been correlated both with mortality and with the development of organ failure in patients with septic shock due to Gram-negative bacteria [1,2]. Infusion of endotoxin in normal volunteers reproduces many of the clinical manifestations of septic shock [3]. In addition to its toxic properties, endotoxin has many potentially beneficial immunologic activities (Table 1). These include enhancement of nonspecific resistance to infection, immune adjuvant effects, and the induction of endotoxin tolerance [4,5]. Accordingly, efforts have been directed towards the development of less toxic derivatives of endotoxin which could possibly be utilized to either antagonize the toxic effects of endotoxin or to take advantage of its beneficial immunologic properties.

• Endotoxin antagonism
• Induction of endotoxin tolerance
• Immunoadjuvancy
• Enhancement of nonspecific resistance to infection
• Reduction of ischemia/reperfusion injury

Table 1. Potential beneficial properties of endotoxin in the treatment of septic shock

The endotoxin molecule consists of three regions [6]. The O-antigen oligosaccharide side chain is specific for any given serotype and is highly variable between organisms. The core polysaccharide is structurally less variable and can be divided into an O-chain-proximal outer core and a lipid A-proximal inner core. Endotoxins incorporating the complete O-specific side chains and the complete core component are termed wild type or smooth endotoxin. Those forms of endotoxin lacking the O-side chain are referred to as rough mutants.

Although both the oligosaccharide side chains and the core polysaccharide component have independent biologic activity, the lipid A component is considered the toxic portion of the molecule. Lipid A also has immunogenic properties and induces anti-lipid A antibodies that cross react widely among lipid A fractions of different gram-negative organisms. The structure of the lipid A molecule consists of diphosphated diglucosamine residues with attached ester and amide-linked fatty acid chains. The ester linked fatty acids chains are commonly fourteen to sixteen carbons in length. The amide-linked fatty acids are even numbered and β-hydroxyl substituted.

Several factors affect the biologic activity of lipid A. These include its solubility, the macromolecular environment in which the lipid A is released, and the conformation of the molecule [6]. Alterations in the number and distribution of the acyl chains, number and location of charges in the backbone, number of hydroxyl groups, and the number of phosphates, also effect the potency of specific lipid A molecules. The molecular structure of lipid A expressing the greatest biologic activity consists of a biphosophorlyated diglucosamine backbone with an asymmetrical distribution of six acyl groups twelve to fourteen carbons in length. Lipid A from *E. coli* combines these features and is the most potent naturally occurring form of lipid A [7] (Figure 1).

Various efforts have been directed towards identifying nontoxic analogs of lipid A (Figure 1). One goal has been the development of molecules with antagonist activity that might be utilized in patients with septic shock. A second goal has been the development of derivatives with the beneficial immunologic activities of lipid A without its associated toxicity. These efforts have taken three general experimental approaches. The first is to chemically modify the native toxic lipid A so as to derive a molecule with attenuated toxicity. The second approach has been to identify naturally occurring lipid A molecules with potential antagonist properties and limited toxicity. Third, a variety of lipid A partial structures with varying degrees of immunologic activity have been synthesized chemically.

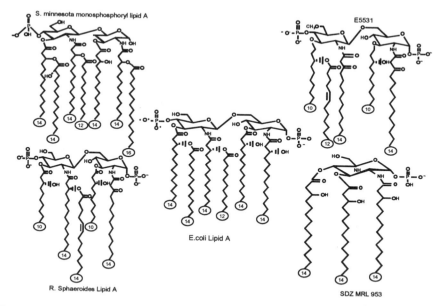

Figure 1. *Proposed structures for asymmetrical E. coli lipid A, S. minnesota monophosphoryl lipid A, R. sphaeriodes lipid A, synthetic SDZ MRL 953, and synthetic E5531.*

Monophosphoryl lipid A is an example of a chemical modification of a native molecule. Acid hydrolysis of the native *S. minnesota* lipid A results in loss of the phosphate groups at the reducing end of the molecule and significantly attenuated toxicity [8]. Additional chemical modification in the length of fatty acid chains associated with monophosphoryl lipid A produces even greater reductions in toxicity [9]. *R. sphaeroides* lipid A, a penta-acylated lipid A with substituted fatty acid chains in two positions, is an example of a native form of lipid A with reduced toxicity that antagonizes the effects of other forms of lipid A [10]. E5531 and SDZ MRL 953 are examples of synthetic compounds with reduced toxicity and possible antagonist properties. E5531 is synthetic product in which the chemical structure of *R. capsulatum* lipid A has been modified by substituting ether linkages in place of ester linkages and a methyl group for a hydroxyl group [11]. SDZ MRL 953 is a synthetic monosaccharide precursor of lipid A with three acyl groups [12].

The agonist (toxic) properties of different lipid A analogs are considerably less than that of native endotoxin. Monophosphoryl lipid A and lipid IV$_A$, a biphosphate terta-acyl lipid A, require 10^4 and 10^5 times the dose of *S.*

typhimurium endotoxin to elicit the same level of human monocyte tumor necrosis factor (TNF)-α release [13]. In animals, the lethal doses of monophosphoryl lipid A are 10^3 to 10^5 times those of control *E. coli* or *S. typhimurium* endotoxin depending on the species tested [14]. *R. sphaeriodes* lipid A has minimal agonist properties when studied in isolated macrophages. At concentrations 10^4 times that of *E. coli* endotoxin, *R. sphaeriodes* lipid A-induced TNF-α release from isolated monocytes was measurable but significantly attenuated [15]. In galactosamine sensitized mice, the toxic doses of *R. sphaeriodes* lipid A were 10^4 times those of *S. abortus-equi* endotoxin [10]. Doses of E5531 10^5 times that of *E. coli* endotoxin were found to be completely devoid of agonist activity in isolated monocytes and elicited no TNF-α release [11]. SDZ MRL 953 was found to be 10^3 fold less potent than synthetic lipid A in inducing TNF-α release from isolated macrophages and was less toxic by a factor of 10^5 in galactosamine sensitized mice [16,17].

Several of the lipid A analogs have also been tested in humans. The standard endotoxin dose used in clinical studies to examine the immunologic and physiologic effects of endotoxin is 4ng/kg of *E. coli* endotoxin [3,18] . This dose of endotoxin causes mild pyrexia, tachycardia and cytokine release. When monophosphoryl lipid A was tested in normal volunteers, a dose of 20 ug/kg was tolerated with modest symptoms and release of proinflammatory cytokines which was less than that seen with the much lower doses of endotoxin [19]. SDZ MRL 953 was tested in patients with cancer in doses as high as 30μg/kg [20]. Fever was the most common symptom and only slight elevations of TNF-α, interleukin (IL)-1β and IL-8 were observed. Recently another synthetic analog of lipid A , ONO-4007 has also been tested in patients with cancer for possible use as a chemotherapeutic agent. In that trial, doses of 100 mg caused mild fever and rigors in association with modest increases in TNF-α [21].

The potential utility of lipid A analogs in patients with septic shock has involved two different approaches. The first approach is the possible application of these agents to directly antagonize the effects of endotoxin in patients with Gram-negative sepsis. This approach is based on the structural similarity between the lipid A analogs and endotoxin. The hypothesis is that the administration of a non-toxic lipid A analog will result in competitive antagonism at cellular receptors, thereby attenuating or blocking endotoxin induced release of inflammatory mediators.

The ability of lipid A analogs to acutely block the effects of lipid A varies between molecules. Blocking experiments typically involve isolated cells or animal models where the analog of lipid A is administered just prior to challenge with endotoxin. Monophosphoryl lipid A failed to inhibit endotoxin-stimulated human monocyte TNF-α production despite weight based concentrations of 1,000:1 (analog:endotoxin) [13]. In contrast, monophosphoryl lipid A inhibited human neutrophil priming by LPS at relative concentrations of 1:1 and 1:2 when added prior to endotoxin stimulation. [22]. In a parallel experiment, monophosphoryl lipid A, administered just prior to endotoxin infusion, completely blocked the hypotension and decrease in cardiac output associated with endotoxemia [23]. At a ratio of 100:1 lipid IV$_A$ produced 90% inhibition of endotoxin stimulated human monocyte TNF-α release when added simultaneously with endotoxin [12]. *R. sphaeriodes* lipid A in ratio of 10:1 inhibited endotoxin stimulated murine monocyte TNF release by greater than 90% [24]. In mice, *R. sphaeriodes* lipid A injected simultaneously with endotoxin at a ratio of 100:1, inhibited TNF-α release by more than 80% [25]. Protection from lethality has also been reported when *R. sphaeriodes* lipid A was administered 1-2 hours prior to endotoxin in galactosamine sensitized mice [24]. E5531 inhibited human monocyte TNF-α, IL-1β and IL-6 release from human monocytes in response to incubation with a variety of gram-negative bacteria [11]. Similar antagonism was observed when human monocytes were incubated with *E. coli* endotoxin. In mice, E5531, when administered simultaneously with a lethal dose of *E. coli* endotoxin in ratios of 3:1 to 30:1, afforded complete protection from mortality and resulted in dose-related decreases in TNF-α release [11].

E5531 has also been tested as an endotoxin blocking agent in humans. In a recent study, E5531 was infused into normal volunteers just prior to endotoxin challenge [25]. Dose-dependent decreases in endotoxin related constitutional symptoms and cardiovascular responses were observed. These changes were coupled with significant decreases in endotoxin-stimulated TNF-α and IL-6 release. Clinical trials of E5564, a stable derivative of E5531, are currently being considered for the treatment of sepsis.

The mechanism underlying the attenuation of endotoxin mediated stimulation by lipid A analogs appears to be competitive antagonism. Endotoxin stimulates monocytes by binding initially to lipopolysaccharide binding protein (LBP) and this complex then binds to the CD14 surface receptor. Subsequent activation of TLR4, a member of the Toll-like receptor family of proteins, leads to activation of nuclear factor-κB (NF-κB) and its translocation from the cytoplasm into the nucleus where it upregulates proinflammatory cytokine gene expression. Studies with *R. sphaeriodes* lipid A indicate that it blocks the binding of endotoxin to both the LBP and the CD14 receptor thereby blocking NF-κB activation [26]. E5531 has also been reported to inhibit binding of radiolabled endotoxin to human monocytes and block subsequent NF-κB activation [11]. In addition, E5531 antagonism of TLR4-mediated NF-κB activation by endotoxin has been demonstrated [27].

The antagonist activity of the lipid A analogs is considered specific for endotoxin. When lipid IV_A was tested in isolated monocytes, no effect was seen on subsequent phorbol myristate acetate (PMA) induced TNF-α release [28]. Similarly, *R.sphaeriodes* lipid A did not inhibit monocyte prostaglandin (PG)E_2 release in response to PMA, nor did it inhibit the release of TNF-α from *Staph. aureus* stimulated monocytes [28]. Specificity for endotoxin has also been demonstrated using E5531. Although E5531 was effective in blocking endotoxin induced neutrophil superoxide production, it did not affect PMA- induced neutrophil superoxide release. E5531 was also ineffective in inhibiting the generation of nitric oxide (NO) from interferon (IFN)-γ stimulated murine macrophages [11].

Of interest is the observation that E5531 antagonized lipoteichoic acid induced monocyte TNF-α release [29]. This antagonism appears to be related to the avidity of E5531 for monocyte CD14 and TLR4 receptors. In addition to being an important receptor for endotoxin induced monoctye activation, CD14 serves as a cell activating receptor for lipoteichoic acid, peptidogylcans and other Gram-positive bacterial toxins [30]. The TLR4 receptor has also been implicated in the activation of macrophages by lipoteichoic acid [31]. The possible implications of these interactions for the use of lipid A analogs as antagonists in Gram-positive infections remains to be determined.

The second use of lipid A analogs in patients with sepsis is based on the phenomena of endotoxin tolerance [4]. Small doses of endotoxin induce resistance to subsequent large does of endotoxin in both experimental animals and humans. This state is known as endotoxin tolerance and can be induced by serologically unrelated forms of endotoxin. The induction of macrophage hyporesponsiveness appears to be the major factor contributing to endotoxin tolerance [32]. The induction of endotoxin tolerance is dose related and dependent on the agonist activity of the tolerance-inducing agent. Increasing the tolerance-inducing doses progressively decreases cytokine release and the systemic response from subsequent endotoxin challenge. Similarly, multiple dosing also increases the degree of tolerance that is induced. While the mechanisms underlying endotoxin tolerance are being defined, they appear in part to be related to the release of immunosuppressive substances such as interleukin-10 and transforming growth factor-α by the initial doses of the tolerance-inducing agent [33]. Suppression of NF-κB activation also appears to be a factor contributing to the development of endotoxin tolerance [34].

The induction of endotoxin tolerance typically involves the administration of small doses of a lipid A analog for one to three days prior to challenge with either endotoxin or bacteria. Monophosphoryl lipid A has been studied extensively as a tolerance-inducing agent. Experiments in mice, rats and pigs have demonstrated almost complete protection from lethal endotoxemia [35-37]. Significant decreases in the endotoxin-induced release of proinflammatory cytokines have been demonstrated in each of these models. Monophosphoryl lipid A has also been tested in cecal ligation and perforation, a model of localized sepsis. Although decreases in sepsis induced cytokine production have been observed, these changes have not been consistently associated with reductions in mortality from peritonitis [36,38,39].

Other lipid A analogs have also been tested in tolerance-inducing experiments. *R.sphaeriodes* lipid A injected 48 hours prior to endotoxin challenge reduced TNF-α release and decreased mortality from 100 to 20 % [40]. SDZ MRL 953 was tested in murine models of endotoxemia and bacteremia [41,412]. In myelosuppressed mice, injection of SDZ MRL 953 one day prior to *E coli* bacteremia decreased mortality form 90 to 10 %. Similar protection was afforded in endotoxic shock [41].

Both monophosphoryl lipid A and SDZ MRL have also been tested in humans in efforts in induce endotoxin tolerance. Monophosphoryl lipid A was injected in normal volunteers twenty-fours prior to infusion of *E. coli* endotoxin. Systemic manifestations of endotoxemia and peak levels of TNF-α, IL-6 and IL-8 were all significantly reduced [19] (Figure 2). Using a different a protocol, seven daily doses of SDZ MRL 953 were administered to cancer patients followed by challenged with *S. abortus equi* endotoxin. Again, significant decreases in the release of the proinflammatory cytokines TNF-α, IL-8, IL-1β, IL-6 and IL-8 were observed [20].

Endotoxin possesses other properties that might be of potential benefit in patients with severe infection. Injection of small doses of endotoxin increases the nonspecific resistance to bacterial infections including Gram-positive infections [5]. The mechanisms contributing to this resistance are unclear and may be related to a generalized decrease in sensitivity to the effects of proinflammatory cytokines and Gram-positive toxins induced by endotoxin [43]. Indeed, prior exposure to endotoxin has been reported to be protective against subsequent exposure to lethal does of TNF-α [44]. Monocytes from human volunteers with prior exposure to endotoxin demonstrated an attenuated release of IL-1β in response to both endotoxin and toxic shock-syndrome toxin [45]. Of interest in this regard is the observation that the administration of monophosphoryl lipid A twenty-four hours prior to challenge with lethal doses of *Staph. aureus*, staphylococcal enterotoxin B and toxic shock toxin was associated with significant protection and increases in survival [46]. In the same report, the administration of monophosphoryl lipid A twenty-four hours prior to lethal infusion of TNF-α also increased survival from 20 to 100 %. Finally, the protection afforded when SDZ MRL was administered 24 hours prior to gram-negative bacterial challenge in myelosuppressed mice was also observed to extend to challenge with *Staph. aureus* bacteremia [41].

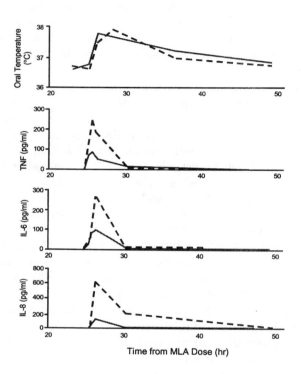

Figure 2. Responses of temperature, tumor necrosis factor (TNF), interleukin (IL)-6, and IL-8 in monophosphoryl lipid A (MLA) treated (solid line) and vehicle control pretreated subjects (dashed line) challenged with EC-5 endotoxin. Peak TNF, IL-6 and IL-8 levels are all significantly lower ($p<0.05$) in MLA subjects. The area under the fever curve is also significantly less ($p<0.05$) in MLA treated subjects. (From [19] with permission)

Another potential benefit of endotoxin is the protection afforded against subsequent oxidative injury. In early studies, endotoxin was reported to protect animals against oxygen toxicity [47]. Subsequent studies have demonstrated a benefit of endotoxin in reducing reperfusion injury [48]. Monophosphoryl lipid A has been tested extensively in experimental models and has been reported to decrease cardiac ischemic/reperfusion injury [49]. The mechanisms contributing to this protective effect involve activation of myocardial inducible nitric oxide synthase (iNOS) coupled with activation of myocardial potassium ATP channels [49]. To the extent that oxidative injury plays a role in septic shock, this mechanism might also be important in reducing organ injury.

Although lipid A analogs may potentially be of therapeutic benefit for patients with septic shock, there are several limitations to consider in the possible clinical application of these agents. The first is the issue of dosing. Dosing requirements for either antagonism or the induction of tolerance are proportional to the patients exposure to endotoxin. Efforts to either block the effects of endotoxin in patients with septic shock, or to induce tolerance in patients at risk for septic shock, would requires doses of lipid A analogs larger than those previously tested which could be associated with significant toxicity. A second issue is timing. When lipid A analogs are used as antagonists they must be administered immediately before an anticipated exposure to Gram-negative organisms. Their benefit is likely to be considerably reduced, when administered hours after septic shock has developed. In the induction of tolerance, determining the ideal timing of tolerance-inducing regimens requires the identification of a group of patients with a relatively defined period of high risk for developing septic shock.

A third issue relates to the concept of trying to induce tolerance to endotoxin and potentially other inflammatory mediators in patients at risk for septic shock. Several studies have demonstrated that the course of patients with septic shock is complicated by immune dysfunction evidenced by monocyte hyporesponsiveness to endotoxin and other inflammatory stimuli [50-52]. This form of endotoxin tolerance is related to the release of anti-inflammatory substances in septic shock and is associated with decreased monocyte HLA-DR expression and impaired antigen presentation [51-53]. Persistence of monocyte hyporesponsivness in septic patients is a characteristic of nonsurvivors [50,53]. Accordingly, in attempting to induce endotoxin tolerance this immunosuppression could be potentiated with possible adverse clinical outcomes.

The final issue is related to the ability of these agents to either block endotoxin or induce tolerance in localized forms of sepsis. The protective effects of nontoxic derivatives of lipid A have been demonstrated in primarily endotoxemia models with limited experience in models of primary bacteremia. When they have been tested in models of localized sepsis, which are more typical of the clinical setting in which sepsis occurs, the results have been less encouraging [36,39].

CONCLUSION

Non-toxic derivatives of lipid A have a potential therapeutic role in septic shock as endotoxin antagonists and as tolerance-inducing or immunoprophylactic agents. Limited experience suggests that particularly as immunoprophylactic agents they may have a role not only in Gram-negative sepsis but also in Gram-positive sepsis. However, several important issues remain to be addressed before experimental data and preliminary observations in humans are translated into clinically effective therapeutic options.

REFERENCES

1. Danner R, Elin R, Hosseini J, Wesley R, Reillly J, Parrillo J.   Endotoxemia in human septic shock. Chest 1991; 99:169-175
2. Parsons P, Worthen S, Moore E, Tate R, Henson P. The association of circulating endotoxin with the development of the adult respiratory distress syndrome. Am Rev Respir Dis; 1989:140:294-301
3. Suffredini A, Fromm R, Parker M et al. The cardiovascular response of normal humans to the administration of endotoxin. N Engl J Med 1989;321:280-287
4. Greisman S. Induction of endotoxin tolerance. In: Nowotny A (ed):Beneficial Effects of Endotoxins. Plenum Press, New York 1983, pp: 149-178
5. Parant M. Effect of LPS on nonspecific resistance to bacterial infections. In: Nowotny A (ed) Beneficial Effects of Endotoxins. Plenum Press, New York 1983 pp: 179-196
6. Morrison D, Silverstein R, Luchi M, Shnyra A. Structure-function relationships of bacterial endotoxins. Infect Dis Clin 1999; 13:3133-340
7. Rietschel E, Kirkae T, Schade F et al. Bacterial endotoxin:molecular relationship to structure activity and function . FASEB J 1994;8:217-225
8. Qureshi N, Mascagni P, Ribi E, et al. Monophosphoryl lipid A obtained from lipopolysaccharide of *Salmonella minnesota* R595. Purification of a dimethyl derivative by high performance liquid chromatography and complete structural determination. J Biol Chem 1985; 260 5271-5278
9. Johnson D, Keegan D, Sowell C, et al. 1-O-Desacyl monophosphoryl lipid A derivatives:synthesis and immunostimulant activities. J Chem Med 1999;42:4640-4649
10. Srittmatter R, Weckesser P, Salimath P, et al. Nontoxic lipopolysaccharide from *Rhodopseudomonas sphaeroides* ATCC 17023. J Bacteriol. 1983; 155:153-158
11. Christ W, Asano O, Rodidoux A et al. E5531, a pure endotoxin antagonist of high potency. Science 1995; 268:80-83
12. Stern A, Englehardt R Goelnbock D, et al. SDZ MR1 953, a lipid A analog as selective cytokine inducer. In: Levin J Alving C, Munford R (eds) Bacterial Endotoxins:Lipopolysaccharides from Genes to Therapy. Wiley-Liss, New York, pp: 549-565
13. Kovach N, Yee E, Munford C et al. Lipid VA inhibits synthesis and release of tumor necrosis factor induced by lipopolysaccharide in human whole blood ex vivo. J Exp Med 1990; 172:77-84
14. Takayama K, Qureshi N, Ribi E. Separation and characterization of toxic and nontoxic forms of lipid A. Rev Infect Dis 1984; 6:439-443
15. Takayama., Qureshi N, Beutler B Kirkland T. Diphosphoryl lipid A from *Rhodopseudomonas shaeroides* ATCC 17023 blocks induction of cachectin in macrophages by lipopolysaccharide. Infect Immun 1989; 57:1336-1338

16. Pera P, Manthey C, Stutz P et al. Induction of early gene expression in murine macrophages by synthetic lipid A analogs with differing endotoxin potential. Infect Immmun 1993; 61:2015-2023

17. Lam C. Schutze E, Hildebrandt J et al. SDZ MRL 953, a novel immunostimulatory monosaccharide lipid A analog with an improved therapeutic window in experimental sepsis. Antimicrob agents Chemothr 1991; 335:500-505

18. Michie HR, Manogue K, Spriggs D et al. Detection of circulating tumor necrosis factor after endotoxin administration in human septic shock. N Engl J Med 1988; 318:1481-1486

19. Astiz M, Rackow E, Still G et al. Pretreatment of normal humans with monophosphoryl lipid A induces tolerance to endotoxin:A prospective, double-blind, randomized, controlled trial. Crit Care Med 1995; 23:9-17

20. Kiani A, Tschiersch A, Gaboriau E et al. Downregulation of the proinflammatory cytokine response to endotoxin by pretreatment with the nontoxic lipid A analog SDZ MRL 953 in cancer patients. Blood 1997; 90:1673-1683

21. De Bobo S, Dalgleish A, Carmicheal J et al. Phase I study of ONO-4007, a synthetic analogue of the lipid A moiety of bacterial lipopolysaccharide. Clin Can Res 2000; 6:397-405

22. Heiman D, Astiz M, Rackow E et al. Monophosphoryl lipid A inhibits neutrophil priming by lipopolysaccharide. J Lab Clin Med 1990; 116:237-241

23. Rackow E, Astiz M, Kim Y et al. Monophosphoryl lipid A blocks the hemodynamic effects of lethal endotoxemia. J Lab Clin Med 189; 113:112-117

24. Qureshi N, Takayama K Kurtz R. Diphosphoryl lipid A obtained form the nontoxic lipopolysacchride of *Rhodpseudomonas sphaeroides* is an endotoxin antagonist in mice. Infect Immun 1991; 59:441-444

25. Bunnel E, Lynn M, Habet K et al. A lipid A analog E5531 blocks the endotoxin response in human volunteers with experimental endotoxemia. Crit Care Med 2000; 28:2713-2720

26. Qureshi N, Jarvis B, Takayama K et al. Natural and synthetic LPS and Lipid A analogs or partial structures that antagonize or induce tolerance to LPS. Prog Clin Biol Res 1998; 397:289-300

27. Chow J, Young D, Golenbock D et al. Toll-like receptor-4 mediates lipopolysaccharide-induced signal transduction. J Biol Chem 1999; 274:10689-10692

28. Golenbock D, Hampton R, Qureshi N, et al. Lipid A-like molecules that antagonize the effects of endotoxins on human monoctyes. J Biol Chem 266; 29:1940-19498

29. Kawata T, Bristol J, Rossignol D, et al. E5531, a synthetic non-toxic lipid A derivative blocks the immunobiological activities of lipopolysaccharide. Br J Pharmacol 1999; 127:853-862

30. Dziarski R, Ulmer A, Gupta D. Interactions of CD14 with components of gram-positive bacteria. Chem Immunol 2000; 74:83-107

31. Takeuchi O, Hoshino K, Kawai T, et al. Differenctial roles of TLR2 and TLR4 in recognition of gram-negative and gram-positive bacterial cell wall components. Immunity 1999; 11:443-451

32. Freudenberg M, Galanos C. Induction of tolerance to lipopolysaccharide (LPS)-D galactosamine lethality by pretreatment with LPS is mediated by macrophages. Infect Immun 1988; 56:1352-1357

33. Randow F, Syrbe U, Meisel C, et al. Mechanism of endotoxin densitization:Involvement of interleukin-10 and transforming growth factor-α. J Exp Med 1995; 181:1887-1892

34. Blackwelll T, Blackwell T, Christman J. Induction of endotoxin tolerance depletes nuclear factor-κB and suppresses its activation in rat alveolar macrophages. J Leukoc Biol 1997; 62:885-891

35. Madonna G, Peterson J, Ribi E, et al. Early-phase endotoxin tolerance. Induction by a detoxified lipid a derivative, monophosphoryl lipid A. Infect Immun 1986;52:6-11.

36. Astiz M. Saha D, Brooks K, et al. Comparison of the induction of endotoxin tolerance in endotoxemia and peritonitis by monophosphoryl lipid A and lipopolysaccharide. Circ Shock 1993; 39:194-198

37. Carpati C, Astiz M, Rackow E, et al. Monophosphoryl lipid A attenuates the effects of endotoxic shock in pigs. J Lab Clin Med1992; 119:346-353

38. Salowski C, Detore G, Ranks A, et al. Pulmonary and hepatic gene expresssion following cecal ligation and puncture: Monophosphoryl lipid A prophylaxis attenuates sepsis-induced cytokine and chemokine expression and neutrophil infiltration. Infec Immun1998; 66:3569-3578

39. Astiz M, Saha D, Carpati C, et al. Induction of endotoxin tolerance with monophosphoryl lipid A in peritonitis:importance of localized therapy. J Lab Clin Med 1994; 123:89-93

40. Carpati C, Astiz M, Saha D, Rackow E. Diphosphoryl lipid A from *Rhodopseudomonas sphaeroides* induces tolerance to endotoxic shock in the rat. Crit Care Med 1993; 21:753-758

41. Lam C, Schutze E, Liehl E, Stutuz P. effect of SDZ MRL 953 on the survival of mice with advanced sepsis that cannot be cured by antibiotics alone. Antimicorb Agents Chemother 1991; 35:506-511

42. Lam C, Schutze E, Hildebrandt J, et al. SDZ MRL 953, a novel immunostimulatory monosaccharide lipid A analog with an improved therapeutic window in experimental sepsis. Antimicrob Agents Chemother 1991; 35:500-505

43. Carvaillon JM. The nonspecific nature of endotoxin tolerance. Trends In Microbiology 1995; 3:320-324

44. Granowitz E, Porat R, Mier J, et al. Intravenous endotoxin suppresses the cytokine response of peripheral blood mononuclear cells of healthy humans. J Imunol 1993; 151:1637-1645

45. Fraker D, Stovroff M, Merino M, et al. Tolerance to tumor necrosis factor in rats and the relationship to endotoxin tolerance and toxicity. J Exp Med 1988; 168:95-105

46. Astiz M, Galera A, Saha D, et al. Monophosphoryl lipid A protects against gram-positive sepsis and tumor necrosis factor. Shock 1994;4:271-274

47. Frank L, Yam J, Roberts R. The role of endotoxin in protection of adult rats from oxygen-induced lung toxicity. J Clin Invest 1978; 61:269-277

48. Brown J, Grosso M, Terada L et al. Endotoxin increases endogenous myocardial catalase activity and decreases ischemia-reperfusion injury of isolated rat hearts. Proc Natl Acad Sci USA 1989; 86:2516-2520

49. Elliot G. Monophosphoryl lipid A induces delayed preconditioning against cardiac ischemia-reperfusion injury. J Mol Cell Cardiol 1998; 30:3-17

50. Munoz C, Carlet J, Fitting C, et al. Dysregulation of in vitro cytokine production by monocytes during sepsis. J Clin Invest 1991; 88:1747-1754

51. Ertel W, Kremer J, Kenney J, et al. Downregulation of proinflammatory cytokine release in whole blood from septic patients. Blood 1995; 85:1341-1347

52. Astiz M, Saha D, Lustbader D, et al. Monocyte response to bacterial toxins, expression of surface receptors and release of anti-inflammatory cytokines during sepsis. J Lab Clin Med 1996; 1298:584-600

53. Volk H, Reinke P, Krausch D, et al. Monocyte deactivation-rationale for a new therapeutic strategy in sepsis. Intensive Care Med 1996; 22:S474-S481

49

VACCINES AGAINST BACTERIAL ENDOTOXINS

Apurba K. Bhattacharjee
Alan S. Cross
Steven M. Opal

Sepsis due to bacterial infections continues to cause substantial morbidity and mortality despite effective antibiotic therapy and modern intensive care. It is estimated that there are 500,000 cases of sepsis per year in the United States with a crude mortality of 35 % [1]. Half of all cases of sepsis are caused by Gram-negative bacilli and half of these are associated with positive blood cultures [2]. The progression of multiple drug resistant organisms among Gram-negative bacteria emphasizes the need to develop anti-sepsis vaccines that will provide protection against infection by a wide variety of Gram-negative pathogens. It has been well documented that lipopolysaccharide (LPS) or endotoxin is the toxic moiety of Gram-negative bacteria responsible for deleterious pathophysiological responses in sepsis patients [3,4]. Therefore, various reagents are being developed to neutralize the effects of endotoxin. Anti-endotoxin reagents such as bactericidal permeability increasing protein (BPI) [5], endotoxin neutralizing protein [6], polymyxin B-IgG conjugate [7], and CAP18-IgG conjugate [8], are being developed for possible therapeutic use in sepsis patients. Two anti-lipid A monoclonal antibodies HA1A [9] and E5 [10] that were tested in clinical trials failed to show significant protection of sepsis patients. Anti-endotoxin vaccines are being developed using core glycolipid of Gram-negative bacteria as antigens. If successful, these vaccines may provide a new modality of intervention against Gram-negative bacteremia and sepsis.

ANTI-ENDOTOXIN STRATEGIES FOR THE TREATMENT OF SEPSIS

A number of excellent reviews has been published on this subject in recent years [11-14]. LPS or endotoxin is an integral component of the cell wall of Gram-negative bacteria [15]. Lipid A is the toxic part of LPS responsible for many of its pathophysiological activities [16]. The O-polysaccharide component of the outer surface of LPS varies among different strains of the same species. For example, there are more than 100 serotypes of *Escherichia coli* based on the structure of O-polysaccharide [17]. The core oligosaccharide region of LPS from Gram-negative bacteria is relatively conserved [18]. Therefore, in order to raise cross-protective antibodies, attempts have been made to use rough mutants of Gram-negative bacteria that lack O-polysaccharide side chain as candidate vaccines.

Early work by Braude and colleagues [19] with a mutant strain of *E. coli* O111:B4 (J5 mutant, Rc chemotype) and by McCabe and colleagues [20] with *Salmonella minnesota* (Re mutant) indicated that antibodies against these rough mutants protected animals against challenge with heterologous smooth Gram-negative bacteria. This early work led to a clinical trial by Ziegler et al. showing that polyclonal antiserum raised in human volunteers against killed whole cell *E. coli* J5 vaccine protected patients from mortality with Gram-negative sepsis [21]. A number of subsequent studies using anti-J5 sera or intravenous immunoglobulin (IVIG) prepared from such sera showed limited or no protection from death due to sepsis [22-25].

These studies failed to provide a clear mechanism of action for any protective effect of the experimental antisera. These results led many investigators to question the therapeutic rationale for this anti-endotoxin treatment approach. In a recent study, Bhattacharjee et al. showed that antibodies produced in rabbits against killed whole cell *E. coli* J5 vaccine, when passively infused at onset of fever, protected neutropenic rats against lethal challenge with *Pseudomonas aeruginosa* 12:4:4 (Fisher immunotype 6). They also showed that *E. coli* J5 LPS-specific IgG prepared from such sera protected 80 % of neutropenic rats in a dose-dependent manner [23] . These authors then developed a subunit LPS vaccine consisting of deacylated LPS from *E. coli* J5 complexed with purified outer membrane protein from group B *Neisseria meningitidis*. Immune rabbit sera produced in rabbits using this subunit vaccine, as well as IgG prepared from such sera, when passively transferred, protected neutropenic rats against lethal challenge with *P. aeruginosa* 12:4:4. [24]. A phase I clinical study in human volunteers with this vaccine showed a modest increase in anti-J5 LPS antibody (Cross, A.S. et al unpublished results). Further evaluation of sera from these human volunteers is in progress.

DESIRABLE PROPERTIES OF A SUCCESSFUL ANTI-ENDOTOXIN VACCINE

A successful anti-endotoxin vaccine should be well defined, non-toxic in the human host, and should elicit high-titer broadly cross-protective antibodies against sepsis caused by a variety of Gram-negative bacteria that are frequently encountered in hospitalized patients. Although lipid A is the most conserved structure of LPS that is common to many Gram-negative bacteria, a number of clinical trials using anti-lipid A monoclonal antibodies failed to show significant protection against Gram-negative sepsis [25-27]. The failure of these anti-lipid A monoclonal antibodies has been attributed to the failure of these antibodies to bind to lipid A in the intact organism, due to the fact that the lipid A is shielded by the O-antigen in smooth bacteria [28]. Other studies have shown that generation of a neoantigen by acid hydrolysis of lipid A is required for reactivity with anti-lipid A monoclonal antibodies [29].

The inner core structures of LPS from Gram-negative bacteria are relatively conserved. Therefore, LPS from deep rough mutants of Gram-negative bacteria are attractive candidates for the development of vaccines that may elicit cross-protective antibodies. The *E. coli* J5 LPS has a core structure that is common to a number of Gram-negative bacteria [11]. To reduce the pyrogenicity of this LPS, Bhattacharjee et al. partially deacylated the LPS and prepared a vaccine formulation using meningococcal group B outer membrane protein as an adjuvant and complexing agent. This vaccine was non-pyrogenic in human volunteers at a dose of 25 microgram (highest dose tested) and elicited modest antibody response to J5LPS in a phase I clinical trial (Cross, A.S. et al unpublished results). Lugowski et al. prepared covalent conjugates of core oligosaccharides (OS) derived from rough mutants *E. coli* R1, R2, R3, and J5 and *Salmonella* Ra, with tetanus toxoid. They immunized rabbits with these vaccines in Freund's complete adjuvant and showed that these antibodies reacted with conserved core oligosaccharide epitopes of smooth LPS of identical or related core types in ELISA and immunoblot assays [30]. These authors also showed that anti-OS R1 antiserum reacted with a free form of smooth LPS and inhibited their TNF stimulation activity *in vitro* and *in vivo* [31]. Active immunization of mice protected 40-100 % of the mice against *P. aeruginosa* challenge [32]. More recently, this group demonstrated that a similarly prepared covalent conjugate vaccine of *E. coli* R4 core oligosaccharide induced antibodies that bound optimally to OS of identical or related core type. This antibody reacted with LPS present on live, intact smooth bacteria and mediated the uptake and killing of bacteria by macrophages [33].

Multiple, different Ra core LPS chemotypes (*E. coli* K12, *E. coli* R1, *P. aeruginosa* PAC608, *Bacteroides fragilis*) were recently incorporated into multilamellar liposomes in an effort to prepare an anti-endotoxin vaccine with broad-reactivity and reduced toxicity [34]. These investigators found that the liposome encapsulation of LPS reduced the ability of LPS to induce tumor necrosis factor (TNF) and nitric oxide (NO) *in vitro* from human monocytes and mouse macrophages compared with the native LPS [35]. This vaccine induced antibodies that recognized heterologous Gram-negative bacteria and protected mice from lethal challenge with *E. coli* O18 LPS.

DEVELOPMENT OF CROSS-PROTECTIVE ANTI-ENDOTOXIN VACCINE

It has been suggested that antisera to rough mutants of *E. coli* J5 (Rc chemotype) or *S. minnesota* R595 (Re chemotype) do not provide significant broad spectrum protection against Gram-negative sepsis [36]. The experimental evidence in favor of this opinion has been the failure of several recent clinical trials using anti-J5 or anti-R595 sera or using immunoglobulins made from such sera, to provide protection against sepsis. These authors also suggested that protection observed in some earlier studies using such antisera were probably due to non-specific factors such as polyclonal stimulation due to the mitogenic action of LPS on B cells, presence of small amounts of endotoxin, and presence of acute-phase reactants in sera. The use of inadequate control groups in human studies and use of systematically biased animal models in animal protection experiments have also been mentioned as important concerns. Cross et al. have indicated that previous clinical studies may have failed because insufficient amounts of antibody were administered early in the course of sepsis [37]. These authors have suggested that the provision of high levels of antibody by active immunization with core glycolipid (CGL) vaccine and /or polyvalent-specific vaccines for the prophylaxis of sepsis, with passive supplementation at the onset of sepsis, may be more beneficial.

Nnalue et al. have described a broadly reactive monoclonal antibody directed against the inner core heptose disaccharide of *Salmonella* LPS [38, 39]. This antibody (MASC1-MM3) showed binding to 123 of 126 clinical isolates of *Salmonella* and 11 of 73 *E. coli* strains. Di Padova et al. have reported a broadly cross-protective monoclonal antibody (WN1 222-5) which showed broad-spectrum binding activity against many strains of *E. coli, Citrobacter, Enterobacter* and *Klebsiella* isolates [40]. This monoclonal antibody of the IgG2a class did not bind to lipid A but bound to *E. coli* J5 LPS and has been shown to have inner core specificity. These authors later showed that WN1 222-5 monoclonal antibody and its chimerized version SDZ 219-800 (human IgG1), protected D-galactosamine-sensitized mice against lethal challenge with LPS of *E. coli* serotypes O18, O127 and O111, but failed to provide protection in a peritonitis model [41]. These studies indicate that antibodies to common core epitopes can protect against heterologous Gram-negative bacteria in at least in some experimental models of sepsis.

We have shown that a polyclonal antibody raised against *E. coli* J5 LPS (Rc chemotype) protects neutropenic rats against challenge with heterologous *P. aeruginosa* 12:4:4 by passive transfer [24], and against challenge with *P. aeruginosa* 12:4:4 and *K. pneumonia* K2 by active immunization [42]. The presentation of a common core epitope in a vaccine formulation must be such that it elicits broadly cross-protective antibodies in the human host. The vaccine must present core glycolipid epitopes in a conformation that is preserved in heterologous smooth LPS serotypes with complete O-specific side chains. This may require further fine tuning of the vaccine formulation in terms of its antigenic components as well as its adjuvant component(s). The actual proof of success will come from human studies that demonstrate protection against Gram-negative sepsis. It will be important to develop *in vitro* correlates of protection against Gram-negative sepsis in order to evaluate various vaccine formulations prior to testing these vaccines in human volunteers. Clinically relevant animal models that mimic human sepsis should be used to test vaccine candidates as well.

TYPE SPECIFIC VACCINES

With the recognition that there was a multiplicity of serotypes among Gram-negative bacteria, efforts at vaccine development against Gram-negative bacterial sepsis focused on highly conserved epitopes in the endotoxin core rather than on the O side chain or capsular-polysaccharide (CPS). Many studies, however, documented that of the >100 serotypes of *E. coli,* only a limited number of O serogroups were associated with bacteremia Similarly, of the >80 CPSs of *Klebsiella* approximately one third were associated with >60% of invasive disease. Consequently, Cryz and colleagues at the Swiss Serum and Vaccine Institute and Walter Reed Army Institute of Research developed polyvalent vaccines against *E. coli*, *Klebsiella* and *P. aeruginosa.* Type-specific polysaccharides from eight *Pseudomonas* serotypes were conjugated to *Pseudomonas* exotoxin A. This conjugation process resulted in the detoxification of the toxin A. In pre-clinical studies these vaccines induced antibodies that were highly effective in neutralizing the activity of toxin A, long believed to be an important virulence determinant of this organism. These experimental vaccines promoted opsonophagocytosis of target bacteria *in vitro* and protected animals from lethal infection [43].

A twelve-valent *E. coli* vaccine was made by similarly conjugating the O polysaccharides to *Pseudomonas* toxin A. This vaccine also induced antibodies that mediated bacterial killing in conjunction with white blood cells and complement, and protected animals against lethal infection [44]. In the case of *Klebsiella*, 23 different CPSs were combined into a formulation similar to the licensed pneumococcal vaccine. Anti-CPS antibodies also were functionally active both *in vitro* and *in vivo*. In separate phase I clinical trials, each of these three type-specific polyvalent vaccines was well tolerated and immunogenic. A follow-up study was performed in which both *Klebsiella* and *Pseudomonas* vaccines were simultaneously administered to the same volunteers. In addition to showing the safety of this strategy, there was no evidence of antigenic competition. The immunogenicity of this 32 valent vaccine was similar to the immunogenicity of each vaccine given alone [45]. Based on these studies, these vaccines were used to immunize over 2,000 healthy volunteers, who then underwent plasmapheresis. The material was then processed into an IVIG for ultimate use in a multi-center clinical trial. Pharmacokinetic and safety studies were performed with this hyperimmune IVIG in both healthy volunteers and patients residing in the intensive care unit (ICU). This study revealed that the hyperimmune IVIG was well tolerated. Following infusion of the IVIG, levels of type-specific antibody increase 2-4 fold over baseline when given at 100 mg/kg as a single infusion. Surprisingly, in healthy volunteers antibody levels against specific antigenic components of the vaccine did not return to pre-infusion levels until nearly 80-days following its administration. In patients the levels remained elevated above baseline throughout the 36-day sampling period. This apparent persistence of antibody in the circulation was surprising and its mechanism has not been defined.

Following these preliminary studies, a multi-center study was conducted by the VA Cooperative Studies Group to determine whether single 100 mg/kg or 300mg/kg doses of IVIG upon entry into ICUs could prevent the development of type-specific bacteremia. This study of nearly 3,000 patients failed to demonstrate that this strategy was effective. While there were too few cases of bacteremia in this study to reach the study end-points, further analysis did reveal some potential insights for future study. It appeared that there were fewer infections in the IVIG treatment group during the first week after infusion but this was no longer evident in the second and third weeks of follow-up. Secondly, patients who may have had an infection incubating at the time of infusion, as evidenced by a positive culture within 48-hours of infusion, were prospectively anticipated and prospectively defined as a 'treatment' group. While there were too few infections to achieve statistical significance, there was a trend toward fewer infections in the IVIG-treated group (McClain et al., unpublished data). Together, these data suggest that high levels of antibody at the time of encounter with a pathogen may provide some benefit. However, this potential advantage decreases with a longer interval between IVIG infusion and acquisition of infection. It may be more cost effective and potentially beneficial to do a treatment trial as opposed to a prophylaxis study.

CONCLUSION

The use of vaccines that induce antibodies to either highly conserved epitopes in the LPS core or to serotype-specific antigens (O-polysaccharide or CPS) remains a viable strategy for the prevention and/or treatment of sepsis. Unfortunately, despite decades of intensive efforts, there is little data that demonstrates a consistent clinical benefit from this vaccine approach. The potential pitfalls are many: developing a relatively non-toxic, reproducible vaccine that is sufficiently immunogenic that it can induce antibodies in a reasonably rapid period of time and in the target (i.e., immunocompromised or trauma patients) patient populations; in the case of anti-core LPS antibodies, identifying critical epitopes to which the antibodies may bind; demonstrating a mechanism of action that would also permit clinicians to monitor patient risk and/or vaccine efficacy (short of mortality). Even if these concerns are satisfied, the antibodies must be delivered and maintained in sufficient amounts such that there is not consumption of antibody below those levels necessary for successful therapy. This latter consideration has not been given sufficient attention in clinical trials reported to date.

REFERENCES

1. Rangel-Frausto SM. The epidemiology of bacterial sepsis. Infect Dis Clin North Am 1999; 13:299-312
2. Wenzel RP. The mortality of hospital-acquired bloodstream infections: Need for a new vital statistic? Int J Epidemiol 1988; 17:225-227
3. Parillo JE, Parker MM, Natanson C. Septic shock in humans. Ann Intern Med 1990; 113:227-242
4. Suffredini AF, Forman RE, Parker MM. The cardiovascular response of normal humans to the administration of endotoxin. N Engl J Med 1989; 321:280-287
5. Bauer RJ, Wedel N, Havrilla N, et al. Pharmacokinetics of a recombinant modified amino terminal fragment of bactericidal/permeability-increasing protein (rBPI21) in healthy volunteers. J Clin Pharmacol 1999; 39:1169-1176

6. Weiner DL, Kuppermann N, Saladino RA, et al. Comparison of early and late treatment with a recombinant endotoxin neutralizing protein in a rat model of *Escherichia coli* sepsis. Crit Care Med 1996; 24:1514-1517

7. Drabick JJ, Bhattacharjee AK, Hoover DL, et al. Covalent polymyxin B conjugate with human immunoglobulin G as an antiendotoxin reagent. Antimicrob Agents Chemother 1998; 42:583-588

8. Fletcher MA, Kloczewiak MA, Loiselle PM, et al. A novel peptide-IgG conjugate, CAP18(106-138)-IgG, that binds and neutralizes endotoxin and kills gram-negative bacteria. J Infect Dis 1997; 175:621-632

9. Ziegler EJ, Fisher CJJ, Sprung CL, et al. Treatment of gram-negative bacteremia in septic shock with HA1A human monoclonal antibody against endotoxin: a randomized, double-blind, placebo-controlled trial. N Engl J Med 1991; 325:429-436

10. Bone RC, Balk RA, Fein AM. A second large controlled clinical study of E5, a monoclonal antibody to endotoxin: Results of a prospective, multicenter, randomized, controlled trial. Crit Care Med 1995; 23:994-1006

11. Bhattacharjee AK, Cross AS. Vaccines and antibodies in the prevention and treatment of sepsis. Infect Dis Clin North Am 1999; 13:355-369

12. Hellman J, Warren HS. Endotoxin Strategies. Infect Dis Clin North Am 1999; 13:373-386

13. Verhoef J, Hustinx WMN, Frasa H, et al. Issues in the adjunct therapy of severe sepsis. J Antimicrob Chemother 1996; 38:167-182

14. Lynn WA. Anti-endotoxin therapeutic options for the treatment of sepsis. J Antimicrob Chemother 1998; 41:71-80

15. Raetz CRH. Biochemistry of endotoxins. Annu Rev Biochem 1990; 59:129-170

16. Raetz CRH, Ulevitch RJ, Wright SD, et al. Gram-negative endotoxin: an extraordinary lipid with profound effects on eukaryotic signal transduction. FASEB J 1991; 5:2652-2660

17. Kenne L, Lindberg B. Bacterial polysaccharides. In: Aspinall GO (ed) Polysaccharides. Vol. 2. Academic Press, New York 1983, pp:287-364

18. Holst O, Brade H. Chemical structure of the core region of lipopolysaccharides. In: Morrison DC, Ryan JL (eds) Bacterial Endotoxic Lipopolysaccharides: Molecular Biochemistry and Cellular Biology. Vol I. CRC Press, Boca Raton 1992, pp:135-152

19. Braude AI, Douglas H. Passive immunization against the local Shwartzman reaction. J Immunol 1972; 108:505-512

20. McCabe WR, Greely A. Immunization with R mutants of S. minnesota. I. Protection against challenge with heterologous gram-negative bacilli. J Immunol 1972; 108:601-610

21. Ziegler EJ, McCutchan JA, Fierer J, et al. Treatment of gram-negative bacteremia and shock with human antiserum to a mutant Escherichia coli. N Engl J Med 1982; 307:1225-1230

22. Calandra T, Glauser MP, Schellekens J, et al. Treatment of gram-negative septic shock with human IgG antibody to *Escherichia coli J5*: A prospective, double-blind, randomized trial. J Infect Dis 1988; 158:312-319

23. Bhattacharjee AK, Opal SM, Palardy JE, et al. Affinity-purified *Escherichia coli* J5 lipopolysaccharide-specific IgG protects neutropenic rats against Gram-negative bacterial sepsis. J Infect Dis 1994; 170:622-629

24. Bhattacharjee AK, Opal SM, Taylor R, et al. A noncovalent complex vaccine prepared with detoxified *Escherichia coli* J5 (Rc chemotype) lipopolysaccharide and *Neisseria meningitidis* group B outer membrane protein produces protective antibodies against Gram-negative bacteremia. J Infect Dis 1996; 173:1157-1163

25. McCloskey RV, Straube RC, Sanders C, et al. Treatment of septic shock with human monoclonal antibody HA-1A. A randomized, double-blind, placebo-controlled trial. Ann Intern Med 1994; 121:1-5

26. Bone RC, Balk RS, Fein AM, et al. A second large controlled clinical study of E5, a monoclonal antibody to endotoxin: results of a prospective, multicenter, randomized, controlled trial. Crit Care Med 1995; 23:994-1006

27. Warren HS, Danner RL, Munford RS. Anti-endotoxin monoclonal antibodies. N Engl J Med 1992; 326:1153-1157

28. Galanos C, Freudenberg MA, Jay F, et al. Immunogenic properties of lipid A. Rev Infect Dis 1984; 6:546-552

29. Brade L, Engel R, Christ WJ, et al. A nonsubstituted primary hydroxyl group in position 6' of free lipid A is required for binding of lipid A monoclonal antibodies. Infect Immun 1997; 65:3961-3965

30. Lugowski C, Jachymek W, Niedziela T, et al. Serological characterization of anti-endotoxin sera directed against the conjugates of oligosaccharide core of Escherichia coli type R1, R2, R3, J5 and Salmonella Ra with tetanus toxoid. FEMS Immunol Med Microbiol 1996; 16:21-30

31. Lugowski C, Niedziela T, Jachymek W. Anti-endotoxin antibodies directed against Escherichia coli R1 oligosaccharide core-tetanus toxoid conjugate bind to smooth live bacteria and smooth lipopolysaccharides and attenuate their tumor necrosis factor stimulating activity. FEMS Immunol Med Microbiol 1996; 16:31-38

32. Stanislavsky ES, Makarenko TA, Kholodkova EV, et al. R-form lipopolysaccharides (LPS) of gram-negative bacteria as possible vaccine antigens. FEMS Immunol Med Microbiol 1997; 18:139-145

33. Lugowski C, Czaja J, Jachymek W, Niedziela T, Lakomska J. Serological characterization of anti-endotoxin serum directed against the conjugate of oligosaccharide core of Escherichia coli type R4 with tetanus toxoid. J Endotoxin Res 2000; 6:166 (Abst)

34. Bennett-Guerrero, E, McIntosh TJ, Barclay GR, et al. Preparation and preclinical evaluation of a novel complete core LPS vaccine. J Endotoxin Res 2000; 6:168 (Abst)

35. Eldridge C, Stewart J, Bennett-Guerrero E, Poxton IR. The biological activity of a liposomal complete core LPS vaccine. J Endotoxin Res 2000; 6:133 (Abst)

36. Griesman SE, Johnson CA. Evidence against the hypothesis that antibodies to the inner core of lipopolysaccharides in antisera raised by immunization with enterobacterial deep-rough mutants confer broad-spectrum protection during Gram-negtive bacterial sepsis. J Endotox Res 1997; 4:123-153

37. Cross AS, Opal SM, Bhattacharjee AK, et al. Immunotherapy of sepsis: flawed concept or faulty implementation. Vaccine 1999; 17:S13-S21

38. Nnalue NA, Lind SM, Lindberg AA. The disaccharide L-a-D-heptose 1-7-L-a-D-heptose 1- of the inner core domain of Salmonella lipopolysaccharide is accessible to antibody and is the epitope of a broadly reactive monoclonal antibody. J Immunol 1992; 149:2722-2728

39. Nnalue NA. α-GlcNAc-1-2-α-Glc, the Salmonella homologue of a conserved lipopolysaccharide motif in the Enterobacteriaceae, elicits broadly cross-reactive antibodies. Infect Immun 1998; 66:4389-4396

40. Di Padova FE, Brade H, Barclay GR, et al. A broadly cross-protective monoclonal antibody binding to Escherichia coli and Salmonella lipopolysaccharides. Infect. Immun. 1993; 61:3863-3872

41. Bailat S, Heuman D, Le Roy D, et al. Similarities and disparities between core-specific and O-side-chain-specific antilipopolysaccharide monoclonal antibodies in models of endotoxemia and bacteremia in mice. Infect Immun 1997; 65:811-814

42. Cross AS, Opal SM, Warren HS, et al. Active immunization with a detoxified Escherichia coli J5 lipopolysaccharide group B meningococcal outer membrane protein complex vaccine protects animals from experimental sepsis. J Infect Dis 2001; 183 :1079-1086

43. Cryz SJJ, Lang AB, Sadoff JC, et al. Vaccine potential of Pseudomonas aeruginosa O-polysaccharide-toxin A conjugates. Infect Immun 1987; 55:1547-1551

44. Cross AS, Artenstein A, Que JO, et al. Safety and immunogenicity of a polyvalent *Escherichia coli* vaccine in human volunteers. J Infect Dis 1994; 170:834-840
45. Edelman R, Taylor DN, Wasserman SS, et al. Phase I trial of a 24-valent Klebsiella capsular polysaccharide vaccine and an 8-valent Pseudomonas O-polysaccharide conjugate vaccine administered simultaneously. Vaccine 1994; 12:1288-1294

INDEX